Cardiology
1985

Cardiology: 1985

Printed in the United States of America

First Edition

International Standard Book Number: 0-914316-48-6

International Standard Serial Number: 0275-0066

Cardiology
1985

WILLIAM C. ROBERTS, MD, Editor
Chief, Pathology Branch
National Heart, Lung, and Blood Institute
National Institutes of Health, Bethesda, Maryland, and
Clinical Professor of Pathology and Medicine (Cardiology)
Georgetown University, Washington, D. C.
Editor-in-Chief, The American Journal of Cardiology

DEAN T. MASON, MD
Physician-in-Chief
Western Heart Institute
St. Mary's Hospital and Medical Center
San Francisco, California
Editor-in-Chief, American Heart Journal

CHARLES E. RACKLEY, MD
Chairman, Department of Medicine
Anton and Margaret Fuisz
Professor of Medicine
Georgetown University Medical Center
Washington, D. C.

JAMES T. WILLERSON, MD
Professor of Medicine
Chief, Division of Cardiology
Department of Medicine
University of Texas Health Science Center
Dallas, Texas

THOMAS P. GRAHAM, JR, MD
Professor of Pediatrics
Chief, Division of Pediatric Cardiology
Department of Pediatrics
Vanderbilt University
Nashville, Tennessee

ALBERT D. PACIFICO, MD
Professor and Director
Division of Cardiothoracic Surgery
University of Alabama Medical Center
Birmingham, Alabama

ROBERT B. KARP, MD
Chief, Cardiac Surgery Section
Department of Surgery
University of Chicago Medical Center
Chicago, Illinois

Contents

Preface

Cardiology 1985 is the fifth book to be published in this series. *Cardiology 1981* summarized 446 articles; *Cardiology 1982*, 665 articles; *Cardiology 1983*, 721 articles; *Cardiology 1984*, 809 articles, and *Cardiology 1985*, 761 articles. Although the number of summaries in *Cardiology 1985* are 6% fewer than the previous year, the average length of each summary is a bit longer. Additionally, *Cardiology 1985* contains 156 figures and tables, a 25% increase over the 117 published in *Cardiology 1984*.

The number of articles summarized by each of the 7 authors is tabulated below. Rackley's submissions were from *Circulation*; Mason's, from *The American Heart Journal*, and Willerson's, from *The Journal of the American College of Cardiology*. Roberts' contributions were from *The American Journal of Cardiology*, *The American Journal of Medicine*, *Annals of Internal Medicine*, *Archives of Internal Medicine*, *Archives of Pathology & Laboratory Medicine*, *British Heart Journal*, *Journal of the American Medical Association*, *Lancet*, *Mayo Clinic Proceedings*, *The New England Journal of Medicine*, and *Science*. Graham's, Pacifico's, and Karp's contributions also were from several journals. The summaries from each contributor were submitted to me, edited, and organized into the 9 chapters.

A book of this type is made possible because of unselfish contributions from several individuals, none of whom are rewarded by authorship. I am

CARDIOLOGY 1985

AUTHOR	CHAPTER NUMBER									TOTALS
	1	2	3	4	5	6	7	8	9	
WCR	91	58	60	38	35	28	2	26	36	374 (49.14%)
DTM	30	24	27	5	4	3	5	6	7	111 (14.59%)
CER	30	18	9	3	6	8	0	14	13	101 (13.27%)
JTW	27	10	8	1	10	8	0	4	2	70 (9.20%)
TPG, Jr	0	0	1	0	1	0	44	0	0	46 (6.04%)
ADP	0	0	0	0	0	0	31	0	0	31 (4.07%)
RBK	9	4	2	0	5	0	1	0	7	28 (3.68%)
TOTALS	187	114	107	47	61	47	83	50	65	761 (100%)

especially indebted to Marjorie Hadsell who typed superbly all 374 summaries contributed by me. Margaret M.M. Moore organized the figures and tables for photography. Joanie Mok typed the large table of contents. Rachell Van Eron, Leslie Silvernail, Barbara Hassler, Belinda Lambert, Evelyn Woods, and Sue Long also typed many summaries. Ann K. Bradley managed to carry the 24-pound package of summaries, references, figures and tables from Bethesda to New York. We hope the efforts from all of us are useful to you the reader.

WILLIAM C. ROBERTS, MD
EDITOR

Coronary Heart Disease

DETECTION

In a single county in Minnesota

Since 1968, a >20% decrease in the mortality of CAD has been observed in the USA and questions have been raised over the possible factors that have contributed to this decline. Studies of autopsy results could provide an important documentation for the incidence of CAD in the population during such a period of surveillance. Elveback and Lie[1] from Rochester, Minnesota, examined autopsy records of all persons >30 years old who died and underwent autopsy in Olmsted County (includes Rochester) from 1950 through 1979 and included 5,558 autopsies with an autopsy rate of approximately 50%. The hearts of 530 subjects were reexamined for the severity of CAD, and this determination was compared with the recorded grade. After both record and specimen reviews, the 3 major coronary arteries were graded according to the percent reduction in luminal area. Grades 4 and 5, which included luminal area reduction from 76–100%, were designated as significant CAD, and 94–99% of diagnoses were confirmed on reexamination. The percentage of persons with significant CAD increased during the period 1950–1969 and remained high in the 1970s (Fig. 1-1). Cohort analysis showed an increase in the disease in all age groups except in the 30–49 year old age group for the later decades of birth. Thus, this study revealed no change in the prevalence of LV scars over a period in which the mortality for CAD was reduced by 20%.

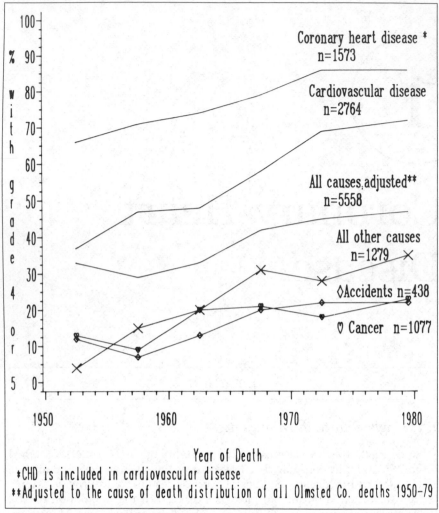

Fig. 1-1. Prevalence of CAD at autopsy, corrected for underreporting, by cause of death, and for each 5-year period from 1950–1979. Note that CHD is included as a cardiovascular disease. Reproduced with permission from Elveback and Lie.[1]

Recall of diagnosis

In a study of the prevalence of CAD in middle-aged men in 24 British towns, Shaper and associates[2] asked subjects whether a doctor had ever told them that they had any form of cardiovascular disease. Their recall of various diagnoses was related to evidence of CAD obtained by an administered questionnaire on chest pain and ECG: 21% of men recalled a diagnosis of cardiovascular disease, in 25% of whom it was CAD. There was a 6-fold increase in the prevalence of recall of a diagnosis of CAD over the age range studied. Only a third of the men with possible AMI on questionnaire recalled such a diagnosis having been made by a doctor. Only half of those with a definite

AMI on an ECG could recall a diagnosis of CAD. Even in severe (grade 2) angina, 40% could not recall being told that they had CAD. Overall, only 1 in 5 of those regarded as having CAD was able to recall such a diagnosis having been made by a doctor, and these were likely to be those most severely affected.

Blood leukocyte count

Previous studies have shown that the total leukocyte count is positively correlated with the future occurrence of AMI. Cigarette smokers are known to have a higher white blood cell (WBC) count than nonsmokers. Kostis and associates[3] from New Brunswick, New Jersey, studied the relation of the WBC to the presence and severity of CAD as determined by coronary angiography in 573 patients who did not have evidence of infection or recent AMI. Cigarette smokers had a higher WBC and red-blood cell (RBC) counts than nonsmokers. Patients with CAD had higher WBC and RBC counts than those with normal angiograms. A positive correlation between WBC and the severity of CAD was noted. Multiple regression showed an independent contribution of WBC count in predicting severity of CAD, after accounting for the effects of age, sex, serum total cholesterol, and triglyceride levels. When cigarette smoking was entered into the equation, the contribution of WBC count in predicting the severity of angiographic CAD became weaker. Similar relations were seen when only cigarette smokers were analyzed and when patients with a history of remote AMI were excluded. In nonsmokers, these associations became either insignificant or much weaker. Thus, the relation of WBC and RBC counts to CAD is mainly due to the elevation of WBC and RBC and the increase of CAD risk induced by cigarette smoking.

Importance of distinguishing from aortic dissection

Thrombolytic therapy is being considered more frequently in the treatment of AMI. Angiographic evidence for thrombolysis has been documented in >60% of patients receiving intracoronary streptokinase (STK). For dissolution of intracoronary thrombi, intravenous STK can be administered rapidly and does not require cardiac catheterization. The major disadvantage of the intravenous route without catheterization is that because information about cardiac enzyme levels is unavailable, the early diagnosis of AMI and the decision to infuse the thrombolytic agent depend entirely on the history, physical examination, and ECG. Unfortunately, chest pain suggestive of AMI may be due to a cardiovascular disorder in which thrombolysis is contraindicated. Statler and associates[4] from Washington, D.C., in a 9-month period performed emergency cardiac catheterization in all patients admitted to their hospital with suspected AMI. Entry criteria for acute catheterization included a history compatible with AMI, age <75 years, pain <24 hours in duration, ST- and T-wave abnormalities, and no contraindication to STK administration. Fifty-three patients with AMI received intracoronary STK. Three patients with severe chest pain and ECG changes suggesting AMI were candidates for the administration of STK but were discovered to have acute dissection of the aorta, a contraindication to administration of STK therapy.

Exercise (treadmill) stress testing

Chronotropic incompetence has been found to be an important predictor of CAD. Few data, however, define the normal heart rate response to progressive exercise and allow a clear definition of chronotropic incompetence. Accordingly, Wiens and associates[5] from St. Louis, Missouri, evaluated 312 patients who underwent an exercise stress test and coronary angiography. The exercise heart rates of 140 normal subjects were used to define the normal mean heart rate at progressive work loads. Two standard deviations of the mean were chosen to represent a normal response at various levels of exercise. Analysis of the exercise heart rates in 172 patients who had CAD revealed 16 patients who had a peak exercise heart rate <2 SD of the mean. Of the 16 patients, 5 had 1-vessel, 5 had 2-vessel, and 6 had 3-vessel CAD. Of 65 patients who had no significant ST-segment shift and who did not reach 85% of age-predicted heart rate, 13 (20%) had an inappropriately low heart rate for the work load performed. Each of the 13 patients had CAD. Of the 172 patients with CAD, those with chronotropic incompetence exercised further than the patients who did not have chronotropic incompetence (9.4 ± 2.1 -vs- 7.0 ± 3.4 METs, p < 0.01). Thus, chronotropic incompetence is a relatively infrequent occurrence in an exercise test population; however, this finding, when present, is relatively specific for CAD and may be useful in detecting patients with CAD who have an indeterminate exercise test.

Unlike the predictive value of a diagnostic test, which depends on the prevalence of disease in the population tested, its sensitivity and specificity have been assumed to be constants. This assumption was examined by Hlatky and associates[6] from Durham, North Carolina, in patients who had both exercise ECG and cardiac catheterization. The effects on sensitivity of factors from clinical history, catheterization, and exercise performance were defined by multivariable logistic regression analysis in 1,401 patients with CAD; effects on specificity were defined by a similar analysis in 868 patients without CAD. Five factors had significant, independent effects on exercise ECG sensitivity: maximal exercise heart rate, number of diseased coronary arteries, type of angina, and the patient's age and sex. Only maximal exercise heart rate had a significant, independent effect on exercise ECG specificity. Thus, the sensitivity and specificity of exercise ECG vary with clinical history, extent of CAD, and treadmill performance; the sensitivity and specificity of other diagnostic tests may also vary.

Quyyumi and associates[7] from London, England, utilized ST segment/heart rate slope during exercise testing to predict the presence and severity of CAD. Exercise tests were performed in 78 patients presenting with chest pain to determine the maximum ST segment/heart rate slope. In 21 (27%) patients the ST segment/heart rate slope could not be calculated in any ECG lead. In the remaining 57 (73%) patients the maximum ST segment/heart rate slope accurately predicted the presence or absence of CAD in 44 patients (sensitivity 90%, specificity 40%). In addition, the extent of CAD was accurately predicted in 24 patients (sensitivity 42%). Thus, the maximum ST segment/heart rate slope did not perfectly predict either the presence or the severity of significant CAD.

Hamby and coworkers[8] in Roslyn, New York, evaluated the utility of a markedly positive ischemic exercise stress test (>2 mmHg ST-segment depression) in identifying severe CAD in 120 patients. Twenty-seven patients were asymptomatic (group A); 36 patients (group B) had type I angina; and 57 patients (group C) had angina with only minor limitations (type II angina). Patients in group B had symptoms only with strenuous, rapid, or prolonged exertion and patients in group C required only slight limitation of ordinary activity to prevent angina. All patients underwent exercise stress testing (Bruce protocol) within 2 months of cardiac catheterization. There were no significant intergroup differences in exercise variables, including time of onset of ischemia, maximal heart rate achieved, rate-BP product, duration of exercise, or mean change in BP. Two patients in group A had normal coronary arteriograms. Comparison of the remaining asymptomatic patients in group A with patients in groups B and C failed to demonstrate differences in the number of coronary arteries involved, LM CAD, coronary score, or the adequacy of collateral circulation. Triple vessel CAD was present in 57% of the patients and LM CAD in 16% of the total group. In this study the only exercise variable useful in identifying patients with severe CAD was an abnormal exercise BP response. In addition, patients whose stress test was terminated at an early exercise level because of symptoms or profound ST-segment changes (>2 mm ST-segment depression) tended to have more severe CAD than patients who exercised beyond that exercise level with similar findings.

Chaitman and associates[9] from Montreal, Canada, studied 83 men who had a chest pain syndrome, no prior history of AMI, and exercise-induced horizontal or downsloping ST-segment depression ≥0.2 mV. The 38 patients unable to complete Bruce stage II had a significant increased risk of coronary (0.97 -vs- 0.71) and multivessel (0.88 -vs- 0.61) disease (p < 0.01) compared with the pretest risk; data obtained from exercise-reperfusion thallium scintigraphy and cardiac fluoroscopy did not alter the risk of single or multivessel CAD. The 45 patients who had ST depression ≥0.2 mV and a peak work capacity≥Bruce stage III did not have a significant increased risk of single (0.76) or multivessel CAD (0.44). When both exercise-reperfusion thallium scintigraphy and cardiac fluoroscopy were abnormal in this latter patient subgroup, the posttest risk of multivessel CAD was increased from 0.44-0.82 (p < 0.03); when both tests were normal, no patient had multivessel CAD (p < 0.03) and only 0.18 had CAD. Thus, cardiac fluoroscopy and exercise thallium scintigraphy increase the diagnostic content of the strongly positive exercise ECG, particularly in men who have a peak work capacity≥Bruce stage III.

Sami and associates[10] from Rochester, New York, studied retrospectively the prognostic significance of exercise-induced ventricular arrhythmia in patients with stable CAD who were included in the multicenter patient registry of the Coronary Artery Surgery Study. The population is composed of 1,486 patients selected from 1975–1979 and followed an average of 4.3 years. All underwent a standard Bruce exercise test and had CAD confirmed by cardiac catheterization at entry. Patients were classified into groups I or II, depending on whether they had minimal or significant CAD. (Significant CAD was defined as ≥70% diameter reduction in any major coronary artery or ≥50% narrowing in the LM artery.) They were further subclassified into groups A or B, depending on whether or not they had exercise-induced ventricular arrhythmia. Groups 1A (16 patients) and 1B (229 patients) had similar clinical and angiographic characteristics except for the average EF, which was 50% for group 1A and 64% for group 1B. Group IIA (130 patients) had a

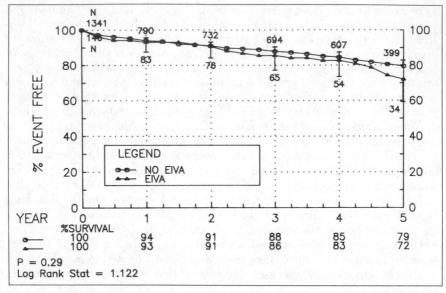

Fig. 1-2. Five-year cumulative event-free survival of all patients. End point is cardiac event (death or rehospitalization) for patients who had exercise-induced ventricular arrhythmia (EIVA) -vs- those who had no arrhythmia during exercise or recovery (no EIVA).

Fig. 1-3. Annual incidence of coronary events in patients with increase in R-wave amplitude (R↑) compared with those with a decrease (R↓). The former group showed twice the number of coronary events of the latter.

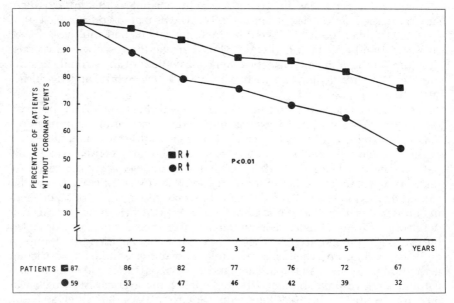

higher prevalence of previous AMI, a lower mean EF, and a higher proportion of patients with at least 2 coronary arteries significantly narrowed than group IIB (1,111 patients). The 5-year event-free survival was not influenced by the presence of exercise-induced ventricular arrhythmia; it was 76 and 88% in groups 1A and 1B, respectively (NS), and 71 and 76% in groups IIA and IIB, respectively (NS) (Fig. 1-2). Using a stepwise Cox regression analysis of selected clinical and angiographic risk factors, the only independent significant risk factors that were found for cardiac events in this patient population were the number of coronary arteries significantly narrowed and the LV EF.

To assess the predictive value of coronary events reflected by changes in R-wave amplitude after exercise, Poyatos and associates[11] from Buenos Aires, Argentina, studied 146 patients with angiographically documented CAD. All patients were followed up for 6 years, during which time AMI and death of cardiovascular origin were considered end points. The incidence of events in patients in whom R-wave amplitude decreased (normal response) and in those in whom R-wave amplitude did not change or increased (abnormal response) were compared. The incidence of coronary events in patients with a normal response was 23% and in those with an abnormal response, 45.8%. Correlating the results with several noninvasive and angiographic variables, an abnormal R-wave response showed a significantly higher rate of events in the subsets of patients with prior AMI, absence of cardiomegaly, maximal functional capacity lower than 4 METs, maximal heart rate >140 beats/min and abnormal LV function (Fig. 1-3). Thus, the changes in R-wave amplitude after exercise is a variable that should be taken into account when assessing the risk of future events in patients with CAD.

The ability of R-wave amplitude augmentation during exercise to differentiate CAD patients from normal subjects requires clarification. To study whether different heart rates achieved at peak exercise by normal subjects and patients with CAD affect the results of R-wave amplitude analysis, de Caprio and associates[12] from Naples, Italy, evaluated R-wave amplitude at progressively increasing heart rate steps in 60 normal subjects with negative exercise tests, in 130 patients with CAD, in 88 patients with true positive and 42 with false negative exercise tests, and in 43 patients with no CAD and false positive exercise tests. This investigation showed that the sensitivity and specificity of R-wave amplitude changes were heart rate dependent, the former decreasing and the latter increasing with progressively increasing heart rate steps. Mean values of R-wave amplitude variations did not discriminate among the 4 groups for heart rate up to 150 beats/min. Significant differences were found between normal subjects and CAD patients, both with true positive and false negative stress tests, at heart rate >150 beats/min (Fig. 1-4). False positive patients had mean R-wave amplitude responses similar to those found in normal subjects. It was concluded that quantitative R-wave amplitude analysis is useful in exercise treadmill ECG diagnosis of false negative and false positive patients at heart rate >150 beats/min.

Roberts and colleagues[13] from San Diego, California, evaluated the clinical practice of estimating oxygen uptake from treadmill time. Patients with CAD and normal subjects had their oxygen uptake measured during treadmill testing. Continuous expired gas analysis was performed to see if the gas exchange anaerobic threshold could explain the difference between meas-

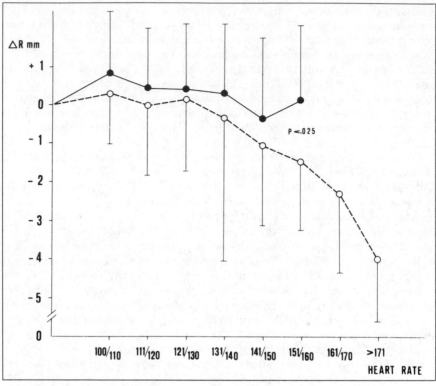

Fig. 1-4. Exercise-induced R-wave changes (mean ± SD) at progressively increasing heart rate steps (beats/min) in normal subjects (open circles) and true positive patients (closed circles). Reproduced with permission from de Caprio et al.[12]

ured and estimated oxygen uptake. Below the gas exchange anaerobic threshold, normal subjects and patients had similar oxygen uptakes for a given workload. However, at workloads above this threshold, patients had approximately 1 MET lower oxygen uptake than normal subjects. Regression equations relating treadmill time to oxygen uptake are specific to groups of patients or individuals due to differences in anaerobic threshold. In addition, the use of standard workloads to predict aerobic capacity depends on the rate at which oxygen uptake obtains a steady state value. These findings should be considered in clinical practice when attempting to estimate aerobic capacity from treadmill testing.

Specchia and colleagues[14] from Pavia, Italy, performed a mental arithmetic stress test in 122 consecutive patients undergoing diagnostic coronary arteriography. Twenty-two patients showed significant ST-segment abnormalities during the test (group 1). Of these patients, 20 performed a bicycle exercise test, which was positive in all of them. Seventy patients had a negative mental stress but a positive exercise test (group 2), and in 30 patients both tests were negative (group 3). There were no patients with a positive mental stress test and a negative exercise test. Mental stress induced a significant increase in heart rate and systolic BP in the 3 groups of patients. Group 1 patients, however, achieved higher values of double product during mental stress and had a shorter exercise duration than groups 2 and 3 patients. The extent of CAD was similar in groups 1 and 2, whereas group 3 patients had a significantly lower prevalence of ≥2-vessel CAD. To investigate the pathogenetic mechanism of mental stress-induced myocardial ischemia, great cardiac vein flow was measured by means of the thermodilution technique in 4 patients with isolated LAD CAD who showed ST-segment depression in anterior leads in response to mental stress. In 3 patients without vasospastic angina the calculated coronary resistance decreased during mental stress as a result of a normal vasodilatory response to the increased myocardial oxygen consumption induced by the test. By contrast, in 1 patient with variant angina, coronary resistance increased, suggesting coronary vasoconstriction. These findings demonstrate that mental arithmetic stress testing may induce significant ST-segment abnormalities in patients with CAD. Such patients respond to mental stress with a disproportionate increase in myocardial oxygen consumption and have decreased exercise capacity. Although coronary resistance generally decreases during mental stress-induced myocardial ischemia, coronary vasoconstriction may occur in patients with variant angina.

Isometric (handgrip) exercise

Isometric handgrip is a potentially useful stress test for the noninvasive detection of CAD and ischemia may be due to a modest increase in myocardial oxygen demand (systolic BP, heart rate, and inotropic state) in the setting of markedly diminished coronary flow reserve. Brown and coworkers[15] from Seattle, Washington, studied the mechanisms of myocardial ischemia during isometric exercise handgrip that was sustained for 4.5 minutes at 25% of maximum by 11 patients with significant coronary stenosis during cardiac catheterization. After recovery, handgrip was repeated with simultaneous infusion of nitroglycerin directly into the diseased artery. The cardiovascular response was assessed by hemodynamic and computer-assisted measurements of stenosis. During the first handgrip test PA wedge pressure rose 56% (15–23 mmHg), the heart rate-systolic BP product rose 33%, and the diseased epicardial arteries constricted. Luminal area in the stenotic segment was reduced by 35%, resulting in a 243% increase in estimated stenotic flow resistance (Fig. 1-5). During handgrip with intracoronary nitroglycerin, the BP-rate product again increased 33%, but relative to resting control, PA wedge pressure decreased 4 mmHg in association with a 32% increase in luminal area of the stenosis and a 28% reduction in flow resistance (all values significantly different from the response to handgrip alone). These investigators concluded that coronary vasoconstriction, not increased BP-rate product, is a dominant mechanism for ischemic LV dysfunction during isometric exercise in patients with significant CAD. The effectiveness of nitrates and calcium slow-channel blocking drugs in relieving ischemia associated with dynamic exercise may be explained in part by the demonstrated capacity of these drugs to block stenotic vasoconstriction and cardiovascular states associated with sympathetic activation.

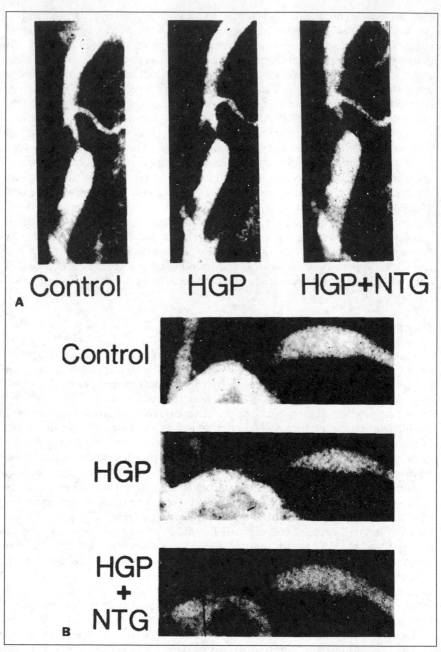

Fig. 1-5. A: Angiographic responses of a significant stenosis of the right coronary artery during the testing sequence of control, handgrip, and handgrip plus intracoronary nitroglycerin. B: Similar responses for a severe stenosis of the LAD coronary artery. In each case, both the normal and the diseased portions of these arteries constrict with handgrip and dilate with handgrip plus nitroglycerin. Reproduced with permission from Brown et al.[15]

Cold pressor test

Gondi and Nanda[16] from Rochester, New York, assessed the feasibility and value of the cold pressor test during real-time 2-D echo in patients with suspected CAD and normal resting LV wall motion. Twenty patients were studied without knowledge of angiographic findings that demonstrated no significant CAD in 7 (group 1) and significant CAD in 13 (group 2). The increments in physiologic parameters (heart rate, systolic BP, and double product) were not significantly different in both groups. Cold pressor test-induced wall motion abnormalities were identified by echo in 9 patients in group 2 and in 1 patient in group 1 (sensitivity 69%, specificity 86%). No patient in this study developed chest pain, ST changes, or ectopic activity during the test. Therefore 2-D echo combined with cold pressor test is valuable in identifying patients with CAD who show no LV asynergy at rest.

Radionuclide angiography with exercise

Higginbotham and associates[17] from Durham, North Carolina, evaluated 264 patients with CAD and an EF at rest <0.50 to determine whether an exercise-induced decrease in EF in patients with CAD and LV dysfunction at rest represents ischemia or a nonspecific response of a compromised left ventricle to exercise stress. A control group of 48 patients with idiopathic dilated cardiomyopathy and a similar degree of ventricular dysfunction also were evaluated. The EF response in patients with CAD was further compared with the angiographic extent of CAD, severity of angina, frequency of chest pain, and ECG ST-segment depression during exercise and long-term prognosis. The LV EF decreased by ≥0.01 and ≥0.05 during exercise in 48 and 28%, respectively, of the patients with CAD compared with only 8 and 2%, respectively, of those with cardiomyopathy. When exercise was limited by fatigue at a submaximal heart rate, LV EF decreased in 25% of the patients with CAD but in none with cardiomyopathy. Patients with CAD whose EF decreased during exercise had a significantly greater incidence of 3-vessel CAD, exercise-induced chest pain, or ST-segment depression, and late mortality than did patients whose EFs did not decrease. These data suggest that in patients with CAD and LV dysfunction at rest, a decrease in EF is more likely to indicate ischemia than a nonspecific LV response to exercise stress. A decrease in LV EF of ≥0.05 and a decrease in LV EF during submaximal exercise appear to be specific manifestations of ischemia and to identify a subgroup of patients with a high prevalence of multivessel CAD and an increased risk of death during follow-up on medical therapy.

Osbakken and associates[18] from Boston, Massachusetts, performed exercise thallium-201 scintigrams and gated radionuclide ventriculograms in 120 patients with a chest pain syndrome undergoing cardiac catheterization. Eighty-six patients had CAD and 34 did not. Sensitivity and specificity of thallium-201 scintigrams with exercise were 76 and 68%, respectively, and for gated radionuclide ventriculograms, 80 and 62%, respectively (p, NS). The use of propranolol decreased the specificity of thallium scans (propranolol, 42%; no propranolol, 87%; p < 0.05). Thallium-201 scintigrams and gated radionuclide ventriculograms were both sensitive in detecting coronary arterial stenoses in 20 patients with a prior AMI, angina, and an abnormal

ECG with exercise. However, the sensitivity of the thallium-201 scintigram significantly decreased as the number of diseased arteries decreased. Sensitivity and specificity of both thallium-201 scintigrams and radionuclide ventriculograms were low in 57 patients with atypical angina, no history of prior AMI, and equivocal stress ECG (thallium, 61 and 63%, respectively; gated radionuclide ventriculograms, 61 and 67%, respectively). Diagnostic accuracy was 81% for thallium-201 scintigrams when the ECG and thallium scan interpretation were included and 83% for radionuclide ventriculograms when regional wall motion, EF, and pulmonary blood volume were included. These data suggest that thallium-201 scintigraphy and gated radionuclide ventriculography have comparable diagnostic accuracy for the identification of ventricular dysfunction occurring as a consequence of significant CAD.

The development of ischemia in patients with CAD produces abnormalities in contractile performance during systole and in relaxation and filling of the ventricles during diastole. Poliner and coworkers[19] from Houston, Texas, characterized diastolic and systolic parameters of LV performance from high frequency time-activity curves in 10 normal volunteers, in 25 patients with normal coronary arteries, and in 50 patients with CAD at rest, and during 3 stages of exercise RNA. In the normal volunteers, EF was 65% at rest and 78% with exercise (Fig. 1-6). In patients with normal coronary arteries, EF was 64% at rest and 72% with exercise. Patients with CAD, resting EF was 60% and during exercise, 61%. Peak diastolic filling rate in the first half of diastole, peak systolic ejection rate, and times to peak rates and to end-systole were measured. In the normal subjects resting peak diastolic filling rate was 3.1 end-diastolic counts/second, and it increased in all subjects with exercise to 3.6. In patients with normal arteries and those with CAD, peak diastolic filling rate was 2.3 at rest and with exercise increased to 3.2 in patients with normal coronary arteries and decreased to 1.7 in those with CAD. Peak systolic ejection rate decreased from 2.5–1.9 with exercise in patients with CAD. The sensitivity of wall motion and EF response to exercise for detection of CAD in patients was 62%, with no false positive results. Sensitivity and specificity of peak systolic ejection rate were 66% and 67%, respectively. Peak diastolic filling rate exercise/rest ratio was >1 for patients with normal and ≤1 for patients with CAD, with sensitivity of 98% and specificity of 94%. Thus, this study demonstrates that alteration of peak diastolic filling rate during exercise is a sensitive and specific indicator of CAD.

Tamaki and coworkers[20] from Kyoto, Japan, used stress thallium-201 myocardial distribution in 104 patients to evaluate the sensitivity of emission transaxial tomography in identifying important CAD. Initial uptake and percent washout of thallium were assessed by the circumferential profile curves of the 3 short-axis sections and 1 middle right anterior oblique long-axis section. Quantitative tomographic analysis showed abnormal distribution in all but 2 patients (98%) with angiographically documented CAD, whereas qualitative analysis showed abnormality in 76 of the patients (93%). Quantitative analysis demonstrated better sensitivity (91%) in the detection of CAD than qualitative analyses (80%) (p < 0.01), particularly for patients with 3-vessel CAD (p < 0.05). Quantitative analysis demonstrated high sensitivity for identification of important CAD in the right coronary artery (96%), LAD (90%), and LC (88%) compared with qualitative analysis (88, 83, and 63%, respectively; p < 0.05), while maintaining similar specificity (92% for quantitative and 93% for qualitative analyses). These data indicate that quantita-

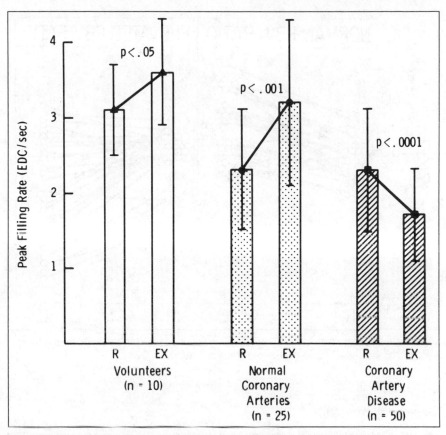

Fig. 1-6. Peak diastolic filling rate during early diastole increases with exercise (EX) in normal volunteers and in patients with normal coronary arteries. Peak filling rate decreases in patients with ischemic heart disease. Reproduced with permission from Polner et al.[19]

tive analysis of stress thallium emission tomography provides improved sensitivity for the detection of CAD in patients with 3-vessel CAD and those with moderate CAD.

Brown and coworkers[21] from Boston, Massachusetts, evaluated the influence of proximal right CAD and RV afterload on RV EF responses to exercise in 64 patients evaluated at rest and during supine exercise with gated radionuclide ventriculography and coronary arteriography. No patient had a history of previous RV AMI and none had valvular or congenital heart disease, acute or chronic lung disease, or CHF. The RV afterload response to exercise was estimated from determinations of exercise-induced changes in pulmonary blood volume, previously shown to correlate with exercise-induced changes in PA wedge pressure. Nine patients had isolated proximal right CAD of $\geq$50% luminal diameter. Isolated left CAD was found in 25 patients, including 24 with important stenoses of the LAD coronary artery and 4 with stenoses of the LC. Twenty patients had both right and left coronary arterial stenoses. Ten patients had no significant stenoses and served as control subjects. The data obtained in this study demonstrate that RV EF decreased from rest to exercise (48 ± 5–$42 \pm 9\%$; $p < 0.001$) in patients with an elevated

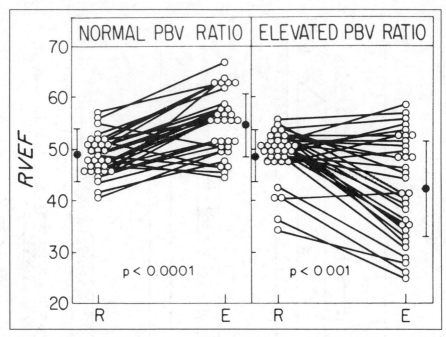

Fig. 1-7. Relation of RV EF response to pulmonary blood volume (PBV) changes from rest (R) to exercise (E). Reproduced with permission from Brown et al.[21]

Fig. 1-8. Combined influence of coronary artery anatomy and pulmonary blood volume (PBV) response to exercise (E) on RV EF reserve. R: rest; LCA: left coronary artery; RCA: right coronary artery. Reproduced with permission from Brown et al.[21]

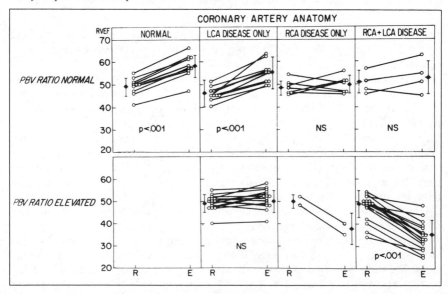

pulmonary blood volume ratio, but increased from 48 ± 5–54 ± 6% (p < 0.001) in patients with a normal pulmonary blood volume ratio. The RV EF was unchanged in patients with isolated proximal right coronary artery stenoses (rest 49 ± 3%, exercise 47 ± 7%), and the RV EF decreased in patients with combined significant right and left coronary stenoses and increased in patients with isolated left coronary artery stenoses. In patients with normal pulmonary blood volume ratio, RV EF with exercise did not change significantly in those with proximal right coronary artery stenoses, but increased significantly in patients with isolated left coronary arterial stenoses. In patients with an elevated pulmonary blood volume ratio, RV EF during exercise decreased significantly in those with proximal right coronary artery stenoses but was unchanged in patients with isolated left coronary artery stenoses. These data suggest that the RV EF response to exercise is influenced by right coronary arterial stenoses and alterations in pulmonary blood volume that reflect increases in PA wedge pressure and RV afterload (Figs. 1-7, 1-8). These data also indicate that RV EF should be evaluated in patients with potential abnormalities in either of these variables, if one hopes to detect such persons using radionuclide ventriculography.

Radionuclide angiography without exercise

Serial thallium-201 imaging after intravenous administration of dipyridamole, a potent vasodilator, has provided an alternative approach to exercise stress for detecting CAD. Since accuracy of qualitative interpretation is limited by the experience of the observers, quantitative techniques for image interpretation may improve diagnostic accuracy of the test. After dipyridamole, experimental studies have quantitatively demonstrated a slower rate of myocardial thallium-201 clearance from zones distal to coronary artery stenosis compared with normal zones. To determine if criteria based on such canine myocardial thallium-201 clearance rates could be applied clinically, Okada and associates[22] from Boston, Massachusetts, studied 40 patients with and 26 patients without CAD by serial thallium-201 images obtained for 2–5 hours after dipyridamole. Regions of interest were manually placed over 6 LV segments in 2 projections for each of 3 imaging times. The myocardial thallium-201 clearance rate was calculated for each of the 6 segments and, using the clearance rate criterion found in canine studies, was considered abnormal if <6.5% per hour. Using this criterion alone, 22 of 26 patients (85%) without CAD had normal and 30 of 40 patients (75%) with CAD had abnormal myocardial thallium-201 clearance rates. Quantitative analysis of regional inhomogeneity in tracer distribution (normal was ≥25% difference between segments) was negative in 24 of 26 patients (92%) without CAD and positive in 20 of 40 patients (50%) with CAD. When both clearance rate and regional inhomogeneity were considered, 21 of 26 patients (81%) without CAD had negative and 36 of 40 patients (90%) with CAD had positive results. Thus, postdipyridamole myocardial clearance rate criteria derived from canine studies can be applied to clinical quantitative thallium imaging for CAD detection.

Exercise thallium scintigraphy has proved to be a sensitive method for detecting CAD. However, early redistribution of thallium and inadequate exercise can reduce its sensitivity. Mason and colleagues[23] from Maywood, Illinois, infused dobutamine in incremental doses (5, 10, 15, and 20 µg/kg/min) in 24 patients being evaluated for chest pain. Thallium scintigraphy was completed during the maximum dose of dobutamine tolerated and repeated 4 hours later. Significant CAD was present in 16 patients; the remaining 8 had normal coronary arteries. Exercise ECG was obtained in 23 patients. During dobutamine thallium scintigraphy, reversible perfusion defects occurred in 15 of 16 CAD and in 1 of 8 non-CAD patients, resulting in a sensitivity of 94% and a specificity of 87%. Exercise ECG had a sensitivity of 60% and a specificity of 63%. It was concluded that dobutamine thallium scintigraphy is a sensitive method for detecting significant CAD and appears to provide a more sensitive screening test than exercise ECG, dobutamine thallium scintigraphy is especially useful in patients who cannot exercise, and because imaging occurs during dobutamine infusion, the problem of early redistribution may be mitigated.

Abnormalities in LV relaxation and diastolic filling are prominent in patients with CAD and may play a pathophysiologic role by reducing coronary perfusion and ventricular compliance for the subsequent elevation in filling pressure. Pouleur and coworkers[24] from Brussels, Belgium, computed local myocardial LV wall stress in 9 subjects and in 22 patients with CAD. In normal left ventricles the rate of decrease in isovolumic local stress was not significantly different from the rate of decrease in isovolumic pressure and the residual wall stress at the end of isovolumic pressure was uniformly low. In patients with CAD, the residual wall stress was increased both in infarcted areas and in noninfarcted areas perfused by stenosed arteries. The rate of decrease in local stress in infarcted areas paralleled the rate of decrease in pressure, but in ischemic areas the rate of decrease in stress was significantly slower than the rate of decrease in pressure. These investigators concluded that in patients with CAD indexes based only on the analysis of decreases in isovolumic pressure underestimate the severity of local impairments in relaxation rate and cannot be used to predict the level of residual diastolic wall stress.

Diastolic LV filling has been reported to be impaired in patients with CAD without evidence of a previous AMI. To study the relation between global and regional LV filling, Yamagishi and coworkers[25] from Kumage Gun, Japan, conducted resting gated radionuclide ventriculographic studies in 15 control subjects (group I) and 22 patients with isolated LAD CAD (group II). None had had a previous AMI. A computer program subdivided the LV image into 4 regions. The time-activity and first-derivative curves of the global and regional left ventricle were computed. In the global left ventricle, the normalized peak filling rate (PFR) was decreased and the ratio of the time to PFR to the diastolic time (TPFR/DT) was greater in group II than in group I. In the regional left ventricle in the side perfused by the stenosed vessel PFR was slightly decreased in the apical but not in the septal region; TPFR/DT was greater in the apical and in the septal region in group II. In the normally perfused lateral side, there were no significant differences in PFR or in TPFR/DT between groups I and II. Total Δt/DT, which was defined as the ratio of the sum of the absolute values of the time differences from global PFR to regional PFR to the DT, was significantly greater in group II. This indicates the existence of asynchronous diastolic filling in the different regions of the left ventricle in group II. A negative correlation existed between total Δt/DT and global PFR. Thus, in patients with single vessel CAD, asynchronous diastolic filling recurred due to the filling disturbance in the affected regions, which may cause impairment of the filling of the global left ventricle.

Pace stress testing

The ECG changes during grading-induced tachycardia have been considered unreliable as a test for the presence of CAD because of poor sensitivity and specificity. As a result, atrial pacing has not been widely used as an alternative to exercise testing. The limited value of the pacing stress test, however, may be related to technical aspects, such as the duration of pacing in ECG monitoring. Heller and associates[26] from Boston, Massachusetts, studied this problem by performing standard exercise stress test and graded tachycardia-induced atrial pacing studies in 22 patients undergoing coronary cineangiography. A 12 lead ECG recorder was used for both tests. Pacing tachycardia was terminated when 85% of maximal predicted heart rate had been achieved or when significant ischemic chest pain accompanied by diagnostic ECG changes occurred. The ECG was considered positive if at least 1 mm of horizontal or downsloping ST-segment depression was present. Six patients with normal or minimally diseased coronary arteries were compared with 16 patients with significant CAD. Of the patients without significant CAD, 5 (83%) had a negative ECG during both exercise and pacing. Of 16 patients with CAD, the ECG was positive for ischemia in 10 patients (63%) during exercise, in 15 (94%) during atrial pacing, and in 12 (80%) after pacing. When the presence or absence of ECG changes was compared between the exercise and the pacing tests, there was a concordance of 90%. Two patients without significant CAD (33%) had chest pain during both exercise and pacing. Among patients with CAD, 7 (44%) had chest pain during exercise and 8 (50%) had chest pain during atrial pacing. Thus, the sensitivity and specificity of ECG changes during atrial pacing compare favorably with those produced by exercise testing. The ECG changes with pacing are reliable for assessing the presence or absence of CAD. Graded tachycardia induced by atrial pacing may be of particular value in patients unable to complete an exercise tolerance test.

Heller and associates[27] from Boston, Massachusetts, evaluated 22 patients undergoing cardiac catheterization to determine the value of pacing thallium imaging compared with standard exercise thallium imaging in the detection of significant CAD. In these studies, positive ischemic ECG changes (>1 mm ST-segment depression) were found in 11 of 16 patients with CAD during exercise and in 15 of the 16 patients during atrial pacing. One of 6 patients with normal or trivial CAD had a positive ECG with each test. Exercise thallium imaging was abnormal in 13 of 16 patients compared with 15 of 16 during atrial pacing. False positive thallium scintigrams with exercise testing were found in 3 of 6 patients without CAD; atrial pacing was associated with a false positive in 2 of the same patients. Redistribution of the thallium-201 occurred in 85% of patients with exercise testing and in 87% of patients during atrial pacing. There was a good correlation in the location of thallium defects produced by exercise testing and atrial pacing. These data suggest that atrial pacing may be used as an alternative to exercise testing with thallium-201 imaging in the detection of patients with significant CAD.

Echocardiography

Berberich and associates[28] from Los Angeles, California, evaluated the ability of echo measurements of LV end-systolic dimension and fractional shortening before and immediately after maximal upright exercise to identify ventricular dysfunction suggestive of CAD. Exercise testing was done in the supine position in 11 normal volunteers, 35 patients with CAD, and 17 patients without CAD. An exercise-induced decrease in end-systolic dimension ($\geqslant 3$ mm) and increase in fractional shortening ($\geqslant 5\%$) persisted for $\geqslant 3$ minutes in the immediate postexercise period in the normal volunteers. Abnormal responses were found in 16 (94%) of the 17 patients with CAD and only 2 (6%) of 35 patients without CAD. Therefore, postexercise echo allows the detection of ventricular dysfunction in some patients with important CAD.

Contrast angiography

To assess visual interpretation of the coronary arteriogram as a means of predicting the physiologic effects of coronary obstructions, White and associates[29] from Iowa City, Iowa, compared caliper measurements of the degree of coronary stenosis with the relative hyperemic response of coronary flow velocity studied with a Doppler technique at operation, after 20 seconds of coronary arterial occlusion. In 39 patients (44 vessels) with isolated, discrete coronary narrowings varying in severity from 10–95% in diameter, measurement of the percentage of stenosis from coronary angiograms was not significantly correlated with the reactive hyperemic response. Results were the same for obstructions in the LAD, diagonal, and right coronary arteries (Fig. 1-9). Underestimation of narrowing severity occurred in 95% of arteries with >60% stenosis of the diameter by arteriography. Both overestimation and underestimation of narrowings <60% were common. These results, together with the high interobserver and intraobserver variability of standard visual analysis of angiograms, suggest that the physiologic effects of most coronary narrowings cannot be determined accurately by conventional angiographic approaches. The need for improved analytic methods for the physiologic assessment of angiographically detected coronary narrowings is apparent.

Paulin and Sandor[30] from Boston, Massachusetts, disagreed with the analysis of the data in Fig. 1-9 of White and associates[29] and suggested the following alternative interpretation. The data point at 10% stenosis is an outlier. Grouping the remaining observations to form a histogram (bin width, 10%), a justifiable procedure in light of the clustered presentation of the data and the considerable error of the measuring technique, the value of the correlation is >70%, rather than the authors' 25%, assuming (as they did, unjustifiably) a linear relation between hyperemia and percent stenosis. Furthermore, grouping of the data into 2 segments of higher and lower reactive hyperemia values results in a stenosis value of approximately 55%, i.e., a figure considered to be a rough divider between clinically unimportant and important narrowings for at least the past 2 decades. Either way the study does not permit a conclusion about which of the 2 methods better describes or quantitates the regional abnormality of the coronary circulation. Obviously, the coronary arteriogram is more practical than the ultrasonic determination of reactive hyperemia, which so far requires surgical exposure of the heart.

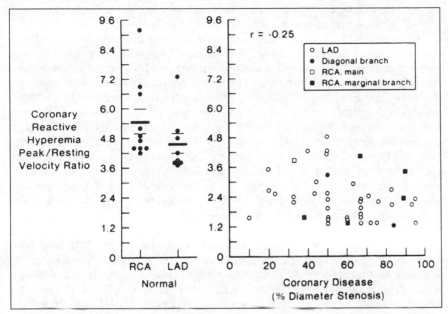

Fig. 1-9.   Relation between the measured percentage of vessel diameter stenosis for the most severe lesion assessed from the coronary angiogram and the coronary reactive hyperemic response (ratio of peak/resting velocity) obtained from Doppler velocity recordings at the time of open heart surgery, for all vessels studied. The left panel shows reactive hyperemic responses in normal coronary vessels, and the right panel shows responses in abnormal vessels. RCA = right coronary artery; "diagonal branch" refers to the branch of the LAD artery. Reproduced with permission from White et al.[29]

Trask and coworkers[31] from Durham, North Carolina, evaluated the accuracy of interpretation of coronary cineangiography in comparison to post-mortem findings in 27 patients who died within 6 months of cardiac catheterization. Coronary cineangiography was interpreted by 2 independent observers and the postmortem evaluation of the coronary arteries included a study of the entire coronary artery tree sectioned at 2–3 mm intervals. In postmortem studies, a fine colloidal suspension of barium sulfate and gelatin was injected at a 100 mmHg pressure over a 20-minute period after which radiographs were obtained. Then, the location and severity of stenotic lesions were recorded on diagrams identical to those used for the cineangiography. Two patients in this study had normal coronary arteries, and the remaining 25 patients had significant CAD, defined as ≥75% reduction in luminal diameter. Of the 326 coronary segments that could be evaluated postmortem, 15% could not be evaluated cineangiographically. Overall accuracy for the 2 observers in detecting significant CAD was 89 and 88%, with an accuracy of 96 and 100% for the LM, 91 and 93% for the LAD, 84 and 86% for the right, and 89 and 79% for the LC coronary artery. The angiographers agreed in their assessments in 86% of the 340 coronary segments. Interobserver agreement was better for the LM, right, and LAD coronary arteries than for the LC (p < 0.05). Accurate interpretation occurred in 93% of 244 segments that were adequately opacified and assessed by both angiographers. These data suggest that cineangiography may be used to evaluate coronary anatomy with a high degree of accuracy and minimal interobserver variability.

The results of previous work from the laboratory of Harrison and colleagues[32] from Iowa City, Iowa, have shown a poor correlation between percent stenosis (determined visually with calipers) and the coronary reactive hyperemic response (an index of maximal coronary vasodilator capacity) determined during cardiac surgery. Thus, the investigators sought to determine whether other parameters of severity could predict the reactive hyperemic response and the hemodynamic significance of coronary narrowings in humans. Twenty-three patients with narrowings in the proximal LAD coronary artery were studied. To account for differences in expected vessel size, patients with large diagonal branches >50% of the diameter of the LAD coronary artery arising before the narrowing were excluded. Computer-assisted quantitative coronary angiography was used to measure percent diameter stenosis, percent area stenosis, and minimal stenosis cross-sectional area. With a pulsed Doppler velocity probe, reactive hyperemic responses were recorded after a 20-second coronary occlusion of the LAD coronary artery at surgery before cardiopulmonary bypass and were quantitated by the peak resting velocity ratio. Percent area stenosis ranged from 7–54% for arteries with normal reactive hyperemic responses and from 27–94% for vessels with abnormal reactive hyperemic responses. With both percent diameter stenosis and percent area stenosis, there was substantial overlap between arteries with normal and abnormal reactive hyperemic responses. In contrast, 9 of 9 arteries with normal reactive hyperemic responses had narrowings, minimal cross-sectional areas of >3.5 mm², and 13 of 14 arteries with abnormal reactive hyperemic responses had minimal cross-sectional areas of <3.5 mm². The investigators concluded that the hemodynamic significance of a coronary stenosis in patients with coronary atherosclerosis is not accurately predicted by percent area or percent diameter stenosis, even when the angiograms are analyzed with quantitative coronary angiography (Fig. 1-10), and minimal cross-sectional area can identify arteries with normal versus abnormal reactive hyperemic responses and thus can be used to predict the hemodynamic significance of stenosis of the proximal LAD coronary artery.

Feit and associates[33] from New York City reviewed 402 consecutive abnor-

Fig. 1-10. Hypothetical explanation for this study's findings. Both vessels would appear to contain 50% lesions at coronary angiography. The hemodynamic significance of the superimposed lesion on the right is greater than that of the lesion on the left. CSA: cross-sectional area. Reproduced with permission from Harrison et al.[32]

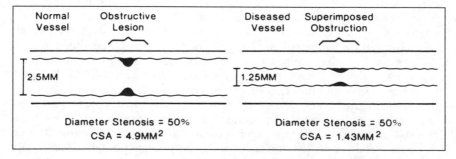

Normal Vessel	Obstructive Lesion		Diseased Vessel	Superimposed Obstruction
2.5MM			1.25MM	
Diameter Stenosis = 50% CSA = 4.9MM²			Diameter Stenosis = 50% CSA = 1.43MM²	

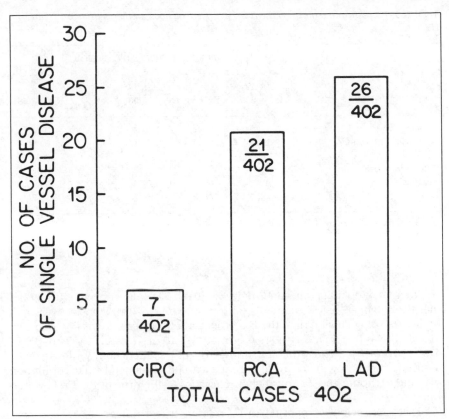

Fig. 1-11. Number of times single-vessel CAD was found in a particular artery. The difference in occurrence of circumflex coronary artery (CIRC) -vs- right coronary artery (RCA) single-vessel disease is significant at p = 0.0081 (chi-square test).

mal and coronary angiographic results in men from 1981–1982. All angiographic findings of single-artery CAD were carefully reviewed. In only 1 of 7 cases of isolated LC narrowing was the right coronary artery nondominant; in all other cases of single-vessel LC or right CAD, the size of the arteries appeared equivalent (Fig. 1-11). There was no unusual anatomic findings present in any of the 54 cases of single-vessel CAD. The probability that the difference in frequency of single-vessel LC -vs- right CAD could be explained by chance in <81%.

Moise and associates[34] from Montreal, Canada, found a new coronary artery occlusion in 98 (31%) of 313 consecutive patients with CAD treated medically and who underwent cardiac catheterization twice, 39 ± 25 months apart. Multivariate logistic regression displayed 8 independent predictors of new occlusion. Four were available at the time of the second angiogram: the interval between the 2 studies, a decrease in EF, the appearance of BBB, and an interim AMI. Four other predictors were found at the time of the first angiogram: 2 angiographic characteristics, 1 related to the severity (presence of an ≥80% luminal diameter narrowing of an artery supplying a nonakinetic LV segment) and 1 to the extent (count of the lesions narrowed ≤75%) in luminal diameter in a 15-segment coding system of CAD, and 2

TABLE 1-1. *Comparison of present series. Reproduced with permission from Harris.*[35]

	PERCENT OF COMPLICATION		
COMPLICATION	ARMY (N = 995)	CASS* (N = 7,553)	SCA* (N = 53,581)
Death	0.30	0.20	0.14
Myocardial infarction	0.10	0.25	0.07
CVA*	0.30	0.09	0.07
Ventricular fibrillation	0.60	0.63	0.32†
Vascular	1.41	0.74	0.57
Total	2.71	1.91	1.17

* CASS = Collaborative Study of Coronary Artery Surgery; SCA = Society for Cardiac Angiography (Kennedy); CVA = cerebrovascular accident.
† Estimates from data given.

risk factors: smoking status and male sex. The 140 male smokers with ≥80% diameter stenosis or ≥4 segments with moderate (≤75%) stenosis were at a higher risk of occlusion than the 173 other patients after intervals of <2 years (13 of 53 -vs- 7 of 74), 2–4 years (23 of 40 -vs- 10 of 47) and >4 years (27 of 47 -vs- 18 of 54). Thus, the appearance of a new occlusion, while strongly associated with new myocardial damage, can be predicted by a combination of 2 angiographic and 2 clinical characteristics at the time of the first evaluation.

Factors previously reported to be related to complications of coronary angiography have included: patient volume, angiographic approach, arterial in-time (the total time that a catheter was present in the arterial tree), presence of LM CAD, 3-vessel CAD, systemic hypertension, and decreased cardiac output. Harris[35] from San Francisco, California, evaluated complications of coronary angiography in 5 Army medical centers. His analysis was a bit different from previous studies. Harris attempted to determine whether 14 factors were associated with increased risk in 95 patients undergoing coronary angiography. The study found consistently increased risk for women, for patients having lengthier procedures, and for patients studied at 1 of the 5 centers. No evidence of increased risk was found for 11 other factors, including 2 related to operator experience. A strong risk of complications, not previously observed or hypothesized in advance, was noted for vascular complications in women studied by the brachial technique. Harris also compared the frequency of complications in his study with those of the previously published coronary artery surgery study and also the study reported by J. W. Kennedy (Complications Associated with Cardiac Catherization in Angiography. Catherization and Cardiovascular Diagnosis 8:5–11 1982) (Table 1-1).

Digital angiography

To assess the ability to detect coronary arterial narrowings from computer-acquired angiograms, Tobis and associates[36] from Irvine, California, identified and measured focal coronary narrowings from digital subtraction angiograms and compared the results with those obtained from standard

35 mm cine film angiograms. Both cine and digital angiograms were obtained sequentially using selective intracoronary artery injection of standard amounts of iodinated contrast media. Digital images were obtained at 8 frames/second with a $512 \times 512 \times 8$ bit pixel matrix. Modifications in the imaging chain for computer acquisition included a slower pulsed radiographic mode, a progressive scan camera, and initial storage of the images on an 80 megabyte digital hard disk. Postprocessing computer algorithms were used to enhance the unsubtracted digital images; these included single-frame, mask-mode subtraction, vessel boundary edge enhancement, and 4-fold pixel magnification. In 19 patient studies, 32 arteries were reduced more than 25% in diameter according to at least 1 of 4 observers on either the digital or cine film angiograms. There was no significant difference in the mean percent diameter narrowing for all the narrowings between the digital angiograms ($53 \pm 31\%$) and the cineangiograms ($52 \pm 31\%$). In addition, a 2-way analysis of variance yielded no significant difference between the amount of variability in the measurements between the cine film and the digital technique. This similar variability persisted when subsets of patients based on the degrees of stenosis were considered (e.g., only narrowings from 50–90% diameter reduction). Because digital acquisition permits immediate playback with image enhancement and greater ease of coronary artery quantification, digital angiography may have widespread clinical use for the detection and quantitation of CAD.

Nuclear magnetic resonance

Higgins and colleagues[37] from San Francisco, California, defined cardiac anatomy by gated nuclear magnetic resonance (NMR) imaging at a magnetic field strength of 3.5 kGauss in 8 normal subjects and 10 patients with chronic myocardial infarctions. Multisectional imaging was performed with the spin echo technique and encompassed most of the left ventricle in an imaging time of 5–12 minutes. In all subjects internal cardiac structure was well delineated without the use of any type of contrast medium. The myocardial wall-blood interface was sharply defined, resulting in visualization of trabeculations, papillary muscle, and chordal structures in both ventricles. In patients with CAD, the extent of postinfarctional wall thinning, aneurysm, and mural thrombus was depicted on NMR images. Images obtained with the second spin echo demonstrated high signal intensity in regions of the LV chamber adjacent to the site of aneurysm or healed AMI. This finding suggested stasis of blood in a region of akinesis or dyskinesis. This study shows that gated NMR is feasible as a technique for imaging the human heart and is capable of demonstrating a variety of LV abnormalities associated with healed AMI.

PROGNOSIS

By exercise testing

To determine prospectively whether the severity of reversible LV ischemia provides prognostic information in mildly symptomatic patients with CAD and preserved LV function at rest (EF > 40%), Bonow and associates[38] from

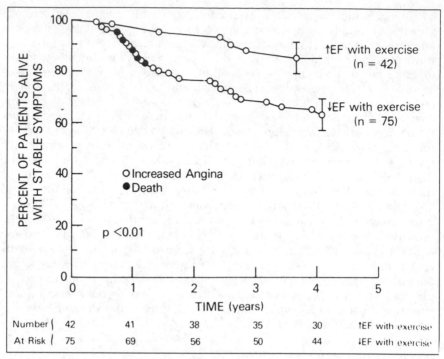

Fig. 1-12. Influence of EF response to exercise on subsequent mortality and increased angina requiring operation. The life-table curve for patients with an increase in EF with exercise is compared with the curve derived for patients with a decrease in EF. The number of patients with potential follow-up at each year is indicated for each group. I bars means ±SE. (p < 0.01 by the Mantel-Haenszel test). Reproduced with permission from Bonow et al.[38]

Bethesda, Maryland, studied 117 patients by exercise ECG and RNA. No patient had stenosis of the LM coronary artery. Mortality during subsequent medical therapy was significantly associated (by univariate life-table analysis) with 3-vessel CAD and the magnitude of the EF during exercise (Fig. 1-12). In patients with 3-vessel disease who had both ST-segment depression of ≥1 mm and a decrease in EF during exercise, in association with an exercise tolerance of ≤120 watts, the probability of survival at 4 years was only 71 ± 11% (Fig. 1-13). All deaths occurred in this subgroup. Thus, objective evidence of LV ischemia during exercise and exercise capacity identify 1 subgroup of minimally symptomatic patients with 3-vessel disease with an excellent prognosis and another subgroup at relatively high risk of dying during subsequent medical therapy.

Weiner and coworkers[39] from Boston, Massachusetts, attempted to identify important noninvasive and invasive predictors of survival in patients with symptomatic CAD who were able to undergo exercise testing and subsequently managed with medical treatment. Four thousand eighty-three patients were evaluated and 30 variables were selected for analysis. The data obtained in this study demonstrate that 7 variables were independent predictors of survival (Table 1-2). Patients at highest risk were those with either significant CHF or ≥1 mm ST-segment depression at a low exercise load. When all 30 variables were analyzed conjointly, the LV contraction pattern

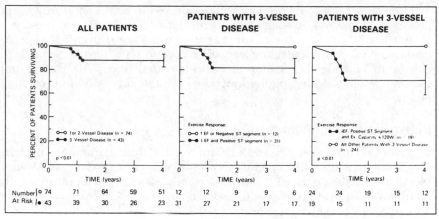

Fig. 1-13. Influence of anatomic severity of CAD, reversible ischemia, and exercise capacity on survival. Survival curves are shown for patients with 3-vessel disease compared with those with 1- or 2-vessel disease, patients with 3-vessel disease and an increase in EF or a negative ST-segment response to exercise compared with those with 3-vessel disease and both a decreased EF and a positive ST-segment response with exercise, and patients with 3-vessel disease and a decrease in EF during exercise, a positive ST-segment response, and exercise capacity of 120 W or less compared with all other patients with 3 vessel disease. The number of patients with potential follow-up at each year is shown for each group. (p < 0.01 by Mantel–Haenszel test.) Reproduced with permission from Bonow et al.[38]

TABLE 1-2. *Predictors of survival by multivariate analysis (method 1). Reproduced with permission from Weiner et al.[39]*

COVARIATES	COEFFICIENT	95% CONFIDENCE INTERVALS	CHI-SQUARE	p VALUE
Clinical and exercise variables				
Congestive heart failure score	0.51	0.35, 0.67	40.27	0.00001
Gender	−1.27	−1.83, −0.71	21.36	0.00001
Final exercise stage	−0.30	−0.44 − 0.16	16.01	0.0001
Cardiac enlargement	0.36	0.12, 0.60	8.60	0.0034
Age	0.03	0.01, 0.05	7.90	0.0049
Prior AMI	0.46	0.10, 0.82	6.66	0.0099
ST-segment response	0.21	0.01, 0.41	4.09	0.0431
Clinical exercise and angiographic variables				
LV score	0.10	0.05, 0.15	16.72	0.0001
# of vessels diseased	0.22	0.07, 0.37	8.92	0.0028
Gender	−0.90	−1.55, −0.25	7.63	0.0057
Diuretic therapy	−0.54	−0.12, −0.96	6.51	0.0107
Peak heart rate	−0.009	−0.001, −0.017	4.74	0.0295
Digitalis therapy	−0.51	−0.03, −0.99	4.40	0.0360
Final exercise stage	−0.18	−0.01, −0.35	4.09	0.0432

and number of diseased coronary arteries proved to be the most important predictors of survival. Among 572 patients with 3-vessel CAD and preserved LV function, the probability of survival at 4 years ranged from 53% for patients only able to achieve a low level of exercise to 100% for patients able to exercise to a high level. Therefore in patients with defined CAD, clinical and exercise variables describing the functional LV state are useful in predicting prognosis.

By radionuclide angiography

Pryor and associates[40] from Durham, North Carolina, examined 6 variables in 386 patients with CAD followed up to 4.5 years. Of the 6 RNA variables analyzed, the exercise EF was most closely associated with future events (cardiovascular death or nonfatal AMI), followed by EF at rest, wall motion abnormalities, and exercise time. Once exercise EF was known, no other RNA variable contributed independent information about the likelihood of future events. The exercise EF also described much of the prognostic information about coronary arterial anatomy. Of their 386 patients, 27 cardiovascular deaths and 45 total cardiac events occurred during the follow-up period (mean duration, 2 years). Seven of the 27 deaths and 22 of the 45 events occurred in patients with a rest EF≥50. All 386 patients included in this study had coronary narrowing ≥75% in diameter of ≥1 major coronary artery and all had stable symptoms, usually only angina pectoris.

Of isolated LC coronary arterial narrowing

Isolated narrowing of the LC coronary artery is uncommon and its features have not been well documented. Since percutaneous coronary angioplasty is now performed in many patients with single vessel disease, Dunn and colleagues[41] from Sydney, Australia, reviewed clinical characteristics of 84 patients with isolated LC narrowing. A total of 66 patients had angina pectoris and 60 had had an AMI. Risk factors averaged 2.2 per patient. In the 84 patients there were 103 discrete LC stenoses, of which 51 were central and 52 were peripheral and 48 were total and 55 were subtotal. The LV function was normal in 21 patients and abnormal in 63 patients, but the mean LV EF of the group was normal at 59 ± 12%. Eighty-two patients had an abnormal ECG: there were Q waves in 25, RV pattern in 43, ST-T wave abnormalities in 19, left BBB in 2, and pacemaker rhythm in one. Inferior abnormalities on the ECG correlated with peripheral stenoses, and lateral abnormalities on ECG correlated with central stenoses. The RV pattern of true posterior AMI was seen in both central and peripheral stenoses. In the 32 patients who underwent thallium scanning, lateral defects were more common with central stenoses, but posterolateral defects occurred similarly in central and peripheral stenoses. Prognosis remained good. There were 2 deaths during the mean follow-up time of 17 months, and the cumulative survival rate was 100% at 12 months, 98% at 24 months, and 98% at 30 months. Thus, these statistics on isolated LC CAD should be taken into consideration when coronary angioplasty is contemplated in this particular anatomic group.

With "LM equivalent" narrowing

Califf and associates[42] from Durham, North Carolina, evaluated clinical characteristics in nonsurgical prognosis of 55 patients with "LM equivalent"

CAD defined as: (1) ⩾75% diameter reduction of the LAD before the takeoff of any large septal perforator or anterolateral (diagonal) branches; (2) ⩾75% diameter reduction of the LC before takeoff of any large marginal branch; and (3) absence of ⩾50% stenosis of the LM coronary artery. Compared with nonsurgically treated patients with ⩾75% stenosis of the LM artery, patients with LM equivalent CAD had a shorter duration of symptoms (median, 51 -vs- 66 months) and more often had a Q wave on the ECG (60 -vs- 39%). Survival in patients with LM equivalent CAD (78% at 1 year and 55% at 5 years) was better than that in patients with LM disease with nonsurgical therapy (65% at 1 year and 40% at 5 years) (p = 0.02) (Fig. 1-14), although the rate of freedom from cardiovascular events was not significantly different (Fig. 1-15). Compared with other nonsurgically treated patients with 2- or 3-vessel CAD involving the LAD and LC (28 and 42%, respectively, with progressive angina), patients with LM equivalent CAD had more severe anginal

Fig. 1-14. Survival rate of patients with LM disease compared with that in patients with LM equivalent ("LME") disease. Bars represent 2 SE of the estimate of the end point of interest. The numbers accompanying each survival curve represent the patients free of the event of interest at each yearly interval. The actual survival rates for each yearly interval are listed below the figure.

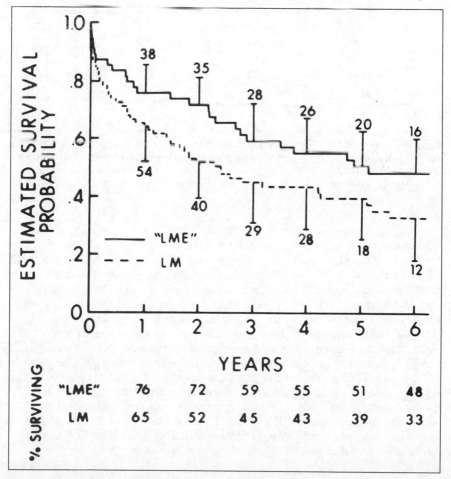

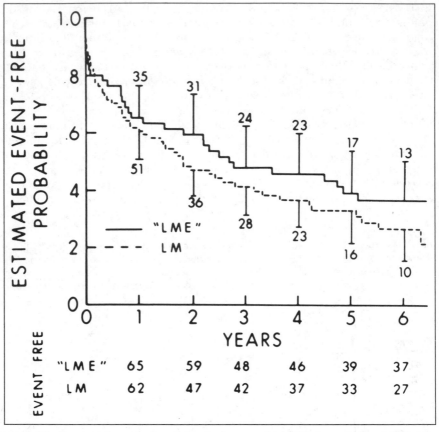

Fig. 1-15. Freedom from cardiovascular death or nonfatal AMI (event-free probability) in patients with LM and LM equivalent ("LME") disease. Bars represent 2 SE of the estimate of the end point of interest. The numbers accompanying each survival curve represent the patients free of the event of interest at each yearly interval. The actual event-free rates for each yearly interval are listed below the figure.

symptoms (55% with progressive angina) and a longer duration of symptoms (medians of 20 months in 2-vessel CAD, 36 months in 3-vessel CAD, and 51 months in LM equivalent CAD). In patients without LM disease, the presence of LM equivalent CAD was a significant univariable prognostic factor (chi-square = 7.1; p = 0.008), but the presence of concomitant right CAD was a more powerful prognostic factor (chi-square = 16.6; p < 0.0001). In multivariable analysis the state of the LV function, the anginal symptoms, and the presence of extracardiac vascular disease were more closely related to survival than the specific cardiac anatomy. The ratio of fatal to nonfatal cardiac events in follow-up was 12:1 in LM disease, 5:1 in LM equivalent CAD, 2.8:1 in 3-vessel non-LM equivalent CAD, and 1.7:1 in 2-vessel non-LM equivalent CAD. These results support the concept that the likelihood of a cardiac event is related to the number of lesions at risk of occlusion, whereas the likelihood that a cardiac event will be fatal is related to the amount of myocardium distal to the occlusion.

Of proteinuria

Despite considerable clinical experience with proteinuria, its prognostic meaning in the ambulatory general population is poorly documented. From a 16-year study of 5,209 men and women in the Framingham cohort, Kannel and associates[43] from Boston, Massachusetts, found that proteinuria, even in casual urine specimens, carries substantial risk, with the mortality rate increased 3-fold. Proteinuria was 3 times as common in hypertensive persons and also occurred to excess in diabetic patients and in persons with cardiac enlargement. In the absence of these factors, proteinuria was so uncommon that its risk could not be accurately assessed. Among persons with these associated risk factors, those with proteinuria have higher death rates than those without proteinuria. In men, overall mortality and cardiovascular mortality rates remained significantly increased even when other contributors to risk were taken into account. Proteinuria in the ambulatory general population is not a benign condition and carries a serious prognosis. It appears to reflect widespread vascular damage.

PROGRESSION OF NARROWING

The timing of repeat coronary arteriography in patients with chronic chest pain after initial coronary arteriogram is a common clinical problem. Especially troublesome are patients found to have normal arteries or nonobstructive intraluminal disease on the first study. To aid in the elucidation of this problem, Haft and Bachik[44] from Newark, New Jersey, studied the incidence of progression of CAD in symptomatic patients from serial coronary arteriograms in 27 patients with normal coronary arteries on initial study, in 17 patients with minimal disease (narrowings $\leq$20%), and in 125 patients with severe disease (narrowings >50%) on the first arteriogram. Interval between arteriograms ranged from 9 months to 13 years. Progression (new lesions or further narrowing $\geq$15%) was seen in normal patients less frequently (15%) than either the minimal disease patients (59%) or severe disease patients (60%) ($p < 0.001$). The incidence of progression was the same in both groups. These data suggest that patients with normal coronary arteries rarely progress to severe narrowing and then only rarely in <4 years. However, minimal narrowing is a serious finding on arteriography and progresses to obstruction frequently in symptomatic patients. Thus, the finding of minimal disease is important, carries a far worse prognosis than normal coronary arteries, and repeat arteriography is warranted at short periods (even within 2 years) when there is persistent recurrent chest pain.

In the National Heart, Lung and Blood Institute Type II Coronary Intervention Study, Brensike and colleagues[45] from Bethesda, Maryland, and Pittsburgh, Pennsylvania, placed patients with type II hyperlipoproteinemia and CAD on a low fat, low cholesterol diet and then randomly allocated them to receive either 6 g cholestyramine 4 times a day or placebo. This double-blind study evaluated the effects of cholestyramine on the progression of CAD as assessed by angiography. Diet alone reduced the LDL cholesterol 6% in both groups. After randomization, LDL cholesterol decreased another 5% in the placebo group and 26% in the cholestyramine-treated groups. Coronary angiography was performed in 116 patients before and after 5 years of treatment: CAD progressed in 49% (28 of 57) of the placebo-treated patients -vs- 32% (19 of 59) of the cholestyramine-treated patients. When only definite progression was considered, 35% (20 of 57) of the placebo-treated patients -vs- 25% (15 of 59) of the cholestyramine-treated patients had definite progression (NS). When this analysis was performed with adjustment for baseline inequalities of risk factors, effect of treatment was more pronounced. Of lesions causing ≥50% stenosis at baseline, 33% of placebo-treated and 12% of cholestyramine-treated patients manifested progression. Similar analyses with other end points (percent of baseline lesions that progressed, narrowings that progressed to occlusion, narrowings that regressed, size of lesion change, and all cardiovascular end points) all favored the cholestyramine group but were not statistically significant. Thus, although the sample size does not allow a definite conclusion to be drawn, this study suggests that cholestyramine treatment retards the rate of progression of CAD in patients with type II hyperlipoproteinemia.

Between January 1, 1970, and May 1, 1980, Moise and coworkers[46] from Montreal, Canada, obtained data on 313 consecutive patients with at least 1 stenosis ≥50% of a major coronary artery documented by cardiac catheterization to determine the clinical and angiographic factors associated with progression of CAD. In these patients, a second coronary arteriographic study was performed at least 3 months later and without interim CABG or PTCA. The interval between the 2 coronary arteriograms ranged from 3–119 months (mean, 39 ± 25, SD). Among these patients, 181 had repeat cardiac catheterizations for stable angina pectoris, 52 for unstable angina pectoris, and 80 for various other reasons. The analyses of the coronary arteries included a definition of the percent diameter narrowing in 15 coronary artery segments as established by a consensus of 3 observers unaware of the clinical diagnosis; a definition of coronary segment size distal to the region of stenosis; a determination of progression of coronary stenoses defined as a ≥20% increase in stenosis in a segment narrowed ≥50% or a ≥30% increase in stenosis in a segment with <50% initial obstruction. From these data, the extent and severity of CAD were computed. Left ventriculography also was performed and LV EF was calculated. The patients consisted mainly of relatively young individuals (mean age, 48 years) with a good LV EF (mean, 59%). Only 14% of the patients had significant 3-vessel CAD. Multivariate logistic regression identified 4 independent predictors of progression of CAD: the interval between studies ($p < 0.0001$), unstable angina pectoris ($p < 0.0001$), relatively extensive CAD ($p = 0.0001$), and relatively young age ($p = 0.0026$) (Tables 1-3 and 1-4). In 74 patients aged ≤50 years with moderately extensive CAD at the first evaluation, the probability of progression of CAD between 2 and 4 years and after 4 years was 80 and 90%, respectively. These data suggest that one may stratify patients according to risks for progression of CAD based on the clinical and angiographic findings.

TABLE 1-3. *Clinical predictors of progression of disease. Reproduced with permission from Moise et al.*[46]

VARIABLES	PROGRESSION (N = 139)	NO PROGRESSION (N = 174)	p VALUE
Age (yr)	46.7 ± 7.5*	48.5 ± 7.8*	0.05
Duration of the disease (mo)	28 ± 38*	33 ± 38*	NS
Cholesterol levels † (mg/dl)	237 ± 38*	239 ± 53*	NS
Interval between studies (mo)	47 ± 25*	32 ± 22*	< 0.001
	No. (%)	No. (%)	
Previous AMI	68 (49)	81 (46)	NS
Positive family history	77 (55)	97 (55)	NS
Hypertension	41 (29)	50 (28)	NS
Smokers	108 (78)	129 (74)	NS
CHF			
1st catheterization	1 (1)	1 (1)	NS
2nd catheterization	18 (13)	6 (3)	0.01
Angina at rest			
1st catheterization	47 (34)	46 (26)	NS
2nd catheterization	70 (50)	54 (31)	< 0.001
Progression of angina functional class	64 (46)	59 (34)	< 0.05
Interim AMI	36 (26)	29 (17)	0.05
Unstable angina at 2nd catheterization	40 (29)	12 (7)	< 0.001

* Mean ± SD.
†Data available for 289 patients.

TABLE 1-4. *Angiographic predictors of progression. Reproduced with permission from Moise et al.*[46]

	PROGRESSION (N = 139)	NO PROGRESSION (N = 174)	p VALUE
# diseased vessels	1.43 ± 0.87*	1.56 ± 0.86*	NS
Friesinger score	7.0 ± 2.6*	7.5 ± 3.0*	NS
Gensini score	32 ± 27*	39 ± 34*	< 0.05
# severe (80–99%) stenoses	0.66 ± 0.84*	0.83 ± 0.91*	NS
Extent score	3.91 ± 2.11*	3.05 ± 1.78*	< 0.001
EF	58 ± 11*	59 ± 11*	NS
Change in EF	−5 ± 12*	−3 ± 10*	NS
	No. (%)	No. (%)	
Use of nitroglycerin			
1st catheterization	73 (52)	93 (53)	NS
2nd catheterization	73 (52)	65 (37)	< 0.01
New akinesia	32 (23)	21 (12)	0.01
New occlusion	49 (35)	49 (28)	NS

* Mean ± SD.

BLOOD LIPIDS

Results of the Lipid Research Clinics Primary Prevention Trials

Plasma total and LDL cholesterol levels may be reduced by diets and drugs. However, before such treatment can be advocated with confidence and before it can be concluded that cholesterol plays a causal role in the pathogenesis of CAD, it is desirable to show that reducing cholesterol levels safely reduces the risk of CAD. Many clinical trials of cholesterol lowering have been conducted, but their results, although often encouraging, have been inconclusive. The most appropriate clinical trial of the efficacy of cholesterol lowering would be a dietary study, because of the links between diets high in saturated fat and cholesterol typical of most industrialized populations, high plasma total and LDL cholesterol levels, and a high incidence of CAD. This type study, however, would cost an estimated $500 million to $1,000 million. Accordingly, the Lipid Research Clinics (LRC) Coronary Primary Prevention Trial (CPPT) was initiated in 1973 as an alternative test of the efficacy of reducing cholesterol levels. The choice of hypercholesterolemic men at high risk of CAD events developing reduced the necessary sample size to a feasible level. Women were not recruited because of their lower risk of CAD. The use of the drug cholestyramine resin permitted a double-blind design. This drug was selected on account of its known effectiveness in reducing total cholesterol and LDL cholesterol levels, the availability of a suitable placebo, its nonabsorbability from the gastrointestinal tract, its few systemic effects, and its low level of significant toxicity.

The report of the LRC program appeared in January 1984,[47,48] and this is probably the most important article on cardiovascular disease published in 1984. The LRC CPPT was a multicenter, randomized, double-blind study that tested the efficacy of cholesterol lowering in reducing the risk of CAD in 3,806 asymptomatic middle-aged men with type II hyperlipoproteinemia. The treatment group received the bile acid sequestrant cholestyramine resin and the control group received a placebo for an average of 7.4 years. Both groups followed a moderate cholesterol-lowering diet. The cholestyramine group experienced average plasma total and LDL cholesterol reductions of 13.4 and 20.3%, respectively, which were 8.5 and 12.6% greater reductions than those obtained in the placebo group. The cholestyramine group experienced a 19% reduction in risk (p < 0.05) of the primary end point—definite CHD death or definite nonfatal AMI or both—reflecting a 24% reduction in definite CAD death and a 19% reduction in nonfatal AMI (Fig. 1-16). The cumulative 7-year incidence of the primary end point was 7% in the cholestyramie group -vs- 8.6% in the placebo group. In addition, the incidence rates for new positive exercise tests, angina, and CABG were reduced by 25, 20, and 21%, respectively, in the cholestyramine group. The risk of death from all causes was only slightly and not significantly reduced in the cholestyramine group. The magnitude of this decrease (7%) was less than for CAD end points because of a greater number of violent and accidental deaths in the cholestyramine group. The LRC CPPT findings show that reducing total cholesterol by lowering LDL cholesterol levels can diminish the incidence of CAD

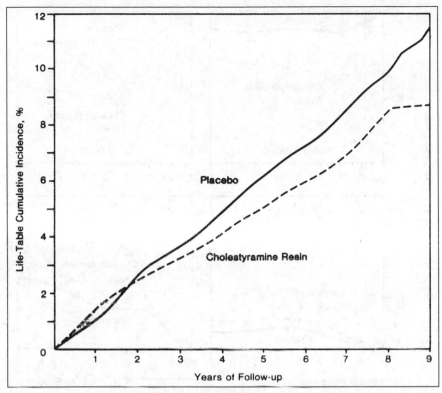

Fig. 1-16. Life-table cumulative incidence of primary end point (definite CAD death and/or definite nonfatal AMI) in treatment groups, computed by Kaplan-Meier method. N = total number of Lipid Research Clinics Coronary Primary Prevention Trial participants at risk for their first primary end point, followed at each time point. Reproduced with permission from the Lipid Research Clinics Program.[47]

morbidity and mortality in men at high risk for CAD because of raised LDL cholesterol levels (Fig. 1-17). This clinical trial provides strong evidence for a causal role for these lipids in the pathogenesis of CAD.

A 19% lower incidence of CAD was observed in the cholestyramine-treated men compared with the men receiving placebo, and this lower incidence of CAD was accompanied by mean decrease of 8 and 12% in plasma total cholesterol and LDL cholesterol relative to levels in placebo-treated men.[48] When the cholestyramine treatment group was analyzed separately, a 19% reduction in CAD risk also was associated with each decrement of 8% in total cholesterol or 11% in LDL cholesterol levels (p < 0.001). Moreover, CAD incidence in men sustaining a decrease of 25% in total cholesterol or 35% in LDL cholesterol levels, typical responses to the prescribed dosage (24 g/day) of cholestyramine resin, was half that of men who remained at pretreatment levels. Adherence to medication was associated with reduced incidence of CAD only when accompanied by decreases in total cholesterol and LDL cholesterol levels. Small increases in HDL cholesterol levels, which accompanied cholestyramine treatment, independently accounted for a 2% reduction in CAD risk. Thus, the reduction of CAD incidence in the cholestyramine group

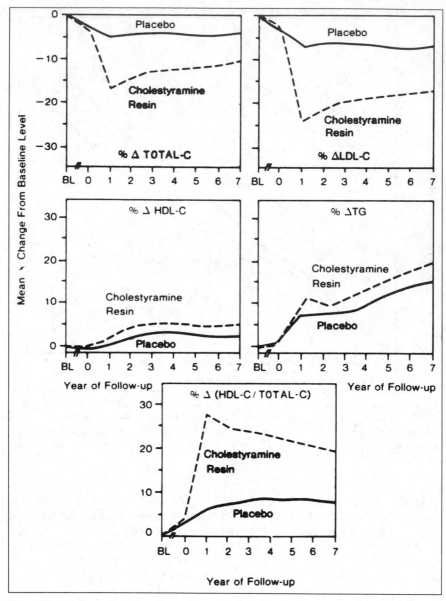

Fig. 1-17. Changes from baseline values of total cholesterol, LDL and HDL cholesterol, triglycerides and the ratio of HDL/total cholesterol. Reproduced with permission from Lipid Research Clinics Program.[47]

seems to have been mediated chiefly by reduction of total cholesterol and LDL cholesterol levels.

The LRC CPPT results give a clear and consistent picture of the relation of its primary end point, CAD incidence, to changes in cholesterol levels. Whether one examines baseline data prospectively, relates post-treatment cholesterol change, or compares the cholestyramine and placebo groups as randomly assigned, the result is the same: a decrement of 22.3 mg/dl (10.4%) in LDL cholesterol levels is associated with a 16–19% reduction in CAD risk (internal consistency). The results of observational studies and other trials of cholesterol lowering, including those of both secondary and primary prevention of CAD and those of both diet and drugs, are consistent with this finding (external consistency). The predicted and observed CAD incidence in men maintaining a 25% decrease in total cholesterol or a 35% decrease in LDL cholesterol levels, responses often achieved by men taking 24 g of cholestyramine resin daily, was about half that of men with no cholesterol lowering. Thus, the benefit of effective cholesterol-lowering therapy in men with type II hyperlipoproteinemia with regard to incidence of CAD is of great potential clinical as well as statistical significance.

The results of this study were presented at a news conference and reported in virtually every newspaper and major magazine in the country. The findings should affect profoundly the practice of medicine in this country.

In a letter to the editor in *Lancet* Tunstall-Pedoe[49] commented on the LRC trial. It was pointed out that the 14,100 man-years of cholestyramine treatment, involving 82 tons of cholestyramine, would cost 8 million pounds in the UK at today's prices. The 8 fatal coronary events prevented would cost about 1 million pounds each. The equivalent figure for all definite coronary events would be 2,000 pounds each. The cost of cholestyramine would have to change by several orders of magnitude to make it a best buy, even if it were desirable on all other grounds.

Relation between lipids and angiographically defined CAD in Japanese men

Kanamori and associates[50] from Sapporo, Japan, studied the relation between the severity and extent of CAD and the lipid profiles in 120 Japanese men who underwent coronary angiography. Analysis of the lipid quartile distribution showed that the percentage of patients with significant CAD increased as the total cholesterol increased and HDL cholesterol decreased. In addition, as the number of coronary arteries with marked narrowing increased, the total cholesterol and total cholesterol/HDL cholesterol increased while HDL cholesterol decreased. However, within this population, triglyceride level, high BP, and cigarette smoking were not significantly associated with coronary angiographic findings.

Changes with age

Miller[51] from London, England, in an attempt to identify the biochemical basis of the age-related increase in LDL concentration in adults collated the data on LDL apoprotein B metabolism in healthy subjects aged 20–75 years, presented in 29 publications since 1972. Additionally, data from 15 reports on LDL metabolism in patients with heterozygous familial hypercholesterolemia also were analyzed. In the pooled data from healthy subjects the plasma concentrations of LDL cholesterol, LDL apoprotein B, and triglyceride were all positively associated with age. On average, LDL cholesterol increased by 1.4 mg/dl and LDL apoprotein B by 0.8 mg/dl/year. Body weight also increased with age (Fig. 1-18). Similar correlations were present in the patients with familial hypercholesterolemia. These results provide persuasive

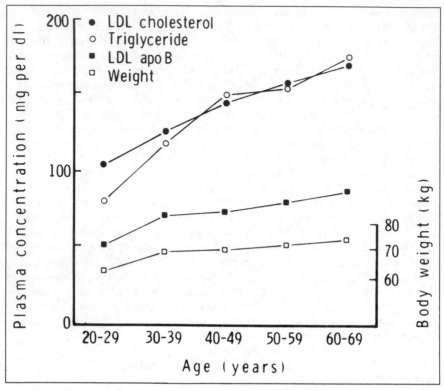

Fig. 1-18. Relation of plasma triglyceride, LDL cholesterol, and LDL apoprotein B concentrations and of body weight to age in healthy men and women. Reproduced with permission from Miller.[51]

evidence that the fractional rate of catabolism of LDL increases with increasing age because of a decline in the activity of LDL receptors. In contrast, the production rate of LDL seems to vary little throughout the age range examined. However, in countries where symptomatic and fatal CAD is infrequent, the plasma LDL concentration does not increase with age. Thus, the decline in LDL receptor activity observed in Western countries might not be an inevitable consequence of aging but might result rather from an interaction between age and an environmental factor or element of lifestyle and therefore potentially avoidable.

Effect of eating eggs

Sacks and associates[52] from Amherst, Massachusetts, and Seattle, Washington, fed 17 lactovegetarian college students 400 kcal of test foods per day containing 1 extra large egg for 3 weeks and similar isocaloric eggless foods for an additional 3 weeks in addition to their usual diet in a randomized double-blind crossover trial. Ingestion of the eggs increased dietary cholesterol from 97–418 mg/day. Mean plasma LDL cholesterol was 12% higher and mean plasma apoprotein B was 9% higher when eggs were being consumed than during the eggless period. Mean plasma HDL cholesterol, apoproteins A-I and A-II, VLDL cholesterol, and total triglycerides did not change significantly. Thus, ingestion of egg seems selectively to raise cholesterol and protein in LDL particles in the plasma of free-living normal persons. Plasma LDL may be more sensitive to cholesterol at low intakes than at moderate to high intakes.

Effect of alcohol

HDL and plasma may be divided into 2 subfractions: less dense HDL_2, the concentration of which appears to be negatively associated with CAD, and more dense HDL_3, which is reportedly unrelated to CAD. Alcohol consumption correlates with both reduced CAD and increased plasma HDL cholesterol concentrations; however, the relation of moderate alcohol intake to HDL_2 and HDL_3 is obscure. To study the effect of alcohol on these HDL subfractions, Haskell and associates[53] from Stanford and Berkeley, California, randomly assigned 24 men who were moderate drinkers to an abstention group (n, 12) or a control drinking group (n, 12). After 6 weeks, concentrations of HDL cholesterol and HDL_3 mass were decreased in abstainers but not in drinkers, whereas HDL_2 mass was unchanged. Resumption of drinking increased the levels of HDL cholesterol and HDL_3 mass without affecting HDL_2 mass. These data suggest that the association of alcohol with CAD is not mediated by increases in plasma HDL_2 levels. Furthermore, the HDL_3 fraction may not be "inert" with respect to CAD, or the association of alcohol with CAD may operate through mechanisms unrelated to HDL.

Effect of diabetes mellitus

Diabetes mellitus is frequently associated with elevated concentrations of total plasma triglyceride in LDL cholesterol and reduced concentrations of HDL cholesterol. Whereas normal women usually have less arteriosclerotic vascular disease then men, diabetic women lose this protection and have prevalence rates of arteriosclerotic disease that approach or equal those of men. It is not known whether lipid abnormalities are greater in diabetic women than in men, or whether these abnormalities may explain the differences in the risk of arteriosclerosis. Walden and associates[54] from Seattle, Washington, studied sex differences in the serum lipid abnormalities associated with diabetes mellitus in 111 patients with insulin-dependent diabetes and in 270 patients with noninsulin-dependent diabetes who were compared with 586 nondiabetic controls. Relative to control levels, the increases in triglycerides were 17–34 mg/dl greater in diabetic women than in diabetic men. The median LDL cholesterol concentration in noninsulin-dependent diabetics was 1–4 mg/dl lower than the control level in women and 16–22 mg/dl lower in men, and was 30 mg/dl higher than control in insulin-dependent diabetic women and similar to control in insulin-dependent diabetic men. The decrease in median HDL cholesterol in noninsulin-dependent diabetics was 2–7 mg/dl greater in women than in men, and the increase in HDL cholesterol in insulin-dependent diabetics was 3 mg/dl less in women than in men. The investigators concluded that diabetes has a greater adverse effect on triglyceride and lipoprotein cholesterol concentrations in diabetic women than in diabetic men and that this may explain the greater increase in risk of arteriosclerosis in diabetic women. This article was followed by an editorial entitled "Exercise and Sudden Cardiac Death: Protection or Provocation?" by Thompson and Mitchell.[55]

Cardiovascular features of homozygous familial hypercholesterolemia

Familial hypercholesterolemia (FH) is characterized by an autosomal codominant inheritance, an abnormality in LDL receptor function, elevated plasma cholesterol levels, and premature atherosclerosis. Sprecher and associates[56] from Bethesda, Maryland, studied 16 patients with homozygous FH to correlate the extent of their atherosclerotic disease with their lipid levels and receptor function. The age range was 3–38 years (mean, 12), and at the last examination, 6–43 years (mean, 20). The mean pretreatment total plasma cholesterol concentration for all patients was 729 ± 58 mg/dl (±SEM), and the mean LDL cholesterol level was 672 ± 58 mg/dl (normal, 60–176). The HDL cholesterol was 28 ± 3 mg/dl (normal, 30–74). In the 7 patients with FH who had symptoms of myocardial ischemia (group I) the mean pretreatment LDL cholesterol value (817 ± 62 mg/dl) was higher than that of the 9 asymptomatic patients (group II; 560 ± 74 mg/dl). In group I, 5 of 7 patients had left or right coronary ostial narrowing and 3 had significant LV outflow obstruction. Most coronary arterial narrowing occurred in the right and LAD coronary arteries and the least amount in the LC coronary artery. A femoral bruit was the physical finding that correlated best with the group I population; brother and sister pairs revealed a milder clinical course for the female. Seven of the 16 patients have survived into their third decade without symptoms. Comparison of these persons with those in whom angina developed reveals a marked heterogeneity in their clinical course, which appears to be associated with receptor negative/defective status.

Roberts[57] from Bethesda, Maryland, in an editorial pointed out that in most Western countries the "normal" levels of total cholesterol (TC) is considered to be excessively high. In the USA, the average plasma TC level of persons 20 years of age is about 160 mg/dl, but thereafter the level progressively increases. The increase is not as high today as it was a decade ago. The average plasma TC of adults >40 years old in the USA is down to 210 mg/dl from about 225 mg/dl a decade ago, and the average of patients in coronary care units with AMI is about 225 mg/dl. All these figures, however, are considered "normal" in most laboratories in the USA. In the Clinical Chemistry Laboratory of the Clinical Center (i.e., the Hospital) of the National Institutes of Health, the "normal" range for serum TC is stated to be 163–263 mg/dl. The upper limit in some laboratories is 300 mg/dl. For laboratories, particularly those of prominent research institutions, to present values of this level as normal prevents attempts of physicians and of patients to make efforts to lower the plasma TC to levels at which signs and symptoms of organ ischemia do not occur, and that level, for practical purposes, is <150 mg/dl. I (WCR) consider any plasma TC level >150 mg/dl to be elevated.

If the upper limit of the normal plasma TC level is considered to be 250 or 300 mg/dl, hypercholesterolemia does not become a greater risk factor for development of symptomatic or fatal cardiovascular atherosclerosis than does systemic hypertension or cigarette smoking. In areas of the world, however, where the frequency of systemic hypertension and cigarette smoking is high but the level of plasma TC is low, i.e., <150 mg/dl, the occurrence of symptomatic or fatal CAD is virtually nonexistent. About 15 years ago, I (WCR) visited Kampala, Uganda, and examined many aortas, coronary arteries, and circles of Willis at necropsy. Other than a few small yellow dots or streaks that produced virtually no luminal narrowing, these arteries were free of atherosclerotic plaques. Yet, the frequency of systemic hypertension in this central African population was extremely high—indeed, hypertension was their most common cardiovascular condition—and a high percentage of the hearts were heavier than normal, presumably the result of the systemic hypertension. I was also impressed with the high frequency of cigarette smoking among the population. In Central Africa, many adults have plasma TC levels of about 100 mg/dl, a value >100% less than the average plasma TC level in adult Americans. In my view, evidence is lacking to implicate either systemic hypertension or cigarette smoking as an accelerator of atherosclerosis in the absence of hypercholesterolemia if the normal plasma TC level is defined as a level <150 mg/dl; if the TC level, however, is >150 mg/dl, as is the situation in 95% of adults >40 years of age in the USA, both systemic hypertension and cigarette smoking are highly atherogenic.

In contrast to the levels in Central Africa where symptomatic and fatal coronary heart disease is virtually nonexistent, only 5% of Americans >40 years have plasma TC levels <150 mg/dl. Thus, to perform studies on meaningful numbers of adults >40 years of age in the USA with plasma TC levels <150 mg/dl (ideal normal value) and compare findings to those with levels 160–260 mg/dl (usual values) is virtually impossible. In contrast to the 5% of middle-aged and older adult Americans with plasma TC levels <150 mg/dl, 5% of American adults >40 years have plasma TC levels >265 mg/dl and about 1 in a million have plasma TC levels >600 mg/dl and normal plasma triglyceride levels.

High density lipoproteins

Glueck and associates[58] from Cincinnati, Ohio, studied black male and female juveniles and adult black males and found higher levels of HDL cholesterol than in whites, differences that potentially "protect" them against augmented CAD morbidity and mortality, given an excess of certain CAD risk factors among blacks, particularly systemic hypertension. The loss of the "protective" HDL cholesterol difference in adult black females appeared most likely to be due to their pandemic obesity. Inasmuch as blacks smoke more cigarettes, are more likely to have diabetes mellitus, and are more often treated with antihypertensive agents, these factors tended to reduce black-white differences in HDL cholesterol. Black-white differences in alcohol intake and habitual and leisure-time physical activity were not found likely, in the aggregate, to affect black-white differences in HDL cholesterol. It thus seems likely that, whereas environment has a substantial effect on HDL cholesterol for blacks and whites, there may be a "genetic" factor accounting for higher levels of HDL cholesterol in blacks.

HDL cholesterol is inversely associated with risk of heart attack. Sex hormones have been suggested as possible factors contributing to the gender difference of CAD risk. Little is known about how endogenous sex hormone concentration might be related to HDL cholesterol. This relation was examined by Dai and associates[59] from Pittsburgh, Pennsylvania, and Greenville, North Carolina, in 225 men participating in the Multiple Risk Factor Intervention Trial. Plasma testosterone concentration was positively correlated with HDL cholesterol and the change in testosterone concentration was also positively correlated with change in HDL cholesterol. The relation between testosterone and HDL cholesterol could not be fully explained by age, relative weight, alcohol consumption, and cigarette smoking in the cross-sectional study. However, when this relation was examined longitudinally, the partial correlation between changes in testosterone and HDL cholesterol did not quite achieve statistical significance ($0.05 < p < 0.10$). The biologic process that relates HDL cholesterol to testosterone is not known. The results suggest an inverse relation between plasma estradiol concentration and LDL cholesterol, but no statistical significant correlation with HDL cholesterol. In addition, there was no association noted in the current research between estradiol concentrations and the known determinants of HDL cholesterol.

Effects of physical training

To ascertain whether older (masters) athletes have a more favorable plasma lipoprotein/lipid profile than sedentary men of similar age, Seals and associates[60] from St. Louis, Missouri, studied 14 endurance trained masters athletes (mean age, 60 ± 2 years), 12 older, untrained and not lean men (mean age, 62 ± 1 years), 9 older, untrained and lean men (mean age, 61 ± 2 years), 15 young endurance-trained athletes (mean age, 26 ± 1 years) and 15 young untrained men (mean age, 28 ± 1 years). The athletes had higher values for maximal oxygen uptake and lower levels of body fatness compared with the untrained men, regardless of age. The HDL cholesterol was markedly higher in the masters athletes than in the other groups (66 -vs- 42–55 mg/dl) (Table 1-5). The total cholesterol and LDL cholesterol concentrations of the masters athletes generally were higher than those of the younger groups, similar to those of the older lean men, and lower than those of the older and not lean men. The total/HDL cholesterol ratios were similarly low (2.8–3.4) for the athletes and the young untrained men compared with the older untrained men (4.0–5.6). Thus, some older endurance ath-

TABLE 1-5. *Plasma lipid concentrations for the 5 subject groups.*

	#	TOTAL CHOLES-TEROL (mg/dl)	LDL CHOLES-TEROL (mg/dl)	HDL CHOLES-TEROL (mg/dl)	TOTAL/HDL CHOLES-TEROL (U)	TRIGLYC-ERIDES (mg/dl)
Masters athletes	14	192 ± 8	112 ± 6	66 ± 3‡	3.0 ± 0.1	72 ± 4
Young athletes	15	151 ± 6*	85 ± 5*	55 ± 2	2.8 ± 0.1	57 ± 5
Young untrained	15	165 ± 11*	100 ± 10	50 ± 2	3.4 ± 0.2	74 ± 6
Older untrained, lean	9	175 ± 9	113 ± 8†	45 ± 4†	4.0 ± 0.3‡	87 ± 11
Older untrained, not lean	12	220 ± 9‡	141 ± 9‡	42 ± 4†	5.6 ± 0.4‡	184 ± 20‡

* Significantly different (p < 0.05) from masters athletes.
† Significantly different (p < 0.05) from young athletes.
‡ Significantly different (p < 0.05) from all other groups.

letes have markedly higher HDL cholesterol levels and lower total/HDL cholesterol ratios compared with their sedentary peers. This favorable plasma lipoprotein profile may indicate a reduced risk of developing CAD for older men who exercise regularly.

Seals and associates[61] from St. Louis, Missouri, determined the effects of low and high intensity tolerance and plasma lipids in 11 healthy men and women (mean age, 63 ± 1 years) who participated in a 12-month endurance training program. Plasma glucose, insulin, and C-peptide concentrations were measured for 3 hours after ingestions of 100 g of glucose, and the total areas under the respective curves were calculated. Total plasma lipids and lipoprotein concentrations were determined during fasting. Maximal oxygen uptake increased 12% during 6 months of low intensity training; a further 18% increase occurred during an additional 6 months of high intensity training. Glucose tolerance, which was normal initially, was not significantly changed after training. However, the total area for insulin was 8% lower after low intensity training, and 23% lower after high intensity training, compared with before training. C-peptide concentrations were similarly reduced. Plasma lipid and lipoprotein concentrations were unchanged after low intensity training, but high intensity training resulted in an increase in HDL cholesterol and a reduction in triglycerides. These results demonstrate that older persons respond to prolonged, high intensity endurance training with an increase in sensitivity to insulin and a favorable alteration in their plasma lipoprotein/lipid profile.

The finding that high doses (160 mg) of zinc lowered HDL cholesterol prompted Crouse and associates[62] from Albuquerque, New Mexico, to study the effect of low dose zinc supplementation on lipoprotein values in sedentary and endurance-trained men. Twenty-one endurance-trained and 23 sedentary men received either placebo or 50 mg of zinc sulfate daily for 8 weeks. Despite the fact that plasma zinc increased 15%, fasting plasma HDL cholesterol, total cholesterol, LDL cholesterol, and triglyceride levels did not change in response to zinc ingestion. The researchers concluded that low dose zinc supplementation does not affect lipid or lipoprotein values in either endurance-trained or sedentary men.

Goldberg and associates[63] from Portland, Oregon, prospectively studied lipid and lipoprotein levels in previously sedentary men (mean age, 33 years) and women (mean age, 27 years) undergoing 16 weeks of weight-training exercise. Women demonstrated a 10% reduction of cholesterol, 18% decrease in LDL cholesterol, and 28% lowering of triglycerides. The ratios of total/HDL cholesterol and LDL/HDL cholesterol were reduced 14 and 20%, respectively. Among men, LDL cholesterol was reduced 16%, whereas the ratios of total/HDL cholesterol and LDL/HDL cholesterol were lowered 21 and 29%, respectively. Weight-training exercise appears to result in favorable changes in lipid and lipoprotein levels in previously sedentary men and women.

Herbert and associates[64] from Providence, Rhode Island, studied the HDL metabolism of 5 trained men who ran 16 km daily and in 5 inactive men. Runners were leaner and their aerobic exercise capacity was much greater. The mean HDL cholesterol level was 65 mg/dl in the runners and 41 mg/dl in the controls. The lipid-rich HDL species accounted for a much higher proportion of the HDL in runners (49 -vs- 29%). Tracer studies of radioiodinated autologous HDL demonstrated that runners did not produce more HDL protein, but rather catabolized less. The mean biologic half-life of HDL proteins was 6.2 days in the runners compared with 3.8 days in the sedentary men. The activity of lipoprotein lipase was 80% higher in the postheparin plasma of the runners, whereas the activity of hepatic triglyceride hydrolase was 38% lower. Thus, the prolonged survival of plasma HDL proteins in runners may result from augmented lipid transfer to HDL by lipoprotein lipase or diminished HDL clearance by hepatic lipase.

Treatment

Dujovne and associates[65] from Kansas City, Kansas, compared the hypercholesterolemic and adverse effects of colestipol (20 g/day) and colestipol (10 g/day) combined with probucol (1 g/day) in a double placebo, diet-controlled, crossover trial that lasted 19 months in 22 hypercholesterolemic patients who had LDL cholesterol levels >180 mg/dl after 3 months of diet and placebo treatment. Uniformity of diet and physical activity were monitored throughout the study. Compared with baseline values after 3 months on diet-placebo treatment, "combined" therapy reduced LDL cholesterol by more than 20% in 15 patients, more than 25% in 9 patients, and more than 45% in 2 patients. Treatment with half-dose colestipol and probucol resulted in the greatest mean LDL cholesterol reduction, from 239 mg/dl during diet-placebo period to 170 mg/dl; the difference was not statistically significantly different from the reduction to 180 mg/dl with 20 g of colestipol alone. Fifteen patients showed the greatest reduction in LDL cholesterol after combined therapy. Probucol produced statistically significant reductions in VLDL and HDL cholesterol. The major gastrointestinal side effects of single therapy with colestipol (constipation) and probucol (diarrhea) were ameliorated or abolished by concomitant administration. Probucol and colestipol coadministration allowed a 50% reduction in the colestipol dosage, with similar efficacy and improved tolerability and reduced mean serum LDL cholesterol with a frequency and magnitude rarely seen with other hypocholesterolemic treatments. Hypercholesterolemic persons who cannot tolerate full doses of resins may receive equal benefit by half the dose if probucol is added to the regimen.

Follick and associates[66] from Providence, Rhode Island, examined the short- and long-term effects of weight loss on HDL and LDL cholesterol levels in 42 women who completed a 14-session behavioral weight loss program. Lipid values were determined from samples taken before treatment, after treatment, and at 6-month follow-up. There were significant changes in plasma lipid levels, but the short- and long-term effects differed. Both total and LDL cholesterol levels decreased during treatment and remained lower at follow-up (Table 1-6). However, HDL cholesterol level and the HDL/LDL ratio did not change during treatment but increased significantly above pretreatment levels at follow-up. Furthermore, long-term changes occurred in the body mass index even after correction for initial values. These results show that weight loss can, in the long term, have a potentially beneficial impact on lipoprotein levels in women.

The National Institutes of Health, Bethesda, Maryland, convened a Consensus Development Conference on hypertriglyceridemia on September 27–29, 1983.[67] After 1.5 days of expert presentation of the available data, a consensus panel consisting of lipidologists, cardiologists, primary care physicians, epidemiologists, and experts in exercise considered the evidence and

TABLE 1-6. *Means for weight and plasma lipid values.* Reproduced with permission from Follick et al.*[66]

MEASURE	PRETREATMENT	POST-TREATMENT	FOLLOW-UP
Weight (kg)	66.8a	62.5b	64.1c
	(9.0)	(8.8)	(9.4)
Body mass index	0.256a	0.241b	0.248c
(kg/cm^2 × 100)	(0.037)	(0.035)	(0.041)
Cholesterol	212.0a	200.6b	202.6b
(mg/dl)	(49.1)	(46.9)	(46.1)
Triglycerides	82.1a	76.0ab	70.3b
(mg/dl)	(45.5)	(38.7)	(43.9)
HDL cholesterol	64.0a	62.0a	67.3b
(mg/dl)	(15.2)	(14.9)	(17.2)
LDL cholesterol	131.4a	123.4b	121.3b
(mg/dl)	(44.5)	(43.3)	(42.6)
HDL/LDL	0.556a	0.571a	0.643b
	(0.28)	(0.27)	(0.36)

* Standard deviations appear in parentheses. Means that do not share a common letter designation differ at $p < 0.05$ or better.

agreed on answers to the following questions: 1) What is hypertriglyceridemia? 2) What is the evidence that plasma triglycerides are associated with disease? 3) What patients with hypertriglyceridemia are candidates for therapy? 4) What can be achieved with dietary and other therapies? 5) What should be the guidelines for dietary and drug therapy? and 6) What should be the direction for future research? Careful evaluation of existing data indicates that in the presence of normal cholesterol levels, mild elevations of plasma triglyceride levels do not necessarily increase the risk for cardiovascular disease. When triglyceride levels are <250 mg/dl, risk generally does not exceed that of other Americans, and changes in lifestyle are unnecessary beyond those recommended for the general public. The same can be said for many normocholesterolemic persons with borderline hypertriglyceridemia who have no risk factors for or family history of cardiovascular disease. However, triglyceride levels in the range of 250–500 mg/dl can be a marker for secondary disorders for a subset of patients with genetic forms of hyperlipoproteinemia who are at increased risk and who need specific therapy. Dietary intervention is the primary approach to therapy in these patients, but drugs have a role in selected persons not responding to dietary management. Finally, the danger of pancreatitis is present in frank hypertriglyceridemia (triglyceride level, >500 mg/dl), and the lowering of triglyceride levels by diet and, if necessary, by drugs is indicated.

Briones and associates[68] from Rochester, Minnesota, administered colestipol, the nonabsorbable bile acid sequestrant resin, to 16 patients with primary hypercholesterolemia and compared its effect on serum lipids, lipoprotein fractions, and circulating platelet aggregate ratios and platelet aggregation in response to adenosine diphosphate to that of sitosterols. Cholesterol absorption and sterol balance studies were done in 4 of the subjects during the following treatment periods: diet alone, colestipol, and sitosterols. Total serum cholesterol was significantly reduced by colestipol but only slightly decreased by sitosterols. Combination treatment with colestipol and sitosterols was associated with a smaller decrease in serum cholesterol than was demonstrated with colestipol alone. Serum triglycerides tended to increase during colestipol therapy (this increase was not clinically significant) but showed a minimal nonsignificant decrease with sitosterols treatment. Colestipol decreased cholesterol absorption, whereas sitosterols slightly increased it. Fecal sterol excretion was increased with colestipol treatment but was minimally affected by administration of sitosterols. LDL and HDL cholesterol levels significantly decreased with colestipol treatment. The circulating platelet aggregate ratio was significantly lower in the group of patients with hypercholesterolemia who received colestipol initially than in control subjects, but platelet aggregation in response to adenosine diphosphate was not significantly different between these two groups. No significant change in platelet aggregation was noted during colestipol or sitosterols treatment despite a significant decrease in total serum cholesterol levels with colestipol therapy, a suggestion that the platelet and lipid abnormalities are not interrelated.

Illingworth[69] from Portland, Oregon, treated 12 patients with severe heterozygous familial hypercholesterolemia with mevinolin and colestipol who had severe heterozygous familial hypercholesterolemia and in whom other hypolipidemic drug therapy had failed to reduce serum cholesterol levels to <300 mg/dl. In 10 patients receiving 80 mg/day of mevinolin, plasma total cholesterol concentrations decreased 33% (487 ± 27–326 ± 16 mg/dl) (Fig. 1-19). Additional therapy with colestipol resulted in a further 18% decrease to 269 ± 13 mg/dl. Concentrations of LDL cholesterol decreased in parallel. Plasma concentrations of HDL cholesterol did not change significantly, but the LDL/HDL ratio decreased from 8.2 in patients on diet only to 3.8 in patients treated with mevinolin and colestipol. In 7 patients treated with 40 mg/day of mevinolin, concentrations of LDL cholesterol decreased by 33%; combined therapy resulted in a further 20% decrease, a 46% reduction from the level achieved with diet alone. No consistent side effects were noted in up to 24 months of therapy. Thus, combined therapy with mevinolin and colestipol promises to be effective for heterozygous familial hypercholesterolemia.

In man epidemiologic, metabolic, and genetic studies have long demonstrated an association between the plasma lipoproteins and CAD. Currently, the bile acid sequestrants cholestyramine and colestipol and the B complex vitamin niacin are considered the hypocholesterolemic drugs of choice for patients with type II hyperlipoproteinemia, but tolerance, side effects, and costs remain problems in patient compliance. The oral administration of neomycin or niacin as single drug therapy can significantly lower total and LDL cholesterol concentrations in patients with type II hyperlipoproteinemia. Unfortunately, in most patients treated with 1 of these drugs as sole therapy plasma lipid and lipoprotein concentrations do not become normal. Hoeg and coworkers[70] from Bethesda, Maryland, determined the effect of combined neomycin and niacin treatment on the plasma lipoprotein concentration in 25 type II hyperlipoproteinemic patients in a double-blind, randomized, placebo-controlled, crossover clinical trial. Neomycin was well tolerated by all 25 patients and significantly reduced the cholesterol concentrations but, in contrast, 11 patients were unable to continue niacin because of adverse side effects. In the 14 patients treated with both neomycin and niacin, niacin further lowered the concentrations of total and LDL cholesterol

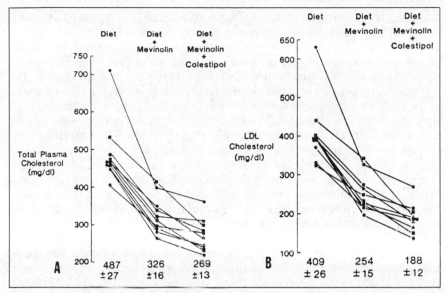

Fig. 1-19. Changes in the concentrations of total (A) and LDL cholesterol (B) in 10 patients with heterozygous familial hypercholesterolemia during sequential therapy with diet, mevinolin (80 mg/day), and mevinolin and colestipol. The values in each panel represent the means of 2 separate determinations obtained under steady state conditions. Mevinolin was taken as 40 mg twice daily and colestipol as 20 g/day (bullets), except in 3 patients, 1 of whom received 15 g/day (solid triangles) and the other 2 10 g/day (open triangles). Four patients were on concurrent therapy for hypertension (squares). The numbers at the bottom represent the mean ± SE for all 10 patients. (To convert milligrams of cholesterol per deciliter to millimoles per liter, multiply by 0.026; to convert milligrams of triglycerides per deciliter to millimoles per liter, multiply by 0.0113.) Reproduced with permission from Illingworth.[69]

by 18 and 25%, respectively, and increased HDL cholesterol by 32% compared with that in the patients receiving neomycin plus placebo. During the study, in 80% of all the study patients and in 92% of the patients who complied with the combined regimen the total and LDL concentrations became normal. No serious or irreversible adverse side effects were detected during combined neomycin and niacin treatment. These results indicate that the lipoprotein concentrations in most type II hyperlipoproteinemic patients can be safely normalized by either therapy with neomycin only or by combined treatment with neomycin and niacin.

Familial hypercholesterolemia is characterized by a marked elevation of plasma LDL level due to impaired receptor-mediated catabolism of this lipoprotein by peripheral tissues, and the high LDL level enhances development of CAD and increases the risk of AMI and coronary death. Partial ileal bypass is effective in reducing circulating cholesterol levels and Koivisto and Miettinen[71] from Helsinki, Finland, studied the 10-year effects of this procedure on serum lipids and lipoproteins in 27 patients with heterozygous familial hypercholesterolemia. The ileal bypass patients were compared with conservatively treated case controls matched for age, sex, serum cholesterol level, relative body weight, BP, cigarette smoking habits, and also for the existence of diabetes mellitus and CAD. Serum triglycerides were initially slightly higher in the patients undergoing ileal bypass. During the 10-year follow-up,

8 surgically treated and 7 control patients had fatal or nonfatal AMI. Of these, all but 1 man who underwent surgery had manifest CAD at entry. Male sex, smoking, triglyceride levels, and angina were significant predictors of new coronary events. The decrease in serum cholesterol levels in patients who underwent ileal bypass and had fatal AMI was smaller than in the corresponding subjects without events. The serum lipid levels of the survivors at the end of the 10-year follow-up showed that ileal bypass, compared with the conservative treatment, led to a decrease in total serum cholesterol, LDL cholesterol, and LDL apoprotein B levels. Higher serum HDL and HDL_2 cholesterol levels were observed. Most ileal bypass patients remained hypercholesterolemic and their LDL cholesterol levels and their LDL apoprotein B levels were still elevated. This study indicates that over the long term, ileal bypass could not normalize plasma lipid levels in patients with heterozygous familial hypercholesterolemia and that a combination of surgery with hypolipidemic drugs may be needed.

Cardiac transplantation for end-stage heart disease would be futile in patients with homozygous familial hypercholesterolemia unless the metabolic processes responsible for the rapidly progressive atherosclerosis in such patients could be counteracted. Starzl and associates[72] from Pittsburgh, Pennsylvania, and Dallas, Texas, performed orthotopic transplantation and the liver was replaced with a liver of the same donor in a girl aged 6 years 7 months with severe heart disease secondary to homozygous familial hypercholesterolemia. In the first 10 weeks after transplantation, the serum cholesterol decreased from the preoperative level of >1,000 to 270 mg/dl. The operation took 16 hours. The removed heart had advanced atherosclerotic and valvular disease and the excised liver was normal by gross and histologic examination. Good cardiac and hepatic function was achieved from the grafts. Standard hepatic function tests were normal from the second postoperative week on. Immunosuppression was continued with 300 mg/day cyclosporine and 7.5 mg/day prednisone. At 4 months, the patient remained well with normal cardiac and liver function. Plasma cholesterol and triglyceride concentrations remained the same as at 10 weeks.

To evaluate the effects of a high complex carbohydrate, low lipid diet on the management of CAD, Ribeiro and associates[73] from Boston, Massachusetts, evaluated 32 patients who had participated in a diet and exercise program, and compared the results with 40 patients who had been managed only with exercise. After a follow-up period of 10–16 weeks, the patients on the diet-exercise program showed significant reduction in body weight (-6 ± 2 kg, mean $\pm$ SD), serum cholesterol (-43 ± 41 mg/dl), and triglycerides (-51 ± 70 mg/dl), whereas patients who were managed only with exercise had no significant changes in weight or serum lipids. Both the diet-exercise and the exercise groups showed significant improvement in working capacity and reduction in resting systolic BP. Patients on the diet-exercise program had significantly less angina (21.9%) occurring on the exercise test after the program compared with before, even though the same double product was reached. Multiple logistic regression analysis of the data for patients with angina on the exercise test demonstrated that the only significant (p = 0.004) contributor for reduction in angina was the dietary intervention. Beta blocking drugs did not affect the results. Although randomized controlled trials must be run in order to ascertain the significance of this finding, this study strongly suggests that a low lipid, high carbohydrate diet is a useful addition to exercise in the management of patients with CAD.

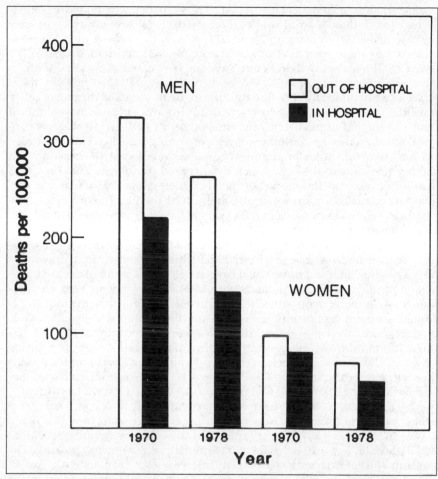

Fig. 1-20. Age-adjusted death rates for CAD by location for 1970 and 1978, Minneapolis-St. Paul Metropolitan area, men and women aged 30–74 years (Minnesota Heart Survey).

By 1979, mortality rates for CAD had declined for 14 consecutive years in the USA. Preliminary data indicate a continued decline (Fig. 1-20). Gillum and associates[74] from Minneapolis, Minnesota, reviewed published reports in the last 5 years regarding the continual decline. These investigators attributed the decline to reduction in population levels of systemic hypertension and cigarette smoking, and improved medical care for AMI. They did not find data that indicated contribution to the decline by change in other risk factors, emergency medical services, medical care of chronic CAD, or other changes in the physical and social environment.

CIGARETTE SMOKING

With use of 24-hour ambulatory ECG monitoring, Davis and associates[75] from Perth, Australia, studied the effect of 1-hour of cigarette smoking on cardiac rhythm in 70 patients with CAD. Fifteen patients had no arrhythmia; 37 had fewer than 2 atrial or VPC/hour with atrial premature complexes possibly related to smoking in 2 and VPC related to smoking in 1. Nineteen subjects had more than 2 VPC/hour (range, 4–368) and had 16 ± 29 VPC/hour (±SD) less during than before smoking (p < 0.05), associated with an increase in heart rate of 4.6 ± 6.8 beats/min (p < 0.01). In none of the 9 subjects with unifocal VPC did multiform beats develop during or after smoking, whereas 3 of 10 subjects with multiform VPC had only unifocal beats during and immediately after smoking. In 1 of these 19 subjects, frequent atrial premature complexes developed during smoking. One other subject had frequent atrial premature complexes unaffected by smoking and another had sinoatrial block, which disappeared during smoking on 1 of 3 monitorings. In conclusion, no sustained or high grade ventricular arrhythmia was provoked by smoking; although atrial premature complexes may have been related to smoking in a few persons, the frequency and complexity of VPC tended to be reduced in these subjects with CAD.

To investigate the effects of cigarette smoking on the coronary vasculature, Martin and associates[76] from Philadelphia, Pennsylvania, measured coronary sinus flow and myocardial oxygen delivery at rest and during incremental atrial pacing in 10 patients with CAD. Measurements were then repeated while the patients smoked 2 unfiltered, high nicotine cigarettes. Although smoking significantly increased the heart rate at rest and double product, coronary sinus flow did not change significantly (141 ± 32 -vs- 146 ± 28 ml/min). At the lowest equivalent pacing rate before and during smoking, the double products were comparable. However, coronary sinus flow was reduced by smoking (146 ± 28 -vs- 159 ± 28 ml/min) and coronary vascular resistance was increased (0.96 ± 0.15 -vs- 0.83 ± 0.13 mmHg ml^{-1} min). The double products were also comparable at the peak pacing rate before and during smoking. Nonetheless, the coronary sinus flow was again lower (167 ± 23 -vs- 227 ± 41 ml/min) and the coronary vascular resistance was higher (0.77 ± 0.10 -vs- 0.63 ± 0.09 mmHg ml^{-1}) during smoking. The transmyocardial arteriovenous oxygen difference was unchanged by smoking; therefore myocardial oxygen delivery was reduced in proportion to the reductions in coronary sinus flow. Thus, cigarette smoking appears to alter acutely the ability of the coronary vasculature to regulate flow in accordance with the oxygen requirements of the myocardium.

Nicod and coworkers[77] from Dallas, Texas, studied 38 smokers (26 men and 12 women; mean age, 50 years) with CAD to determine the influence of smoking on hemodynamic and serologic responses. Systemic and coronary hemodynamics and serologic variables were measured before and after smoking 2 cigarettes in 8–10 minutes in 21 patients or 8–10 minutes without smoking (17 patients, control group). No variable changed in the control group. However, smoking increased heart rate-systolic BP product, cardiac output, and maximal first derivative of LV pressure without significantly changing the coronary sinus concentration of thromboxane B$_2$ or 6-keto-PGF$_{1\alpha}$, the stable metabolites of thromboxane A$_2$ and prostacyclin, respectively. Smoking did not increase coronary flow in 6 of 11 patients with > 70% stenosis of the proximal LAD or LC coronary artery, or both, whereas it did increase coronary flow in all 10 patients without proximal stenoses. Ten smokers underwent atrial pacing for 5 minutes followed 15 minutes later by atrial pacing for 5 minutes during smoking to determine whether smoking altered the response of coronary blood flow to increased myocardial oxygen demand. In 5 patients without proximal left coronary stenoses, coronary flow increased with pacing and with pacing and smoking. However, in 5 patients with proximal stenoses, coronary flow increased with pacing but it did not change with pacing and smoking. These data indicate that in smokers with CAD, myocardial oxygen demand is increased during smoking. However, in persons with severe proximal stenoses of the left coronary artery, it may cause either no change or a decrease in coronary flow. Thus, the influence of smoking on coronary vascular responses appears to be influenced by the location and severity of CAD.

Klein and coworkers[78] from New York City evaluated the acute changes in coronary blood flow and resistance that occur in response to cigarette smoking in 16 patients (group I) with CAD and 6 patients (group II) without angiographically detectable significant CAD. Each patient was either a present or past chronic cigarette smoker. Nitrates, beta blocking agents, and calcium antagonists were discontinued for 8–12 hours before cardiac catheterization. Patients did not smoke for at least 1 hour before the cardiac catheterization. Seven patients (group IA) had severe ($\geq$75%) proximal left coronary stenoses and 9 patients (group IB) had significant distal narrowings with $\leq$50% proximal stenoses. Patients in group I had a smaller increase in coronary sinus blood flow than did patients in group II ($p < 0.05$). Coronary resistance increased in patients overall in group I, but decreased in patients in group II ($p < 0.05$). Patients in group IA had a greater increase in coronary resistance compared with those in group IB (7.0 ± 4.2% -vs- a decrease of 0.9 ± 2.6%) ($p < 0.001$). These data suggest that smoking increases coronary resistance in patients with CAD, especially in those with a severe proximal stenosis.

Hartz and associates[79] from Milwaukee, Wisconsin, investigated the possibility that cigarette smoking has an association with left ventricular wall motion abnormalities that is independent of its known association with CAD. They studied 4,763 men aged 35–74 years who had coronary angiography and ventriculography. Three kinds of wall motion abnormalities were evaluated: hypokinesis in 1–4 ventricular segments, hypokinesis in 5–6 ventricular segments (diffuse hypokinesis), and akinetic or dyskinetic wall motion in at least 1 segment. Among men younger than age 55 years, the relative risk of diffuse hypokinesis was 2.8 (1.1–7.0) for heavy cigarette smokers compared with nonsmokers. Adjusting for the degree of coronary narrowing or eliminating subjects with a history of AMI did not change this relative risk. Among men aged $\geq$55 years, the relative risk (odds ratio for heavy smokers compared with nonsmokers) was not significant (0.6–2.3). Regardless of age, the relative risk of akinesis or dyskinesis, adjusted for coronary stenosis, was significant: 1.8 (1.3–2.7) for men <55 and 1.6 (1.1–2.2) for men $\geq$55 years. These results suggest that cigarette smoking is related to both wall motion abnormalities and transmural AMI and that the relations are largely separate from the association of cigarette smoking with CAD.

PHYSICAL ACTIVITY

Many epidemiologic studies have suggested that personal athleticism alters trends in lifestyle and CAD. Paffenbarger and associates[80] from Boston, Massachusetts, Stanford, California, and Findley, Ohio, analyzed 572 first heart attacks among 16,936 Harvard alumni (1962–1972) and 1,413 total deaths (1962–1970) and found that habitual postcollege exercise, not student sports play, predicted low CAD risk. Sedentary alumni, even exvarsity athletes, had high risk. Sedentary students becoming physically active alumni acquire low risk. Exercise benefit is independent of contrary lifestyle elements—smoking, obesity, weight gain, hypertension, and adverse parental disease history—in affecting CAD incidence. Hypertension was clinically the strongest predictor of coronary attack, but inadequate exercise was strongest on a community basis. Exercise level was inversely related to total, cardiovascular, and respiratory mortality, but less related to cancer or unnatural deaths. The current exercise revolution may improve lifestyle, cardiovascular health, and longevity.

FAMILY HISTORY

Although a family history of CAD is a well-accepted risk factor for cardiovascular disease, only 3 prospective studies in men have examined the predictive strength of a positive family history after adjusting for other heart disease risk factors. Barrett-Connor and Khaw[81] from San Diego, California, analyzed a 9-year follow-up of 4,014 men and women from 40–79 years old who resided in Rancho Bernardo, California, and who reported no known cardiovascular disease in response to a standardized interview. At baseline, 38% of this group reported a family history of a heart attack in a parent, sibling, or child; 15% of those with a positive family history in a first-degree relative indicated that the heart attack had occurred before the relative was 50 years old. Younger men (<60 years) with a positive family history at any age had significantly higher mean BP and total plasma cholesterol levels; older men were likely to have diabetes mellitus. Younger women with a positive family history were more likely to smoke cigarettes and older women had higher cholesterol levels and were more likely to use exogenous estrogens. The independent contribution of a positive family history of heart attack to subsequent cardiovascular death was determined by the Cox model after adjusting for age, systolic BP, total plasma cholesterol level, obesity, cigarette smoking, personal history of diabetes mellitus, and estrogen use in women. In men, but not in women, a positive family history of heart attack was independently predictive of death from all causes and from cardiovascular disease and CAD. Significant differences were restricted to younger men; those with a positive family history had a 5-fold excess risk of cardiovascular death independent of other risk factors. With a family history of premature heart attack, <50 years was not predictive of mortality in men or women. Thus, the differences between younger and older men probably reflect survivorship, but the differences between men and women remain unexplained.

FIBRINOGEN

To study the possible risk factors for cardiovascular disease, Wilhelmsen and colleagues[82] from Goteborg, Sweden, collected data on plasma levels of coagulation factors, BP, serum cholesterol, and cigarette smoking habits in a random sample of 792 men with a mean age of 54 years. During nearly 14 years of follow-up, AMI occurred in 92 men, stroke in 37, and death from causes other than AMI or stroke in 60. The BP, degree of smoking, serum cholesterol, and fibrinogen level measured at the baseline examination proved to be significant risk factors for AMI by univariate analyses during follow-up, and BP and fibrinogen were risk factors for stroke. Fibrinogen and smoking were strongly related to each other. The relation between fibrinogen and AMI, and between fibrinogen and stroke, became weaker when BP, serum cholesterol, and smoking habits were taken into account, but was still significant for stroke. Although causality cannot be inferred from these data, it is possible that the fibrinogen level plays an important part in the development of stroke and AMI.

VASECTOMY

In a historical cohort study Massey and associates[83] from multiple medical centers identified, located, and, if living, interviewed 10,590 vasectomized men from 4 cities, along with a paired neighborhood control for each. The times between procedure data and interview or death ranged from <1–41 years, (median, 8 years) and with 2,318 pairs having ≥10 years of follow-up. Participant reports of diseases or conditions that might possibly be re-

Fig. 1-21. Estimated probability of postbaseline survival free of any disease or death from cardiovascular core for vasectomized (V) and nonvasectomized (NoV) subjects. Reproduced with permission from Massey et al.[83]

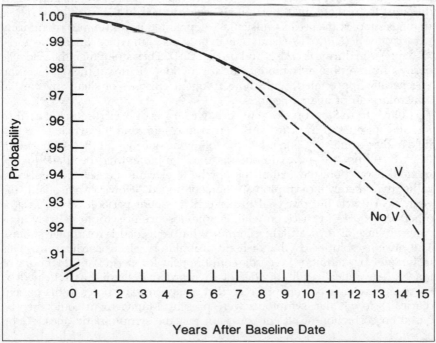

lated to vasectomy through an immunopathologic mechanism were validated by direct contact with physicians and review of medical records. Results of this study do not support the suggestions of immunopathologic consequences of vasectomy within the period of follow-up (Fig. 1-21). Except for epididymitis-orchitis, the incidence of diseases for vasectomized men was similar or lower than for their paired controls. This was true not only of individual diseases but also for conditions in which a particular immunopathologic mechanism (antibodies, immune complexes, or sensitized cells) might conceivably operate.

SILENT MYOCARDIAL ISCHEMIA

Deanfield and associates[84] from London, England, investigated episodes of transient ST-segment depression during ordinary daily life in 30 patients with stable angina pectoris secondary to CAD. Each patient underwent positron tomography, recording the regional myocardial uptake of rubidium-82, pain, and ST-segment changes before, during, and after 59 technically satisfactory exercise tests, 35 cold pressor tests, and 22 episodes of unprovoked ST depression. Exercise resulted in 53 episodes of ST depression with angina and in 5 episodes without pain. After cold pressor tests, there were 3 episodes of ST depression and pain and 12 of painless ST depression. Only 9 episodes of unprovoked ST depression were accompanied by pain. Tomography showed independent evidence of ischemia in 63 (97%) of the total 65 episodes of ST depression with angina and in all 30 episodes of painless ST depression. In each patient perfusion defects occurred in the same myocardial segment during painful and painless ST depression, and responses were significantly different from those in 16 normal subjects studied in the same way. These findings support the use of transient ST depression in continuous monitoring to assess the activity of CAD, but only in patients with typical angina pectoris, ST depression during exercise, and proved CAD. They strengthen the evidence derived from ambulatory monitoring for a wider picture of the disease than is generally appreciated, with more frequent episodes of silent myocardial ischemia than of angina pectoris.

Cohn[85] from Stonybrook, New York, wrote an editorial discussing asymptomatic episodes of myocardial ischemia in response to the article by Deanfield and associates.[84] Cohn asked the following question. If these abnormalities are still present, how can one say that the patient has been adequately treated? Should not the goal of therapy be to eleviate the ischemic episodes rather than merely the symptoms? Cohn continued: "However reasonable the goal, clearly it is not practical to perform frequent periodic stress tests or other procedures to check on whether the absence of symptoms truly indicates absence of myocardial ischemia. What is needed is a simpler system. The obvious solution is the 24-hour ambulatory electrocardiogram. This technique, by definition, records continuously for periods of 24 hours or longer. Theoretically, all episodes of myocardial ischemia, as reflected by ST-segment changes, would be recorded by appropriate notes in the patient diaries as to whether symptoms were present. Management could then be based on correction of all episodes, not just the symptomatic ones." Cohn

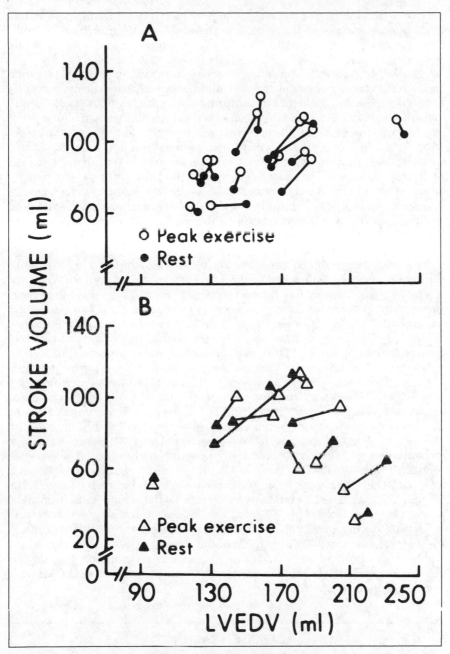

Fig. 1-22.   Left ventricular end-diastolic volume (LVEDV) and stroke volume relation (Frank-Starling mechanism) in patients with normal (A) and abnormal (B) LV exercise reserve. In patients whose LV exercise reserve was normal, peak exercise stroke volume was higher than the resting level. Left ventricular end-diastolic volume did not change. In patients whose LV exercise reserve was abnormal, the average stroke volume at peak exercise did not change from the resting level. In this group, stroke volume tended to be lower in patients with a larger end-diastolic volume than that in patients with a smaller end-diastolic volume. Reproduced with permission from Ehsani et al.[87]

proposed that the goal of therapy is the reduction in total numbers of ische-mic episodes and not just reduction in the number of symptomatic events. Why 1 episode of myocardial ischemia is asymptomatic and another is not remains unclear.

Ellestad and Kuan[86] from Long Beach, California, investigated whether naloxone, a specific antagonist, could initiate anginal pain during exercise-induced myocardial ischemia in asymptomatic patients with angiographi-cally defined CAD. A single-blind trial was conducted in 10 men with a prior positive exercise ECG. Multistage treadmill exercise tests were performed twice within a week. On the second test, patients received naloxone, 2 mg intravenously, by a syringe infusion pump. Exercise was terminated because of fatigue in 6 patients and completion of the protocol in 4. No patient reported chest pain during exercise. Naloxone did not significantly alter exer-cise duration, heart rate, BP, and ST-segment changes compared with control testing. Thus, the researchers concluded that endorphins do not play a signif-icant role in the recognition of anginal pain in patients who have asympto-matic exercise-induced ischemia.

Maximal oxygen uptake capacity (VO_2max) is generally lower in patients with CAD than in age-matched healthy subjects, and many of these patients also exhibit impaired LV function in response to exercise. Recent studies have described a poorer correlation between VO_2max and LV performance. To examine the relation between VO_2max and LV systolic function in patients with CAD, Ehsani and colleagues[87] from St. Louis, Missouri, studied 27 pa-tients at an average age of 50 years who were asymptomatic and unable to attain true VO_2max, which was defined by the leveling-off criterion or a respiratory exchange rate of ≥ 1.15 or both. The LV EF was determined by gated cardiac blood pool imaging. In patients whose EF decreased with exer-cise, VO_2max was 21 -vs- 27 ml/kg/min in those whose EF increased. Systolic BP and end-systolic volume relation was shifted upward and to the right in the former group in response to peak exercise (Fig. 1-22). In contrast, the pressure and volume relation was shifted upward and to the left in patients whose EF increased with exercise. The EF at rest did not correlate with VO_2max. There was a significant but weak correlation between peak exercise EF and VO_2max. The LV exercise reserve, that is, the change in EF from rest to exercise, correlated with VO_2max, maximal oxygen pulse, and maximal heart rate during treadmill exercise. Maximal heart rate during treadmill exercise correlated with VO_2max. Thus, these data suggest that impaired LV function can limit VO_2max and that maximal heart rate and LV exercise reserve are among the variables affecting VO_2max in patients with CAD who are not limited by angina.

EXERCISE TRAINING

To determine whether or not regular exercise could alter myocardial per-fusion or function, Froelicher and associates[88] from San Diego, California, randomized 146 male volunteers with stable CAD to either a supervised exer-cise program (72 patients) or to a usual care program (74 patients). Subjects underwent exercise tests initially and 1 year later. Significant differences between the 2 groups included improved aerobic capacity, thallium ischemia scores, and ventricular function in the exercise intervention group. It was not possible to classify the conditions of patients as to the likelihood of improvement or deterioration. This study demonstrated changes in myocardial perfusion and function in a select group of middle-aged men with CAD who underwent a medically appropriate exercise program lasting 1 year, but these changes were relatively modest.

Beta blocking agents are widely used in the treatment of patients with CAD. Their negative chronotropic and inotropic actions may alter the effects of physical training in cardiac rehabilitation programs. Therefore in a study carried out by Vanhees and associates[89] from Leuven, Belgium, resting and exercise cardiac output, stroke volume, heart rate, and arteriovenous oxygen content difference were measured before and after training in 15 male patients with CAD, who were treated with beta blockers, and in a control group of 14 patients not treated with beta blocking agents. At the end of a 3-month training period, oxygen uptake at peak exercise increased similarly in the 2 groups, 37 and 34%, respectively; this was related to increases in stroke volume and heart rate, and therefore cardiac output, and to increases in arteriovenous oxygen content difference. The effects were similar whether or not the patients were treated with beta blockers. Also, at rest and submaximal exercise, beta blockade did not affect the training-induced changes of cardiac output, heart rate, and arteriovenous oxygen content difference. In both groups heart rate decreased with training while stroke volume and cardiac output increased significantly. It was concluded that beta blockade did not significantly alter the hemodynamic effects of training.

Exercise training in patients with CAD produces 2 major results: increased work capacity and a relative bradycardia at any given workload, and these changes are qualitatively similar to those observed in normal subjects. To test the hypothesis that physical conditioning may improve LV function in patients with CAD, Williams and colleagues[90] from Durham, North Carolina, performed first-pass radionuclide ventriculography in 53 patients at rest and during upright bicycle exercise before and after 6–12 months of exercise training. The peak bicycle workload achieved before the onset of fatigue, dyspnea, or angina increased by an average of 22% after training, and mean heart rate at a workload equal to the pretraining maximum workload was decreased by 10 beats/min after training. Of 21 subjects with angina or exertional ST-segment depression before training, 15 (71%) were able to exercise to the same workload without manifestations of ischemia after training. Whereas neither mean resting LV EF nor LV EF at peak exertion was significantly altered, mean LV EF at the pretraining maximum workload was increased from 0.50–0.54 after training. A significant correlation between the magnitude of training bradycardia and the increment in LV EF at the pretraining maximum workload was observed. The investigators concluded that the relative bradycardia comparable exercise workload is produced by exercise conditioning and is associated with improvements in LV performance as assessed by the LV EF. This observation is compatible with the hypothesis that training bradycardia in conditioned subjects with CAD is associated with lower myocardial oxygen demand and lesser degrees of ischemia at comparable workloads. Training effects on ventricular afterload or on intrinsic contractile performance of the heart cannot be excluded.

ANGINA PECTORIS

Coronary reserve

The mechanism for angina pectoris in patients with LV hypertrophy secondary to systemic hypertension and with normal coronary arteries remains unexplained. Opherk and colleagues[91] from Heidelberg, West Germany, measured coronary blood flow using the argon method in 12 control subjects and in 16 patients with systemic hypertension at rest and after intravenous administration of dipyridamole. In patients with systemic hypertension, coronary blood flow response to dipyridamole was markedly reduced compared with control values. During coronary vasodilation, a linear correlation between coronary resistance and LV end-diastolic pressure was demonstrated. The LV biopsy specimens did not reveal alterations in myocardial microvasculature. Although the increase in LV end-diastolic pressure did not seem sufficient to account for the reduction in coronary reserve by >40%, this hemodynamic abnormality could reflect the additional influence of compliant abnormalities in the presence of hypertrophy. Another mechanism may have been the failure of the growth of coronary resistant vessels to keep pace with the increase in LV mass. The investigators interpret these findings to suggest that reduction of coronary reserve may be an important contributor to the pathogenesis of angina pectoris in these patients, since arteriographic and biopsy material failed to reveal abnormalities in large and small coronary arteries.

Left ventricular function

Narahara and associates[92] from Dallas, Texas, studied 30 consecutive patients with unstable angina during pain-free intervals with gated RNA. The initial study was performed within 18 hours of admission to the coronary care unit. A second study was performed near the time of hospital discharge, after stabilization with medical therapy. Three months thereafter patients were categorized according to their worst anginal status after hospital discharge. Fifteen patients were New York Heart Association functional class I or II (group A); 15 patients were in functional class III or IV (group B). The LV EF was similar at the time of initial study ($56 \pm 2\%$ and $56 \pm 4\%$ for groups A and B, respectively). At the time of hospital discharge, EF had increased to $60 \pm 2\%$ ($p < 0.01$) in group A, and in group B it had decreased to $48 \pm 3\%$ ($p < 0.005$). End-systolic volume index in group B increased from $37 \pm 6–43 \pm 6$ ml/M^2 ($p < 0.005$) at the time of the follow-up study. There were no significant intergroup differences in the amount of nitrates or beta blockers received by the patients during the 2 scintigraphic examinations. Eleven group B patients subsequently underwent CABG; a significant increase in EF and a significant decrease in end-systolic volume index were noted when these patients were restudied an average of 3.2 months after CABG. This study suggests that changes in LV function during unstable angina pectoris are common and may be detected by serial gated RNA. The direction of the change in EF was associated with the severity of angina in the follow-up period. A decrease in EF and an increase in end-systolic volume index from admission to follow-up study were associated with an unfavorable clinical outcome and may represent clinically silent ischemic depression of LV function.

Hakki and associates[93] from Philadelphia, Pennsylvania, examined rest thallium-201 perfusion pattern during angina-free periods in 40 patients with rest angina pectoris secondary to CAD (≥70% diameter narrowing). Seventeen patients had previous Q-wave myocardial infarction. The perfusion defects were considered fixed or reversible, depending on the absence or presence of redistribution in the 4-hour delayed images. There were 40 perfusion defects (26 fixed and 14 reversible) in 27 patients, whereas 13 patients had normal scans. Reversible perfusion defects were present in 10 patients (25%). Of the 26 fixed perfusion defects, 17 did not have corresponding Q waves. Occluded vessels (63%) had more perfusion defects than vessels with subtotal occlusion (30%) (p < 0.01). The perfusion defect size was larger in patients with lower EF than in patients with higher EF. These findings indicate that 1) perfusion defects are common in patients with rest angina and are reversible in 25% of patients, indicating reduced regional coronary blood flow; 2) the degree of stenosis affects the presence of perfusion defect; 3) fixed defects may be present without corresponding Q waves; and 4) global LV function is related to the size of perfusion defects.

Angiographically detected intracoronary thrombus

To examine the role of intracoronary thrombus in unstable angina, Zack and associates[94] from St. Louis, Missouri, reviewed the coronary arteriograms of 83 patients with unstable angina (group I) and 37 patients with stable angina (group II) for angiographic evidence of thrombus. Groups I and II patients were similar with respect to mean age, presence of single and multiple vessel CAD, and past history of AMI. Group I patients had no ECG or creatine kinase enzyme evidence of AMI. The angiographic criteria for thrombus included an intracoronary filling defect, intraluminal staining, and total coronary artery occlusion with convex dye outline. Thrombus was found in 10 of 83 patients in group I (12%) -vs- 0 of 37 patients in group II (p < 0.05). These findings suggest that in some patients coronary artery thrombosis plays an important role in the pathogenesis of unstable angina.

Role of heart rate

Chierchia and associates[95] from London, England, monitored 11 patients with chronic stable angina, off medication apart from nitroglycerin, by ECG during normal, unrestricted daily activity. Computerized ECG analysis demonstrated during 33 24-hour periods of monitoring, 278 episodes of transient ischemic ST-segment depression of which 52 were associated with angina. In the 15 minutes preceding the onset of ischemia, heart rate did not increase in 164 episodes, increased slightly (≥5 beats/min) in 61, and increased moderately or markedly (≥10 beats/min) in 53. Findings were similar when episodes with or without angina or of different severity were analyzed separately. In all patients, periods of sinus tachycardia exceeding the control rate by >30 beats/min and lasting >10 minutes, often occurred in the absence of angina or ST-segment depression. Also, in 65% of the ischemic episodes, heart rate at the beginning of the ST change was either below or <10 beats/

min above the modal value of the 24-hour heart rate. This suggests that increased myocardial demand is not necessarily the only or the most common cause of acute ischemia in patients with chronic effort angina during unrestricted daily activity. Factors that only transiently interfere with myocardial oxygen supply are probably important in this syndrome.

Effect of low fat, low caloric diet

Thuesen and associates[96] from Aarhus C, Denmark, treated 8 patients with exertional angina pectoris for 3 months with a low fat, low caloric diet. Serum cholesterol was reduced by 28% and body weight by 8 kg on average. The effect of the dietary intervention was assessed by a heart metabolic study during pacing-induced tachycardia. After dietary treatment, coronary sinus blood flow and myocardial oxygen consumption were considerably reduced, but pacing time before angina developed was increased. Other improvements were a reduction in lactate release during pacing, a reduction in citrate release during recovery, a reduction in alanine output during rest and recovery, and a lower uptake of glutamate. The results suggest a beneficial effect of low fat, low calorie dietary treatment on myocardial energy metabolism in patients with exertional angina pectoris.

Thromboxane release

To determine thromboxane A_2 (TXA_2) release in CAD, Mehta and associates[97] from Gainesville, Florida, measured its stable metabolite thromboxane B_2 (TXB_2) by radioimmunoassay in 20 patients. In 15 patients with stable disease (last angina episode >96 hours before study), coronary venous TXB_2 concentrations were lower than in aortic blood (mean, 109 ± 36 -vs- 194 ± 40 pg/ml; p < 0.001). In contrast, in 5 other patients with spontaneous angina, coronary venous TXB_2 concentrations were higher than aortic TXB_2 concentrations during the angina episode (mean, 1,716 ± 316 -vs- 875 ± 388 pg/ml; p < 0.02). Plasma TXB_2 levels were in the normal range (mean, 175 ± 35 pg/ml) in patients with stable angina but significantly (p < 0.02) higher in patients with spontaneous angina. With atrial pacing to the point of chest pain or ECG changes in patients with stable CAD, aortic TXB_2 concentrations increased in 10 of 13 patients (mean, 283 ± 70 pg/ml; p < 0.02). Coronary venous TXB_2 concentrations increased in 7 patients at peak pacing rates (mean, 223 ± 76 pg/ml) and in 3 other patients after termination of pacing. These data indicate that release of TXA_2 is much greater during spontaneous angina than with pacing stress in patients with CAD. TXA_2 released during spontaneous or pacing-induced angina may modulate coronary and systemic vascular tone. Enhanced TXA_2 activity may either precede or follow myocardial ischemia and could be a factor in the initiation and propagation of the ischemic episode.

Prostaglandin E_1 infusion

Intermittent vasospasm, platelet aggregation, or both may play an important role in producing transient coronary artery obstruction leading to an unstable ischemic syndrome. To determine whether intravenous infusion of prostaglandin E_1 (PGE_1), a known coronary vasodilator and inhibitor of platelet aggregation, produces salutary effects in unstable angina, Siegel and associates[98] from Los Angeles, California, evaluated its effects in 19 patients with an unstable acute ischemic syndrome. The PGE_1 produced a significant decrease in the number of episodes of rest angina ($p < 0.001$) and eliminated the need for intravenous nitroglycerin and morphine in 10 patients. These salutary clinical effects were associated with a significant ($p < 0.05$) reduction in mean arterial pressure, mean PA pressure, mean PA wedge pressure, and the double product, without a reduction in the endocardial perfusion gradient (aortic diastolic BP to mean PA wedge pressure). Adverse effects were generally minor and easily controlled. Thus, PGE_1 infusion may be of value in the treatment of acute unstable ischemic syndromes.

Frequency of CAD when angina is the initial symptom of myocardial ischemia

Connolly and associates[99] from Rochester, Minnesota, examined retrospectively the resting ECG at the time of initial diagnosis of angina pectoris, which was the initial manifestation of CAD during a 26 year period (1950–1975) in 1,154 Rochester residents. The finding of a normal resting ECG at the time of the initial diagnosis of angina pectoris was associated with a good prognosis (Fig. 1-23). Survival at 5 years was equal to that expected for the given age and sex distribution under a cohort life table for the Minnesota white population. In contrast in those patients who had an abnormal ECG at the time of diagnosis of angina pectoris, the observed survival rate was 80% of that expected at 5 years.

Fig. 1-23. Graph showing survivorship of 683 patients with a normal ECG at time of diagnosis of angina and of 471 patients with an abnormal ECG. Relative survival is shown at right for comparison. Reproduced with permission from Connolly et al.[99]

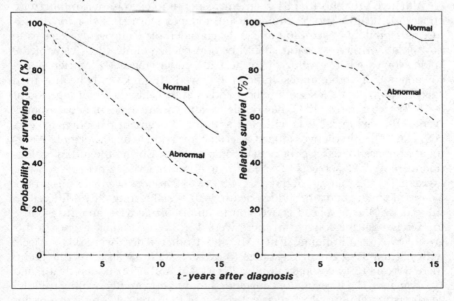

Relation of severity of symptoms of myocardial ischemia to prognosis

To determine if severity of angina was related to the extent of CAD or prognosis, the participants of the Veterans Administration Cooperative Study of Surgery for CAD evaluated 345 patients by a systematic patient-administered angina questionnaire at entry into a large-scale randomized study of medical -vs- surgical treatment of stable angina pectoris.[100] Severity of angina was numerically scored; scores were based on frequency of pain, rest pain, amount of daily medication, and level of daily activity. Severity scores were separated into mild, moderate, and severe groups of approximately equal numbers and correlated with number of coronary arteries narrowed, presence of LM CAD, EF <50%, abnormalities of LV function, 3-vessel CAD with abnormal LV function, increased heart size by chest radiograph, a non-invasive measure of prognosis, and mortality. Severity of angina was not significantly related to any of these variables except for the presence of LM CAD (p = 0.046) and increased heart size by chest radiograph (p = 0.001), both of which had low prevalence rates. Severity of angina at baseline was not related to 7-year survival of inpatients treated medically or surgically. Severity of angina at baseline, however, did predict 1- to 2-year survival in medically treated patients. Similarly, the severity of angina at 1 year and at 5 years predicted survival in the subsequent 4 at 5 years in the medical group. Thus, in patients with stable angina, severity of symptoms as defined by a systematic questionnaire was not highly related to extent of CAD or long-term prognosis. Increasing severity of angina, however, may be associated with lower survival rate in medically treated patients.

Exercise testing

Although an abnormal ST-segment response to exercise in an otherwise apparently healthy subject represents an independent risk factor for the future development of symptomatic CAD, considerable controversy exists as to how an abnormal test result should be approached clinically in view of the known low predictive value of the test for underlying CAD. McHenry and coworkers[101] in Indianapolis, Indiana, followed 916 apparently healthy men aged 27–55 years with serial medical and exercise evaluations for a period of 8–15 years to determine: 1) the prevalence and specific types of new coronary events observed in subjects with and without ST-segment responses to exercise; and 2) the predictive value of a serial conversion to an abnormal ST-segment response to exercise for new coronary events. During the initial evaluation there were 23 subjects (2.5%) with an abnormal ST-segment response to exercise. During follow-up, there were 9 (39%) coronary events in this group: 8 cases of angina and 1 of sudden death. With serial testing, an additional 38 subjects (5%) experienced conversion to an abnormal ST-segment response to exercise. During follow-up, there were 12 (32%) coronary events in this group: 10 cases of angina, 1 of AMI, and 1 other. There were 833 subjects with normal ST-segment responses to exercise with all tests. In this group there were 44 (5%) coronary events: 25 cases of AMI, 7 of sudden death, and 12 of angina. The investigators concluded that in apparently healthy middle-aged men an abnormal ST-segment response to exercise is predictive of angina pectoris but not of AMI or sudden cardiac death as an initial coronary event.

Butman and coworkers[102] from Long Beach, California, determined the prognostic value of submaximal exercise testing in 125 hospitalized patients with unstable angina pectoris. Exercise testing was performed after exclusion of AMI and a pain-free period of at least 3 days. No complications were noted during or immediately after exercise testing. Positive tests (angina or ≥ 1 mm ST-segment depression, or both) were found in 60 patients (48%). During a 1-year follow-up period, 52 (87%) of these patients had an unfavorable outcome, including the development of severe angina, recurrent unstable angina, CABG, AMI, or cardiac death compared with 19 (29%) of the 65 patients with a negative test (p < 0.001). Sensitivity and specificity of exercise testing in predicting prognosis were 73 and 85%, respectively. Positive submaximal exercise tests had a predictive value of 87% and a negative test had a predictive value of 71%. These findings were not significantly affected by beta blocking agents or digitalis. Thus, these data suggest that in patients with unstable angina pectoris submaximal exercise testing after stabilization of the patient is useful in predicting prognosis in the subsequent 1 year.

Ambulatory monitoring

Continuous monitoring of the ECG in patients with angina pectoris and CAD has shown episodes of asymptomatic ST-segment depression, suggesting frequent silent myocardial ischemia during normal daily life. Interpretation of this finding depends on whether similar changes occur in normal subjects. Accordingly, Deanfield and associates[103] from London, England, performed in 80 asymptomatic normal volunteers (20 from each decade between 20 and 50 years and 20 >50 years old) frequency-modulated ambulatory ECG recordings and in 20 patients with noncardiac pain, negative exercise and provocative tests, and angiographically normal coronary arteries. Treadmill exercise testing was performed in all subjects >40 years old. Episodes of T-wave change were identified in 53 subjects. Five subjects <40 years of age had episodes of ST elevation that were prolonged; they usually occurred at night. In 3 patients they could be reproduced by postural change. Only 2 subjects, both >40 years of age, had planar ST depression during tachycardia; 1 subject had a positive exercise test response. No patient with normal coronary arteries had significant ST depression. Tachycardia was frequently associated with upsloping ST depression (36%), which was more common in younger subjects. Five subjects also showed isolated single complexes with ST depression during baseline instability. With use of frequency-modulated recordings, transient ST depression of ≥ 0.1 mV that lasted ≥ 80 ms and >30 seconds in duration was rare in a normal population. This finding supports the use of this signal to follow the activity of CAD out of the hospital, specifically in patients with typical angina and proved CAD.

Ventricular arrhythmias during coronary angiography

Nishimura and associates[104] from Rochester, Minnesota, found 39 patients aged 37–79 years (mean, 57) who had sustained VT or VF during coronary angiography from 1978–1983. During that period 7,915 patients

TABLE 1-7. *Ventricular arrhythmia during catheterization in patients undergoing coronary angiography*

	# Cases
Type of arrhythmia	
Ventricular tachycardia	12
Ventricular tachycardia → ventricular fibrillation	4
Ventricular fibrillation	23
Artery injected	
Right coronary artery*	24
Left coronary artery	10
Graft	5
Onset of ventricular arrhythmia†	
During injection	6
Less than 10 seconds after injection	29
10 seconds to 1 minute after injection	2

* One patient had a conus branch injected.
† No data for 2 patients.

had undergone coronary angiography. Of the 39 patients, 9 had atypical chest pain and 30 had angina pectoris. Fifteen had had previous AMI and 1 patient, VT or VF. Resting ECGs revealed a prolonged QT interval in 14. A normal EF was found in 79%. Coronary angiography revealed that 10 patients had 3-vessel CAD, 15 had 1- or 2-vessel CAD, and 14 had normal coronary arteries. The VT or VF was seen with injection of contrast medium into the right coronary artery in 24, the left coronary artery in 10, and vein bypass grafts in 5 patients (Table 1-7). Of the episodes of VT or VF, 67% occurred after injection of contrast medium into a minimally diseased coronary artery. In patients in whom VT or VF occurred after injection into a minimally diseased coronary artery, the arrhythmia was preceded by bradycardia, usually with pronounced widening of the QRS and QT intervals. This response was significantly different from that in patients in whom VT or VF occurred after injection into a coronary artery with significant stenosis; in these patients VT or VF was initiated by a single VPC on a T wave. The VT or VF was successfully cardioverted in all instances, without further arrhythmias.

Variables predictive of successful medical therapy

Although many patients with unstable angina respond to medical management while in a coronary care unit, there remains a high incidence of subsequent failure of medical therapy with and incidence of AMI or death from 20–30% and an additional 30–40% incidence of persistent severe angina over 2–3 years. Identification at the time of presentation of the patient likely to fail medical therapy would be useful in considering CABG. Since coronary arterial spasm may have a significant role in the pathophysiology of unstable angina in some patients, calcium-channel blockers may be of particular benefit in the medical therapy of unstable angina. Ouyang and colleagues[105] from Baltimore, Maryland, entered 138 patients into a randomized, double-blind study of the efficacy of adding nifedipine to conventional treatment of unstable angina with nitrates and beta blockers and followed these patients for 18 months. Of these patients, 104 underwent coronary arteriography. A multivariate Cox's hazard function analysis was applied to variables selected from the history, ECG changes during chest pain, and from scintigraphic and coronary arteriographic data to determine those variables most predictive of response to medical therapy. The percentage of LV myocardium supplied by arteries with ≥70% luminal stenosis was found to be the most significant variable in influencing failure of medical therapy defined as sudden death, AMI, or need for CABG. The second most powerful variable was whether or not the patient received nifedipine that reduced by half the relative risk of failing medical therapy. Cigarette smoking and the presence of global ST-segment changes during ischemia were the next important influential variables. After 18 months, the nifedipine group had fewer patients failing medical therapy with fewer patients undergoing CABG. However, nifedipine did not appear to prevent AMI or death. Actuarial curves confirmed that medical therapy was significantly less successful in the presence of increasing numbers of significantly stenotic vessels. Nifedipine did prove beneficial in patients with ≥2 stenotic arteries and in whom ≥50% of the myocardium were supplied by vessels with ≥70% stenosis. Although patients with advanced CAD have the greatest likelihood of unfavorable outcomes, this study suggests that the addition of nifedipine is of significant benefit. Such patients can be identified at the time of presentation by diffuse ECG changes accompanying angina and additional data obtained from coronary arteriography.

Nitroglycerin

Cutaneous application of nitroglycerin (NTG) as a 2% ointment has long been recognized as an effective method of prolonged NTG administration. The need for multiple applications each day has tended to limit its use. Cutaneous patch devices designed to provide continuous 24-hour administration of NTG have recently become available. The rationale for their clinical use has been based heavily on comparisons of blood levels achieved after NTG patch applications to those produced 6 hours after reference doses (typically, 0.5 inch) of 2% NTG ointment. Data documenting the antianginal effects of NTG patches and the comparative magnitude and duration of these antianginal effects are limited. Additionally, the relation of blood levels of NTG to clinical effects is complex and incompletely understood. Reichek and associates[106] from Philadelphia, Pennsylvania, performed a blinded, randomized trial of the acute effects of both low dose and maximal tolerance dose NTG patches and placebo on exercise tolerance in 14 patients with CAD and typical exertional angina pectoris. The bicycle exercise protocol was used in sublingual NTG administered as a positive control. In 7 patients, low dose patches produced no statistically significant effect on exercise tolerance at 4, 8, and 24 hours after administration (Fig. 1-24). Comparable doses of sublingual and oral isosorbide dinitrate, NTG ointment, and transmucosal NTG in previous studies have produced effects similar to those of conventional doses of sublingual NTG. Maximally tolerated doses of 2 types of NTG patches were then tested. The first (n, 8; mean NTG dose delivered, 25 mg) produced increases in exercise tolerance of 82 and 72 seconds at 4 and 8 hours, respectively (both p < 0.01), but was ineffective at 24 hours. The second patch type (n, 5; mean NTG dose delivered, 22 mg) was also ineffective at 24 hours.

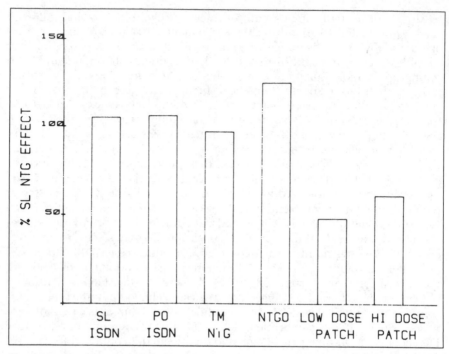

Fig. 1-24.   Data from 4 published studies of sublingual (SL) and oral (PO) isosorbide dinitrate (ISDN), transmucosal (TM) nitroglycerin (NTG), and NTG ointment (NTGO) are compared with those obtained in the present study with low and high dose patches. Results from each study are expressed as the ratio of the peak effect of the long-acting nitrate tested to that of sublingual NTG (mean doses, 0.35 mg), multiplied by 100 and expressed as a percentage. Only low and high dose patches produced peak effects that were clearly smaller than those of sublingual NTG. Peak effects were noted 10 minutes after sublingual ISDN, 1 hour after PO ISDN and NTGO, 8 hours after low dose NTG patches, and 4 hours after high dose NTG patches.

Furthermore, even at maximal doses, peak effects on exercise tolerance were about half those of sublingual NTG. Thus, NTG patches, even at maximal doses, appear to have smaller therapeutic effects than other long-acting nitrates and are ineffective at 24 hours. These results suggest rapid attenuation of NTG effect during prolonged maintenance of constant blood levels.

Parker and Fung[107] from Kingston, Canada, and Amherst, New York, assessed in 11 patients with chronic stable angina pectoris the hemodynamic and antianginal efficacy of transdermal NTG patches. In 11 patients, acute dosing, with 10, 20, and 30 cm^2 of transdermal NTG (designed to deliver 5, 10, and 15 mg transdermal NTG over 24 hours) improved treadmill walking time 2 and 4 hours after application, but no clinical effects were seen at 24 hours (Fig. 1-25). In a second study in 6 patients with doses of 30, 60, and 90 cm^2 of transdermal NTG treadmill walking time was improved at 2 and 4 hours, but no changes were seen at 24 hours except with the 90 cm^2 preparation. After daily therapy with 30 cm^2 patches of transdermal NTG for 1–2 weeks, exercise tolerance was similar to that seen during daily placebo therapy. These results suggest that transdermal NTG patches are of inadequate size to produce 24-hour antianginal protection. During sustained therapy,

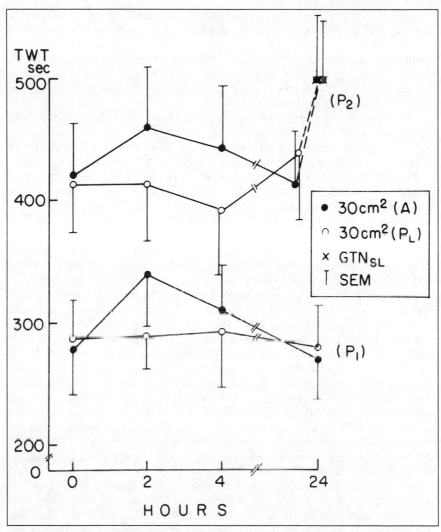

Fig. 1-25.   Treadmill walking time (TWT) to the onset of angina (P$_1$) and to the development of moderate angina (P$_2$) before (0) and 2, 4, and 24 hours after the acute application of 30 cm^2 of active (A) and placebo (P$_L$) nitroglycerin (GTN) patches. The changes in TWT to P$_1$ and P$_2$ were significantly greater than control at 2 and 4 hours, but not at 24 hours. Significant increases in TWT to P$_2$ occur after 0.6 mg of sublingual (SL) nitroglycerin.

tolerance develops to the antianginal efficacy of this form of NTG administration.

Parker and associates[108] from Kingson, Canada, applied 100 mg of transdermal isosorbide dinitrate (ISDN) and matching placebo to 12 patients with chronic stable angina pectoris and then did hemodynamic and exercise tests. Compared with placebo, there were no changes in systolic BP or heart rate at rest or during exercise; but treadmill walking time to the onset of angina and to the development of moderate angina was significantly prolonged at 2, 4, and 8 hours but not at 24 hours after drug application. Patients subsequently received these same treatment regimens for 7–10 days and underwent repeat exercise testing. During this sustained phase of the investigation, treadmill walking time to the onset of angina and to the development of moderate angina was similar at 4, 8, and 24 hours after application of ISDN and placebo. Thus, transdermal ISDN in a dose of 100 mg is effective for 8 hours during acute therapy, but during sustained therapy tolerance developed and no antianginal effects of ISDN persisted.

Abrams[109] from Albuquerque, New Mexico, wrote an editorial commenting on the articles by Reichek and associates[106] and by Parker and associates.[107,108] Abrams related the history of transdermal NTG, indicating that it began with independent marketing in 1982 by 3 American drug houses. From evaluation of the reports on transdermal NTG available to this time, Abrams concluded the following: 1) the actions of transdermal NTG discs in angina pectoris are modest using conventional dosage, but transdermal NTG is more effective at higher doses. Available evidence suggests that the anti-ischemic actions of the disc systems are not as potent as administration of sublingual NTG or other long-acting nitrate formulations. There is little evidence for an antianginal effect at 24 hours. 2) Transdermal NTG works in CHF. The dose-response relations are not well worked out, but high dose transdermal NTG therapy is probably necessary to increase cardiac output and decrease systemic vascular resistance. The effects of transdermal NTG may persist for a full 24 hours in CHF, but this is not fully resolved by the available data. 3) Nitrate tolerance appears to be an important phenomenon complicating the use of transdermal NTG therapy and may prove to be the limiting factor precluding the use of sustained 24 hours/day nitrate therapy. 4) High dose transdermal NTG administration is necessary to produce a clinical effect in many patients, and 15–30 mg of NTG per 24 hours is clearly effective in angina and CHF. Thus, physicians must be prepared to increase transdermal NTG dosage until a definite clinical response has been achieved. Pharmaceutical companies are actively working on transdermal NTG formulations that will increase the overall surface area of the discs and are also studying methods of enhancing NTG absorption across the skin. As with other forms of nitrate therapy, side effects may be a limiting factor, and the clinical experience with high dose transdermal NTG is limited. 5) More studies on transdermal NTG are required. Whether transdermal NTG will achieve the promise of once daily nitrate delivery is not clear. Nevertheless, approaches to provide ⩾24 hours of a bioactive drug through the skin with a single dosing unit clearly represents an idea whose time has come.

In a randomized, single-blind, crossover study, Dalal and Parker[110] from Kingston, Canada, studied 10 patients with stable, exercise-induced angina pectoris during sustained therapy with oral ISDN. Circulatory changes and exercise performance were evaluated before and 6 hours after therapy with oral ISDN. One-half hour after this therapy, sublingual ISDN or NTG was administered and exercise testing repeated. Treadmill walking time 6 hours after oral ISDN was similar to the control value. Subsequent administration of sublingual ISDN improved walking time from 429 ± 156–513 ± 166 seconds (p <0.005), whereas NTG improved it from 411 ± 159–480 ± 158 seconds (p < 0.005). The improvement in walking time with ISDN (23%) and NTG (18%) and the absolute walking times were not different. The standing systolic BP decreased from 124 ± 23–112 ± 22 mmHg (p <0.02) after therapy with sublingual ISDN and 122 ± 23 to 110 ± 24 mmHg (p <0.005) after administration of NTG. This study demonstrates that during sustained ISDN therapy, walking time returns to control values by 6 hours; administration of either sublingual ISDN or NTG results in significant circulatory changes and improvement in walking time; and the changes in circulatory and exercise variables after administration of NTG in patients taking sustained ISDN therapy cannot be taken as evidence of an absence of cross-tolerance between these agents.

Marzullo and coworkers[111] from Pisa, Italy, determined the influence of ISDN on myocardial perfusion and ventricular function using thallium-201 perfusion studies and equilibrium radionuclide ventriculography in 15 patients with angina at rest but no previous AMI. Transient thallium-201 perfusion defects occurred in all patients during angina at rest and coronary vasospasm was documented in 9 of these individuals. Radionuclide ventriculograms performed at control, during the ischemic episodes, and after intravenous ISDN (3–5 mg) demonstrated a LV EF averaging 65 ± 11% at control, decreasing during angina at rest to 49 ± 14% (p <0.01), and increasing after ISDN to 66 ± 12%. Only 9 patients demonstrated a reduction in LV EF during ischemia and in 2 more it changed by <5% from control values. Regional wall motion abnormalities were found in all patients during ischemic episodes and they resolved after ISDN administration. These data suggest that angina at rest may occur in the absence of a significant change in global LV EF. The data also indicate that ISDN may reverse global and segmental ventricular dysfunction occurring with rest angina.

Sasayama and coworkers[112] from Kyoto, Japan, used biplane cine-ventriculography to establish the effects of sublingual NTG in 13 patients with CAD. Six patients were considered responders, as is evident from a significant increase in LV EF (40 ± 5–52 ± 4%, p <0.001), whereas the other 7 patients were considered nonresponders and did not demonstrate any change in EF. Contractile pattern of the regional myocardium over the entire ventricular surface was analyzed using a computer-generated 3 D model. Thirty-two points at equal angles around the center of gravity of the end-diastolic cavity were generated to form a border image. This process was repeated for 16 successive cross sections that would allow reconstruction of the ventricular surface by a sequence of 32 by 16 points. Regional wall motion was expressed as a percent change in radial length drawn from the center of gravity. Significant heterogeneity in regional ventricular functional response to NTG was found. Among the responders, the normally contracting area was significantly increased (p <0.001), usually caused by a greater improvement in segmental shortening. In the nonresponders, a lessening of the severe dysfunction of a given area was associated with significant deterioration of segmental shortening in another normal contracting area. These data indicate that the response to sublingual NTG in patients with CAD is variable; some patients improve their global and regional ventricular function, whereas others do not. These results may be explained by either a beneficial effect of NTG on coronary collateral perfusion or a failure of such an effect to occur.

Propranolol and acebutolol

To determine if propranolol given twice daily (bid) was as effective as 4 times daily (qid) for treatment of stable angina pectoris, Beller and associates[113] in a multicenter study randomized 78 patients with exercise-induced ST-segment depression of 1.5 mm or more to qid, bid, daily, and placebo groups. All patients received 5 tablets/day, and propranolol groups received 80, 160, and 320 mg/day on successive weeks. At weekly visits, patients underwent treadmill exercise testing before the 8:00 am dose and at 2 and 9 hours afterward. Exercise duration (seconds) was significantly improved at the final visit compared with baseline by bid (120 ± 36, mean ± SEM) and qid (100 ± 37; n, 17) regimens, but not by the daily (30 ± 33; n, 18) and placebo regimens (27 ± 37; n, 17). There was a significant decrease from baseline in the magnitude of ST depression at the final visit, measured at maximal common exercise duration in bid (−0.96 ± 0.20 mm), qid (−0.84 ± 0.20 mm), and daily (−0.58 ± 0.18 mm) groups, but not in the placebo group (0.03 ± 0.2 mm). Hourly heart rate by Holter monitoring was reduced in all 3 propranolol groups; however, the mean serum propranolol level was significantly lower just before the first dose in the daily group (56 ± 20 ng/ml) compared with the bid and qid groups (146 ± 22 and 119 ± 28 ng/ml) with 320 mg/day. Thus, propranolol administered bid and qid had similar efficacy in improving exercise duration in patients with angina compared with propranolol given daily or placebo. All dose regimens reduce exercise ST depression.

Acebutolol is a new beta antagonist that has intrinsic sympathomimetic and cardioselective properties. In a study performed by Kaul and associates[114] from Los Angeles, California, the agent's effects on the ischemic consequences after supine bicycle exercise were compared with those of propranolol in 16 patients with chronic stable CAD using a double-blind placebo crossover protocol and equilibrium RNA. In 8 patients (group I), the LV EF at peak exercise decreased under control conditions. During chronic acebutolol therapy (400 mg thrice daily), the exercise-induced LV EF (means ± 1 SD) was significantly higher (37 ± 16% -vs- 42 ± 14%; p < 0.05). The corresponding values during placebo and during propranolol (80 mg thrice daily) were 39 ± 12% -vs- 43 ± 15% (p = 0.07). In 8 patients (group II) in whom supine bicycle exercise produced increases in LV EF, both acebutolol (59 ± 5% -vs- 54 ± 4%) and propranolol (58 ± 6% -vs- 54 ± 5%) attenuated the increases. In neither group was the resting LV EF reduced by acebutolol or propranolol. These findings show that acebutolol and propranolol are approximately equipotent in minimizing the LV RNA manifestations of myocardial ischemia induced by supine bicycle exercise.

Diltiazem

In a study by Hossack and colleagues[115] from Seattle, Washington, the efficacy of diltiazem (360 mg/day) was compared with placebo in 15 men with exertional angina during a 21-week study. Symptom-limited exercise testing was used to evaluate the effects of the drug. Analysis of variance indicated the increases in the values of 3 time-related variables (time to onset of angina, time to onset of 1 mm ST depression, and total duration of exercise) were highly significant (all p < 0.001). The increase from the second week of placebo to the last week of diltiazem was 4.1 minutes for time to angina, 2.4 minutes for time to 1 mm ST depression, and 2.3 minutes for total duration. In addition, the differences between mean values of these variables for placebo and corresponding diltiazem period at weeks 3 and 4 were significant (p < 0.01, p < 0.01, p < 0.05) and for diltiazem week 20 and placebo week 21 were significant (p < 0.005, p < 0.01, p < 0.005). Weekly angina frequency was reduced from a mean of 17 episodes/week during placebo to 1 episode/week during diltiazem (p < 0.001). Submaximal pressure-rate product was reduced significantly during diltiazem (p < 0.001), and the ECG evidence of myocardial ischemia was reduced by diltiazem at submaximal (p < 0.02) and maximal exercise (p < 0.001). The drug was well tolerated and appears to be effective monotherapy for exertional angina.

Although the mechanism of action of diltiazem in patients with exertional angina is related in part to a reduction in submaximal myocardial oxygen demand, other studies have suggested that it may improve myocardial blood flow during exertion. To determine mechanisms of benefit from diltiazem, Hossack and colleagues[116] from Seattle, Washington, studied 13 patients with CAD by sustained isometric handgrip exercise and repeated the procedure during intravenous infusion of diltiazem. Cardiovascular responses to handgrip, diltiazem, their combination, and nitroglycerin were assessed by hemodynamic and ECG measurements and by computer-assisted measurements of normal and diseased segments of epicardial coronary arteries. Handgrip produced increases in heart rate of 12%, PA pressure of 19%, and PA wedge pressure of 33%. Diltiazem produced significant reductions in heart rate of 7% and aortic pressure of 14%. The PA pressure and PA wedge pressure were unchanged by diltiazem. Diltiazem did not prevent the increase in heart rate or in aortic or PA wedge pressure associated with handgrip. Diltiazem prolonged AV conduction from 0.18–0.20 second. Compared with control values, nitroglycerin reduced aortic pressure by 14%, PA pressure by 38%, and PA wedge pressure by 42%. Heart rate remained unchanged. The constriction of 20% of lumen area of normal coronary arterial segments during handgrip was effectively prevented by infusion of diltiazem. Nitroglycerin produced a significantly greater increase of 20% in diameter of normal coronary arterial segments than diltiazem and tended to have a more favorable effect than diltiazem on stenosis of minimum area and flow resistance. The handgrip-induced constriction of minimum area and increase in stenosis flow resistance were prevented during diltiazem infusion. Diltiazem is a minimal epicardial coronary dilator compared with nitroglycerin, the drug effectively blocking sympathetically mediated constriction of normal and diseased coronary epicardial coronary arteries in human beings. Thus, in addition to reducing myocardial oxygen demand by lowering heart rate and BP, diltiazem virtually prevents alpha mediated vasoconstriction of normal and diseased segments of epicardial coronary arteries.

Kenny and associates[117] from London, England, evaluated the effects of diltiazem in 11 patients with stable angina pectoris and confirmed obstructive CAD at rest and during rapid atrial pacing. Symptomatic, metabolic, coronary, and systemic hemodynamic indices were monitored at rest and during pacing-induced ischemia. At rest, after the administration of intravenous diltiazem, potent vasodilator effects were observed with a significant decrease in mean BP and an increase in cardiac index. Importantly, however, the systemic vasodilator effect of diltiazem was associated with no significant increase in heart rate. During pacing, there was similar decrease in mean BP after diltiazem, and mean pacing time to angina increased significantly. Three patients did not develop angina on repeat pacing. Coupled with an improved pacing time to angina, there was a significant improvement in myocardial lactate extraction during pacing, changing from lactate production to lactate extraction after diltiazem. This study confirms the antianginal effects of diltiazem and suggests that this agent may have advantages in the management of angina pectoris. The results suggest that diltiazem may exert its beneficial effect not only by reducing afterload reduction, but also by a direct metabolic effect on the myocardium.

Khurmi and associates[118] from Harrow, England, assessed by multistage graded exercise tests the long-term efficacy of diltiazem, 360 mg/day in 17 patients with grades II or III stable exertional angina pectoris (Canadian Cardiovascular Society criteria). The study was carried out in placebo-controlled, double-blind, dose titration protocol and all 17 patients received long-term therapy. Exercise tests were performed at the end of 2 weeks of placebo treatment and after 6, 18, 26, 40, and 52 weeks of diltiazem. All patients had angina during treadmill testing with placebo and the mean ($\pm$SEM) exercise time was 5.8 $\pm$ 0.7 minutes. This increased to 10.8 $\pm$ 1.0 minutes after 6 weeks, 11.3 $\pm$ 1.1 minutes after 18 weeks, 11.4 $\pm$ 1.1 minutes after 26 weeks, 12.9 $\pm$ 1.2 minutes after 40 weeks, and 11.6 $\pm$ 1.3 minutes after 52 weeks of continuous diltiazem therapy (p $<$ 0.001 -vs- placebo at all stages). Four patients were withdrawn after 26 weeks of treatment; 1 patient underwent CABG and 3 patients required the addition of beta adrenoreceptor blocking agents. In 1 patient an irritant rash developed on the torso, legs, and arms after 39 weeks of diltiazem and disappeared after discontinuation of the drug. One patient complained of swelling and stiffness of the fingers and 3 patients complained of shoulder and elbow pain. Another patient had an AMI after 8 weeks of diltiazem treatment and died. No other adverse effects were observed during this study. These findings suggest that diltiazem in a dose of 360 mg/day possesses a powerful and sustained antianginal effect and merits a place as a primary therapeutic agent in the management of chronic stable angina pectoris.

Nifedipine

Little information is available on the effects of calcium blocking agents such as nifedipine on LV function, particularly during upright dynamic exercise. Nelson and associates[119] from Leeds, England, evaluated the immediate effects of sublingual nifedipine (20 mg) in 18 men with stable exercise-related angina pectoris and angiographically confirmed CAD, stratified at the time of LV angiography according to the degree of LV dysfunction supine at rest (group 1: n, 9, LV end-diastolic pressure <20 mmHg; Group 2: n, 9, end-diastolic pressure >20 mmHg). At rest, in the upright position in both groups, nifedipine reduced the systemic vascular resistance, the systemic arterial mean, and diastolic pressures and increased cardiac output. Heart rate increased only in group 1. During upright bicycle exercise in all 18 patients, compared with control measurements, systemic BP and vascular resistance were similarly reduced, whereas exercise cardiac output response and LV filling pressure did not change after nifedipine. Heart rate was increased in group 1 and decreased in group 2. Stroke volume during exercise after nifedipine decreased in group 1 and increased in group 2 compared with control measurements. These results indicate that the major hemodynamic effect of nifedipine was systemic arteriolar dilation. In group 1, failure of the reduction in LV pressure work to improve cardiac output and stroke volume during exercise may reflect some degree of negative inotropic activity of the drug, particularly in view of the evidence of reflex sympathetic stimulation of the heart (tachycardia). However, patients in group 2 with more severe impairment of LV function showed no hemodynamic evidence of further cardiac depression after nifedipine. These results indicate that nifedipine did not further impair cardiac pumping activity, even in patients with severe LV dysfunction.

Gottlieb and coworkers[120] from Baltimore, Maryland, evaluated the consequences of acute nifedipine withdrawal in 81 patients with prior unstable angina pectoris. Thirty-nine patients underwent CABG for uncontrolled angina or LM CAD. All 81 patients had completed a prospective, double-blind, randomized trial of nifedipine -vs- placebo for rest angina. In this study, no significant difference between patients withdrawn from nifedipine or placebo was found with regard to the frequency of perioperative AMI hypotension requiring balloon counterpulsation, vasopressor or vasodilator requirements, or the frequency of significant arrhythmias. An additional 42 patients completed 2 years on a protocol consisting of nitrates and propranolol in addition to nifedipine or placebo. During 66 hours of continuous monitoring after withdrawal of nifedipine or placebo, heart rate and BP were unchanged. An increase in the frequency of angina at rest occurred in 5 patients who had continued to experience rest angina before drug withdrawal. No patient with lesser degrees of angina experienced new onset of rest angina during drug withdrawal and no patient had an AMI. Thus, these data indicate that there is no early adverse effect of acute nifedipine withdrawal in patients similar to those studied in this evaluation.

Nicardipine

Khurmi and coworkers[121] from Harrow, England, evaluated a new calcium blocker, nicardipine, in 39 patients with chronic stable angina pectoris in 2 different placebo-controlled single- and double-blind crossover trials with long-term follow-up using quantitated exercise testing and ambulatory ST-segment monitoring. The first study established the minimal effective dose of nicardipine and the second evaluation determined the effects of 3 different dose levels. Treadmill exercise testing was performed at the end of each 2-week treatment period. The data obtained indicate that the mean exercise time was increased from 6.8 ± 0.7 minutes on placebo to 7.0 ± 0.8 minutes during treatment with nicardipine, 60 mg/day; exercise time increased to 8.7 ± 0.8 and 9.2 ± 0.9 minutes with 90 and 120 mg/day, respectively ($p < 0.001$). Heart rate increased with nicardipine from 75 ± 2–88 ± 3 beats/min at the maximal dose. Time to exercise-induced ECG evidence of ischemia was prolonged from 4.8 ± 0.6 minutes during placebo to 6.7 ± 0.8 at the peak dose of nicardipine ($p < 0.001$). Improvement noted after 2 weeks of nicardipine, 120 mg daily, was maintained during a 6-month follow-up. Few important side effects were noted. Thus, nicardipine appears to be an effective antianginal agent with an optimal dose of 90–120 mg/day in patients with chronic CAD.

Bepridil

Narahara and associates[122] from Dallas, Texas, evaluated 20 patients with chronic stable angina pectoris utilizing bepridil, a new calcium channel blocker, in a single-blind trial that was placebo controlled within patients. Of the 20 patients, 13 also underwent rest and exercise gated blood pool scintigraphy to assess the effects of the agent on LV performance. Mean anginal frequency was significantly reduced, from 7.3–3.1 episodes/week. Total work performed increased from 410–581 kpm and exercise time increased from 5.3–6.6 minutes. Supine resting LV end-diastolic volume index, end-systolic volume index, stroke volume index, cardiac index, and EF were not altered by bepridil. During supine exercise, EF decreased from 60–55% during placebo therapy. Despite an increase in total work, the mean EF increased from 60–62% during exercise with bepridil therapy. Maximal exercise stroke volume index and cardiac index were significantly greater during bepridil therapy. Exercise resulted in new or increased LV wall motion abnormalities in 7 of 13 patients during placebo therapy. During bepridil therapy, only 4 new or increased wall motion abnormalities were noted despite the increase in total work performed. Thus, bepridil is an effective antianginal agent. The drug allows an increase in exercise work load and preserves LV performance. DiBianco and associates[123] in a prospective multicenter, placebo-controlled, dose-ranging study compared bepridil with placebo in 77 patients with confirmed CAD and chronic stable angina pectoris. After 2 weeks of placebo (phase 1), bepridil was given for 3 phases (2, 3, and 4) at total daily dosage of 200, 300, and 400 mg. The study was completed after final reintroduction of placebo (phase 5). Within each phase once and twice daily regimens of bepridil were randomly compared. Bepridil (300 mg/day) reduced anginal frequency 68%, from 8.5 ± 1.1 (SEM) to 2.7 ± 0.7 attacks/week and nitroglycerin tablet use, 76% (p < 0.001). Bepridil improved exercise duration 26%, from 6.9 ± 0.4–8.7 ± 0.5 minutes (p < 0.001) and exercise work, 52%, from 2.7 ± 0.3–4.1 ± 0.4 kpm $\times 10^{-3}$ (p < 0.001) on a standardized treadmill protocol. Resting and peak exercise heart rate and BP were unaffected by bepridil. The antianginal effects were similar with either once or twice daily treatment schedules. Minor side effects of nausea, epigastric discomfort, and tremor were infrequent and there were no major side effects. The results of this large but preliminary, single-blind and short-term study suggest that bepridil is an effective and well-tolerated antianginal agent when administered once daily.

Drug comparisons

To determine whether cigarette smoking affects the results of drug treatment for angina, Deanfield and associates[124] from London, England, studied 10 cigarette smokers with angina who were given placebo, nifedipine (60 mg/day), propranolol (240 mg/day), and atenolol (100 mg/day), each for 1 week. The 4-week double-blind study was repeated with the same randomly determined order of drug sequences after all 10 subjects had stopped smoking. Before and after the subjects stopped smoking, all 3 drugs significantly reduced the frequency of angina, as measured with angina diaries, and improved the results of maximal exercise testing and 48-hour ambulatory monitoring of ST segments. However, during the nonsmoking phase of the study, there was an overall decline in the frequency of angina and an improvement in performance on exercise testing compared with the smoking period, although the results of 48-hour ambulatory monitoring remained unchanged. The improvement after patients stopped smoking was greater during treatment with nifedipine than during administration of the other 2 drugs or placebo. Blood levels of propranolol were increased when patients stopped smoking; levels of nifedipine and atenolol were unchanged. The data show that smoking had direct and adverse effects on the heart and interfered with the efficacy of all 3 antianginal drugs, but with nifedipine the most.

Anderson and colleagues[125] from Salt Lake City, Utah, studied the effects of oral diltiazem (120 mg), propranolol (100 mg), and placebo on exercise performance and LV function before and during symptom-limited supine bicycle exercise by means of multigated RNA in 12 patients with documented, symptomatic CAD. A double-blind, randomized crossover protocol was used. Diltiazem increased EF at submaximal exercise (+7.0 absolute percentage points, p < 0.02) and maximal exercise (+8.1 percentage points, p < 0.01). Exercise EF was increased by 13.6 percentage points (p < 0.02) in patients with decreased ventricular function (resting EF < 50%). Propranolol had no effect on exercise EF at any stage, even when patients with EF < 50% were excluded. The increase in total exercise time was significant after diltiazem (+27%, p < 0.01) but not after propranolol (+16%; p, NS). Propranolol decreased both resting (−9 beats/min, p < 0.01) and exercise heart rates (−27 beats/min, p < 0.001), whereas diltiazem had no significant effect. Propranolol decreased resting diastolic BP (−8 mmHg, p < 0.02), exercise systolic (−27 mmHg, p < 0.001) and diastolic (−9 mmHg, p < 0.01) BP, and rest (p < 0.01) and exercise (p < 0.001) double product. Diltiazem decreased resting systolic BP (−9 mmHg, p < 0.01) and both resting (−8 mmHg, p < 0.001) and exercise (−9 mmHg, p < 0.01) diastolic BP. Diltiazem decreased double product at submaximal (p < 0.005) but not maximal exercise. Angina restricted exercise in 4 patients after diltiazem compared with 8 and 7 patients after placebo and propranolol, respectively (p < 0.05). Thus, diltiazem improved exercise performance by RNA during symptom limited supine bicycle ergometry to a greater extent than did propranolol or placebo, and this effect was most apparent in those with decreased LV function.

O'Hara and associates[126] from Harrow, England, compared 2-dose levels of diltiazem with propranolol in the management of chronic stable angina pectoris. Two groups of patients were treated for alternate periods of 4 weeks with each drug in a double-blind crossover study with computer-assisted maximal treadmill tests and ambulatory ST-segment monitoring for evaluation of efficacy and safety. In 12 patients who received diltiazem, 180 mg/day, the time to development of angina increased from 5.9 ± 0.7 minutes (±SEM) during placebo treatment to 8.3 ± 0.8 minutes during diltiazem treatment and to 9.2 ± 0.8 minutes with propranolol, 240 mg/day. Three patients became angina-free when they were treated with both drugs. Among 12 patients who received diltiazem, 360 mg/day, 1 patient became angina-free during treatment with both drugs and 1 became angina-free with diltiazem only. The mean exercise time increased from 5.8 ± 0.7 minutes with placebo to 8.6 ± 1.0 minutes with diltiazem, 360 mg/day, and to 8.2 ± 0.6 minutes with propranolol, 240 mg/day. Analysis of variance showed no difference in efficacy between the 2 doses of diltiazem or between the 2 drugs. Ambulatory heart rate was reduced both during the day and at night with both drugs and significantly more with propranolol than with diltiazem treatment. Except for 1 patient in whom a rash developed when given diltiazem, 180 mg/day, and another who had both a rash and first-degree heart block with diltiazem, 360 mg/day, both drugs were well tolerated. Thus, diltiazem in a daily dose of 180 or 360 mg/day is as effective as propranolol for the treatment of chronic stable angina.

Chaitman and associates[127] from Montreal, Canada, compared exercise tolerance 1, 3, and 8 hours after 80 mg of propranolol, 120 mg of diltiazem and 20 mg of nifedipine, and after 20 minutes of 0.6 mg of sublingual nitroglycerin with placebo in 15 men who had chronic stable angina pectoris. Three hours after drug ingestion, the exercise time was prolonged by 72 ± 26, 162 ± 27, and 161 ± 30 seconds (p < 0.05) for propranolol, diltiazem, and nifedipine, respectively, and by 123 ± 35 seconds (p < 0.001) 20 minutes after sublingual nitroglycerin compared with placebo. The onset of ST-segment depression ≥1 mm was delayed by 120 ± 34, 203 ± 29, and 189 ± 35 seconds (p < 0.05) and by 79 ± 23 seconds (p < 0.05), respectively. After propranolol, the peak rate-BP product decreased compared with placebo (15 ± 1 U [10^{-3}]-vs-20 ± 2 U, p < 0.01). In contrast, the peak rate-pressure product was greater after diltiazem and nifedipine than after placebo (22 ± 1 U, p < 0.05, and 24 ± 1 U, p < 0.01). The maximal increase in exercise tolerance was most marked for each drug at 3 hours, but was also significant at 1 hour for nifedipine and at 8 hours for diltiazem. At 3 hours, an increase in exercise time of (more than) 2 minutes was observed in 4 of 6 patients who had plasma propranolol concentrations > 40 ng/ml, 8 of 9 who had a plasma diltiazem concentration > 150 ng/ml, and in 7 of 7 who had a plasma nifedipine concentration > 90 ng/ml. Thus, in patients with chronic stable angina pectoris, propranolol decreases myocardial oxygen demand to a greater extent than diltiazem, nifedipine, and nitroglycerin. Each drug increases exercise tolerance, although the timing of the antianginal effect of the drugs differ. Diltiazem showed a prolonged improvement in exercise tolerance up to 8 hours after administration.

Effect of medical and surgical therapy on resting LV function

Detre and associates[128] from Washington, D.C., summarized as part of the Veterans Administration Cooperative Study the effect of CABG and medical therapy on 5-year resting LV function in 194 randomized patients with stable angina pectoris. The 92 medical and 102 surgical patients were comparable at entry; 28% of the medical and 30% of the surgical patients had a baseline EF of <50%. There was no significant change in mean EF between baseline and 5-year values in either treatment group. The baseline and 5-year values were 56 and 58% in each treatment group. Intervening AMI had an adverse effect in medically treated patients (59–46%) and in surgically treated patients with late AMI (58–47%). Perioperative AMI was not associated with a decrease in EF. These findings extend the similar results of previous short-term studies of the effect of CABG on resting LV function to 5 years and provide data in a comparable medical control group.

VARIANT ANGINA and/or CORONARY SPASM

Comparison with fixed coronary narrowing

To determine if the clinical features of variant angina are predictive of the severity of underlying CAD, Bott-Silverman and associates[129] from Cleveland, Ohio, compared 43 patients with variant angina who had less than 50% fixed coronary luminal diameter narrowing (group 1) with 65 patients with variant angina who had ≤70% diameter narrowing (group 2). Statistically significant differences were found in 3 clinical features between groups 1 and 2: 1) a more than 3 month history of angina at rest before diagnosis (80 -vs-23%); 2) an abnormal ECG at rest (19 -vs- 48%); and 3) an abnormal stress test (26 [8 of 30] -vs- 84% [15 of 18]). However, these features were not clinically reliable in separating patients with variant angina with and without fixed severe obstructions because of overlap between the 2 groups. No difference was found between the 2 groups in age, sex, predominant symptom at the time of catheterization, history of exertional angina, syncope with angina, prolonged angina, previous myocardial infarction or risk factors for coronary artery disease. There was also no difference in the location of ST elevation or occurrence of major arrhythmias during angina. Thus, among patients with Prinzmetal's variant angina, those with normal or mildly abnormal coronary arteriograms cannot be differentiated reliably by clinical features from those with fixed severe coronary obstructions. Coronary arteriography should be performed to define the underlying coronary anatomy and to determine optimal therapy in patients with variant angina.

Circadian variation

Waters and associates[130] from Montreal, Canada, assessed circadian variation in disease activity in 13 hospitalized patients with variant angina pectoris. Over 14 hours, all anginal attacks were noted, a continuous Holter ECG was recorded, and 2 ergonovine tests were performed 12 hours apart, 1 at 4 am and the other at 4 pm. Only 2 patients gave a clear-cut history of more frequent nocturnal or early morning attacks. During the study period, 1.8 ± 1.6 am and 0.62 ± 1.2 pm angina episodes per patient were reported (p < 0.02), but a circadian pattern was apparent in only 4 patients. However, Holter analysis revealed 5.3 ± 13.8 am and 2.6 ± 8.5 pm episodes of ST elevation per patient (p < 0.05) and 8.1 ± 13.9 am and 3.2 ± 8.5 pm episodes of ST elevation, ST depression, or T-wave pseudonormalization (p < 0.01). Ten of 11 patients with Holter abnormalities had more frequent am than pm attacks (p < 0.01). ST elevation developed during all 13 of the 4 am and 12 of 13 of the 4 pm ergonovine tests. In 10 cases the ergonovine threshold at which the attack occurred was lower in the morning, in no case was it lower in the afternoon, and in 3 patients the morning and afternoon doses were identical (p < 0.01). Thus, circadian variation in disease activity both for spontaneous and provoked attacks is present in most patients with variant angina, even though it is often not clinically apparent.

Transient right ventricular ischemia

Although coronary vasospasm is a well-recognized cause of transient ischemia at rest, evidence for RV involvement has been limited to hemodynamic monitoring in affected patients. Parodi and colleagues[131] from Pisa, Italy, described their clinical experience with 4 patients with varying angina caused by spasm of the right coronary artery who were assessed for evidence of RV involvement. The patients were suspected of having predominant RV ischemia on the basis of a normal thallium-201 scan, LV EF, regional wall motion assessed by equilibrium RNA, 2-D echo findings, and LV hemodynamics. All procedures were performed during transient ST-segment elevation in the inferior leads of the ECG. A RV ischemia was documented in 4 patients by first-pass RNA studies and phase analysis and in 3 patients by simultaneous right and left hemodynamic monitoring. Clinical findings from these 4 patients were compared with those from 4 other patients with similar ECG changes, coronary anatomic distribution, and documented right coronary spasm but with evidence of LV involvement as documented by abnormal thallium-201 scintigraphy, RNA, 2-D echo, and LV hemodynamics during ischemic episodes. These preliminary data indicate the existence of prevalent RV ischemia during variant angina caused by right coronary artery vasospasm. This condition should be suspected whenever typical anginal symptoms or ischemic ECG changes are accompanied by normal thallium-201 scintigraphic findings or normal LV function as assessed by RNA, echo, and left hemodynamic monitoring. First-pass RNA study and phase analysis of RNA represent suitable techniques for detecting transient RV dysfunction.

Heart rate and BP changes

Araki and associates[132] from Fukuoka, Japan, examined responses of heart rate and BP to transient myocardial ischemia in patients with variant angina. Heart rate changes during ST-segment elevation were examined by means of a Holter ECG monitoring system. All 27 ST-segment elevations from 10 patients with anterior ischemia were accompanied by an increase in heart rate by 12 ± 2 beats/min (mean $\pm$ SEM, $p < 0.001$) at peak ST-segment elevation. With inferior ischemia in 9 patients, heart rate decreased significantly by 4 ± 1 beats/min (n, 28; $p < 0.001$). However, 9 of these 28 ST-segment elevations showed a biphasic response of heart rate, i.e., an initial increase and subsequent decrease. Such heart rate changes were not different between ST-segment elevations with and without chest pain. With chest pain, systolic BP increased in anterior ischemia by 42 ± 5 mmHg (n, 10; $p < 0.001$) but decreased in inferior ischemia by 22 ± 8 mmHg (n, 7; $p < 0.05$). It was concluded that a different cardiovascular reflex occurs in response to inferior-vs-anterior ischemia and it is independent of chest pain.

U-wave inversion

Matsuguchi and associates[133] from Fukuoka, Japan, studied the prevalence and clinical significance of transient U-wave inversion in 43 patients with variant angina. Twenty-four patients (group A) had ST-segment elevation in the anterolateral and 19 patients (group B) had this finding in the inferoposterior leads of the ECG during spontaneous angina. In no patient was U-wave inversion present on the resting 12-lead ECG in the absence of anginal attack. During anginal attacks, U-wave inversion developed in association with ST-segment elevation in 16 patients (66.7%) of group A but in no patient of group B. To exclude the possibility that a transient increase of systolic BP during angina caused U-wave inversion, treadmill exercise testing was done in the 16 patients after the discontinuation of antianginal drugs. In 12 of the 16 patients, exercise testing did not produce angina or U-wave inversion despite a marked elevation of systolic BP. These results indicate that transient U-wave inversion frequently develops with anterolateral ischemia but not with inferoposterior ischemia during attacks of variant angina. It is likely that transient U-wave inversion was caused by myocardial ischemia but not by an increase of BP during angina.

Changes in LV mechanics

In a study carried out by Distante and colleagues[134] from Pisa, Italy, 55 ischemic attacks at rest with ST-segment elevation were recorded by 2-D echo in 20 patients with Prinzmetal's angina. Eighteen ischemic attacks were recorded starting from intravenous injection of ergonovine maleate and 37 spontaneous ischemic attacks were recorded from onset of either anginal pain or ECG changes or from the basal state. In each ischemic attack at least 1 of the following transient alterations was observed by 2D echo during ST elevation: 1) regional hypokinesia, akinesia, or dyskinesia; 2) step sign, i.e., a sharp demarcation between an akinetic or dyskinetic area and an adjacent normal or hypercontracting region; and 3) geometric changes in LV shape, i.e., globular appearance in diastole and hourglass silhouette in systole. Regional myocardial asynergy was detected earlier than onset of pain (which was not present in 21 [38%] ischemic episodes) or ST-segment elevation on ECG, as documented in 40 ischemic episodes (16 induced and 24 spontaneous) in which echo monitoring was performed from basal state and carried on up to the appearance of ischemia. All described mechanical changes were fully reversible after pain subsided and ST segment was back to isoelectric, either spontaneously or with nitrates; furthermore, a contractile rebound phenomenon of the previously ischemic wall was observed in some episodes.

To assess LV function during transient reversible myocardial ischemia underlying variant angina, Distante and associates[135] from Pisa, Italy, recorded M-mode echoes in 12 patients with Prinzmetal's angina during 29 episodes at rest (18 spontaneous and 11 ergonovine-induced). At peak ST-segment elevation, a regional mechanical impairment was observed in the interventricular septum during 23 episodes of angina and in the posterior wall during 6 episodes. In the 18 spontaneous episodes the LV ischemic wall, when compared with the basal state, was found to have a significant reduction in motion ($-76 \pm 9\%$) (mean $\pm$ SEM), in diastolic thickness ($-12 \pm 3\%$), and in percent systolic thickening ($-88 \pm 6\%$). Increase in LV end-diastolic diameter ($+13 \pm 2\%$) and decrease in percent fractional shortening ($-38 \pm 4\%$) were also observed. When ST segment was back to the isoelectric line, a transient overshoot in regional LV function was observed. In induced episodes statistically significant changes could be detected by M-mode echo even before appearance of ST-segment elevation and angina pain. No significant difference was found in type or degree of mechanical impairment between induced and spontaneous episodes. Therefore in patients with

Prinzmetal's angina: 1) M-mode echo allows detection of mechanical changes due to transient myocardial ischemia; and 2) mechanical impairment occurs earlier than clinical (pain) and ECG (ST-segment elevation) signs of transmural ischemia.

Consequences and survival

Mark and colleagues[136] from Durham, North Carolina, studied 109 consecutive patients with variant angina who underwent cardiac catheterization over an 11-year period (Table 1-8). All patients were followed for ≥6 months or until death, and 46 patients (22 treated medically and 24 treated surgi-

TABLE 1-8.   *Baseline characteristics of 109 patients with variant angina grouped according to the presence (n, 85) or absence (n, 24) of significant fixed coronary disease. Reproduced with permission from Mark et al.*[136]

CHARACTERISTIC	SIGNIFICANT CORONARY DISEASE (%)	NO SIGNIFICANT CORONARY DISEASE (%)
Male	81	54
Age ≤50 years	39	67
Historical features		
Duration of angina ≤6 weeks	42	38
Progressive angina	85	75
Preinfarction angina	66	29
Exertional angina	55	54
Nocturnal angina	43	50
Previous AMI	26	13
CHF (NYHA class ≥2)	5	4
Beta blocker therapy on admission	50	48
History of hypertension	45	33
History of diabetes	9	0
History of smoking	87	75
History of syncope	4	4
History of cardiac arrest or VT	15	29
Laboratory findings		
Cardiomegaly on chest x-ray film	11	0
Diagnostic Q waves on ECG	25	4
Anterior ST-segment elevation	57	37
Nonspecific ST-T wave changes on ECG	74	67
# vessels with ≥75% stenosis in total group (n = 109)		
0	22%	
1	33%	
2	25%	
3	20%	
Left main coronary artery disease	3%	

NYHA = New York Heart Association.

cally) were followed for ≥5 years. Of the 62 patients initially treated medically, 14 had nonfatal AMI (12 within 1 month of catheterization) and 12 died (6 within 6 months). Survival probabilities at 1, 3, and 5 years was 0.88, 0.84, and 0.77, respectively. Of the 48 surgically treated patients, 4 had nonfatal AMI (3 in the perioperative period) and 3 died (all in the perioperative period). The survival probability of these patients at 1 year was 0.94 and remained unchanged at 3 and 5 years. The single most important prognostic factor in medically treated patients was the presence or absence of fixed obstructive CAD. AMI-free survival probabilities at 1 and 3 years in the 23 patients without significant CAD were 1.0 and 0.89, compared with 0.51 and 0.46 in the 39 patients with significant CAD. Analysis by the Cox model showed that variant angina patients had a higher probability of death and nonfatal AMI than did those with nonvariant angina if other important prognostic variables were held constant. The major independent prognostic variables for medically treated patients with variant angina were similar to those that were important in medically treated patients with CAD who did not have variant angina. Finally, the investigators examined how well variant angina patients with and without CAD could be distinguished from each other with the use of noninvasive baseline characteristics. Although these 2 groups did have different distributions of some variables, neither univariable nor multivariable techniques were accurate enough to supplant cardiac catheterization for identifying variant angina patients without significant disease.

Alpha adrenergic receptors

Chierchia and coinvestigators[137] from London, England, investigated the possible role of coronary alpha adrenergic receptors in the genesis of coronary spasm in 14 consecutive patients with varying angina. Computerized, beat by beat analysis of the ECG recording during continuous Holter monitoring in 8 patients failed to reveal any increase of heart rate and corrected QT interval in the period preceding the onset of ST-segment changes in 197 episodes of ischemia caused by coronary spasm. In the same patients analysis of the circadian distribution of ischemic episodes revealed a significantly higher incidence in the early morning hours when sympathetic activity is at the lowest level. Provocative testing with cold pressor, phenylephrine or norepinephrine infusion and administration of ergonovine maleate was performed in 12 patients. Ergonovine consistently reproduced coronary spasm in all 12 patients, whereas results of the cold pressor testing were positive in 1 patient. Infusion of phenylephrine or norepinephrine after beta blockade failed to precipitate myocardial ischemia. Infusion of phentolamine at the highest tolerated dose in 5 patients did not reduce significantly the number of ischemic attacks compared with placebo. In contrast to previous reports, these investigators' data would tend to militate against the hypothesis that an increase in sympathetic outflow to the heart plays an important role in the genesis of coronary spasm. The investigators do emphasize that they cannot exclude the possibility of localized alpha stimulation of epicardial arteries. Such careful clinical observations as reported in this study would raise the possibility that alpha stimulation may involve modifications of a single receptor or possible other mechanisms could be responsive.

Role for serotonin in genesis

De Caterina and coworkers[138] from Pisa, Italy, designed a study to test the hypothesis of a possible role of serotonin in the pathogenesis of myocardial ischemia in patients with pure vasospastic angina, since serotonin is known to cause contraction in isolated coronary arteries. This effect, as well as serotonin-induced platelet aggregation, is reduced by ketanserin, a specific S_2-receptor blocker. Five men with >6 episodes a day of myocardial ischemia at rest characterized by ST-segment elevation on the ECG were selected for the study after a 2-day run-in period of continuous ECG Holter monitoring in the absence of any therapy except sublingual nitrates. In a double-blind crossover protocol they received consecutive infusions of 6 hours each of ketanserin (2 mg/h intravenous, preceded by a 10 mg bolus in 3 patients) and placebo in the following sequence: ketanserin-placebo-ketanserin-placebo in the first and placebo-ketanserin-placebo-ketanserin in the second 24-hour period. The efficacy of the infused drug was tested by exposing platelet-rich plasma, obtained from the study patients at a fixed morning time before and during ketanserin infusions, to a series of serotonin concentrations in a conventional aggregometer. A complete suppression of aggregation curves in the range of serotonin concentrations tested resulted during administration of ketanserin. The efficacy of the drug in preventing ischemic episodes was assessed by computing the ischemic episodes recorded by Holter monitoring and nitroglycerin consumption in each 6-hour ketanserin period and in the corresponding placebo period. A total of 171 ischemic periods was recorded, 33 of which were symptomatic. Total numbers of ischemic episodes were 94 during ketanserin and 77 during placebo. No consistent differences in numbers of ischemic episodes and nitroglycerin consumption were observed in the comparison of the corresponding ketanserin and placebo 6-hour periods. Also, severity, as assessed by both nitroglycerin consumption and ST-segment elevation, was not affected by the drug; one patient required nitrate infusion after the first day of the trial owing to a worsening of symptoms. Although the periods of observation are brief in this study, the large number of ischemic episodes, both on and off therapy, support the conclusion of the researchers that it appears unlikely that serotonin can play an important role in vasospastic angina.

Ergonovine induced

Although fixed atherosclerotic obstructions remain the cause of chronic stable angina, transient changes in caliber of coronary stenosis could contribute an important modulatory role in determining the frequency of symptoms. To test this hypothesis, Crea and colleagues[139] from London, England, tested 31 patients with histories typical of exertional angina with ergonovine and compared the ECG and clinical responses to those observed in 7 patients with variant angina. All patients underwent bicycle ergometric exercise testing and coronary angiographic evaluation. For all tests, ST-segment shifts of ≥0.1 mV were considered to be diagnostic of myocardial ischemia. In patients with exertional angina, exercise testing produced diagnostic ST-segment depression in 21 (68%). Ergonovine testing produced diagnostic ST-segment depression in 9 (29%). All 9 patients with positive exercise test results had 2- or 3-vessel CAD, yet the test was negative in 7 other patients with positive exercise test results and similar angiographic finding. Conversely, in the 7 patients with variant angina, results of exercise testing were positive in 5, and ergonovine produced ST-segment elevation in all 7. Coronary angiographic examination showed normal arteries in 2, 1-vessel CAD in 4, and 3-vessel CAD in 1. Results of all ergonovine tests were positive at values of rate-pressure product much lower than those observed during exercise. These investigators concluded it reasonable to postulate that in a sizable proportion of patients with exertional angina and diffuse coronary atherosclerosis, dynamic stenoses can contribute to produce ischemia, although the different ECG response to ergonovine testing suggests that the effects of vasoconstriction are less severe than those in variant angina. These clinical observations support studies on isolated perfuse coronary arteries and the response of thrombus lesions to vasoconstricting substances, particularly histamine and prostaglandin.

Since ergonovine appears to produce coronary contractions by a serotonergic (5-HT) mechanism, Freedman and coinvestigators[140] from London, England, attempted to prevent ergonovine-induced ischemia in patients with vasospastic angina by treatment with ketanserin, a new selective 5-HT blocker. The investigators studied 7 patients with consistently positive results of ergonovine testing with ST-segment elevation in 3 and ST-segment depression in 4 patients. Ergonovine testing was performed before and after a bolus of 10 mg of ketanserin and infusion of 2–4 mg/hour for 8 hours in 6 patients. To assess 5-HT blockade during ketanserin infusion, the constrictor response of hand veins to 5-HT was tested before and after ketanserin. Despite evidence of 5-HT blockade in hand veins, ergonovine-induced ischemia was not prevented by ketanserin in any patient, and there was no significant change in the dose of ergonovine required to provoke ischemia. In 1 patient, 4 spontaneous episodes of ST-segment elevation occurred during infusion of ketanserin. The plasma concentrations of ketanserin at the time of ergonovine testing ranged from 61–127 ng/ml and were well above those that completely inhibit canine coronary 5-HT contractions in vitro. Although human coronary arteries may differ in their responsiveness to 5-HT or ketanserin, these data suggest that ischemia from ergonovine-induced coronary vasospasm is not mediated by 5-HT receptors. Previous studies have eliminated other potential suspects, such as alpha adrenergic stimuli, thromboxane, and prostacyclin deficiency, as potential causes of coronary arterial spasm, and this study, by casting doubts on the role of serotonin, may further narrow the field in the search for the underlying mechanism.

Szlachcic and associates[141] from Montreal, Canada, analyzed the clinical correlates of ventricular arrhythmias during ergonovine-induced episodes of variant angina. Of 95 consecutive patients with active variant angina who underwent ergonovine testing in the coronary care unit while off treatment, 24 (25%) developed serious ventricular arrhythmias: VT in 8, bigeminy in 7, pairs in 5, and frequent VPC in 4. Ergonovine-induced arrhythmias were observed more often in patients with anterior than inferior ST-segment elevation (p < 0.05). ST-segment elevation was significantly higher (10 ± 8 -vs- 3 ± 2 mm) in patients who developed arrhythmias. All ventricular arrhythmias began within 3 minutes after the onset of ST-segment elevation. The intravenous administration of nitroglycerin eliminated arrhythmias in 22 of 24 cases; in only 2 patients did ventricular arrhythmias develop after the administration of nitroglycerin. Serious ventricular arrhythmias were found

during spontaneous variant angina attacks in 14 of 24 patients with ergonovine-induced arrhythmias compared with 16 of 71 patients without ergonovine-induced arrhythmias (p < 0.001). It was concluded that arrhythmias
during ergonovine testing are most often caused by ischemia and not reperfusion, and patients with arrhythmias during ergonovine-induced attacks are
more likely to have arrhythmias during spontaneous attacks.

Calcium antagonist plus isosorbide dinitrate

Winniford and colleagues[142] from Dallas, Texas, assessed the efficacy of
concomitant calcium antagonist and isosorbide dinitrate therapy in patients
with frequent episodes of variant angina and compared such combination
therapy with isosorbide dinitrate alone. Nine such patients (6 men and 3
women, aged 47 ± 9 [mean ± SD] years) were enrolled in a long-term comparison of oral isosorbide dinitrate (117 ± 63 mg/day) alone, verapamil
(453 ± 75 mg/day) plus isosorbide dinitrate (given in the same dose as just
stated), and nifedipine (71 ± 14 mg/day) plus isosorbide dinitrate (given in
the same dose as stated), each administered for 2 months. During isosorbide
dinitrate therapy, these 9 patients averaged 24 ± 37 chest pains/week, consumed 24 ± 47 sublingual nitroglycerin tablets/week, and demonstrated
47 ± 43 episodes/week of transient ST-segment deviations on calibrated 2-
channel Holter monitoring. During therapy with verapamil and isosorbide
dinitrate and nifedipine and isosorbide dinitrate, the frequency of angina
and ST-segment deviations was dramatically reduced (verapamil and isosorbide dinitrate, 3.9 ± 3.6 chest pains/week and 3.6 ± 2.6 ST-segment devia-
tions/week, p < 0.05; nifedipine and isosorbide dinitrate, 3.1 ± 4.0 chest
pains/week and 5.5 ± 6.6 ST-segment deviations/week, p < 0.05). In all respects, verapamil and isosorbide dinitrate and nifedipine and isosorbide dinitrate were similar. Thus, in patients with frequent episodes of variant angina, a calcium antagonist and isosorbide dinitrate combination is much
more effective than isosorbide dinitrate alone in reducing the frequency of
angina and ischemic ECG alterations.

PERCUTANEOUS TRANSLUMINAL CORONARY ANGIOPLASTY

Assessing results

Silverton and associates[143] from Leeds, England, used a new exercise test
to assess the effects of coronary angioplasty in 22 patients. Twenty-five angioplasty procedures were performed and the exercise maximal ST segment/
heart rate (HR) slope was measured before and after operation on 23 occasions; in 2 patients treated for unstable angina the slope was measured only
after the 2 procedures. Successful angioplasty (23 of the 25 procedures) resulted in a significant reduction of the maximal ST/HR slope, usually decreasing by the equivalent of single-vessel disease according to previously published criteria. When angioplasty produced little angiographic change (2 of
25 procedures) the maximal ST/HR slope was not significantly altered. A
second, and successful, angioplasty for these 2 patients led to a significant

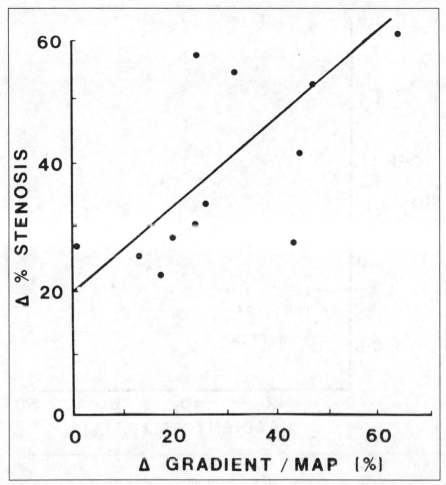

Fig. 1-26. Changes (Δ) in caliper percent stenosis are compared with changes in percent translesional gradient (r = 0.61, p < 0.05, y = 20 + 0.61x); MAP = mean arterial pressure. Reproduced with permission from O'Neill et al.[144]

reduction of the maximal ST/HR slope. Twelve patients were restudied by coronary angiography and exercise testing approximately 6 months after angioplasty. Of these, 6 had experienced recurrent chest pain, and the exercise test successfully identified the 3 who had restenoses and the 3 who did not. Thus, the maximal ST/HR slope was useful as a noninvasive and accurate method for following the progress of individual patients after coronary angioplasty.

O'Neill and coworkers[144] from Ann Arbor, Michigan, attempted to develop criteria that would objectively identify the successfulness of coronary angioplasty. Fifteen patients undergoing clinically indicated PTCA were studied. Patients were chosen on the basis of severe refractory angina and appropriate location and geometry of arterial stenosis. The translesional pressure gradient and coronary vasodilatory reserve were studied. Coronary vasodilatory reserve was measured by a digital radiographic technique that had been

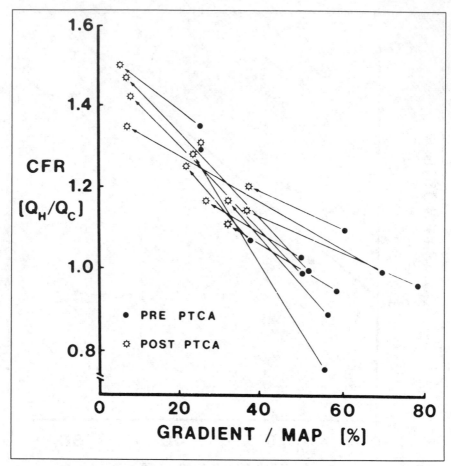

Fig. 1-27. Coronary vasodilatory reserve (CFR) before and after angioplasty (PTCA) compared with translesional gradient before and after angioplasty. • = preangioplasty; ○ = postangioplasty values. MAP = mean arterial pressure; Q = l/myocardial contrast appearance time; Q_C = relative flow, control; Q_H = relative flow, hyperemia. Reproduced with permission from O'Neill et al.[144]

previously validated against directly measured coronary sinus flow. The data obtained indicate that a significant reduction in luminal stenosis from 71 ± 12–34 ± 11% (p < 0.001) was accompanied by a reduction in translesional gradient from 47 ± 19–21 ± 12 mmHg (p < 0.001) and an increase in coronary vasodilatory reserve from 1.03 ± 0.15–1.29 ± 0.13 (p < 0.001). There was a significant correlation between changes in luminal stenosis and changes in translesional gradient (r = 0.61, p < 0.05). However, a change of ≤20% in luminal diameter was accompanied by no change in pressure gradient (Fig. 1-26). There was a significant relation between changes in gradient and in coronary hyperemic reserve (r = 0.77, p < 0.005) (Fig. 1-27). On the basis of these data, the authors proposed that physiologic criteria be used to define the success of PTCA. Specifically, the translesional gradient should be ≤25% of ostial pressure and ≤20 mmHg.

Effect of nitroglycerin on coronary collateral flow and pressure

Feldman and associates[145] from Gainesville, Florida, evaluated coronary collateral function in 21 conscious, unsedated patients by measuring aortic and distal coronary pressures and great coronary vein flow during transient (1 minute) balloon occlusion of the LAD coronary artery during PTCA. Measurements were made before and during administration of nitroglycerin (NTG) intravenously. Clinical, ECG, and hemodynamic events of transient myocardial ischemia occurred in 10 patients before and 7 patients during NTG administration (p = 0.11). The NTG infusion consistently decreased pressure determinants of myocardial oxygen demand without increasing heart rate. The NTG also decreased a calculated coronary collateral resistance index in 13 patients. Responsiveness to NTG did not appear to depend on the presence or absence of collateral vessels detected by angiography or on any other angiographic variable assessed. Measurement of coronary collateral function during coronary angioplasty is a new technique with the potential to assess the ability of interventions to prevent transient myocardial ischemia and improve myocardial perfusion during acute coronary occlusion in humans.

Effect on LV performance, regional blood flow, wall motion, and lactate metabolism

Serruys and coworkers[146] from Rotterdam, The Netherlands, studied the response of LV function, coronary blood flow, and myocardial lactate metabolism during PTCA in patients undergoing PTCA. From 4 to 6 balloon inflation procedures per patient were performed with an average duration per occlusion of 51 ± 12 seconds and a total occlusion time of 252 ± 140 seconds. Analysis of LV hemodynamics in 19 patients showed that the relaxation parameters, peak negative rate of change in pressure, and early time constants of relaxation responded more gradually. These observations suggested a progressive depression of myocardial mechanics throughout the procedure. The LV angiograms in 14 patients indicated an early onset of asynchronous relaxation concurrent with the early response in peak negative dP/dt and the time constant of early relaxation. All hemodynamic functions recovered fully within minutes after the end of PTCA. Mean blood flow in the great cardiac vein and proximal coronary sinus and the hyperemic response were measured in 20 patients. Before PTCA, mean flow in the great cardiac vein was 69 ± 17 ml/min and in the coronary sinus it was 129 ± 34 ml/min. Reactive hyperemia in the great cardiac vein was 55% after the first PTCA and 91% after the third. A more pronounced reaction was observed when the residual functional coronary stenosis was reduced in subsequent dilations. Arteriovenous lactate difference appeared constant during the first 2 occlusions and did not increase during subsequent occlusions. Within minutes after the procedure, lactate balance was again positive, demonstrating the reversibility of the metabolic disturbances after repeated ischemia. These results indicate that there is no permanent dysfunction of global or regional myocardial mechanics, myocardial blood flow, or lactate metabolism after PTCA with 4–6 coronary occlusions of 40–60 seconds.

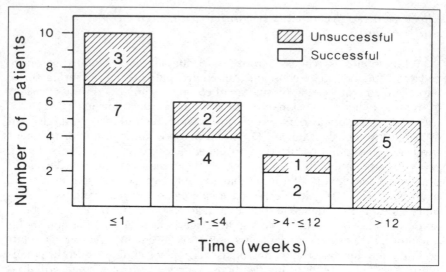

Fig. 1-28. Effect of estimated duration of occlusion (abscissa) on outcome of PTCA in 24 patients. Reproduced with permission from Holmes et al.[147]

For total coronary artery occlusion

Holmes and coworkers[147] from Rochester, Minnesota, studied the feasibility of PTCA alone in a selected group of patients with total coronary artery occlusion without associated AMI in whom the duration of occlusion could be estimated. Twenty-four patients were evaluated to determine whether PTCA might reestablish perfusion. The maximal duration of occlusion was estimated to be ≤1 week in 10 patients, >1–4 weeks in 6 patients, >4–12 weeks in 3 patients, and >12 weeks in 5 patients. In 17 patients, dilation of an occluded LAD coronary artery was attempted. Dilation of an occluded right coronary artery was attempted in 4 patients and of an occluded LC in 3 patients. PTCA was successful in 13 patients (54%), including 59% of patients with an occluded LAD coronary artery, 50% of patients with an occluded right, and 33% with an occluded LC. Successful dilation was associated with a mean decrease in coronary artery stenosis from 100–23%. In the 19 patients whose occlusion was estimated to be 12 week's duration or less, PTCA was successful in 68%. In the 5 patients whose occlusions were estimated to be >12 week's duration, dilation was less successful (p = 0.0006) (Fig. 1-28). These data suggest that in selected patients with symptomatic coronary artery disease and recent coronary artery occlusion without associated myocardial infarction, PTCA may restore perfusion.

Cost -vs- bypass grafting

In some patients with CAD PTCA is widely considered to be an acceptable and less expensive alternative to CABG. Reeder and associates[148] from Rochester, Minnesota, and Tucson, Arizona, compared expenditures related to cardiac care for 79 unselected patients undergoing PTCA with expenditures for 89 unselected patients undergoing elective CABG without a previous attempt at PTCA. All patients had 1-vessel CAD. The mean aggregate 1-year monetary outlay was 15% lower in the PTCA group than in the CABG group. A major component of the expense of PTCA was the treatment of restenosis in the 33% of patients in this group in whom this late complication occurred.

Warfarin and aspirin for prevention of recurrence of stenosis

After such revascularization procedures as CABG and PTCA, several adjunctive therapies have been proposed to prevent thrombus formation with closure of graft or artery. To determine the influence of adjunctive treatment with warfarin or aspirin on recurrence after PTCA, Thornton and colleagues[149] from Atlanta, Georgia, randomized 248 patients after successful PTCA to either 325 mg aspirin daily or to warfarin treatment sufficient to maintain a prothrombin time of 2–2.5 times the control value. The follow-up protocol included stress testing and coronary angiographic examinations 3–6 months after PTCA. All patients were followed for ≥9 months. Of the 122 patients randomized to warfarin, 44 (36%) had recurrent stenoses as opposed to 34 of 126 (27%) patients on aspirin (NS). However, patients with ≥6-month history of angina had a significantly different response to adjunctive therapy in that 19 of 43 (44%) of the warfarin patients compared with 10 of 48 (21%) of the aspirin patients had recurrent stenoses. Thus, warfarin was not shown to be more effective than aspirin as adjunctive therapy after PTCA, whereas aspirin was demonstrated to be superior to warfarin in patients with a longer history of angina.

Repeat angioplasty

Meier and coworkers[150] from Atlanta, Georgia, performed repeat PTCA in 95 patients from among a group of 514 patients undergoing successful PTCA. Recurrent coronary stenosis developed in 171 (33%) of the 514 patients. Repeat PTCA was attempted in 95 patients with a significantly higher primary success rate (97 -vs- 85%, p < 0.001) and a lower complication rate (8 -vs- 15%, p < 0.10) than those associated with the original PTCA. Follow-up evaluation was possible in the 92 patients with successful repeat PTCA. A second recurrence of stenosis occurred in 26% of the patients and a third PTCA was performed in 7. Among these patients, 6 procedures were successful and in short-term follow-up there have been no recurrent stenoses. Thus, these data indicate that PTCA provides a means to treat recurrent coronary stenosis.

Intraoperative balloon-catheter dilation

Faro and associates[151] from Gainesville, Florida, performed in 34 CAD patients with stable angina undergoing CABG supplemental intraoperative coronary artery balloon-catheter dilation. Antegrade or retrograde coronary dilation was performed on 35 arteries at 50 sites using a modified PTCA-type device performed via conventional coronary arteriotomy. The balloon catheter could not be passed through 1 stenotic site. Intimal dissection occurred at 2 sites, with resolution on follow-up studies. There was 1 perioperative AMI, 100% early relief of angina, and 1 operative death. Of 25 distal arterial narrowings studied by angiography early after surgery (mean, 10 days), 15 (60%) were unchanged, 2 (8%) were worse, and 8 (32%) were improved. Discrete narrowings improved more than diffuse narrowings; in 46% of the former there was an increase in luminal diameter, in comparison to only 17% of the latter. During a maximal 34-month follow-up, 2 patients developed recurrent angina and 1 died of CHF. Of 13 distal coronary narrowings studied late after surgery (mean, 1 year), 6 (46%) were unchanged, 3 (23%) were worse, and 4 (31%) were improved. Postoperative serial catheterization (early and late) of 10 distal narrowings revealed that 9 were unchanged and 1 was worse. Adjunctive intraoperative coronary balloon-catheter dilation can be performed safely with acceptable clinical results and the procedure may also allow more complete myocardial revascularization.

American Medical Association's report

This council report should be familiar both to physicians recommending PTCA and to those performing PTCA.[152]

CORONARY ARTERY BYPASS GRAFTING

Results

Cobanoglu and colleagues[153] from Portland, Oregon, examined the urgency of clinical presentation in 3,575 patients having CABG as a determinant of survival. The clinical presentation ranged from unstable through progressive to chronic stable angina. Unstable angina was defined as ischemic myocardial pain: 1) of recent onset with rapid progression; 2) occurring within 3 months of AMI; or 3) at rest. Thirty-six percent of patients with unstable angina had preoperative diagnostic cardiac enzyme elevations or new permanent ECG changes diagnostic of AMI. Additionally, most patients in the unstable group had transient ischemic ECG changes during episodes of pain. Among the 1,404 patients with chronic angina, survival at 1 month was 98% and at 8 years, 79%. Among the 1,008 patients with progressive angina, survival at 1 month was 98% and at 8 years, 80%, and among the 1,163 patients with unstable angina, 1-month survival was 98% and 8-year survival, 89%. Thus, the best long-term results were obtained in patients with an acute clinical presentation. Ventricular function was an important determinant of late survival for the groups with chronic and progressive angina, but it had no affect on the group with unstable angina. For unstable angina, early CABG is further supported by an operative mortality of 1.7% and a rate of perioperative AMI of 3%. Additionally, patients with unstable angina, 92 and 90% who were operated on, were AMI-free at 5 and 8 years, respectively. The lack of effect of LV wall motion abnormalities (dysfunction) in the unstable group might be explained by the fact that any segmental wall abnormality was classified as poor LV function. When the study compared a group of high LV end-diastolic pressure and multiple wall motion abnormalities in the unstable angina group with a second group of no wall motion abnormalities and normal end-diastolic pressure, the survival was the same. An alternative

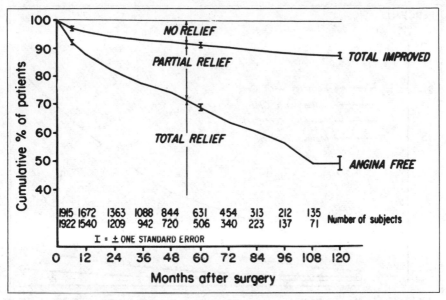

Fig. 1-29. Relief of angina in all male patients presenting with angina preoperatively. Actuarial curves showing percentage of patients totally free of angina (bottom curve) and improved (top curve). The top row of "number of subjects" pertains to the top curve, the bottom row to the bottom curve. Reproduced with permission from Johnson et al.[154]

explanation is that by early CABG in the unstable group, segmental wall dysfunction is transient and the myocardium is salvaged before irreversible damage has occurred. Thus, delaying CABG for a prolonged period in patients with unstable angina may convert a transient LV impairment to a permanent one. The investigators recommended early operation in unstable angina. They demonstrated enhanced survival at 1, 5 and 8 years and suggested that the LV dysfunction seen early may be reversible. These data vary from some other reported series and the variation may depend on definition of terms, such as unstable angina, LV dysfunction, and degree of segmental wall motion abnormalities.

Many studies document the effectiveness of CABG in relieving angina pectoris. However, few have described patterns of prevalence preoperatively and recurrence postoperatively. After excluding those known to be dead and those residing outside the continental USA, Johnson and colleagues[154] from Milwaukee, Wisconsin, attempted to contact all patients who had undergone first CABG by their group. Follow-up was 94%. Women had a higher prevalence of preoperative angina and lesser relief after CABG (p < 0.01). Because of this difference, only men presenting with angina preoperatively were analyzed in detail (Fig. 1-29). In this subgroup, the cumulative percentage of patients with total relief of angina was 87% after the first year; thereafter, the percentage decreased 6%/year. The cumulative percentage of patients improved (those with no angina plus those with less angina than before CABG) was 97% after the first year; thereafter the percentage decreased 0.9%/year. Duration of angina preoperatively had no effect on recurrence unless preoperative duration was less than 6 months. Preoperative LV func-

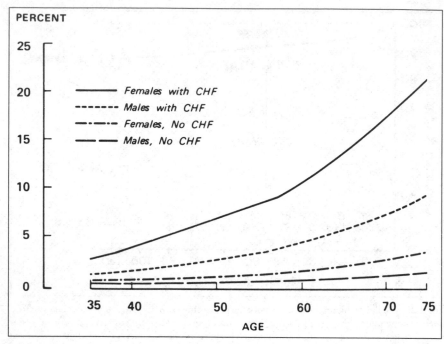

Fig. 1-30. Effect of preoperative CHF on surgical mortality. Reproduced with permission from Cosgrove et al.[155]

tion had little effect on relief of angina postoperatively. In 1.5–2 years after the original study, patients with postoperative angina had twice the mortality rate of those totally free of angina (p = 0.000004). Furthermore, those with angina at rest had twice the mortality rate of those who had angina but never at rest (p = 0.009).

From 1970–1982 24,672 patients underwent primary isolated CABG at the Cleveland Clinic. Cosgrove and associates[155] divided those patients chronologically into 4 groups. Operative mortality was 1.2% for the entire experience and was 1.2, 1.4, 1.6 and 0.8% for groups 1–4, respectively. Mortality in group 4 was significantly lower than in the other 3 groups (p < 0.001). In decreasing order of significance, the risk factors for operative mortality were emergency operation, CHF, LM narrowing, female gender, advancing age, normothermic arrest, number of grafts, poor LV function and incomplete CABG (Fig. 1-30). Cardiac causes accounted for 62% of patient deaths. This gradually decreased from 75% in group 2 to 59% in group 4. Neurologic deficit was the second most frequent cause of death (10%), reaching a high in group 4 (19% of deaths). Throughout the experience preoperative CHF carried an ominous prognosis. Patients with CHF continued to have an operative mortality 10 times that of patients without preoperative CHF. The operative mortality for patients >70 years of age was twice as high as that for younger patients. Cosgrove and colleagues concluded that morbidity and mortality decreased significantly despite increasing risk factors in the population. In the more recent experience CHF replaced emergency operation as the principal risk factor, and LM narrowing, number of grafts, and poor LV function were neutralized as risk factors and cardiac causes of death were decreased and were replaced by other system failure.

FitzGibbon and associates[156] from Ottawa, Canada, reported results of CABG in 118 consecutive patients who did not have angina when selected for surgical treatment during an 8-year period. The patients without angina had not had ischemic cardiac discomfort within 3 months of assessment, but all had had some past symptomatic event or an abnormal ECG suggestive of CAD; 66% had had ≥1 AMI. The surgeons operated on such patients because of the conviction that severe obstructive CAD with grave functional consequences could occur in the absence of angina and that major determinants of prognosis were morphologic and that coronary atherosclerosis must be actively sought when there was reasonable suspicion of its presence. They further suggested that the results of coronary arteriography were better indicators of suitability for surgical treatment than was angina. They compared the 118 patients operated on without angina with a consecutive series of 605 other patients having angina also treated by CABG during the same period. There were striking similarities between the groups with and without angina in age, treadmill test results, extent of CAD, types of operation, perioperative AMI, duration and completeness of follow-up, 1-year and 5-year graft patency rates, and operative and late deaths. Because they demonstrated a close similarity between patients with and without angina, they concluded that there was no reason why the same basic surgical principle of CABG should not be applied equally to each group. There was excellent follow-up in this tightly monitored group of relatively young patients, 80% of whom were active duty uniformed personnel. Mean age of patients with angina was 46 years and those without angina, 45 years. For both groups, mean duration of follow-up was about 6.5 years and in both groups about 93% of patients were surviving at the end of the study. Graft patency was determined in all but 1 of the 623 patients postoperatively and before discharge. Repeat angiography was done in about 90% of the patients at 1 year and about 35% at 5 years. In the angina group early graft patency was 89%, 1-year graft patency was 80%, and 5-year graft patency was 74%. In the group without angina early graft patency was 89%, 1-year patency was 83%, and 5-year patency was 78%; <1% of the total group had internal mammary artery grafts. The investigators argued that angina is but one symptom of CAD. They suggested that since graft patency was excellent, and because 93% of patients survived an average of 6.5 years, and early operative mortality was low, patients with morphologic evidence of CAD need not be symptomatic to be candidates for CABG. Furthermore, if CABG in some way neutralizes the detrimental effects of CAD in patients with angina, it is suggested by these researchers that CABG has similar effects in patients without angina.

The Veterans Administration Coronary Artery Bypass Surgery Cooperative Study Group evaluated long-term survival after CABG in 686 patients with stable angina pectoris who were randomly assigned to medical and surgical treatment at 13 hospitals and followed for an average of 11.2 years.[157] For all patients and for the 595 without LM CAD, cumulative survival did not differ significantly at 11 years according to treatment. The 7-year survival rates for all patients were 70% with medical treatment and 77% with CABG, and the 11-year rates were 57 and 58%, respectively (Fig. 1-31). For patients without LM CAD, the 7-year rates were 72 and 77% in medically and surgically

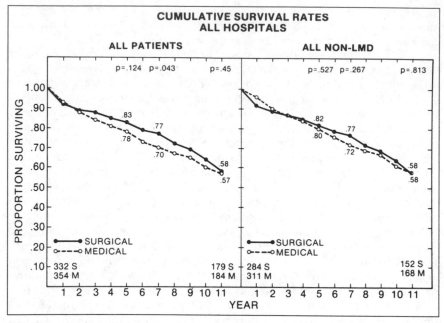

Fig. 1-31. Eleven-year cumulative survival for all patients and for those without LM CAD (non-LMD), according to treatment assignment. Numbers of patients at risk are given at bottom of figure. M = medical; S = surgical. Reproduced with permission from The Veterans Administration Coronary Artery Bypass Surgery Cooperative Study Group.[157]

treated patients, respectively, and the 11-year rates were 58% in both groups (Fig. 1-32). A statistically significant difference in survival suggesting a benefit from CABG treatment was found in patients without LM CAD who were subdivided into high risk subgroups defined angiographically, clinically, or by a combination of angiographic and clinical factors: 1) high angiographic risk (3-vessel CAD and impaired LV function)—at 7 years, 52% in medically treated patients -vs- 76% in surgically treated patients; at 11 years, 38 and 50%, respectively (Figs. 1-33 and 1-34); 2) clinically defined high risk (≥2 of the following: resting ST depression, history of AMI or of systemic hypertension)—at 7 years, 52% in the medical group -vs- 72% in the surgical group; at 11 years, 36 -vs- 49%, respectively; and 3) combined angiographic and clinical high risk—at 7 years, 36% in the medical group -vs- 76% in the surgical group; at 11 years, 24 -vs- 54%, respectively. Survival among patients with impaired LV function differed significantly at 7 years (63% in the medical group -vs- 74% in the surgical group) but not at 11 years (49 -vs- 53%). The surgical treatment policy resulted in a nonsignificant survival disadvantage throughout the 11 years in subgroups with normal LV function, low angiographic risk, and low clinical risk, and a statistically significant disadvantage at 11 years in patients with 2-vessel CAD. The Cooperative Study Group concluded that among patients with stable CAD, those with a high risk of dying benefit from surgical treatment, but beyond 7 years the survival benefit gradually diminishes.

Elayda and coworkers[158] from Houston, Texas, evaluated 1,275 elderly patients (≥70 years) undergoing CABG alone from 1970–1981. Most patients

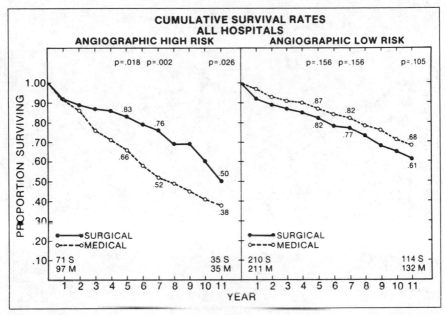

Fig. 1-32. Eleven-year cumulative survival for patients without LM CAD, according to angiographic risk. High risk was defined as 3-vessel disease plus impaired LV function, and low risk as 1-, 2-, or 3-vessel disease plus normal LV function or 1- or 2-vessel disease plus impaired LV function. Numbers of patients at risk are given at bottom of figure. M = medical; S = surgical. Reproduced with permission from The Veterans Administration Coronary Artery Bypass Surgery Cooperative Study Group.[157]

Fig. 1-33. Eleven-year cumulative survival for patients without LM CAD who had 1-, 2-, or 3-vessel disease. Numbers of patients at risk are given at bottom of figure. M = medical; S = surgical. Reproduced with permission from The Veterans Administration Coronary Artery Bypass Surgery Cooperative Study Group.[157]

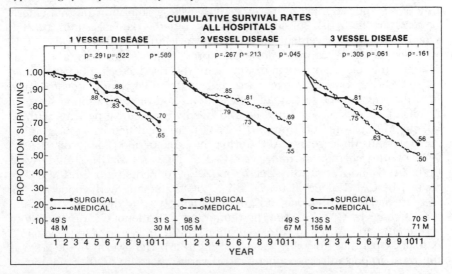

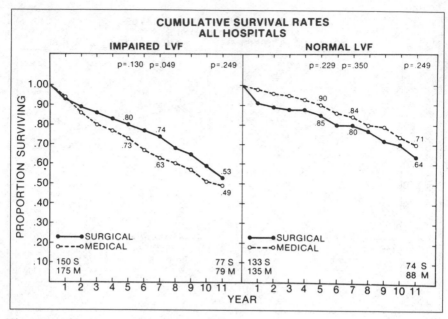

Fig. 1-34. Eleven-year cumulative survival for patients without LM CAD, according to whether LV function (LVF) was impaired or normal. Numbers of patients at risk are given at bottom of figure. M = medical; S = surgical. Reproduced with permission from The Veterans Administration Coronary Artery Bypass Surgery Cooperative Study Group.[157]

had severe, disabling or unstable angina pectoris. In this study the overall early mortality rate was 6%. Mortality rates declined in this patient population from 14% in the period 1970–1975 (n, 158) to 5% in the period 1976–1981 (n, 1,117). An average of 3.1 bypass grafts per patient were implanted. Angina was relieved or decreased in 89% of the patients. The 5-year survival rate was 81% and the 10-year survival rate was 44%, with an average death rate of 3.9 and 5.6% per year, respectively. These data indicate that elderly patients are high risk surgical candidates, but the data also indicate that when medical management fails, CABG is a legitimate alternative.

Information is scanty regarding the prognostic significance of ischemic MR, and the role of surgery in dealing with this risk factor is not established when CABG is done. Pinson and associates[159] from Portland, Oregon, examined the effect of the severity of ischemic MR and the wall motion score on results of operation. One hundred and twenty consecutive patients with ischemic MR operated on from 1970–1983 were identified as a subgroup of 3,454 patients undergoing CABG during the same period (3.5%): 83 patients (69%) with ischemic MR underwent CABG alone and 37 (31%) underwent both CABG and mitral valve operation. All 67 patients with mild MR were treated by CABG alone. Fourteen (67%) of 21 patients with moderate MR were treated by CABG alone and 2 of 32 patients (6%) in the severe MR group were treated by CABG alone. The remaining 37 patients with moderate to severe MR had CABG and valve operations; MVR in 28 and valve repair in 9 patients. Operative mortality was 14% (Fig. 1-35). The severity of the MR was the most important determinant of operative mortality. Other significant

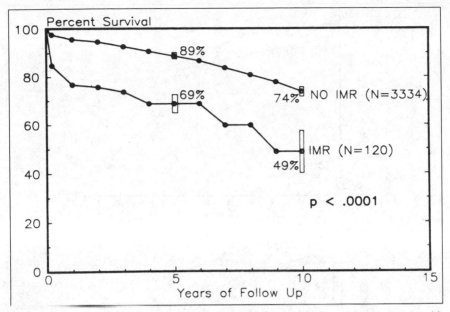

Fig. 1-35.   Overall survival for patients with ischemic MR (IMR) compared with patients with no MR who required coronary bypass. Operative mortality is represented by the first points plotted in time. Bars indicate SE of the cumulative proportions surviving at 5 and 10 years. Reproduced with permission from Pinson et al.[159]

determinants by univariate analysis were preoperative shock, cardiomegaly, CHF, and AMI. Operative survival for mild MR was 96%, for moderate MR, 90%, and for severe MR, 62%. Wall motion score influenced operative survival. The 5-year survival rate for 67 patients with a wall motion score of 5–10 was 83%, and for 45 patients with a higher wall motion score it was 54% (p < 0.05). The operative mortality for CABG alone in the MR patients was 4%. The operative mortality for CABG plus mitral valve operation was 38%. At the same institution in the same period, operative mortality for 620 patients without CAD undergoing MVR alone was 6% and for 70 patients undergoing CABG plus MVR for nonischemic causes, 9%. The negative effect of the ischemic etiology of MR is clearly demonstrated from these data. Others have shown similar results. The common denominator seems to be ischemic myopathy leading to decreased segmental wall motion (increased wall motion score) and mitral valve dysfunction.

In 658 patients who received CABG, Gould and colleagues[160] from Salt Lake City, Utah, investigated the correlation between the degree of early (6 months) graft patency and recurrence of anginal symptoms, late AMI and postoperative coronary-related death. The patients were grouped according to the number of surgically placed grafts, and each group was further subgrouped on the basis of the number of grafts functioning at the early postsurgical follow-up examination. The patients were observed for as long as 13 years. The frequency with which angina returned correlated significantly with the degree of patency within each of the groups (1, 2, 3, or 4 grafts); patients with a higher percentage of patent grafts experienced longer periods of freedom from angina (Fig. 1-36). On the average, patients with all of their

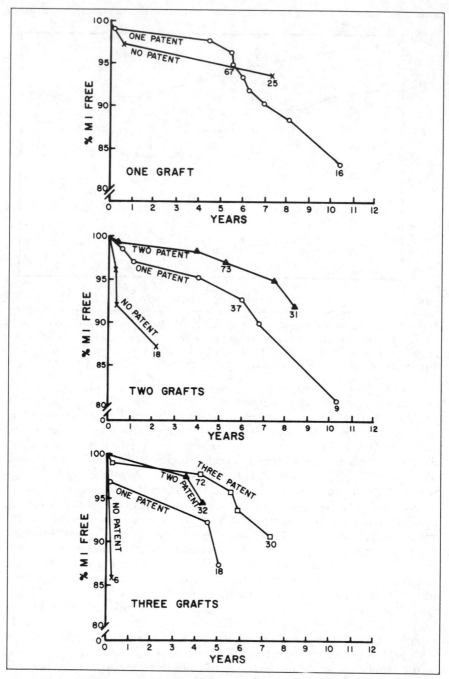

Fig. 1-36. Kaplan-Meier event curves for late AMI. The vertical axis represents the percentage of the subgroup that has remained free of postoperative infarction, and the horizontal axis represents the period of time from surgery until incidence of infarction. The results for the patients with a single graft are shown on the top, those with 2 grafts are in the middle, and those with 3 grafts are on the bottom. The numbers under the curves are the number of patients at risk. Reproduced with permission from Gould et al.[160]

multiple grafts patent had ≥7 years of symptomatic relief than their counterparts with all grafts occluded. Most surprisingly, the rate of the return of angina for those patients who had all grafts patent and were completely revascularized was independent of the number of diseased arteries or the number of grafts placed. The findings for coronary death and postoperative AMI showed similar trends.

Poor LV function before or afterward

Tyras and colleagues[161] from St. Louis, Missouri, examined factors that may influence operative and late survival in patients with severe global impairment of LV contractility undergoing CABG. Of 2,782 patients having CABG from 1970–1979, 196 had severe global impairment of LV wall motion preoperatively (EF <40% in all patients and <30% in 67% of patients). The initial 89 patients (group A) underwent CABG without potassium chloride cardioplegia. The subsequent 107 patients (group B) were given potassium chloride cardioplegia. Group B patients received more grafts per patient (3.1 -vs- 2.5, p < 0.001) and were completely revascularized more often (73 -vs- 58%, p < 0.05). Operative mortality was lower in group B (4 -vs- 12%, p < 0.025) and 5-year cumulative survival was better in group B (89 -vs- 64%, p < 0.0001). Preoperative CHF resulted in higher operative mortality (14 -vs- 5%, p < 0.05) and lower 5-year survival (65 -vs- 82%, p < 0.02). Complete revascularization led to higher 5-year survival (82 -vs- 66%, p < 0.02) but did not alter operative mortality significantly (7 -vs- 9%). Although this study was not randomized and was not concurrent, the data do suggest that in the cardioplegia era CABG is possible in patients with moderately severe LV dysfunction. Most groups subscribe to this notion. At issue at the present time are patients with very severe LV function, EF 20–30% and moderate narrowing of the coronary arteries with small distal vessels. The researchers suggested that CABG in patients with LV dysfunction should be reserved for those with a good chance of complete revascularization, i.e., satisfactory distal vessels.

Freeman and associates[162] from Sydney, Australia, studied the effects of CABG on ventricular performance and long-time clinical status in 18 consecutive patients with disabling angina pectoris and severely depressed LV performance (EF 27 ± 9%). All patients survived CABG. There was no change in LV EF at rest, 29 ± 12%, in the 17 patients who did not have AMI in the perioperative period. However LV EF during peak exercise increased from 22 ± 7–27 ± 14% (p < 0.05). The 17 patients were separated into 2 groups: those who increased their peak exercise LV EF by ≥10% (group A, 8 patients) and those who increased it by <10% (group B, 9 patients). Preoperatively, patients in group A had a higher LV EF at rest (p < 0.001) and smaller end-systolic and end-diastolic volumes at rest (p < 0.001) and during exercise (p < 0.005). Preoperatively, the LV EF in group A decreased with exercise, from 36 ± 4–27 ± 5% (p < 0.01), but was unchanged in group B (19 ± 3 -vs- 17 ± 4% [NS]). After CABG, patients in group A had a smaller increase in end-systolic volume with exercise than those in group B (13 ± 7 -vs- 34 ± 22 ml/M², p < 0.05), but the changes in end-diastolic volume with exercise were not significantly different. At 27 ± 5 months after CABG, 5 of 8 patients in group A were asymptomatic. Of the 9 patients in group B, 2 had died and 5 had recurrence of angina or CHF. In patients with depressed LV function who undergo CABG, improvement in LV performance and long-term clinical status is more likely to occur in patients with less severely impaired LV function at rest and evidence of exercise-induced ischemic dysfunction.

Topol and coworkers[163] from Baltimore, Maryland, evaluated the immediate effects of CABG on regional myocardial function utilizing intraoperative transesophageal 2-D echo in 20 patients using a 3.5 MHz phased array transducer at the tip of a flexible gastroscope. Cross-sectional LV images were obtained at multiple levels before skin incision and were repeated serially before and immediately after cardiopulmonary bypass. In these patients, percent systolic wall thickening was determined for 8 anatomic segments in each patient at similar loading conditions. In the 152 segments analyzed, systolic wall thickening improved from a prerevascularization mean value ($\pm$SEM) of 43 $\pm$ 3% to a postrevascularization mean value of 52 $\pm$ 3% (p < 0.001). Thickening improved most in those segments with the poorest preoperative function (p < 0.001). Subsequent chest wall ECGs obtained 8.4 $\pm$ 2.3 days after operation showed no deterioration or further improvement in segmental function compared with values obtained intraoperatively. These data indicate that regional myocardial function frequently improves immediately after CABG and that some patients with chronic coronary arterial stenoses have subclinical ischemic dysfunction.

Brundage and coworkers[164] from San Francisco, California, evaluated the influence of CABG on LV segmental function in 23 patients with angina (stable in 21, unstable in 2) with reversible asynergy at rest. All patients underwent exercise myocardial perfusion scintigraphy with thallium-201, contrast ventriculography, and coronary arteriography before and after CABG. Selective graft angiography was performed during the postoperative catheterization to determine graft patency. Segmental LV function was quantitated by a regional fraction method. The scintigrams were divided into 5 regions and compared with the corresponding regions of the ventriculogram. Seventy-one of a possible 142 ventricular segments had exercise-induced perfusion defects. Regional EF preoperatively was normal in 42 of the 71 segments and abnormal in 29. After successful CABG, segmental function improved or became normal in 19 of the abnormal segments. Each segment had improved perfusion during exercise after CABG and was supplied by a patent bypass graft. Nine of the 10 segments in which abnormal wall motion persisted postoperatively continued to have exercise-induced perfusion defects and 9 of the 10 segments were supplied by an occluded or stenotic graft or 1 with poor runoff. In the 42 segments with normal wall motion preoperatively, 30 had improved perfusion after surgery and 35 maintained normal function. These data indicate that regional ventricular asynergy at rest is reversed after CABG if improved myocardial perfusion can be documented. These data also suggest that reversible rest asynergy may reflect chronic ischemia or a prolonged effect on regional wall motion from previous ischemic episodes.

Hossack and associates[165] from Denver, Colorado, evaluated 70 patients undergoing CABG for angina pectoris to determine the influence of CABG on subsequent LV function. Postoperative studies were done 6–14 months after CABG. Cardiac output was measured using the direct Fick principle. Postoperatively, there was a 3.1 liters/min increase in cardiac output in men (n, 61) and a 2.0 liters/min in women (n, 9, p < 0.01) at maximal exercise. Patients with complete CABG demonstrated a significantly greater improvement in cardiac output postoperatively than did those with incomplete CABG (p < 0.0001). An increase in heart rate was the major factor responsible for the increased cardiac output with exercise; stroke volume remained at the same preoperative level. The increase in heart rate was found irrespective of the preoperative use of beta adrenergic blocking agents.

Although exercise-based rehabilitation programs have demonstrated improved work capacity, production in incidence of attacks of angina pectoris and reduction in rates of morbidity and mortality, the effect on LV function has remained unclear. Foster and coworkers[166] from Milwaukee, Wisconsin, conducted a prospective randomized trial to evaluate the effects of exercise-based cardiac rehabilitation after CABG on work capacity (measured in METS) and LV function as determined from EF. Twenty-eight patients undergoing CABG were randomly assigned to experimental (aerobic exercise) or control (muscle relaxation and low level exercise) groups. Patients were studied before CABG and the weeks after surgery with first-pass RNA, both while at rest and during maximal upright cycle ergometric exercise. Subsets of patients were also studied at 2, 3, and 4 weeks at a standard work load of 75 watts, and during maximal exercise 1 year after CABG. Work capacity improved in both groups, although significantly more so in the experimental group. The differences between groups were significant by the third week. Peak exercise LV EF increased significantly in both groups from the first to the second week, then decreased at the third week and remained unchanged through the fifth week. Peak exercise LV EF at the third and fifth weeks remained significantly above that observed at week 1. The LV EF responses were not related to the exercise program. During a standard work load, heart rate decreased, BP increased, and LV EF did not change in either group. At the conclusion of the formal protocol at the fourth week, work capacity and LV EF did not change for either group throughout an additional 6 months. The investigators concluded that exercise training significantly enhances both the magnitude and rate of the increase in work capacity after coronary surgery, but that peak exercise LV EF is not influenced by the exercise program.

Flameng and coworkers[167] from Beerse, Belgium, studied histologic and ultrastructural changes in myocardium of 61 consecutive patients with CAD and compromised LV function. The angiographic and ECG changes were examined in patients undergoing CABG. Histologic delineation of myocardium was obtained by analysis of transmural biopsy specimens acquired at CABG. Group I comprised patients with histologic findings associated with severe LAD coronary artery stenosis, without abnormal LV wall motion or EF. The ECG abnormalities were limited to ST-segment changes. Group II patients had severe myocardial cell degeneration with only modest fibrosis associated with severe LAD stenosis and severely impaired LV wall motion. There was a low incidence of myocardial damage on the ECG. Group III patients had important myocardial cell degeneration with severe fibrosis associated with severe LAD stenosis, severely depressed LV wall motion, and significantly impaired EF. In this group there was a high incidence of myocardial damage on ECG. Postoperative follow-up for 24 months showed a survival of 94% in group I, 93% in group II, and 73% in group III. This study demonstrated that the morphologic picture of a certain myocardial zone can be predicted from preoperative and angiographic findings and that reduced contractile function is invariably related to myocardial cell degeneration. The ECG signs of myocardial damage suggest that additional fibrosis and critical CAD are associated with significant endocardial degeneration.

Huikuri and associates[168] from Oulu, Finland, evaluated the LV response to isometric exercise in 20 patients who performed handgrip exercise tests before and 3 months after CABG. Preoperative LV EF decreased during the handgrip test from 0.57 ± 0.08–0.49 ± 0.09 ($p < 0.001$); the ratio between the LV peak systolic pressure (PSP) and end-systolic volume index (ESVI) did not change. In 12 patients with patent grafts, the LV EF after operation did not change (0.54 ± 0.06 at rest and 0.56 ± 0.06 during handgrip exercise) and PSP/ESVI ratio increased from 4.5 ± 1.5–5.6 ± 2.1 mmHg/ml $\cdot$ M^{-2} ($p < 0.001$) during exercise. In 8 patients with occluded grafts, the LV EF after operation decreased from 0.56 ± 0.10–0.48 ± 0.06 ($p < 0.02$), whereas PSP/ESVI did not change during handgrip exercise. Thus, the LV response to isometric handgrip exercise appears to improve after CABG in patients with patent grafts, but not in patients with ≥ 1 occluded grafts.

Kardash and associates[169] from Leeds, England, evaluated the new exercise test, i.e., maximum heart rate of progression of ST-segment depression relative to increases in heart rate (HR) to assess the usefulness of CABG in 46 patients before CABG and in 26 of them 6 months after operation. At each stage of the investigation, the maximal ST/HR slope detected without false results the absence and the number of significantly diseased vessels, as shown by angiocardiography. As in previous findings, the ranges of the maximal ST/HR slope showed no overlap between the 4 groups of patients: those with no significant disease and those with 1-, 2-, or 3-vessel CAD. In each of the 46 patients in whom the maximal ST/HR slope was determined before operation and 3 months afterward the slope was lower after operation than before, indicating improvement. Follow-up examinations showed that the maximal ST/HR slopes accurately detected the number of patent grafts used to bypass significantly narrowed coronary arteries. Furthermore, the development of a significant narrowing or occlusion in any vein graft caused an increase in the maximal ST/HR slope that was equivalent to the value of 1-vessel CAD. It was suggested that the maximal ST/HR slope may be used reliably in individual patients to indicate restoration of adequate blood supply to the myocardium after successful CABG and to detect in the period of 6 months after the operation the degree of severity of CAD whether it is caused by occlusion of the graft or CAD.

Stevens and Hanson[170] from Madison, Wisconsin, compared functional capacity and cardiovascular responses to serial graded treadmill testing in 180 patients who performed prescribed unsupervised exercise and in 24 patients who were referred for supervised exercise after CABG. The groups were men similar in age range, number of bypass grafts, preoperative LV impairment, and number of days hospitalized. All patients received similar predischarge exercise monitoring and began a progressive home walking or cycling program. Initial graded treadmill testing (T1) was performed 44 ± 9 days postoperatively. Both groups were instructed to continue prescribed exercise at 75–85% maximal heart rate for 30–40 minutes 3 days (supervised) or 5 days (unsupervised) per week. The second graded treadmill testing (T2) was performed 115 ± 27 days after CABG. In each group there were significant ($p < 0.01$) increases in exercise capacity and heart rate from T1 to T2. However, there were no significant differences in maximal exercise capacity and heart rate between groups on T1 or T2. Improvement in functional capacity was not influenced by therapeutic beta blockade. These findings indicate that prescribed unsupervised exercise can be performed safely and results in similar functional improvements compared with supervised exercise after uncomplicated CABG.

Complications

Accelerated progression of atherosclerosis is believed to occur in surgically bypassed coronary arteries in which the preoperative degree of coronary narrowing was <50% diameter reduction. To assess the effect of CABG on progression of atherosclerosis in coronary arteries with lesser degrees of narrowing, Cashin and associates[171] from Los Angeles, California, studied 85 men who had undergone CABG. Of the 85, 37 had grafts placed in arteries with minimum (<50% diameter reduction) narrowing preoperatively. In the same 85 men there were 93 coronary arteries with minimal narrowings and these arteries did not have a bypass conduit inserted. Progressive narrowing, defined as further loss of ≥25% of the luminal diameter during an average follow-up of 37 months was >10 times as frequent (38 -vs- 3%) in the bypassed arteries with minimal narrowings compared with the nonbypassed arteries with minimal narrowings (Table 1-9). These findings support the view that minimally narrowed coronary arteries should not by bypassed.

This article by Cashin and associates[171] was followed by an editorial by Loop[172] from Cleveland, Ohio. Loop wrote the following: "The critical question . . . is, what constitutes minimal disease? Cashin and others define it as stenosis of <50%, but 23 of the 37 arteries evaluated were angiographically normal. Normality is not equivalent to minimal disease. One would then ask, 'Why were these vessels bypassed, thereby causing 7 of 23 arteries to acquire new lesions?' Since bypassing of normal coronary arteries is not accepted practice, one must surmise that there was a misinterpretation of the original coronary arteriograms or problems comparing the sequential studies. The initial coronary arteriography was performed in 40 hospitals. It is difficult to match views, angles, the use of nitroglycerin, and injection pressure, and to

TABLE 1-9. *Progression of atherosclerosis in vessels with less than 50% preoperative stenosis. Reproduced with permission from Cashin et al.*[171]

| | DEGREE OF PREOPERATIVE STENOSIS | | | |
| | 0–25% | | 26–49% | |
	BYPASS PRESENT	BYPASS ABSENT	BYPASS PRESENT	BYPASS ABSENT
# vessels	26	85	11	8
% stenosis*				
Before bypass	2.3 ± 1.3	1.2 ± 2.5	36.4 ± 1.5	33.8 ± 1.8
At entry	31.7 ± 7.7	5.2 ± 1.5	60.5 ± 7.8	35.0 ± 7.6
Change	29.4 ± 7.2	4.0 ± 1.3	24.1 ± 8.2	1.3 ± 6.1

* Values are means ±SEM.

ensure minimal interobserver variability, especially in the mild-to-moderate range of stenoses. Computerized techniques for evaluating cineangiographic data with a reproducible accuracy of 150 μm were not used. Most consistent results are obtained by either a consensus panel or a group-opinion panel whose members view pairs of films simultaneously. The current practice among cardiac surgeons is to bypass the moderately obstructed coronary artery—i.e., the artery with an estimated reduction in lumen diameter of 40 to 60%—when it occurs in patients with graftable severe coronary athero-sclerosis. Few surgeons advocate bypassing lesions with less severe estimated narrowing. The justification for bypassing arteries in the 40 to 60% range is based on sequential angiographic examinations. Moderate lesions may progress to the point of total occlusion in a sudden, unpredictable manner precluding appropriate medical or surgical intervention." Loop concluded by supporting Cashin and others' report about the perils of bypassing normal arteries or those with minimal disease. As Sam Rayburn said, "If it ain't broke, don't fix it."

Campeau and associates[173] from Montreal, Canada, examined 82 patients 10 years after saphenous-vein CABG to determine the angiographic status and to relate those findings to the risk factors for CAD. Of 132 grafts shown to be patent 1 year after CABG, only 50 were unaffected at 10 years; 43 were narrowed and 39 were totally occluded. Disease progression in coronary arteries without grafts was also frequent, both in arteries that were normal (15 of 32) and in those with minor narrowings (25 of 53). New narrowing did not develop in 15 patients, whereas they did in 67—in the grafts or the native vessels or both. There was no significant difference between the 2 groups in the incidence of systemic hypertension, diabetes mellitus, or cigarette smoking, whereas plasma levels of VLDL and LDL were higher, and HDL levels were lower in those with new lesions than in those without (Table 1-10). Univariate analysis showed that plasma cholesterol and triglyceride levels were significantly higher at the time of CABG and at the 10-year examination in those with new lesions. Multivariate analysis indicated that among the lipoprotein indexes, levels of HDL cholesterol and plasma LDL apoprotein B best distinguished the 2 groups. The findings indicate that atherosclerosis in these patients was a progressive disease, frequently affecting both the

TABLE 1-10. *Total lipid, lipoprotein lipid, and plasma LDL apoprotein B levels 10 years after surgery.* *Reproduced with permission from Campeau et al.[173]*

	TOTAL CHOLES-TEROL	TRIGLYC-ERIDE	LDL CHOLES-TEROL	LDL APOPROTEIN B	HDL CHOLES-TEROL
Group I	243 ± 43	139 ± 55	153 ± 37	98 ± 17	63 ± 17
# patients	15	15	15	15	15
Group II	278 ± 50	205 ± 110	190 ± 45	149 ± 33	48 ± 10
# patients	67	67	65	65	65
T value	−2.52	−2.25	−2.98	−5.89	4.37
P value	<0.01	<0.05	<0.005	<0.0001	<0.0001

* Plus-minus values are means ±SD. Values are in milligrams per deciliter.

grafts and the native vessels, and that the course of such disease may be related to the plasma lipoprotein levels.

Brindis and associates[174] from San Francisco, California, evaluated 18 patients with perioperative AMI to determine whether graft occlusion was responsible for the disease. Perioperative AMI was recognized by demonstrating elevations in creatine kinase MB isoenzyme, characteristic ECG changes, and in most patients an abnormal pyrophosphate scan. Fourteen patients (78%) had patent grafts and perioperative AMI in the distribution of the grafted vessel. Only 4 patients had an occluded graft in the distribution of the perioperative AMI. There was a significant difference in the degree of CAD in patients with perioperative AMI having significantly greater coronary arterial diameter obstruction (80 ± 11% in native arteries supplying the perioperative infarcted myocardium -vs- 55 ± 12% in the bypassed native coronary arteries supplying noninfarcted myocardium). Thus, most perioperative myocardial infarcts occur for reasons other than coronary arterial graft occlusion. The severity of native coronary arterial obstruction in the grafted vessel and a lack of collateral vessels to the region of perioperative AMI suggest that jeopardized myocardium exists that is not adequately protected intraoperatively in patients with perioperative AMI.

The long-term benefits of CABG in terms of longevity and prevention of major ischemic events in patients who have mild angina is not well defined. The randomized Coronary Artery Surgery Study (CASS) was designed to evaluate this issue.[175] It consists of 780 patients who were considered operable and who had mild stable angina pectoris or who were free of angina after AMI. As a result of the randomization process, there were no significant differences in baseline variables between patients randomly assigned to medical and to surgical therapy. The likelihood of death in the 5-year period after randomization was only 8% in the medical cohort compared with 5% in the surgical cohort (NS). The likelihood of nonfatal Q-wave AMI was 11 and 14%, respectively (NS) (Fig. 1-37). The 5-year probability of remaining alive and free of AMI was 82% in the patients assigned to medical therapy and 83% in the patients assigned to surgery (NS). There were no statistically significant differences in the survival rate or in the AMI rate between subgroups of patients randomly assigned to medical and to surgical therapy when they were analyzed according to initial group assignment, number of diseased vessels, or EF. Therefore, compared with medical therapy, CABG appears neither to prolong life nor to prevent AMI in patients who have mild angina or who are asymptomatic after AMI in the 5-year period after coronary angiography.

The early and late influence of perioperative AMI on survival after coronary artery bypass grafting has in the past been controversial. Schaff and colleagues[176] from the CASS group have supplied important information from a review of 9,777 patients who underwent CABG between 1974 and 1979. Definite or probable perioperative AMI was diagnosed in 561 (6%). The incidence decreased from 6.6% in 1974 to 4.1% in 1971 (p < 0.005). In patients without perioperative AMI actuarial survival including hospital deaths at 1, 3, and 5 years was significantly better than in patients with AMI (96, 94, and 90% -vs- 78, 74, and 69%, p < 0.0001) (Fig. 1-38). This difference persisted among patients dismissed from the hospital. Reduction in late survival among patients with perioperative AMI was due to the poor outcome of those who had complications (5-year survival rates 40% overall and 73% for pa-

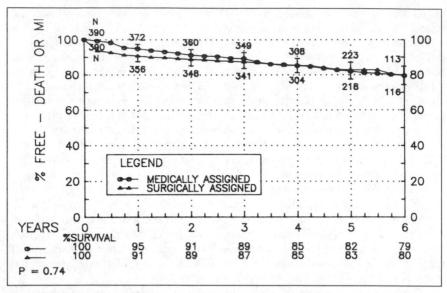

Fig. 1-37. Survival and absence of recognized AMI in patients with CAD who were randomly assigned to medical or surgical therapy (life-table method). The probability of remaining alive and free of myocardial infarction was similar in the medical and surgical groups. Reproduced with permission from CASS Principal Investigators and Their Associates.[175]

tients dismissed from the hospital). Multivariate analysis identified perioperative AMI as an important independent predictor of late survival after CABG. It was surpassed only by LV function (wall motion score), age, and number of associated medical diseases. Although debate on the true incidence of perioperative AMI and the best method for its diagnosis will continue, occurrence of perioperative AMI is clearly detrimental to subsequent survival. In the present study late survival was significantly poorer for patients with perioperative AMI even when patients who died in the hospital were excluded. Several previous studies have not detected a significant influence of perioperative AMI on late survival. The uniformity among the CASS patients for diagnosis of AMI and the number of patients in this study go a long way to settle the question regarding the influence of perioperative AMI. The dissimilarities of various reports can perhaps be explained by the fact that the major portion of the mortality associated with perioperative AMI is in those with complicated AMI and in those with poor LV function.

Certain patients who have undergone CABG have episodes of acute cellulitis, often repeatedly, in the saphenous vein donor extremity. Baddour and Bisno[177] from Memphis, Tennessee, described 9 patients with this entity, 5 of whom had recurrent attacks (2 to >20). The mean interval between CABG and the initial bout of cellulitis was 15 months (range, 2–46 months). A characteristic clinical syndrome was present in most patients: abrupt onset of chills, followed by fever, prostration, and obvious cellulitis. Seven patients also had tinea pedis. The pathogenesis of the entity may involve complex interactions between fungal and bacterial agents.

Kuan and coworkers[178] from Long Beach, California, conducted a retrospective analysis of 365 consecutive patients (75 women and 290 men; mean age, 60 ± 10 years) who had CABG during 1981. This retrospective analysis

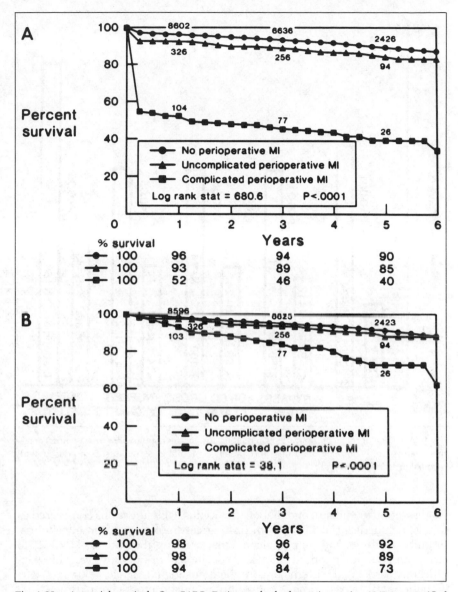

Fig. 1-38. Actuarial survival after CABG. Patients who had a perioperative AMI are stratified according to the presence or absence of complications. A: The important effect of perioperative AMI on early mortality is evident; only 52% of patients were alive 1 year postoperatively in the complicated perioperative AMI group. B: Survivorship includes only patients who were dismissed from the hospital. Late survival for patients with uncomplicated perioperative AMI was virtually the same as that for patients who had no perioperative infarction, but was significantly reduced for patients with complicated perioperative infarction. Reproduced with permission from Schaff et al.[176]

wished to define clinical characteristics and intraoperative variables that might affect morbidity and mortality. Complications of CABG classified as major included: mediastinal hemorrhage, pericardial tamponade, wound dehiscence, sternal osteomyelitis, myocardial infarction, bacterial endocardi-

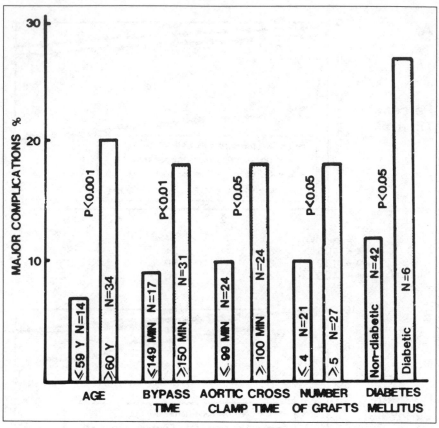

Fig. 1-39. Percent major complications in relation to age, cardiopulmonary bypass time, aortic cross-clamp time, number of grafts, and presence of diabetes mellitus. Reproduced with permission from Kuan et al.[178]

tis, dissecting aneurysm, and diabetes insipidus. Classifications considered as minor included: atrial fibrillation, postpericardiotomy syndrome, cellulitis, thrombophlebitis, and phrenic nerve palsy. Among the patients studied, 48 (13%) had 52 major complications. Those clinical or operative variables significantly associated with major complications included: age >60 years, cardiopulmonary bypass time >150 minutes, aortic cross-clamp time >100 minutes, number of grafts >5, and the presence of diabetes mellitus (Fig. 1-39). Complications were more frequent in women, obese subjects, and those with emergency operation or LV EF <30%, but these associations were not statistically significant.

Effects of aspirin and/or dipyridamole

Chesebro and associates[179] from Rochester, Minnesota, conducted a prospective, randomized, double-blind trial comparing long-term administration of dipyridamole (begun 2 days before operation) plus aspirin (begun 7 hours after operation) with placebo in 407 patients who had undergone CABG. The results at 1 month showed a reduction in the rate of graft occlusion in patients receiving dipyridamole and aspirin. At vein graft angiography performed in 343 patients (84%) 11–18 months (median, 12) after operation, 11% of 478 vein graft distal anastomoses were occluded in the treated group, and 25% of 486 were occluded in the placebo group. The proportion of patients with ≥1 distal anastomoses occluded was 22% of 171 patients in the treated group and 47% of 172 in the placebo group (Fig. 1-40). All grafts were patent within 1 month of operation in 94 patients in the placebo group and in 116 patients in the treated group; late development of occlusions was reduced from 27% in the placebo group to 16% in the treated group. The results show that dipyridamole and aspirin continue to be effective in preventing vein graft occlusion late after operation, and we believe that such treatment should be continued for at least 1 year.

Lorenz and associates[180] from Muenchen, West Germany, studied in a double-blind trial of 83 patients prevention of aortocoronary bypass conduit occlusion by aspirin (ASA, 100 mg/day): 60 (72%) were randomly allocated to ASA or to placebo starting 24 hours after operation, and 90% of grafts in the ASA group and 68% in the placebo group were patent at 4 months. At least 1 anastomosis was occluded in 62% of the patients on placebo and in 27% of those on aspirin (Table 1-11). Ventricular arrhythmias increased after CABG in more patients on placebo (12 of 18) than in patients on ASA (5 of

Fig. 1-40. Occlusion rates for all types of vein grafts. The rates are expressed per distal anastomosis and per patient (proportion with at least one occlusion). Occlusion is shown as events occurring within 1 month (95% confidence limits for the per patient difference, 8–24%), as new events occurring beyond 1 month (in distal anastomoses and patients without occlusion within 1 month of operation) from angiography performed 1 year later (per patient, p = 0.048; 95% confidence limits for the difference, 0–22%), and as events at a median of 1 year after operation (95% confidence limits for the per patient difference, 11–34%). These subsets include only patients who had angiography within 1 month of operation and again 1 year later. Below each percentage is shown the ratio of distal anastomoses or patients with occlusion to total distal anastomoses or patients. Reproduced with permission from Chesebro et al.[179]

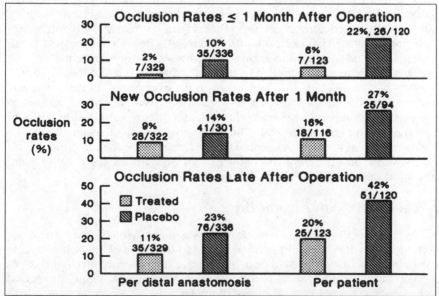

TABLE 1-11. *Bypass status and clinical outcome at 4 months after operation. Reproduced with permission from Lorenz et al.[180]*

	PLACEBO	ASPIRIN	2 p
Grafts occluded	17/53 (32%)	4/40 (10%)	0.012
Distal anastomoses occluded	28/81 (35%)	11/57 (19%)	
Patients with ≥1 occlusions	15/24 (62%)	6/22 (27%)	0.017
Occlusion or event	20/31 (65%)	9/29 (31%)	0.01
Occlusion, event, or drop out	22/31 (71%)	13/29 (45%)	0.025

17). Platelet thromboxane formation on collagen tested before operation was significantly higher in patients in whom bypass occlusion developed (occlusion: 40 ± 19; no occlusion: 25 ± 13 ng/ml). A 100 mg dosage of ASA per day effectively blocked platelet thromboxane formation and thromboxane-supported aggregation on collagen and was safe in the postoperative phase. No side effects were reported. The reduced toxicity with full efficacy favors a low and infrequent dosage of aspirin.

Mechanisms for relief of angina

To determine the physiologic effect of CABG and the mechanisms for pain relief, Ribeiro and associates[181] from London, England, studied 15 patients with exertional angina before and after CABG. Before CABG, conventional tests included exercise studies (all positive) and coronary angiography (all patients had >70% diameter reduction of ≥1 major coronary artery). In addition ambulatory ECG monitoring during 48 hours detected 92 episodes (>1 mm) of ST depression. Regional myocardial perfusion was assessed with positron tomography using rubidium-82 ($t_{1/2}$ 78 s) and this showed reversible inhomogeneity with absolute regional reduction of cation uptake after exercise in all 15 patients. After CABG 10 of the 15 patients had no angina, patent grafts (≥3), no evidence of ischemia during ambulatory monitoring out of hospital, and homogeneous perfusion with reversal of the disturbances in regional myocardial perfusion after exercise. After operation 1 of the 15 patients had no angina and showed silent AMI in the segment that was previously ischemic but supplied by a patent graft. All but 1 of the remaining patients had no angina, patent grafts, but disturbances of regional myocardial perfusion with silent ischemia on exercise. Two patients continued to have asymptomatic and ischemic episodes of ST depression during ambulatory monitoring out of hospital. This physiologic study of regional myocardial perfusion in patients in hospital and in those with ischemia out of hospital showed that 3 different mechanisms may account for the relief of pain: improved perfusion, AMI, and silent ischemia.

Management with carotid bruit

Ivey and colleagues[182] from Seattle, Washington, discussed neurologic complications of cardiopulmonary bypass and the effect of an asymptomatic carotid bruit. During a 31-month period 1,433 consecutive patients were screened for carotid bruit; 9 had a history of transient ischemic attack and reduction in internal carotid artery diameter of >50% according to ultrasonic carotid duplex scanning. All 9 patients underwent carotid arteriography followed by thromboendarterectomy before or simultaneous with cardiopulmonary bypass. There was 1 neurologic complication in that subset. Sixteen patients with asymptomatic carotid bruit had ultrasonic carotid duplex scanning revealing an internal carotid artery lesion of >50% but did not undergo arteriography or thromboendarterectomy. There were no focal neurologic events in this subset. The 66 remaining patients with carotid bruit in whom duplex scanning revealed a carotid artery stenosis of <50% had no further workup or modification of perfusion technique, and there were no focal neurologic events in this group. Thus, there were no focal neurologic events in any of the 82 patients with asymptomatic carotid bruit. The remaining 1,339 patients without carotid bruit had 9 (0.7%) focal neurologic events postoperatively. The investigators concluded that asymptomatic patients with carotid bruit can safely undergo cardiac operations without prior extracranial cerebrovascular arteriography or carotid endarterectomy. Patients with neurologic symptoms before operation should undergo arteriography and either combined or staged operative procedures. Ultrasonic duplex scanning in this study revealed the degree of stenosis in those patients with asymptomatic bruit, but it did not force arteriography and it did not dictate combined or staged carotid thromboendarterectomy. The authors concluded that there would appear to be little justification in placing asymptomatic patients at any higher risk than that of an uncomplicated CABG, and thus invasive (and noninvasive) study of the carotid problem is unnecessary and operative intervention unwarranted.

Fate of arm veins used for grafts

Arm veins have been a common second choice conduit for those patients having insufficient saphenous veins for CABG. Stoney and colleagues[183] from

Fig. 1-41. Cumulative patency rates of arm vein, internal mammary, and saphenous vein grafts. The arm vein grafts show progressive failure with each year. Reproduced with permission from Stoney et al.[183]

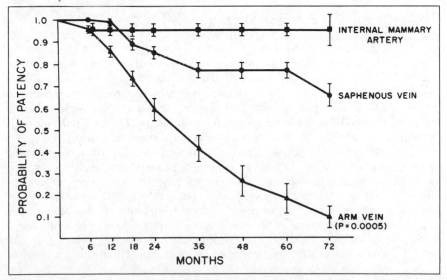

Nashville, Tennessee, reviewed 59 patients with ⩾1 arm veins used for CABG between 1974 and 1982. Postoperative arteriograms were obtained in 28 patients. Of 56 arm veins used, 32 (57%) were patent and 24 (43%) were not at 2 years (Fig. 1-41). Additionally, 7 patent grafts had a localized stenosis. In the same patients, 16 internal mammary grafts also had been used and 15 (93%) were patent. They concluded that arm veins had a high failure rate and were not as dependable as saphenous vein grafts or internal mammary grafts. Other variables, however, such as harvesting technique, may be important. The cephalic vein remains a distant second choice for aortocoronary grafting.

Timolol for prevention of supraventricular tachyarrhythmias after surgery

Supraventricular arrhythmias occur in 20–54% in patients after CABG. White and colleagues[184] from Boston, Massachusetts, randomly assigned 41 patients undergoing CABG to receive prophylactic timolol or placebo, given in a double-blind fashion. Beta adrenergic blocking therapy was stopped at least 1 half-life before CABG. Three to 7 hours after CABG, 0.5 mg of timolol or placebo was given intravenously twice daily in a double-blind manner. When oral medications were resumed postoperatively, 10 mg of timolol twice daily or placebo was continued orally. No patient received digoxin and both groups were comparable for frequency of preoperative supraventricular arrhythmias, LV EF, duration of cardiopulmonary bypass, aortic cross-clamp time, and total duration of monitoring. Analysis of arrhythmias was done by and counts of continuous ECGs, and supraventricular arrhythmias were divided into SVT and AF or flutter. Timolol decreased the frequency of SVT and of AF or flutter. There were no differences in the durations of supraventricular arrhythmias. All 11 episodes of SVT and 11 episodes of AF or flutter with heart rates >200 beats/min occurred in the placebo group. These results suggest that prophylactic use of timolol after CABG is effective and safe therapy for decreasing the frequency and severity of supraventricular arrhythmias.

Intermittent aortic cross-clamping -vs- St. Thomas' Hospital cardioplegia

Myocardial protection was assessed in 72 patients undergoing extensive CABG by Flameng and colleagues[185] from Leuven, Belgium. The patients were allocated at random to 3 surgical techniques: Group I, intermittent aortic cross-clamping at 32°; group II, intermittent aortic cross-clamping at 25°; and group III, St. Thomas Hospital cardioplegia. The EF in all 3 groups averaged about 60%. There were 4.1 grafts per patient in group I, 4.6 grafts per patient in group II, and 4.4 grafts per patient in group III, with ischemic times of 40, 43, and 63 minutes in each group, respectively. Adenosine triphosphate, creatine kinase (CK), and glycogen contents were determined by biopsy specimens taken at the beginning and end of cardiopulmonary bypass. The results show a better preservation of high energy phosphates, glycogen, and ultrastructure in the cardioplegia group compared with the 2 cross-clamp groups. However, severe myocardial damage was never observed. Release of CK-MB was the same in all 3 groups. Functional recovery of the hearts immediately after cessation of cardiopulmonary bypass was better in the cardioplegia group, but the incidence or rhythm disturbances was higher in the cardioplegia group that the other 2 groups (p < 0.05). Clinical outcome in terms of incidence of perioperative AMI, survival, and event-free follow-up was not different among groups. It is concluded that both techniques offered good myocardial protection in extensive CABG. St. Thomas cardioplegia in contrast to intermittent cross-clamping prevents the onset of ischemia-induced deterioration of cardiac metabolism, i.e., destruction of the adenine nucleotide pool.

Comparison with PTCA

Jones and associates[186] from Atlanta, Georgia, studied 339 patients having PTCA (initial first year experience) and compared them with 338 matched patients who had CABG. Patients who underwent PTCA had a shorter duration of angina, a lower frequency of prior AMI, and better LV function (p < 0.01). The PTCA was considered initially successful in 87% (295 of 339) of patients. The most common finding at operation in those who failed PTCA and who underwent urgent or emergency CABG was dissection of atheromatous plaque. Although the cumulative frequency of new Q waves in the entire 18-month PTCA series was low (2.7%), the incidence was high (18%) in those with angioplasty failure and subsequent operation (n, 20) and significantly greater than in patients who had elective CABG (3.6%). Use of inotropic agents and lidocaine for ventricular arrhythmias was significantly higher in patients with unsuccessful PTCA who required operation than in those who underwent elective CABG (10 -vs- 3% and 10 -vs- 1.5%, [p < 0.01]). In an analysis of the investigators' entire experience between October 1980 and June 1982, 777 patients who had PTCA and 2,068 patients who underwent CABG were analyzed for differences in clinical complications and early outcome. Patients who had CABG were significantly older and had a higher incidence of systemic hypertension (46 -vs- 32%), more multivessel disease (80 -vs- 12%), and more LV dysfunction. Emergency CABG was required in 5% of patients after PTCA. There were no deaths after the PTCA procedure and 9 deaths in 1,162 patients who underwent CABG between 1980 and 1981 (hospital mortality, 0.8%).

Usefulness of preoperative insertion of intraaortic balloon

Port and coworkers[187] from Milwaukee, Wisconsin, studied 13 patients with severe CAD at the time of elective preoperative insertion of an intraaortic balloon catheter to test the hypothesis that myocardial blood flow distal to a critical stenosis increases during this form of circulatory assistance. Hemodynamic and myocardial blood flow measurements were made before and during counterpulsation. Myocardial blood flow was estimated utilizing a xenon-133 washout technique. The data obtained indicate that intraaortic balloon counterpulsation did not increase myocardial blood flow or regional flows in the LAD and LC coronary arteries. Intraaortic balloon counterpulsation, however, did decrease heart rate and systolic BP while increasing diastolic arterial BP from 72 ± 10.1–120 ± 21 mmHg. Thus, the beneficial effects of intraaortic balloon counterpulsation in stable patients with severe CAD are more likely due to a reduction in oxygen demand than a primary increase in coronary blood flow.

References

1. ELVEBACK L, LIE JT: Continued high incidence of coronary artery disease at autopsy in Olmsted County, Minnesota, 1950 to 1979. Circulation 70:345–349, Sept 1984.

2. SHAPER AG, COOK DG, WALKER M, McFARLANE PW: Recall of diagnosis by men with ischaemic heart disease. Br Heart J 51:606–611, June 1984.

3. KOSTIS JB, TURKEVICH D, SHARP J: Association between leukocyte count and the presence and extent of coronary atherosclerosis as determined by coronary arteriography. Am J Cardiol 53:997–999, Apr 1, 1984.

4. STATLER LF, LEVINE S, KENT KM, PEARLE DL, GREEN CE, DEL NEGRO A, RACKLEY CE: Aortic dissection masquerading as acute myocardial infarction: implication for thrombolytic therapy without cardiac catheterization. Am J Cardiol 54:1134–1135, Nov 1, 1984.

5. WIENS RD, LAFIA P, MARDER CM, EVANS RG, KENNEDY HL: Chronotropic incompetence in clinical exercise testing. Am J Cardiol 54:74–78, July 1, 1984.

6. HLATKY MA, PRYOR DB, HARRELL FE, CALIFF RM, MARK DB, ROSATI RA: Factors affecting sensitivity and specificity of exercise electrocardiography. Am J Med 77:64–71, July 1984.

7. QUYYUMI A, RAPHAEL MJ, WRIGHT C, BEALING L, FOX KM: Inability of the ST segment/heart rate slope to predict accurately the severity of coronary artery disease. Br Heart J 51:395–8, Apr 1984.

8. HAMBY RI, DAVISON ET, HILSENRATH J, SHANIES S, YOUNG M, MURPHY DH, HOFFMAN I: Functional and anatomic correlates of markedly abnormal stress tests. J Am Coll Cardiol 3:1375–1381, June 1984.

9. CHAITMAN BR, BREVERS G, DUPRAS G, LESPERANCE J, BOURASSA MG: Diagnostic impact of thallium scintigraphy and cardiac fluoroscopy when the exercise ECG is strongly positive. Am Heart J 108:260–265, Aug 1984.

10. SAMI M, CHAITMAN B, FISHER L, HOLMES D, FRAY D, ALDERMAN E: Significance of exercise-induced ventricular arrhythmia in stable coronary artery disease: A coronary artery surgery study project. Am J Cardiol 54:1182–1188, Dec 1, 1984.

11. POYATOS MA, LERMAN J, ESTRADA A, CHIOZZA M, PEROSIO A: Predictive value of changes in R-wave amplitude after exercise in coronary heart disease. Am J Cardiol 54:1212–1215, Dec 1, 1984.

12. DE CAPRIO L, CUOMO S, VIGORITO C, MECCARIELLO P, ROMANO M, ZARRA AMF, RENGO F: Influence of heart rate on exercise-induced R-wave amplitude changes in coronary patients and normal subjects. Am Heart J 107:61–68, Jan 1984.

13. ROBERTS JM, SULLIVAN M, FROELICHER VF, GENTER F, MYERS J: Predicting oxygen uptake from treadmill testing in normal subjects and coronary artery disease patients. Am Heart J 108:1454–1460, Dec 1984.

14. SPECCHIA G, DE SERVI S, FALCONE C, GAVAZZI A, ANGOLI L, BRAMUCCI E, ARDISSINO D, MUSSINI A: Mental arithmetic stress testing in patients with coronary artery disease. Am Heart J 108:56–63, July 1984.

15. BROWN BG, LEE AB, BOLSON EL, DODGE HT: Reflex constriction of significant coronary stenosis as a mechanism contributing to ischemic left ventricular dysfunction during isometric exercise. Circulation 70:18–24, July 1984.

16. GONDI B, NANDA NC: Cold pressor test during two-dimensional echocardiography: usefulness in detection of patients with coronary disease. Am Heart J 107:278–285, Feb 1984.

17. HIGGINBOTHAM MB, COLEMAN RE, JONES RH, COBB FR: Mechanism and significance of a decrease in ejection fraction during exercise in patients with coronary artery disease and left ventricular dysfunction at rest. J Am Coll Cardiol 3:88–97, Jan 1984.

18. OSBAKKEN MD, OKADA RD, BOUCHER CA, STRAUSS HW, POHOST GM: Comparison of exercise perfusion and ventricular function imaging: an analysis of factors affecting the diagnostic accuracy of each technique. J Am Coll Cardiol 3:272–283, Feb 1984.

19. POLINER LR, FARBER SH, GLAESER DH, NYLAAN L, VERANI MS, ROBERTS R: Alteration of diastolic filling rate during exercise radionuclide angiography: a highly sensitive technique for detection of coronary artery disease. Circulation 70:942–950, Dec 1984.

20. TAMAKI N, YONEKURA Y, MUKAI T, KODAMA S, KADOTA K, KAMBARA H, KAWAI C, TORIZUKA K: Stress thallium-201 transaxial emission computed tomography: quantitative versus qualitative analysis for evaluation of coronary artery disease. J Am Coll Cardiol 4:1213–1221, Dec 1984.

21. BROWN KA, OKADA RB, BOUCHER CA, STRAUSS HW, POHOST GM: Right ventricular ejection fraction response to exercise in patients with coronary artery disease: influence of both right coronary artery disease and exercise-induced changes in right ventricular afterload. J Am Coll Cardiol 3:895–901, Apr 1984.

22. OKADA RD, DAI Y-H, BOUCHER CA, POHOST GM: Serial thallium-201 imaging after dipyridamole for coronary disease detection: quantitative analysis using myocardial clearance. Am Heart J 107:475–481, Mar 1984.

23. MASON JR, PALAC RT, FREEMAN ML, VIRUPANNAVAR S, LOEB HS, KAPLAN E, GUNNAR RM: Thallium scintigraphy during dobutamine infusion: nonexercise-dependent screening test for coronary disease. Am Heart J 107:481–485, Mar 1984.

24. POULEUR H, ROUSSEAU MF, VAN EYLL C, CHARLIER AA: Assessment of regional left ventricular relaxation in patients with coronary artery disease: importance of geometric factors and changes in wall thickness. Circulation 69:696–702, Apr 1984.

25. YAMAGISHI T, OZAKI M, KUMADA T, IKEZONO T, SHIMIZU T, FURUTANI Y, YAMAOKA H, OGAWA H, MATSUZAKI M, MATSUDA Y, ARIMA A, KUSUKAWA R: Asynchronous left ventricular diastolic filling in patients with isolated disease of the left anterior descending coronary artery: assessment with radionuclide ventriculography. Circulation 69:933–942, May 1984.

26. HELLER GV, AROESTY JM, MCKAY RG, PARKER JA, SILVERMAN KJ, COME PC, GROSSMAN W: The pacing stress test: a reexamination of the relation between coronary artery disease and pacing-induced electrocardiographic changes. Am J Cardiol 54:50–55, July 1, 1984.

27. HELLER GV, AROESTY JM, PARKER JA, MCKAY RG, SILVERMAN KJ, ALS AV, COME PC, KOLODNY GM, GROSSMAN W: The pacing stress test: thallium 201 myocardial imaging after atrial pacing. Diagnostic value in detecting coronary artery disease compared with exercise testing. J Am Coll Cardiol 3:1197–1204, May 1984.

28. BERBERICH SN, ZAGER JRS, PLOTNICK GD, FISHER ML: A practical approach to exercise echocardiography: immediate postexercise echocardiography. J Am Coll Cardiol 3:284–290, Feb 1984.

29. WHITE CW, WRIGHT CB, DOTY DB, HIRATZA LF, EASTHAM CL, HARRISON DG, MARCUS ML: Does visual interpretation of the coronary arteriogram predict the physiologic importance of a coronary stenosis? N Engl J Med 310:819–24, Mar 29, 1984.

30. PAULIN S, SANDOR T: Estimating the severity of coronary artery stenosis. N Engl J Med 311:409, Aug 9, 1984.

31. TRASK N, CALIFF RM, CONLEY MJ, KONG Y, PETER R, LEE KL, HACKEL DB, WAGNER GS: Accuracy and interobserver variability of coronary cineangiography: a comparison with postmortem evaluation. J Am Coll Cardiol 3:1145–1154, May 1984.

32. HARRISON DG, WHITE CW, HIRATZKA LF, DOTY DB, BARNES DH, EASTHAM CL, MARCUS ML: The value of lesion cross-sectional area determined by quantitative coronary angiography in assessing the physiologic significance of proximal left anterior descending coronary arterial stenoses. Circulation 69:1111–1119, June 1984.

33. FEIT A, KHAN R, EL-SHERIF N, REDDY CVR: Nonrandom occurrence of single-vessel coronary artery disease. Am J Med 77:683–689, Oct 1984.

34. MOISE A, LEPERANCE J, THEROUX P, TAEYMANS Y, GOULET C, BOURASSA MG: Clinical and angiographic predictors of new total coronary occlusion in coronary artery disease: analysis of 313 nonoperated patients. Am J Cardiol 54:1176–1181, Dec 1, 1984.

35. HARRIS JM: Coronary angiography and its complications: the search for risk factors. Arch Intern Med 144:337–341, Feb 1984.

36. TOBIS J, NALCIOGLU O, ISERI L, JOHNSTON WD, ROECK W, CASTLEMAN E, BAUER B, MONTELLI S, HENRY WL: Detection and quantitation of coronary artery stenoses from digital subtraction angiograms compared with 35-millimeter film cineangiograms. Am J Cardiol 54:489–496, Sept 1, 1984.

37. HIGGINS CB, LANZER P, STARK D, BOTVINICK E, SCHILLER NB, CROOKS L, KAUFMAN L, LIPTON MJ: Imaging by nuclear magnetic resonance in patients with chronic ischemic heart disease. Circulation 69:523–531, Mar 1984.

38. BONOW RO, KENT KM, ROSING DR, LAN KKG, LAKATOS E, BORER JS, BACHARACH SL, GREEN MV, EPSTEIN SE: Exercise-induced ischemia in mildly symptomatic patients with coronary-artery disease and preserved left ventricular function: identification of subgroups at risk of death during medical therapy. N Engl J Med 311:1339–1345, Nov 22, 1984.

39. WEINER DA, RYAN TJ, MCCABE CH, CHAITMAN BR, SHEFFIELD T, FERGUSON JC, FISHER LD, TRISTANI F: Prognostic importance of a clinical profile and exercise test in medically treated patients with coronary artery disease. J Am Coll Cardiol 3:772–779, Mar 1984.

40. PRYOR DB, HARRELL FE, LEE KL, ROSATI RA, COLEMAN RE, COBB FR, CALIFF RM, JONES RJ: Prognostic indicators from radionuclide angiography in medically treated patients with coronary artery disease. Am J Cardiol 53:18–22, Jan 1, 1984.

41. DUNN FR, NEWMAN HN, BERNSTEIN L, HARRIS PJ, ROUBIN GS, MORRIS J, KELLY DT: The clinical features of isolated left circumflex coronary artery disease. Circulation 69:477–484, Mar 1984.

42. CALIFF RM, CONLEY MJ, BEHAR VS, HARRELL FE, LEE KL, PRYOR DB, MCKINNIS RA, ROSATI RA: "Left main equivalent" coronary artery disease: its clinical presentation and prognostic significance with nonsurgical therapy. Am J Cardiol 53:1489–1495, June 1, 1984.

43. KANNEL WB, STAMPFER MJ, CASTELLI WP, VERTER J: The prognostic significance of proteinuria: the Framingham study. Am Heart J 108:1347–1352, Nov 1984.

44. HAFT JI, BACHIK M: Progression of coronary artery disease in patients with chest pain and normal or intraluminal disease on arteriography. Am Heart J 107:35–39, Jan 1984.

45. BRENSIKE JF, LEVY RI, KELSEY SF, PASSAMANI ER, RICHARDSON JM, LOH IK, STONE NJ, ALDRICH RF, BATTAGLINI JW, MORIARTY DJ, FISHER MR, FRIEDMAN L, FRIEDEWALD W, DETRE KM, EPSTEIN SE: Effects of therapy with cholestyramine on progression of coronary arteriosclerosis: results of the NHLBI Type II Coronary Intervention Study. Circulation 69:313–324, Feb 1984.

46. MOISE A, THÉROUX P, TAEYMANS Y, WATERS DD, LESPÉRANCE J, FINES P, DESCOINGS B, ROBERT P: Clinical and angiographic factors associated with progression of coronary artery disease. J Am Coll Cardiol 3:659–667, Mar 1984.

47. LIPID RESEARCH CLINICS PROGRAM: The Lipid Research Clinics coronary primary prevention trial results: 1. Reduction in incidence of coronary heart disease. JAMA 251:351–364, Jan 20, 1984.

48. LIPID RESEARCH CLINICS PROGRAM: The Lipid Research Clinics coronary primary prevention trial results: II. The relationship of reduction in incidence of coronary heart disease to cholesterol lowering. JAMA 251:365–374, Jan 20, 1984.

49. TUNSTALL-PEDOE H: Cholesterol lowering and the risk of coronary heart disease (letter). Lancet 1:854–855, Apr 14, 1984.

50. KANAMORI K, NISHIJIMA H, KOJIMA S, MATSUMURA N, SATO I, MURAKAMI M, MINAMI M, YASUDA H: Relationship between lipids and angiographically defined coronary artery disease in Japanese patients. Am Heart J 108:1207–1211, Nov 1984.

51. MILLER NE: Why does plasma low density lipoprotein concentration in adults increase with age? Lancet 1:263–266, Feb 4, 1984.

52. SACKS FM, MILLER L, SUTHERLAND M, ALBERS JJ, SALAZAR J, FOSTER JM, SAMONDS KW, KASS EH: Ingestion of egg raises plasma low density lipoproteins in free-living subjects. Lancet 1:647–649, Mar 24, 1984.

53. HASKELL WL, CAMARGO C, WILLIAMS PT, VRANIZAN KM, KRAUSS RM, LINDGREN FT, WOOD PD: The effect of cessation and resumption of moderate alcohol intake on serum high-density-lipoprotein subfractions. N Engl J Med 310:805–810, Mar 29, 1984.

54. WALDEN CE, KNOPP RH, WAHL PW, BEACH KW, STRANDNESS E: Sex differences in the effect of diabetes mellitus on lipoprotein triglyceride and cholesterol concentrations. N Engl J Med 311:953–959, Oct 11, 1984.

55. THOMPSON PD, MITCHELL JH: Exercise and sudden cardiac death: protection or provocation? N Engl J Med 311:914–915, Oct 4, 1984.

56. SPRECHER DL, SCHAEFER EJ, KENT KM, GREGG RE, ZECH LA, HOEG JM, McMANUS B, ROBERTS WC, BREWER HB: Cardiovascular features of homozygous familial hypercholesterolemia: analysis of 16 patients. Am J Cardiol 54:20–39, July 1, 1984.

57. ROBERTS WC: Extreme hypercholesterolemia-malignant atherosclerosis. Am J Cardiol 54:242–243, July 1, 1984.

58. GLUECK CJ, GARTSIDE P, LASKARZEWSKI PM, KHOURY P, TYROLER HA: High density lipoprotein cholesterol in blacks and whites: potential ramifications for coronary heart disease. Am Heart J 108:815–826, Sept 1984.

59. DAI WS, GUTAI JP, KULLER LH, LAPORTE RE, FALVO-GERARD L, CAGGIULA A: Relation between plasma high-density lipoprotein cholesterol and sex hormone concentrations in men. Am J Cardiol 53:1259–1263, May 1, 1984.

60. SEALS DR, ALLEN WK, HURLEY BF, DALSKY GP, EHSANI AA, HAGBERG JM: Elevated high-density lipoprotein cholesterol levels in older endurance athletes. Am J Cardiol 54:390–393, Aug 1, 1984.

61. SEALS DR, HAGBERG JM, HURLEY BF, EHSANI AA, HOLLOSZY JO: Effects of endurance training on glucose tolerance and plasma lipid levels in older men and women. JAMA 252:645–649, Aug 3, 1984.

62. CROUSE SF, HOOPER PH, ATTERBOM HA, PAPENFUSS RL: Zinc ingestion and lipoprotein values in sedentary and endurance-trained men. JAMA 252:785–787, Aug 10, 1984.

63. GOLDBERG L, ELLIOT DL, SCHUTZ RW, KLOSTER FE: Changes in lipid and lipoprotein levels after weight training. JAMA 252:504–506, July 27, 1984.

64. HERBERT PN, BERNIER DN, CULLINANE EM, EDELSTEIN L, KANTOR MA, THOMPSON PD: High-density lipoprotein metabolism in runners and sedentary men. JAMA 252:1034–1037, Aug 24, 1984.

65. DUJOVNE CA, CHERNOFF SB, KREHBIEL P, JACKSON B, DECOURSEY S, TAYLOR H: Low-dose colestipol plus probucol for hypercholesterolemia. Am J Cardiol 53:1511–1516, June 1, 1984.

66. FOLLICK MJ, ABRAMS DB, SMITH TW, HENDERSON O, HERBERT PN: Contrasting short- and long-term effects of weight loss on lipoprotein levels. Arch Intern Med 144:1571–1574, Aug 1984.

67. CONSENSUS DEVELOPMENT CONFERENCE: Treatment of hypertriglyceridemia. JAMA 251:1196–1200, Mar 2, 1984.

68. BRIONES ER, STEIGER D, PALUMBO PJ, KOTTKE BA: Primary hypercholesterolemia: effect of treatment on serum lipids, lipoprotein fractions, cholesterol absorption, sterol balance, and platelet aggregation. Mayo Clin Proc 59:251–257, Apr 1984.

69. ILLINGWORTH DR: Mevinolin plus colestipol in therapy for severe heterozygous familial hypercholesterolemia. Ann Intern Med 101:598–604, Nov 1984.

70. HOEG JM, MAHER MB, BOU E, ZECH LA, BAILEY KR, GREGG RE, SPRECHER DL, SUSSER JK, PIKUS AM, BREWER HB: Normalization of plasma lipoprotein concentrations in patients with type II hyperlipoproteinemia by combined use of neomycin and niacin. Circulation 70:1004–1011, Dec 1984.

71. KOIVISTO P, MIETTINEN TA: Long-term effects of ileal bypass on lipoproteins in patients with familial hypercholesterolemia. Circulation 70:290–296, Aug 1984.

72. STARZL TE, BAHNSON HT, HARDESTY RL, IWATSUKI S, GARTNER JC, BILHEIMER DW, SHAW BW, GRIFFITH BP, ZITELLI BJ, MALATACK JJ, URBACH AH: Heart-liver transplantation in a patient with familial hypercholesterolemia. Lancet 1:1382–1383, June 23, 1984.

73. RIBEIRO JP, HARTLEY LH, SHERWOOD J, HERD JA: The effectiveness of a low lipid diet and exercise in the management of coronary artery disease. Am Heart J 108:1183–1189, Nov 1984.

74. GILLUM RF, FOLSOM AR, BLACKBURN H: Decline in coronary heart disease mortality: old questions and new facts. Am J Med 76:1055–1065, June 1984.

75. DAVIS MJE, HOCKINGS BEF, EL DESSOUKY MAM, HAJAR HA, TAYLOR RR: Cigarette smoking and ventricular arrhythmia in coronary heart disease. Am J Cardiol 54:282–285, Aug 1, 1984.

76. MARTIN JL, WILSON JR, FERRARO N, LASKEY WK, KLEAVELAND P, HIRSHFELD JW: Acute coronary vasoconstrictive effects of cigarette smoking in coronary heart disease. Am J Cardiol 54:56–60, July 1, 1984.

77. NICOD P, REHR R, WINNIFORD MD, CAMPBELL WB, FIRTH BG, HILLIS LD: Acute systemic and coronary hemodynamic and serologic responses to cigarette smoking in long-term smokers with atherosclerotic coronary artery disease. J Am Coll Cardiol 4:964–971, Nov 1984.

78. KLEIN LW, AMBROSE J, PICHARD A, HOLT J, GORLIN R, TEICHHOLZ LE: Acute coronary hemodynamic response to cigarette smoking in patients with coronary artery disease. J Am Coll Cardiol 3:879–886, Apr 1984.

79. HARTZ AJ, ANDERSON AJ, BROOKS HL, MANLEY JC, PARENT GT, BARBORIAK JJ: The association of smoking with cardiomyopathy. N Engl J Med 311:1201–1206, Nov 8, 1984.

80. PAFFENBARGER RS, HYDE RT, WING AL, STEINMETZ CH: A natural history of athleticism and cardiovascular health. JAMA 252:491–495, July 27, 1984.

81. BARRETT-CONNOR E, KHAW KT: Family history of heart attack as an independent predictor of death due to cardiovascular disease. Circulation 69:1065–1069, June 1984.

82. WILHELMSEN L, SVARDSUDD K, KORSAN-BENGSTEN K, LARSSON B, WELIN L, TIBBLIN G: Fibrinogen as a risk factor for stroke and myocardial infarction. N Engl J Med 311:501–505, Aug 23, 1984.

83. MASSEY FJ, BERNSTEIN GS, O'FALLON WM, SCHUMAN LM, COULSON AH, CROZIER R, MANDEL JS, BENJAMIN RB, BERENDES HW, CHANG PC, DETELS R, EMSLANDER RF, KORELITZ J, KURLAND LT, LEPOW IH, McGREGOR DD, NAKAMURA RN, QUIROGA J, SCHMIDT S, SPIVEY GH, SULLIVAN T: Vasectomy and health: results from a large cohort study. JAMA 252:1023–1029, Aug 24, 1984.

84. DEANFIELD JE, SHEA M, RIBIERO P, DE LANDSHEERE CM, WILSON RA, HORLOCK P, SELWYN AP: Transient ST-segment depression as a marker of myocardial ischemia during daily life. Am J Cardiol 54:1195–1200, Dec 1, 1984.

85. COHN PF: Time for a new approach to management of patients with both symptomatic and asymptomatic episodes of myocardial ischemia. Am J Cardiol 54:1358–1359, Dec 1, 1984.

86. ELLESTAD MH, KUAN P: Naloxone and asymptomatic ischemia: failure to induce angina during exercise testing. Am J Cardiol 54:982–984, Nov 1, 1984.

87. EHSANI AA, BIELLO D, SEALS DR, AUSTIN MB, SCHULTZ J: The effect of left ventricular systolic function on maximal aerobic exercise capacity in asymptomatic patients with coronary artery disease. Circulation 70:552–560, Oct 1984.

88. FROELICHER V, JENSEN D, GENTER F, SULLIVAN M, McKIRNAN MD, WITZTUM K, SCHARF J, STRONG ML, ASHBURN W: A randomized trial of exercise training in patients with coronary heart disease. JAMA 252:1291–1297, Sept 14, 1984.

89. VANHEES L, FAGARD R, AMERY A: Influence of beta-adrenergic blockade on the hemodynamic effects of physical training in patients with ischemic heart disease. Am Heart J 108:270–275, Aug 1984.

90. WILLIAMS RS: Effects of physical conditioning on left ventricular ejection fraction in patients with coronary artery disease. Circulation 70:69–75, July 1984.

91. OPHERK D, MALL G, ZEBE H, SCHWARZ F, WEIHE E, MANTHEY J, WOLFGANG K: Reduction of coronary reserve: a mechanism for angina pectoris in patients with arterial hypertension and normal coronary arteries. Circulation 69:1–7, Jan 1984.

92. NARAHARA KA, HILLERT MC JR, SMITHERMAN TC, BURDEN LL: Alterations in left ventricular function during therapy of unstable angina pectoris: relationship to clinical outcome. Am Heart J 107:261–269, Feb 1984.

93. HAKKI A-H, ISKANDRIAN AS, KANE SA, AMENTA A: Thallium-201 myocardial scintigraphy and left ventricular function at rest in patients with rest angina pectoris. Am Heart J 108:326–332, Aug 1984.

94. ZACK PM, ISCHINGER T, AKER UT, DINCER B, KENNEDY HL: The occurrence of angiographically detected intracoronary thrombus in patients with unstable angina pectoris. Am Heart J 108:1408–1412, Dec 1984.

95. CHIERCHIA S, SMITH G, MORGAN M, GALLINO A, DEANFIELD J, CROOM M: Role of heart rate in pathophysiology of chronic stable angina. Lancet 2:1353–1357, Dec 15, 1984.

96. THUESEN L, THOMASSEN A, NIELSEN TT, BAGGER JP, HENNINGSEN P: Beneficial effect of a low-fat low-calorie diet on myocardial energy metabolism in patients with angina pectoris. Lancet 2:59–62, July 14, 1984.

97. MEHTA J, MEHTA P, FELDMAN RL, HORALEK C: Thromboxane release in coronary artery disease: spontaneous versus pacing-induced angina. Am Heart J 107:286–292, Feb 1984.

98. SIEGEL RJ, SHAH PK, NATHAN M, RODRIGUEZ L, SHELL WE: Prostaglandin E_1 infusion in unstable angina: effects on anginal frequency and cardiac function. Am Heart J 108:863–868, Oct 1984.

99. CONNOLLY DC, ELVEBACK LR, OXMAN HA: Coronary heart disease in residents of Rochester, Minnesota. IV. Prognostic value of the resting electrocardiogram at the time of initial diagnosis of angina pectoris. Mayo Clin Proc 59:247–250, Apr 1984.

100. HULTGREN HN, PEDUZZI P: Relation of severity of symptoms to prognosis in stable angina pectoris. Am J Cardiol 54:988–993, Nov 1, 1984.

101. McHENRY PL, O'DONNELL J, MORRIS SN, JORDAN JJ: The abnormal exercise electrocardiogram in apparently healthy men: a predictor of angina pectoris as an initial coronary event during long-term follow-up. Circulation 70:547–551, Oct 1984.

102. BUTMAN SM, OLSON HG, GARDIN JM, PITERS KM, HULLETT M, BUTMAN LK: Submaximal exercise testing after stabilization of unstable angina pectoris. J Am Coll Cardiol 4:667–673, Oct 1984.

103. DEANFIELD JE, RIBIERO P, OAKLEY K, KRIKLER S, SELWYN AP: Analysis of ST-segment changes in normal subjects: implications for ambulatory monitoring in angina pectoris. Am J Cardiol 54:1321–1325, Dec 1, 1984.

104. NISHIMURA RA, HOLMES DR, McFARLAND TM, SMITH HC, BOVE AA: Ventricular arrhythmias during coronary angiography in patients with angina pectoris or chest pain syndromes. Am J Cardiol 53:1496–1499, June 1, 1984.

105. QUYYUMI P, BRINKER JA, MELLITS ED, WEISFELDT ML, GERSTENBLITH G: Variables predictive of successful medical therapy in patients with unstable angina: selection by multivariate analysis from clinical, electrocardiographic, and angiographic evaluations. Circulation 70:367–376, Sept 1984.

106. REICHEK N, PRIEST C, ZIMRIN D, CHANDLER T, SUTTON MS: Antianginal effects of nitroglycerin patches. Am J Cardiol 54:1–7, July 1, 1984.

107. PARKER JO, FUNG HL: Transdermal nitroglycerin in angina pectoris. Am J Cardiol 54:471–476, Sept 1, 1984.

108. PARKER JO, VANKOUGHNETT KA, FUNG H: Transdermal isosorbide dinitrate in angina pectoris: effect of acute and sustained therapy. Am J Cardiol 54:8–13, July 1, 1984.

109. ABRAMS J: The brief saga of transdermal nitroglycerin discs: Paradise lost? Am J Cardiol 53:220–224, July 1, 1984.

110. DALAL JJ, PARKER JO: Nitrate cross-tolerance: effect of sublingual isosorbide dinitrate and nitroglycerin during sustained nitrate therapy. Am J Cardiol 54:286–288, Aug 1, 1984.

111. MARZULLO P, PARODI O, SCHELBERT HR, L'ABBATE A: Regional myocardial dysfunction in patients with angina at rest and response to isosorbide dinitrate assessed by phase analysis of radionuclide ventriculograms. J Am Coll Cardiol 3:1357–1366, June 1984.

112. SASAYAMA S, NONOGI H, FUJITA M, SAKURAI T, WAKABAYASHI A, KAWAI C, EIIIO S, KUWAHARA M: Three-dimensional analysis of regional myocardial function in response to nitroglycerin in patients with coronary artery disease. J Am Coll Cardiol 3:1187–1196, May 1984.

113. BELLER GA, BITTAR N, COELHO JB, CRADDOCK GB, EXEKOWITZ MD, MURRAY GC, STEEN SN, WAKSMAN JA: Double-blind, placebo-controlled trial of propranolol given once, twice and four times daily in stable angina pectoris: a multicenter study using serial exercise testing. Am J Cardiol 54:37–42, July 1, 1984.

114. KAUL S, HECHT HS, SEIDMAN R, HOPKINS J, SINGH BN: Comparative effects of oral acebutolol and propranolol at rest and during exercise in ischemic heart disease: Double-blind placebo crossover study utilizing radionuclide ventriculography. Am Heart J 108:469–475, Sept 1984.

115. HOSSACK KF, KANNAGI T, DAY B, BRUCE RA: Long-term study of high-dose diltiazem in chronic stable exertional angina. Am Heart J 107:1215–1220, June 1984.

116. HOSSACK KF, BROWN G, STEWART DK, DODGE HT: Diltiazem-induced blockade of sympathetically mediated constriction of normal and diseased coronary arteries: lack of epicardial coronary dilatory effect in humans. Circulation 70:465–471, Sept 1984.

117. KENNY J, DALY K, BERGMAN G, KERKEZ S, JEWITT DE: Beneficial effects of diltiazem in coronary

artery disease. Br Heart J 52:53–56, July 1984.

118. KHURMI NS, BOWLES MJ, O'HARA MJ, SUBRAMANIAN B, RAFTERY EB: Long-term efficacy of diltiazem assessed with multistage graded exercise tests in patients with chronic stable angina pectoris. Am J Cardiol 54:738–743, Oct 1, 1984.

119. NELSON GIC, SILKE B, AHUJA RC, VERMA SP, HUSSAIN M, TAYLOR SH: Hemodynamic effects of nifedipine during upright exercise in stable angina pectoris and either normal or severely impaired left ventricular function. Am J Cardiol 53:451–455, Feb 1, 1984.

120. GOTTLIEB SO, OUYANG P, ACHUFF SC, BAUGHMAN KL, TRAILL TA, MELLITS ED, WEISFELDT ML, GERSTENBLITH G: Acute nifedipine withdrawal: consequences of preoperative and late cessation of therapy in patients with prior unstable angina. J Am Coll Cardiol 4:382–388, Aug 1984.

121. KHURMI NS, BOWLES MJ, SUBRAMANIAN VB, RAFTERY EB: Short- and long-term efficacy of nicardipine, assessed by placebo-controlled single- and double-blind crossover trials in patients with chronic stable angina. J Am Coll Cardiol 4:908–917, Nov 1984.

122. NARAHARA KA, SHAPIRO W, WELIKY I, PARK J: Evaluation of bepridil, a new antianginal agent: Clinical and hemodynamic alterations during the treatment of stable angina pectoris. Am J Cardiol 53:29–34, Jan 1, 1984.

123. DIBIANCO R, ALPERT J, KATZ RJ, SPANN J, CHESTER E, FERRI DP, LARCA LJ, COSTELLO RB, GORE JM, EISENMAN MJ: Bepridil for chronic stable angina pectoris: results of a prospective multicenter, placebo-controlled, dose-ranging study in 77 patients. Am J Cardiol 53:35–41, Jan 1, 1984.

124. DEANFIELD J, WRIGHT C, KRIKLER S, RIBEIRO P, FOX K: Cigarette smoking and the treatment of angina with propranolol, atenolol, and nifedipine. N Engl J Med 310:951–954, Apr 12, 1984.

125. ANDERSON JL, WAGNER JM, DATZ FL, CHRISTIAN PE, BRAY BE, TAYLOR AT: Comparative effects of diltiazem, propranolol, and placebo on exercise performance using radionuclide ventriculography in patients with symptomatic coronary artery disease: results of a double-blind, randomized, crossover study. Am Heart J 107:698–706, Apr 1984.

126. O'HARA MJ, KHURMI NS, BOWLES MJ, SUBRAMANIAN VB, DORE CJ, RAFTERY EB: Comparison of diltiazem at two dose levels with propranolol for treatment of stable angina pectoris. Am J Cardiol 54:477–481, Sept 1, 1984.

127. CHAITMAN BR, WAGNIART P, PASTERNAC A, BREVERS G, SCHOLL JM, LAM J, METHE M, FERGUSON RJ, BOURASSA MG: Improved exercise after propranolol, diltiazem or nifedipine in angina pectoris: comparison at 1, 3 and 8 hours and correlation with plasma drug concentration. Am J Cardiol 53:1–9, Jan 1, 1984.

128. DETRE KM, PEDUZZI P, HAMMERMEISTER KE, MURPHY ML, HULTGREN HN, TAKARO T: Five-year effect of medical and surgical therapy on resting left ventricular function in stable angina: Veterans Administration cooperative study. Am J Cardiol 53:444–450, Feb 1, 1984.

129. BOTT-SILVERMAN C, HEUPLER FA, YIANNIKAS J: Variant angina: Comparison of patients with and without fixed severe coronary artery disease. Am J Cardiol 54:1173–1175, Dec 1, 1984.

130. WATERS DD, MILLER DD, BOUCHARD A, BOSCH X, THEROUX P: Circadian variation in variant angina. Am J Cardiol 54:61–64, July 1, 1984.

131. PARODI O, MARZULLO P, NEGLIA D, GALLI M, DISTANTE A, ROVAI D, L'ABBATE A: Transient predominant right ventricular ischemia caused by coronary vasospasm. Circulation 70:170–177, Aug 1984.

132. ARAKI H, ANAN T, KOIWAYA Y, NAKAGAKI O, TAKESHITA A, NAKAMURA M: Reflex heart rate and blood pressure changes during ST segment elevation in patients with variant angina. Am Heart J 108:1273–1279, Nov 1984.

133. MATSUGUCHI T, KOIWAYA Y, NAKAGAKI O, TAKESHITA A, NAKAMURA M: Transient U wave inversion during variant angina. Am Heart J 108:899–904, Oct 1984.

134. DISTANTE A, ROVAI D, PICANO E, MOSCARELLI E, MORALES MA, PALOMBO C, L'ABBATE A: Transient changes in left ventricular mechanics during attacks of Prinzmetal angina: a two-dimensional echocardiographic study. Am Heart J 108:440–446, Sept 1984.

135. DISTANTE A, ROVAI D, PICANO E, MOSCARELLI E, PALOMBO C, MORALES MA, MICHELASSI C, L'ABBATE A: Transient changes in left ventricular mechanics during attacks of Prinzmetal's

angina: an M-mode echocardiographic study. Am Heart J 107:465–474, Mar 1984.

136. MARK DB, CALIFF RM, MORRIS KG, HARRELL FE, PRYOR DB, HLATKY MA, LEE KL, ROSATI RA: Clinical characteristics and long-term survival of patients with variant angina. Circulation 69:880–888, May 1984.

137. CHIERCHIA S, DAVIES G, BERKENBOOM G, CREA F, CREAN P, MASERI A: Alpha-adrenergic receptors and coronary spasm: an elusive link. Circulation 69:8–14, Jan 1984.

138. DE CATERINA R, CARPEGGIANI C, L'ABBATE A: A double-blind, placebo-controlled study of ketanserin in patients with Prinzmetal's angina: Evidence against a role for serotonin in the genesis of coronary vasospasm. Circulation 69:889–894, May 1984.

139. CREA F, DAVIES G, ROMEO F, CHIERCHIA S, BUGIARDINI R, KASKI JC, FREEDMAN B, MASERI A: Myocardial ischemia during ergonovine testing: different susceptibility to coronary vasoconstriction in patients with exertional and variant angina. Circulation 69:690–695, Apr 1984.

140. FREEDMAN SB, CHIERCHIA S, RODRIGUEZ-PLAZA L, BUGIARDINI R, SMITH G, MASERI A: Ergonovine-induced myocardial ischemia: no role for serotonergic receptors? Circulation 70:178–183, Aug 1984.

141. SZLACHCIC J, WATERS DD, MILLER D, THÉROUX P: Ventricular arrhythmias during ergonovine-induced episodes of variant angina. Am Heart J 107:20–24, Jan 1984.

142. WINNIFORD MD, GABLIANI G, JOHNSON SM, MAURITSON DR, FULTON KL, HILLIS LD: Concomitant calcium antagonist plus isosorbide dinitrate therapy for markedly active variant angina. Am Heart J 108:1269–1273, Nov 1984.

143. SILVERTON NP, ELAMIN M, SMITH DR, IONESCU MI, KARDASH M, WHITAKER W, MARY D, LINDEN RJ: Use of the exercise maximal ST segment/heart rate slope in assessing the results of coronary angioplasty. Br Heart J 51:379–385, Apr 1984.

144. O'NEILL WW, WALTON JA, BATES ER, COLFER HT, AUERON FM, LEFREE MT, PITT B, VOGEL RA: Criteria for successful coronary angioplasty as assessed by alterations in coronary vasodilatory reserve. J Am Coll Cardiol 3:1382–1390, June 1984.

145. FELDMAN RL, JOYAL M, CONTI R, PEPINE CJ. Effect of nitroglycerin on coronary collateral flow and pressure during acute coronary occlusion. Am J Cardiol 54:958–963, Nov 1, 1984.

146. SERRUYS PW, WIJNS W, VAN DEN BRAND M, MEIJ S, SLAGER C, SCHUURBIERS JCH, HUGENHOLTZ PG, BROWER RW: Left ventricular performance, regional blood flow, wall motion and lactate metabolism during transluminal angioplasty. Circulation 70:25–36, July 1984.

147. HOLMES DR, VLIESTRA RE, REEDER GS, BRESNAHAN JF, SMITH HC, BOVE AA, SCHAFF HV: Angioplasty in total coronary artery occlusion. J Am Coll Cardiol 3:845–849, Mar 1984.

148. REEDER GS, KRISHAN I, NOBREGA FT, NAESSENS J, KELLY M, CHRISTIANSON JB, MCAFEE MK: Is percutaneous coronary angioplasty less expensive than bypass surgery? N Engl J Med 311:1157–1162, Nov 1, 1984.

149. THORNTON MA, GRUENTZIG AR, HOLLMAN J, KING SB, DOUGLAS JS: Coumadin and aspirin in prevention of recurrence after transluminal coronary angioplasty: a randomized study. Circulation 69:721–727, Apr 1984.

150. MEIER B, KING SB III, GRUENTZIG AR, DOUGLAS JS, HOLLMAN J, ISCHINGER T, GALAN K, TANKERSLEY R: Repeat coronary angioplasty. J Am Coll Cardiol 4:463–466, Sept 1984.

151. FARO RS, ALEXANDER JA, FELDMAN RL, PEPINE CJ, CONTI CR, KNAUF DG, ROBERTS AJ: Intraoperative balloon-catheter dilatation: University of Florida experience. Am Heart J 107:841–844, Apr 1984.

152. COUNCIL ON SCIENTIFIC AFFAIRS: Percutaneous transluminal angioplasty. JAMA 251:764–768, Feb 10, 1984.

153. COBANOGLU A, FREIMANIS I, GRUNKEMEIER G, LAMBERT L, ANDERSON V, NUNLEY D, GARCIA C, STARR A: Enhanced late survival following coronary artery bypass graft operation for unstable versus chronic angina. Am Thorac Surg 37:52–59, Jan 1984.

154. JOHNSON WD, KAYSER KL, PEDRAZA PM: Angina pectoris and coronary bypass surgery: patterns of prevalence and recurrence in 3105 consecutive patients followed up to 11 years. Am Heart J 108:1190–1197, Nov 1984.

155. COSGROVE DM, LOOP FD, LYTLE BW, BAILLOT R, GILL CC, GOLDING LAR, TAYLOR PC, GOORMASTIC M: Primary myocardial revascularization: trends in surgical mortality. J Thorac Cardiovasc Surg 88:673–684, November 1984.

156. FitzGibbon GM, Keon WJ, Burton JR: Aorta-coronary bypass in patients with coronary artery disease who do not have angina. J Thorac Cardiovasc Surg 87:717–724, May 1984.

157. The Veterans Administration Coronary Artery Bypass Surgery Cooperative Study Group: Eleven-year survival in the Veterans Administration randomized trial of coronary bypass surgery for stable angina. N Engl J Med 311:1333–1339, Nov 1984.

158. Elayda MA, Hall RJ, Gray AG, Mathur VS, Cooley DA: Coronary revascularization in the elderly patient. J Am Coll Cardiol 3:1398–1402, June 1984.

159. Pinson CW, Coganoglu A, Metzdorff MT, Grunkemeier GL, Kay PH, Starr A: Late surgical results for ischemic mitral regurgitation: role of wall motion score and severity of regurgitation. J Thorac Cardiovasc Surg 88:663–672, Nov 1984.

160. Gould BL, Clayton PD, Jensen RL, Liddle HV: Association between early graft patency and late outcome for patients undergoing artery bypass graft surgery. Circulation 69:569–576, Mar 1984.

161. Tyras DH, Kaiser GC, Barner HB, Pennington DG, Codd JE, Willman VL: Global left ventricular impairment and myocardial revascularization: determinants of survival. Ann Thorac Surg 39:47–51, Jan 1984.

162. Freeman AP, Walsh WF, Giles RW, Choy D, Newman DC, Horton DA, Wright JS, Murray IP: Early and long-term results of coronary artery bypass grafting with severely depressed left ventricular performance. Am J Cardiol 54:749–754, Oct 1, 1984.

163. Topol EJ, Weiss JL, Guzman PA, Dorsey-Lima S, Blanck TJJ, Humphrey LS, Baumgartner WA, Flaherty JT, Reitz BA: Immediate improvement of dysfunctional myocardial segments after coronary revascularization: detection by intraoperative transesophageal echocardiography. J Am Coll Cardiol 4:1123–1134, Dec 1984.

164. Brundage BH, Massie BM, Botvinick EH: Improved regional ventricular function after successful surgical revascularization. J Am Coll Cardiol 3:902–908, Apr 1984.

165. Hossack KF, Bruce RA, Ivey TD, Kusumi F: Changes in cardiac functional capacity after coronary bypass surgery in relation to adequacy of revascularization. J Am Coll Cardiol 3:47–54, Jan 1984.

166. Foster C, Pollock ML, Anholm JD, Squires RW, Ward A, Dymond DS, Rod JL, Saichek RP, Schmidt DH: Work capacity and left ventricular function during rehabilitation after myocardial revascularization surgery. Circulation 69:748–755, Apr 1984.

167. Flameng W, Wouters L, Sergeant P, Lewi P, Borgers W, Thone F, Suy R: Multivariate analysis of angiographic, histologic, and electrocardiographic data in patients with coronary heart disease. Circulation 70:7–17, July 1984.

168. Huikuri HV, Korhonen UR, Linnaluoto MK, Takkunen JT: Effect of coronary artery bypass grafting on left ventricular response to isometric exercise. Am J Cardiol 54:514–518, Sept 1984.

169. Kardash MM, Boyle RM, Watson DA, Stoker JB, Mary D, Linden RJ: Assessment of aortocoronary bypass grafting using exercise ST segment/heart rate relation. Br Heart J 51:386–394, Apr 1984.

170. Stevens R, Hanson P: Comparison of supervised and unsupervised exercise training after coronary bypass surgery. Am J Cardiol 53:1524–1528, June 1,1984.

171. Cashin WL, Sanmarco ME, Nessim SA, Blankenhorn DH: Accelerated progression of atherosclerosis in coronary vessels with minimal lesions that are bypassed. N Engl J Med 311:824–828, Sept 27, 1984.

172. Loop FD: Progression of coronary atherosclerosis. N Engl J Med 311:851–853, Sept 27, 1984.

173. Campeau L, Enjalbert M, Lesperance J, Bourassa MG, Kwiterovich P, Wacholder S, Sniderman A: The relation of risk factors to the development of atherosclerosis in saphenous-vein bypass grafts and the progression of disease in the native circulation: a study 10 years after aortocoronary bypass surgery. N Engl J Med 311:1329–1332, Nov 22, 1984.

174. Brindis RG, Brundage BH, Ullyot DJ, McKay CW, Lipton MJ, Turley K: Graft patency in patients with coronary artery bypass operation complicated by perioperative myocardial infarction. J Am Coll Cardiol 3:55–62, Jan 1984.

175. CASS Principal Investigators and Their Associates: Myocardial infarction and mortality in the coronary artery surgery study (CASS) randomized trial. N Engl J Med 310:750–758, Mar 22, 1984.

176. SCHAFF HV, GERSH BJ, FISHER LD, FRYE RL, MOCK MB, RYAN TJ, ELLS RB, CHAITMAN BR, ALDERMAN EL, KAISER GC, FAXON DP, PARTICIPANTS IN THE CORONARY ARTERY SURGERY STUDY (Appendix I): Detrimental effect of perioperative myocardial infarction on late survival after coronary artery bypass. J Thorac Cardiovasc Surg 88:972–981, Dec 1984.

177. BADDOUR LM, BISNO AL: Recurrent cellulitis after coronary bypass surgery: association with superficial fungal infection in saphenous venectomy limbs. JAMA 251:1049–1052, Feb 24, 1984.

178. KUAN P, BERNSTEIN SB, ELLESTAD MH: Coronary artery bypass surgery morbidity. J Am Coll Cardiol 3:1391–1397, June 1984.

179. CHESEBRO JH, FUSTER V, ELVEBACK LR, CLEMENTS IP, SMITH HC, HOLMES DR, BARDSLEY WT, PLUTH JR, WALLACE RB, PUGA FJ, ORSZULAK TA, PIEHLER JM, DANIELSON GK, SCHAFF HV, FRYE RL: Effect of dipyridamole and aspirin on late vein-graft patency after coronary bypass operations. N Engl J Med 310:209–214, Jan 26, 1984.

180. LORENZ RL, WEBER M, KOTZUR J, THEISEN K, SCHACKY CV, MEISTER W, REICHARDT B, WEBER PC: Improved aortocoronary bypass patency by low-dose aspirin (100 mg daily). Lancet 1:1261–1264, June 9,1984.

181. RIBEIRO P, SHEA M, DEANFIELD JE, OAKLEY CM, SAPSFORD R, JONES T, WALESBY R, SELWYN A: Different mechanisms for the relief of angina after coronary bypass surgery: physiological versus anatomical assessment. Br Heart J 52:502–509, Nov 1984.

182. IVEY TD, STRANDNESS D, WILLIAMS DB, LANGLOIS Y, MISBACH GA, KRUSE AP: Management of patients with carotid bruit undergoing cardiopulmonary bypass. J Thorac Cardiovasc Surg 87:183–198, Feb 1984.

183. STONEY WS, ALFORD WC JR, BURRUS GR, GLASSFORD DM JR, PETRACEK MR, THOMAS CS JR: The fate of arm veins used for aorta-coronary bypass grafts. J Thorac Cardiovasc Surg 88:522–526, Oct 1984.

184. WHITE HD, ANTMAN EM, GLYNN MA, COLLINS JJ, COHN LH, SHEMIN RJ, FRIEDMAN PL: Efficacy and safety of timolol for prevention of supraventricular tachyarrhythmias after coronary artery bypass surgery. Circulation 70:479–484, Sept 1984.

185. FLAMENG W, VAN DER VUSSE GJ, DE MEYERE R, BORGERS M, SERGEANT P, VANDER MEERSCH E, GEBOERS J, SUY R: Intermittent aortic cross-clamping versus St. Thomas' Hospital cardioplegia in extensive aorta-coronary bypass grafting: a randomized clinical study. J Thorac Cardiovasc Surg 88:164–173, Aug 1984.

186. JONES EL, MURPHY DA, CRAVER JM. Comparison of coronary artery bypass surgery and percutaneous transluminal coronary angioplasty including surgery for failed angioplasty. Am Heart J 107:830–835, Apr 1984.

187. PORT SC, PATEL S, SCHMIDT DH: Effects of intraaortic balloon counterpulsation on myocardial blood flow in patients with severe coronary artery disease. J Am Coll Cardiol 3:1367–1374, June 1984.

2

Acute Myocardial Infarction and Its Consequences

DIAGNOSIS

Unrecognized AMI

Of patients studied at necropsy with transmural LV scars, only 50% have had during life clinical episodes compatible with AMI. Kannel and Abbott[1] from Framingham, Massachusetts, and Bethesda, Maryland, found that 25% of the participants in the Framingham Study who had myocardial infarcts had clinically silent ones. Among the 5,127 participants, 708 had myocardial infarcts and 25% of them were discovered only through the appearance of new diagnostic evidence during routine biennial ECG examination. Of the unrecognized infarcts, almost half were "silent" and the others caused atypical symptoms. The proportion of all myocardial infarcts that were unrecognized were higher in women and in older men. Unrecognized AMI was uncommon in patients with angina pectoris. Unrecognized AMI was as likely as a recognized one to cause death, CHF, or stroke. Recurrent infarcts were more common in women with recognized than with unrecognized AMI, but this difference was not present in men. Recurrent AMI was more likely to be recognized than was the first AMI.

Association with acute respiratory symptoms

Spodick and associates[2] from Worcester, Massachusetts, studied 150 patients prospectively with AMI and 150 control patients matched for age, sex, and admission date, and found that acute respiratory symptoms occurred in 42 AMI patients and in 23 control patients (p < 0.02). Matched-pair analysis gave an odds ratio for a respiratory syndrome of 2.2:1 for AMI. The statistically significant association of minor respiratory symptoms and the onset of AMI must be further investigated to determine whether there is any pathogenetic relation of respiratory symptoms, presumably viral induced, to the onset of AMI.

Electrocardiographic observations

Mukharji and coworkers[3] from Dallas, Texas, tested the hypothesis that anterior ST-segment depression represents concomitant posterior AMI in 49 patients admitted with a first transmural inferior AMI. In this study, anterior ST-segment depression was defined as $\geqslant 0.1$ mV ST depression in leads V_1, V_2, or V_3 on an ECG recorded within 18 hours of AMI. Serial vectorcardiograms and technetium pyrophosphate scintigrams were obtained: 80% had anterior ST depression (39 of 49 patients). Among these 39 patients, 34% demonstrated vectorcardiographic criteria for posterior AMI and 60% had pyrophosphate evidence of posterior AMI. Anterior ST depression was not sensitive (84%) or specific (20%) in the detection of posterior AMI as defined by pyrophosphate imaging. Eighty-seven percent of patients with persistent anterior ST depression for >72 hours had posterior AMI detected by pyrophosphate imaging. An RV AMI was present on pyrophosphate imaging in 40% of patients, with pyrophosphate changes of posterior AMI. These data indicate that: most patients with inferior AMI have anterior ST-segment depression; early anterior ST-segment depression is not a specific marker for posterior AMI; and standard vectorcardiographic criteria for transmural posterior AMI may be less accurate in patients with concomitant transmural inferior AMI or RV AMI.

Roubin and associates[4] from Sydney, Australia, examined the relation between coronary pathoanatomy and anterolateral ST-segment depression during inferior AMI in 84 consecutive survivors of inferior AMI who underwent prospective coronary angiography a median time of 2 weeks after AMI. Multivessel CAD was defined as $\geqslant 2$ significantly (>70%) stenosed arteries. A QRS scoring system was used to estimate infarct size. Patients with ST depression had more multivessel CAD compared with patients with no ST depression (53 -vs- 6%, p < 0.01), more LAD stenoses (36 -vs- 10%, p < 0.05), and higher QRS scores (5.8 ± 3.2 -vs- 2.6 ± 1.8, p < 0.01) indicating larger infarcts. Patients with ST depression and 1-vessel CAD (47%) had higher QRS scores compared with patients with no ST depression (4.8 ± 2.9 -vs- 2.6 ± 1.8, p < 0.001) and had an increased prevalence of infarct-related arteries with a terminal branch supplying the LV lateral wall or apex. It was concluded that anterolateral ST depression during inferior AMI may indicate the presence of additionally stenosed arteries or that the infarct-related artery has a large vascular territory. The absence of ST depression virtually precludes multivessel CAD.

Many studies have established the usefulness of the 12-lead ECG in localizing the anatomic location of AMI. Likewise LV wall motion abnormalities by angiography have correlated well with the ECG location of AMI. Blanke and associates[5] from New York City and Goettingen, West Germany, did cardiac catheterization and coronary angiography within 6.3 ± 6.0 hours of onset of symptoms of AMI in 152 patients and correlated the ECG abnormalities during the first few hours of AMI with the coronary angiographic data to determine the usefulness of the "admission" ECG in predicting the AMI-related artery. All 152 patients had standard 12-lead ECGs recorded within 1 hour of cardiac catheterization. The ECG abnormalities present were correlated with the infarct-related artery as determined by coronary arteriography. ST-segment elevation was the most common finding in patients with the LAD or right coronary artery as the infarct-related artery. ST-segment depression was the most common abnormality in patients with the LC artery as the infarct-related artery. A classic pattern of anteroseptal AMI was seen in 93% of all patients with the LAD as the infarct-related artery. A classic pattern of inferior AMI was seen in 53% of patients with right or LC narrowing taken as 1 group. The pattern of true posterior and isolated lateral wall AMI in the absence of classic changes in the inferior leads was highly specific and predictive of LC narrowing. In contrast, the pattern of an inferior wall AMI, in the absence of true posterior or lateral wall changes, was highly specific and predictive of right coronary artery narrowing. Fifty-six percent of patients with LC artery as the infarct-related artery presented with nonclassic ECG abnormalities. The ECG patterns in patients with subtotal occlusions were similar to those of patients with total occlusions. Thus, the ECG obtained in the first few hours of AMI is reliable in localizing the LAD as the infarct-related artery. Certain patterns are specific but not sensitive in localizing the right coronary artery as opposed to the LC artery as the infarct-related artery. Presentation with signs and symptoms of AMI and a nonclassic ECG is suggestive of LC narrowing.

Braat and associates[6] from Maastricht, The Netherlands, recorded a right precordial lead V_4R ECG in addition to the standard 12-lead ECG in 84 patients with an inferior wall AMI admitted within 10 hours after the onset of chest pain. The presence or absence of ST-segment elevation in lead V_4R correlated with results of coronary angiography performed 2 to 26 weeks (mean, 10) after AMI. Patients were classified into 3 groups: those with a critical stenosis or occlusion proximal to the first RV branch (27 patients); those with stenosis distal to the RV branch of the right coronary artery (36 patients); and those with stenosis in the LC coronary artery (21 patients). The presence of ST-segment elevation ≥1 mm in lead V_4R had a sensitivity of 100% and a specificity of 87% for occlusion of the right coronary artery above the first RV branch; the predictive accuracy was 92%. Seven of 36 patients with a distal occlusion of the right coronary artery had ST-segment elevation of ≥1 mm in lead V_4R. The absence of ST-segment elevation ≥1 mm in lead V_4R excluded proximal occlusion of the right coronary artery. ST-segment elevation in lead V_4R was not seen either in 29 of 36 patients with a distal occlusion of the right coronary artery or in patients with an occlusion of the LC artery. Recording of lead V_4R within 10 hours after onset of acute inferior wall AMI can give information rapidly about the artery responsible for AMI. This could have implications when emergency procedures (streptokinase infusion, balloon dilation, and emergency surgery) are considered.

Echocardiographic observations

Nador and associates[7] from Milan, Italy, assessed the relation between echo and hemodynamic parameters in 28 patients with AMI who underwent M-mode echo and Swan-Ganz catheterization during the same hospitalization. On mitral valve echo, DE interval was measured and the area enclosed by mitral valve echo during DE interval (DE subarea) was calculated in each echo (Fig. 2-1). The DE subarea/DE interval ratio was computed for each measurement set. Hemodynamic parameters were obtained in the usual fashion. Patients with PA wedge pressure < 18 mmHg showed a DE interval markedly longer than patients with PA wedge > 18 mmHg: 82 ± 15 -vs- 55 ± 10 ms ($p < 0.001$). Patients with cardiac index > 2.2 liters $\min^{-1} m^{-2}$ had a DE subarea/DE interval ratio greater than patients with cardiac index < 2.2 liters $\min^{-1} m^{-2}$: 0.17 ± 0.4 -vs- 0.09 ± 0.02 $dM^2 \sec^{-1}$ ($p < 0.001$). Echo and hemodynamic data were then correlated in the whole study group; the DE interval was significantly ($p < 0.001$) and inversely correlated to PA wedge pressure; stroke index more than cardiac index was correlated ($p < 0.005$) both to DE subarea/DE interval ratio and to DE interval itself; DE interval was not affected by heart rate. Patients were able to be categorized into 4 subsets on the basis of echo measurements. These findings suggest the possibility of providing, through M-mode echo, a noninvasive and accurate evaluation of PA wedge pressure and stroke index.

Kan and associates[8] from Amsterdam, The Netherlands, assessed LV EF by biplane cross-sectional echo in 65 patients with a first AMI on the first

Fig. 2-1. Schematic drawing illustrating DE interval and respective subarea (hatched). Reproduced with permission from Nadar et al.[7]

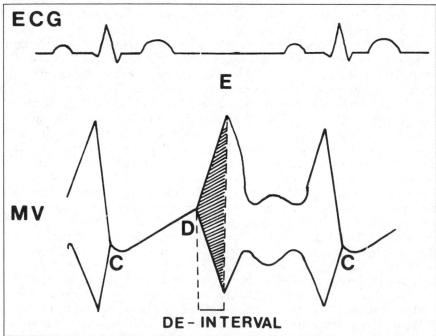

day. In 30 patients (group 1) measurements were repeated on the third day and the other 35 patients (group 2) at 3 months. Changes in EF of ≤0.05 were called insignificant. In group 1 only 2 patients had a decrease of >0.1 between days 1 and 3, and both had an enzymatically confirmed infarct extension. The remaining patients had no complications. In group 2, 11 patients had decreases of >0.1 between day 1 and 3 months; 3 of them had an enzymatically confirmed reinfarction (perioperative in 1) and 4, a possible reinfarction, and in 2, an angiographically confirmed LV aneurysm developed. In 2 no complications occurred. The other complications that occurred were an enzymatically confirmed but small reinfarction, an angiographically confirmed aneurysm, and an uncomplicated CABG in 1 patient each. These 3 patients had a small increase (0.5–0.1) in EF. Reproducibility of the method of measuring the EF was assessed concurrently in 20 outpatients with a previous AMI who were studied twice on the same day (with a 30-minute interval) by 2 different observers. The mean absolute difference in EF between the paired observations was 0: 0.4 ± 0.02 with a range of 0–0.07. Thus, only changes in EF of >0.1 correlated with clinically recognized complications. Changes between 0.05 and 0.1 may be due to spontaneous variability or to the limited reproducibility of the method.

Arvan and Varat[9] from Pittsburgh, Pennsylvania, examined 23 patients with an anterior wall AMI and persistent ST-segment elevations (group I) for wall motion abnormalities using 2-D echo: 22 (96%) had dyskinetic motion of the infarcted wall and 10 (43%) had a LV aneurysm. Among 15 patients who had a chronic anterior wall AMI without ST segment elevation (group II), 13 (86%) had akinesia of the infarcted segment. To document that dyskinetic wall motion caused the persistent ECG ST-segment elevations, 15 patients with an anterior wall AMI (group III) were followed by serial 2-D echo for 2–24 months (mean, 8). Of the 10 patients who had dyskinetic wall motion abnormalities on their initial 2-D echo, persistent ST-segment elevation developed in 9. All 5 patients with akinetic or severely hypokinetic wall motion abnormalities on their first 2-D echo did not show ST-segment elevation on late follow-up surface ECG. Infarct size as determined by peak creatine kinase levels for the former subgroup was greater than that for the latter subgroup (2,243 ± 429 -vs- 899 ± 320 IU, respectively, p < 0.01). Thus, persistent ST-segment elevation after an anterior wall AMI is indicative of dyskinetic wall motion rather than aneurysm formation. Dyskinesia precedes the appearance of ST-segment elevation and is probably responsible for these changes on the surface ECG. Infarct size is larger in persons in whom dyskinetic wall motion abnormalities are likely to develop.

Erlebacher and associates[10] from Baltimore, Maryland, obtained 2-D echoes from 27 patients within 72 hours of the onset of symptoms of transmural anterior wall AMI and from 13 healthy control subjects to evaluate mechanisms of LV dilation. Anterior and posterior endocardial segment lengths at end-diastole were measured with a microprocessor-based graphic system. Papillary muscles were used as internal landmarks to identify the anterior and posterior segments. The anterior ("infarcted") segment length in patients with AMI was 12 ± 2 cm (mean ± SD), whereas in the control subjects anterior segment length was 9 ± 1 cm (p < 0.001). Segment length in the posterior uninfarcted myocardium was not different between patients with infarcts and normal subjects. These data indicate that LV dilation during the first 3 days after transmural anterior AMI is due to dilation of the infarcted segment. The LV enlargement occurring by this mechanism may have significant implications for ventricular mechanics and infarct size estimation.

Van Reet and associates[11] from Houston, Texas, compared the information obtained from 2-D echo and gated radionuclide ventriculography in 93 patients with 95 episodes of AMI. The comparisons were made within 48 hours and at 10 days after AMI. The EF was determined by echo and radionuclide ventriculography and correlated well (r = 0.82) and did not change from the first 48 hours to 10 days after the event. Normal regional wall motion was detected equally well by echo and radionuclide ventriculography for anterior infarcts, but regional wall motion alterations in the inferior or posterior wall segments were better detected by echo (91 -vs- 61%, respectively). In-hospital mortality was 37 and 42% in those patients with an LV EF ≤35% by echo and radionuclide ventriculography and no deaths occurred in patients with an EF >40% by either test. The 1-year mortality rate was lowest in patients with an EF >49% or well-maintained regional wall motion and poorest in those with an EF <36% and marked alterations in regional wall motion by either technique. These data suggest that echo and radionuclide ventriculography provide complementary assessment of LV function and wall motion in patients with anterior wall AMI and that echo appears more sensitive in detecting inferoposterior wall motion abnormalities. Both techniques are capable of predicting some patients at risk for death during an acute event and with a 1-year follow-up.

Radionuclide angiographic observations

Hirsowitz and colleagues[12] from Detroit, Michigan, performed RNA studied in 26 patients with a first AMI, 11 with anterior and 15 with an inferior location. Mean LV EF in anterior AMI (33 ± 7) was lower than in inferior AMI (60 ± 10) (p < 0.001). Mean RV EF in the anterior infarct group was 41 ± 15 and in the inferior AMI group, 34 ± 13 (p, NS). The RV EF was < 40% in 11 of 15 with inferior and 7 of 11 with anterior AMI. The ratio of LV EF/RV EF was 0.84 ± 0.19 in the anterior and 2.13 ± 1.28 in the inferior AMI groups (p < 0.001). The LV EF correlated with RV EF in patients with anterior AMI (r = 0.77; p < 0.05) but not in those with inferior AMI (r = 0.14). The RV regional wall motion abnormalities were observed in the inferolateral zones in 10 of 15 with inferior and in 0 of 11 with anterior AMI (p < 0.001). Inferoseptal wall motion abnormalities were observed in 3 of 15 with inferior and 6 of 11 with anterior AMI (p, NS). The RV dysfunction in inferior AMI is probably an expression of primary RV dysfunction rather than secondary to LV dysfunction; RV dysfunction was proportional to LV dysfunction in the anterior AMI group and was often accompanied by RV septal contraction abnormalities.

Fox and coworkers[13] from St. Louis, Missouri, determined whether coronary thrombi could be detected scintigraphically after AMI using indium-111 labeled platelets and technetium-99m labeled red blood cells. Twenty-four patients were studied, including 9 with suspected AMI evaluated within 9 hours of the onset of symptoms and again 18–24 hours after onset. Eight patients with neurologic symptoms but without cardiac disease and 7 patients with angina but without AMI served as unmatched control subjects.

Foci of net indium accumulation were detected after image processing that incorporated subtraction of blood pool activity. In patients with AMI, distinct foci of net indium accumulation were present in regions corresponding to the coronary artery supplying ischemic zones. This occurred in 7 of 8 patients at the time of the earliest study (5.6 ± 3.3 hours, mean ± SD) and 8 of 9 patients at the time of subsequent imaging (23.6 ± 1.9 hours). Only 1 of the 15 control patients demonstrated a cardiac focus of net indium accumulation. Thus, this method may permit relatively early detection and sequential assessment of coronary artery thrombi large enough to be detected.

Usefulness of computed tomography

Masuda and coworkers[14] from Chiba, Japan, performed conventional and enhanced computed tomographic (CT) examinations in 103 patients with an AMI for evaluation of the diagnostic usefulness of CT. After intravenous bolus injection of contrast material, an initial filling defect and late enhancement of the infarcted myocardium appeared on the CT images. These 2 findings were evidence of AMI; the former was found mostly in patients with recent AMI, and the later was recognized both in those with recent and those with healed AMI. Wall thinning at the site of AMI was found by enhanced CT, mostly in patients with anteroseptal or extensive anterior AMI. An LV aneurysm and LV thrombi were found by enhanced CT in 39 and in 23 of the 103 subjects, respectively, and the sensitivity of CT in detecting intracardiac thrombi was higher than that of 2-D echo. Calcified myocardium and pericardial effusion associated with AMI were also detected by conventional nonenhanced CT. These patients underwent CT scanning with intravenous drip infusion and close ECG monitoring and the time required for an examination was approximately 30 minutes. Side effects were minor. Although cardiac CT may be useful in evaluating patients with AMI, the economy of this technique must be carefully weighed against information from other techniques.

Thromboxane A$_2$

Walinsky and associates[15] from Philadelphia, Pennsylvania, evaluated the presence of thromboxane B$_2$, the stable metabolite of thromboxane A$_2$, early in the course of AMI in both animals and patients. In an open chest model, the LAD coronary artery was isolated and the great cardiac vein was cannulated in 9 dogs. After occlusion of the LAD, there was an increase in thromboxane B$_2$ concentration from 0.77 ± 0.09–1.79 ± 0.46 pmol/ml (p < 0.05) and 1.96 ± 0.48 pmol/ml (p < 0.05) at 1 and 5 minutes, respectively, after coronary occlusion. At 30 and 60 minutes after occlusion, there was no significant increase compared with the baseline. In 17 patients with AMI, the mean thromboxane B$_2$ concentration was 0.96 ± 0.13 pmol/ml at 4.88 ± 0.40 hours after the onset of chest pain. In 12 patients with sequential samples before and after restoration of patency of the occluded artery, the initial concentration was 0.71 ± 0.058 pmol/ml. At 5 minutes after restoration of patency, thromboxane B$_2$ concentration was 1.1 ± 0.17 pmol/ml (p = 0.05). One hour later, a return to baseline occurred (0.82 ± 0.75 pmol/ml). It was concluded that generation of thromboxane A$_2$ occurs during the early stages of AMI and may be important in AMI.

INFARCT SIZE: ASSESSING IT AND FACTORS AFFECTING IT

DePace and associates[16] from Philadelphia, Pennsylvania, determined whether resting ischemia limits the usefulness of the QRS scoring system in predicting LV EF in AMI. These investigators studied 48 patients after AMI by means of 12-lead ECG, thallium-201 scintigraphy, and RNA. The thallium-201 scintigrams showed fixed defects in 25 patients, perfusion defects with partial or complete redistribution in the delayed images in 19 patients, and normal images in the remaining 4 patients. In the 48 patients there was a significant correlation between the QRS score and LV EF (r = −0.67; p < 0.001). Patients with fixed defects had a better correlation than patients with resting ischemia (r = −0.77 -vs- r = −0.60). A QRS score of ≤3 was used to separate patients with LV EF of ≥40% from those with lower LV EF in patients with fixed defects (p = 0.0005), but this cutoff did not categorize patients with resting ischemia as to LV EF. Thus, the presence of rest ischemia in patients with AMI affects the correlation between QRS score and LV EF.

Serial changes in plasma creatine kinase (CK) have been widely used to estimate infarct size in animal and human studies since their development in 1970. The enzymatic estimate of AMI size has correlated with the other clinical parameters, reflecting the extent of myocardial loss, but few direct comparisons have been made with postmortem anatomic measurements. The Multicenter Investigation of Limitation of Infarct Size (MILIS) program provided an opportunity to compare independent estimates of infarct size obtained with the anatomic and enzymatic methods. Hackel and colleagues[17] along with the MILIS study group compared enzymatic estimates of AMI size based on plasma levels of CK-MB with anatomic infarct size in 49 human hearts obtained at autopsy. The patients studied had been enrolled in the MILIS study program within 18 hours of the onset of AMI and were treated at 1 of 5 participating hospitals. Infarct size was estimated from serial measurements of plasma CK-MB made at the core laboratory for CK analysis. Hearts obtained at autopsy were studied independently by the core pathology laboratory without knowledge of the CK-MB levels or clinical results. Data from the 2 laboratories were compared at the data coordinating center. Of 49 hearts, 12 were excluded either because anatomic infarct size could not be established or because the infarct occurring at the time of enrollment in the MILIS study could not be distinguished with certainty from other infarcts. Of the remaining 37 hearts, peak CK-MB level was available in 36, but samples sufficient for estimation of infarct size were available in 25. The overall correlation coefficient was 0.87 for these 25 hearts, indicating that enzymatic estimates of infarct size correlated closely with anatomic measurements (Fig. 2-2). The results indicate that CK estimates of AMI size represent a valid clinical end point for assessing AMI size, and the effect of therapy thereon, in groups of treated and control patients. However, investigators and clinicians must be aware of the vitiating factors of a previous infarction, infarct extension, pharmacologic agents, and reperfusion with wash-out on the enzymatic estimates of AMI size.

Sinusas and associates[18] from Burlington, Vermont, evaluated the pathoanatomic correlates of qualitative assessment of regional wall motion

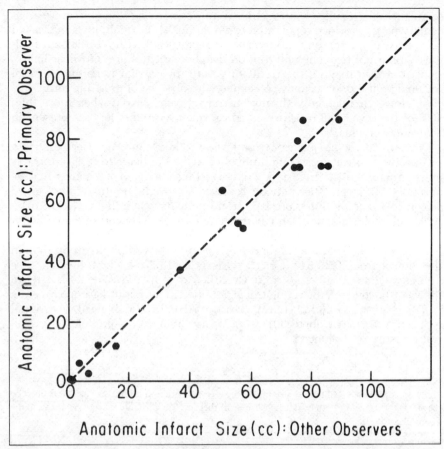

Fig. 2-2   Relation between the official anatomic estimates submitted to the data coordinating center by the primary observer and anatomic estimates of infarct size by independent observers. The dashed line is the line of unity. r (Spearman) = 0.94. Reproduced with permission from Hackel et al.[17]

on routine equilibrium RNA in 62 patients who had RNA within 3 months of death. Of 51 patients with abnormal regional wall motion, 46 (90%) had gross myocardial lesions at autopsy. Of 11 patients with normal regional wall motion, 9 (82%) had normal myocardium. Complete agreement of regional wall motion with postmortem findings in all LV segments occurred in 32% of the patients. Compared with postmortem findings, abnormal regional wall motion on RNA overestimated the number of macroscopically abnormal segments in 21% of the patients and underestimated them in 47%. Of 372 segments analyzed, the overall sensitivity, specificity, and predictive value of abnormal regional wall motion on RNA for detecting gross AMI or fibrosis was 73, 75, and 83%, respectively. There were 35 false positive segments (9%; 15 patients). In 27 of these segments (77%) severe stenosis of the coronary artery supplying the segment or ECG left BBB could explain these findings. There were 61 false negative segments (16%; 30 patients). In 55 of these segments (90%), either nontransmural infarction or masking by severe adjacent asynergy provided a potential explanation. Thus, qualitative analysis of regional wall motion on routine RNA correlates well with postmortem findings. Abnormal regional wall motion usually indicates gross myocardial lesions, but also may be the result of severe myocardial ischemia. Normal regional wall motion usually correlates with absence of gross anatomic disease. However, regional wall motion may appear normal when more than 50% of the myocardium is preserved or when severe asynergy is present in adjacent segments.

Bussmann and associates[19] from Frankfurt am Main, West Germany, in a prospective control study, randomly allocated 29 patients to receive intravenous verapamil (5–10 mg/h) for 2 days starting at a mean of 8 hours after the onset of AMI. Twenty-five patients received no specific treatment and served as controls. The LV filling pressure in all patients was initially <15 mmHg. Age, infarct localization, and hemodynamic values on admission (Swan-Ganz catheter) were comparable in both groups. Maximal creatine kinase (CK) and CK-MB values were markedly lower in the verapamil group than in the control group (CK, 547 -vs- 703 U/liter; CK-MB, 51 -vs- 68 U/liter), as was infarct weight (CK, 48 -vs- 65 gEq; CK-MB, 31 -vs- 49 gEq) (Fig. 2-3). Arterial BP was 10% lower in the verapamil group than in the control group. Systemic vascular resistance and LV filling pressure remained unchanged. Verapamil reduced AMI size by about 30% in patients without LV failure and the arterial pressure was reduced.

Fig. 2-3.   CK and CK-MB infarct size in 54 patients. Reduction in infarct size as determined by CK and CK-MB enzyme activity during verapamil therapy. The differences were clearer with the isoenzyme CK-MB.

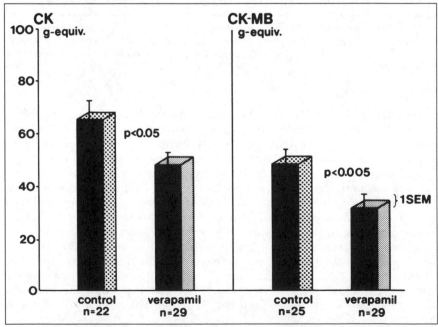

COMPLICATIONS

Atrioventricular block

Feigl and coworkers[20] from Holon, Israel, evaluated 288 patients with inferior AMI to determine the frequency and prognostic significance of AV block. Second- and third-degree AV block was found in 37 patients (14%). Three of the 37 patients died. In the 34 survivors AV block was differentiated into early and late. In 15 patients, second- and third-degree AV block developed within 6 hours of the onset of AMI. In these patients, the AV block disappeared within 24 hours after AMI. Atropine often abolished AV block completely or caused an acceleration of ventricular escape rhythm in these patients. In contrast, in 14 patients second- and third-degree AV block developed later than 6 hours after AMI. It was often followed by long periods of first-degree AV block and the total duration of AV block was >40 hours. Atropine did not abolish AV block in these patients and acceleration of ventricular rates after atropine was slight. These data indicate that the 2 types of AV block appear to have different mechanisms in patients with inferior AMI. Increased vagal tone may be responsible for the first type and metabolic changes due to ischemia, for the second type. Responsiveness to atropine is better in those with early compared with late AV block, and pacing would appear to be rarely indicated.

Sclarovsky and colleagues[21] from Petah-Tiqva, Israel, described 76 patients with inferior AMI and advanced AV block. According to preestablished ECG criteria and time of appearance of the advanced AV block, the patients were divided into 2 groups. The early block group consisted of 31 patients who developed advanced AV block during the hyperacute ECG stage of AMI. Advanced AV block in these patients was characterized by early appearance, short duration, third degree type block, poor response to atropine, and increased need for pacemaker therapy. The late block group consisted of 45 patients who developed advanced AV block during subsequent ECG stages of AMI. Advanced AV block in them was characterized by late appearance, longer duration, second degree type block, positive response to atropine, and diminished need for pacemaker therapy. Morbidity and mortality also differed between both groups. Patients with early block had more syncope (32 -vs- 2%, p < 0.0001), more CHF (36 -vs- 7%, p < 0.005), and more cardiogenic shock (39 -vs- 2%, p < 0.001) than patients with late block. The mortality rate in the early block group was high (23%) and similar to that previously reported, whereas the mortality rate in the late block group was low (7%, p < 0.05) and similar to the mortality rate reported for inferior AMI without advanced AV block. These data identify a subgroup of patients with inferior AMI and advanced AV block, accounting for the high mortality rate.

Strasberg and associates[22] from Tel-Aviv, Israel, studied 139 consecutive patients with a first inferior wall AMI and 26 (19%) developed advanced AV block and 113 (81%) did not. All patients were evaluated by 2-D echo and RNA. Patients with advanced AV block had lower RNA LV EF (51 ± 10 -vs- 58 ± 11%), higher LV wall motion score on 2-D echo (5.6 ± 2.6 -vs- 3.1 ± 2.7, p < 0.001), lower radionuclide RV EF (32 ± 15 -vs- 39 ± 16%, p < 0.001) and higher RV wall motion score on 2-D echo (3.4 ± 1.7 -vs- 1.5 ± 2,

TABLE 2-1. *Clinical and biventricular function data in patients with acute inferior myocardial infarction and with or without advanced atrioventricular block*

			WITHOUT ADVANCED AV BLOCK (N = 113)		WITH ADVANCED AV BLOCK (N = 26)
Sex (# men)			86		17
Age (yr)					
		Mean	60 ± 9	NS	64 ± 11
		Range	35–79		44–84
Radionuclide	LV	mean	58 ± 11	p < 0.01	51 ± 10
ejection		range	32–88		32–68
fraction (%)	RV	mean	39 ± 16	p < 0.001	32 ± 15
		range	4–86		6–64
2-D echo	LV	mean	3.1 ± 2.7	p < 0.001	5.6 ± 2.6
wall motion		range	0–11		0–10
score	RV	mean	1.5 ± 2	p < 0.002	3.4 ± 1.7
		range	0–7		0–7
RV dysfunction			45 pt. (40%)	p < 0.02	20 pts (78%)
Mortality			7 pts	NS	4 pts (15%)

$p < 0.002$) than did patients without AV block (Table 2-1). The incidence rate of RV dysfunction was higher in patients with advanced AV block (78 -vs- 40%, $p < 0.02$), and the mortality rate was also higher (although not significantly) in patients with advanced AV block (15 -vs- 6%). In conclusion, patients with inferior AMI and advanced AV block have larger infarct sizes (as seen on RNA and 2-D echo) and lower RV and LV function than patients without AV block, which may explain the higher mortality rate.

Ventricular tachycardia

Polymorphous VT is believed to be uncommon during AMI. Grenadier and associates[23] from Haifa, Israel, reviewed 771 consecutive patients admitted with AMI for the occurrence of this arrhythmia. Nine patients (1.2%) had polymorphous VT. No patient had any other predisposing factors previously associated with polymorphous VT. The arrhythmia was resistant to multiple drugs, and repeated cardioversion was effective in only 3 patients. Overdrive pacing was ineffective in the 3 patients in whom it was attempted. Verapamil was effective in 3 of 4 patients in whom it was tried. Six patients with polymorphous VT died during hospitalization; the remaining 3 died within 6 months of discharge. It is concluded that, when compared with regular VT, polymorphous VT in AMI carries a poor prognosis. When the arrhythmia occurs in the context of acute ischemia, it appears to be more difficult to treat compared with other predisposing factors. Verapamil, not usually indicated for ventricular arrhythmias, should be tested in a therapeutic trial.

Left ventricular thrombus

Stratton and Ritchie[24] from Seattle, Washington, prospectively studied patients with LV thrombi not caused by healed AMI by indium-111 platelet imaging and 2-D echo to determine the reproducibility of these techniques and the short-term effects of sulfinpyrazone (200 mg 4 times daily), aspirin (325 mg 3 times daily), plus dipyridamole (75 mg 3 times daily), and full-dose warfarin. At baseline, all patients underwent indium-111 platelet imaging and echo, and the results were positive for thrombus. In 6 patients on no antithrombotic drug therapy, repeat platelet scans and echo studies in 6 weeks remained positive and were unchanged. In 7 patients studied on sulfinpyrazone, 3 platelet scans became negative, 2 became equivocal, and 2 were unchanged. The presence and size of thrombus was constant by echo in all 7 patients. Of the 6 patients studied on aspirin plus dipyridamole, 1 platelet scan became negative, those of 3 became equivocal, and 2 were unchanged; all echo findings remained positive, but 1 patient had decreased thrombus size. Among 4 warfarin-treated patients, 3 had resolution of platelet deposition, 1 was unchanged; by echo thrombus resolved in 1 patient, was decreased in size in 1, and was unchanged in 2. These investigators concluded that in the absence of antithrombotic drug therapy, platelet imaging, and echo findings are stable in patients with LV thrombi not caused by AMI. Sulfinpyrazone, aspirin plus dipyridamole, and warfarin all interrupt platelet deposition in some patients with chronic LV thrombi. The hematologic activity of LV thrombus, i.e., the extent of ongoing platelet incorporation, may be inhibited by short-term drug therapy without significant changes in echo-measured thrombus size. Although these findings were obtained in patients with remote AMI whose thrombi were chronic, an important consideration in the implication of this study is that more rapid changes in thrombus mass might be found in recently formed thrombi, such as those associated with AMI.

Johannessen and associates[25] from Bergen, Norway, in a prospective study of 90 consecutive patients with AMI, found 28% by cross-sectional echo to have LV thrombus. All had anterior wall AMI. Of the 28 patients with an inferior wall AMI, none had an LV thrombus. Five (5.5.%) of the 90 patients had a cerebral vascular accident and all had an anterior wall AMI. In 4 of these 5 patients an LV thrombus was confirmed by echo before this cerebral vascular accident. All patients with LV thrombus had apical akinesis.

To test the hypothesis that LV thrombi that project into the lumen and are mobile are more likely to embolize than those that do not have these characteristics, Meltzer and associates[26] from Amsterdam, The Netherlands, and New York City, reviewed retrospectively 2-D echoes of 16 patients with LV thrombi detected during AMI. Ten had evidence of peripheral emboli and 6 did not. Each echo, reviewed without knowledge of the clinical data, was graded as showing a protruding or nonprotruding LV thrombus and the presence or absence of increased mobility. The thrombus projected into the lumen on the echoes of 8 of 10 patients who had had emboli and in 0 of 6 who had not. The thrombus had increased mobility in 4 of 10 patients with emboli and 0 of 6 without. Thus, LV thrombi that project into the lumen and have increased mobility are more likely to embolize than those without these characteristics.

Dressler's syndrome

The post AMI syndrome was described by Dressler in 1956, and numerous studies since then have estimated its incidence at <5% of patients with

AMI. Northcote and associates[27] from Glasgow, Scotland, determined the frequency of Dressler's syndrome in 80 consecutive patients with proved AMI admitted to the coronary care unit and studied prospectively during a 5-month period in 1982 and 1983. Each patient was examined daily during hospital stay and at 3 and 6 weeks after onset of AMI. All patients received anticoagulants unless specifically contraindicated. The anticoagulation consisted of intravenous heparin infusion for 48 hours and continued with oral warfarin. A diagnosis of Dressler's syndrome was made if all of the following conditions developed or persisted for >1 week after onset of AMI: pleural pericardial pain, pericardial friction rub, temperature >37.5°C, and erythrocyte sedimentation rate >40 mm/hour. Of 80 patients admitted to the coronary care unit with AMI, 56 had anterior and 44 had posterior transmural AMI: 23 patients (28%) had post AMI pericarditis and in each patient pericardial friction occurred in the first week after AMI. A diagnosis of Dressler's syndrome was made in 4 patients in the first 6 weeks after AMI. In each patient there had been early post AMI pericarditis. Thus, Dressler's syndrome continues to be a complication of AMI, although aggressive treatment with anti-inflammatory agents for early post AMI pericarditis and more judicious use of anticoagulant drugs may reduce its frequency.

Left ventricular aneurysm

To assess the clinical and prognostic importance of the early appearance of LV aneurysm after AMI, Meizlish and associates[28] from New Haven, Connecticut, used equilibrium RNA to study 51 patients with an initial anterior wall transmural AMI. A functional aneurysm was defined as an area of systolic akinesis or dyskinesis with a distinct diastolic deformity and preserved adjacent wall motion. Functional aneurysms developed in 18 patients (group 1). The LV EF was comparable in this group and in the 33 patients without aneurysm (group 2) (27 ± 10 -vs- 31 ± 12%). One-year mortality was markedly different, with 11 deaths (61%) in group 1 and 3 (9%) in group 2. Six (55%) of the deaths in group 1 were sudden. Patients with a functional aneurysm appearing within 48 hours had the highest risk of dying (8 of 10). Thus, early formation of a functional aneurysm occurs frequently after anterior AMI and carries a high risk of death within 1 year that is independent of EF. In addition, the absence of a functional aneurysm identifies a large group with a low 1-year mortality despite a markedly impaired EF.

Foster and associates[29] from Manchester, England, performed computed tomography (CT) in 20 patients with LV aneurysm documented by LV angiography. Measurements of LV short axis, percentage of nonaneurysmal myocardium, and size of aneurysm were determined by both techniques. Qualitative assessments of LV size together with the anatomic relation of the LV aneurysm also were made. The aneurysm was assessed for resectability by both techniques using these criteria. In all cases there was a distinct and diagnostic change in the contour of the ventricle on CT, and CT indicated 8 aneurysms to be unresectable, which agreed with the angiographic assessment. Of the remaining 12 aneurysms, 7 were considered to be resectable on angiography. Thus, CT appears to be a reliable noninvasive technique for identifying LV aneurysm and a useful screening method for identifying unresectable aneurysm.

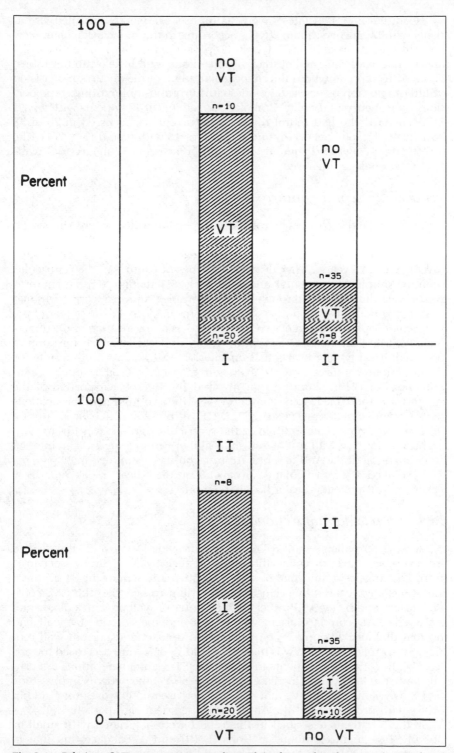

Fig. 2-4. Relation of VT to aneurysm type (I or II) in the combined group of surgical and autopsy patients. Top. Occurrence of VT according to aneurysm type. Bottom. Occurrence of aneurysm type according to presence of VT. Reproduced with permission from Hochman et al.[30]

Hochman and associates[30] from Baltimore, Maryland, classified 73 patients with LV aneurysm into 2 types according to the endocardial characteristics of the aneurysmal wall: type I, 30 patients, in whom the endocardial aneurysmal wall consisted of thick fibrous tissue with little or no thrombus, and type II, those in whom the endocardial lining of the aneurysm consisted of little to no fibrous or elastic tissue with thrombus obliterating some portion of the aneurysmal cavity. Emboli occurred in 5 of 43 patients with type II LV aneurysm who had mural thrombi. Recurrent VT occurred in 20 of 33 patients with type I aneurysm but in only 8 of 43 with type II (Fig. 2-4). The investigators concluded that structural differences in LV aneurysmal walls had functional significance.

Ventricular septal rupture

Edwards and associates[31] from Minneapolis and Rochester, Minnesota, studied at necropsy 53 hearts with rupture of the ventricular septum during AMI: 33 were from men (average age, 76 years) and 20 were from women (average age, 73 years). They described 2 types of rupture of the ventricular septum: simple (28 patients) and complex (25 patients). Simple ruptures were direct through-and-through defects. Complex ruptures were associated with serpiginous dissection tracts remote from the primary site of tear of the ventricular septum. Specimens were classified as to the location of the underlying AMI and the level of the septum (apex to base) at which the rupture occurred. Twenty-nine hearts had an inferior AMI and 24 had an anterior AMI. Complex ruptures occurred in 20 with inferior AMI (69%) and in 5 with anterior AMI (21%). Rupture that involved the inferobasal portion of the septum was more likely to be complex (94%) than rupture in other locations (27%). Significant 3-vessel obstructive CAD was present in 48 hearts. Rupture of a second structure in addition to the ventricular septum was observed in 11 hearts (LV free wall in 9 cases and papillary muscle in 2). The interval from the onset of the AMI to septal rupture could be estimated in 22 patients and averaged 4 days (median, 2.5 days). Complete heart block reportedly occurred in 6 patients during hospitalization.

Right ventricular infarction

Among 69 patients with ST elevations in leads V_1–V_5 and subjected to intracoronary or intravenous thrombolytic therapy, Geft and associates[32] from Los Angeles, California, observed 5 patients in whom the ST-segment elevations were caused by occlusion of the right rather than the LAD coronary artery and by RV AMI rather than LV anterior wall or ventricular septal AMI. The LAD coronary artery was patent and the anterior LV wall had normal thallium-201 uptake, no technetium uptake, and normal wall motion. ST-segment elevation was highest in lead V_1 or V_2 and decreased toward lead V_5. In contrast to patients in whom the ST-segment elevations are usually lowest in lead V_1 and increased toward lead V_5, the patients in this study had R waves in leads V_1–V_5 that did not decrease and Q waves that did not evolve with progression of the AMI. The ST-segment elevations in leads V_1–V_5 in the 5 patients described in this report were associated with small or absent ST-segment elevations in leads II, III, and AVF, suggesting that in other cases of RV AMI, the appearance of ST-segment elevations in leads

V_1–V_5 is blocked by the dominant electrical forces of the LV inferior AMI. This report indicates that the ECG is useful in diagnosing RV AMI and diagnosis of the latter, of course, is important for therapeutic purposes.

Morgera and associates[33] from Trieste, Italy, compared 2 groups of patients with AMI with regard to specificity and sensitivity of ECG criteria characteristic of RV AMI. Group 1 included 21 patients with LV inferior AMI and with a variable degree of RV involvement; group 2 included 9 patients with AMI confined to the LV inferior wall. In both groups the presence of ST elevation ($\geq$0.05 mV) and the morphology of the QRS complex in V_4R, V_3R, and V_1 were assessed in ECGs performed on admission. Also, to evaluate the morphology of the ST segment and QRS complex in right precordial leads in normal subjects, an ECG with 12 standard and 4 right precordial leads (V_6R–V_3R) was performed in 82 subjects (group 3) without clinical and ECG evidence of heart disease. In normal subjects an rS pattern was always present in V_3R and frequently (91%) in V_4R. On the contrary, the presence of QS or QR complexes in both V_4R and V_3R was a specific marker for RV necrosis (specificity, 100%; sensitivity, 78%) (Fig. 2-5). The presence of injury and necrosis waves in V_4R or V_4R–V_3R during LV inferior AMI is a useful diagnostic criterion in that it ensures a highly specific diagnosis of RV AMI in (most) (76 and 71%, respectively) patients with autopsy evidence of RV involvement.

A high incidence of AV nodal block is anticipated in patients with LV inferior wall AMI accompanied by RV involvement, because right coronary artery occlusion would be proximal to the AV node branch. Braat and colleagues[34] from Maastricht, The Netherlands, in 67 consecutive patients with LV inferior wall AMI, performed technetium-99m pyrophosphate scintigraphy 36–72 hours after the onset of chest pain to detect RV involvement. All patients were continuously monitored during at least 3 days to detect rhythm and conduction disturbances. In 29 patients RV involvement was diagnosed by scintigraphy. None of these 29 patients had clinical signs of right-sided CHF. Fourteen of the 19 patients showing AV nodal conduction disturbances

Fig. 2-5. Typical ECG pattern of left inferior infarction associated with RV AMI. Reproduced with permission from Morgera et al.[33]

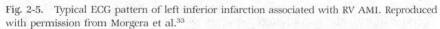
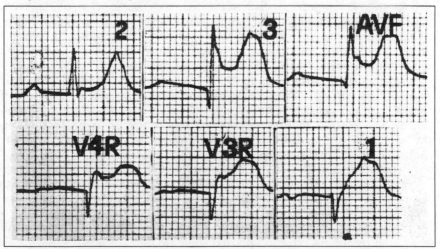

in the setting of LV inferior wall AMI also had RV involvement. Therefore the incidence of high degree AV nodal block in patients with RV involvement (14 of 29 patients) was 48% compared with only 13% (5 of 38) in patients with LV inferior AMI without RV involvement.

Hypotension in LV inferior AMI may be due to extensive RV involvement. Jugdutt and associates[35] from Edmonton, Canada, studied 24 patients with LV inferior AMI and hypotension (systolic BP < 100 mmHg) within 48 hours of admission, by 2-D echo. The extent was measured of regional RV and LV asynergy (akinesis or dyskinesis) in parasternal short-axis sections at mitral, chordal, midpapillary and low papillary muscle levels. Initial right-sided heart catheterization revealed predominant RV dysfunction in 16 patients (group 1) and predominant LV dysfunction in 8 patients (group 2). For all patients, the initial 2D echo revealed: (1) biventricular asynergy involving the posterior RV wall, posterior LV wall, and posterior portion of the ventricular septum; (2) a wide range of values for the extent of asynergy (RV, 21–90%; LV, 19–48%); and (3) a direct correlation between peak creatine kinase levels and percentage of LV asynergy (r = 0.80; p < 0.001) or percentage of RV plus LV asynergy (r = 0.72; p < 0.001). Although the extent of LV asynergy was similar in the 2 groups (34 -vs- 34%, NS), the extent of RV asynergy was greater in group 1 than in group 2 (57 -vs- 30%, p < 0.001). More important, the ratio of RV/LV asynergy was greater for group 1 than group 2 (1.75 -vs- 0.89, p < 0.001), and this difference in ratios between the 2 groups also was found in 2D echo studies at 10 days and 6 months. A RV/LV asynergy ratio value of 1.1 provided clear separation between the groups. Thus, the RV/LV asynergy ratio on an initial 2D echo can clarify the clinical syndrome of hypotension in patients with LV inferior AMI. An increased asynergy ratio might identify those patients with predominant RV involvement.

Jugdutt and colleagues[36] from Edmonton, Canada, studied 17 patients with predominant RV AMI by 2-D echo. The RV AMI was defined by inferior AMI on ECG with clinical RV failure without LV decompensation. On initial 2D echo, all had abnormal wall motion, defined as akinesis plus dyskinesis, in the inferior RV wall, inferior portion of the ventricular septum, and inferior LV wall. The extent of RV -vs- LV abnormal wall motion in short-axis sections at mitral, chordal, and papillary levels was 58 -vs- 29%, 56 -vs- 38%, and 59 -vs- 38%, respectively. The calculated topographic extent of abnormal wall motion was greater in the right than in the left ventricle (58 -vs- 36%, p < 0.05), and the corresponding RV/LV ratio (1.65) exceeded (p < 0.001) unity. Peak creatine phosphokinase levels correlated significantly (p < 0.001) with the topographic extent of LV abnormal wall motion (r = 0.79) or RV plus LV abnormal wall motion (r = 0.75). Although all patients had dilated RV cavities, 8 also had dilated LV cavities. Serial studies detected the cause of mechanical complications, mural echo densities suggesting thrombi, and persistent abnormal wall motion in survivors. Thus, 2D echo provided important data concerning clinical course, and assessment of RV and LV abnormal wall motion confirmed predominant RV involvement.

Hypotension and shock associated with heart block and other forms of AV dissociation frequently accompany RV AMI. Such patients do not invariably improve with ventricular pacing. Love and associates[37] from Worcester, Massachusetts, evaluated the relative effects of AV dissociated rhythms (ventricular pacing or nodal rhythm) and AV synchronous rhythms (atrial pacing, AV sequential pacing, or return to normal sinus rhythm) in 7 patients with RV

AMI complicated by AV dissociation, who had hypotension or shock. Hemo-dynamic monitoring demonstrated the characteristic features of RV AMI in all patients. Restoration of AV synchrony resulted in a highly significant ($p\leqslant0.001$) increase in systolic BP (88 ± 17–133 ± 22 mmHg), cardiac output (3.8 ± 0.9–5.7 ± 0.9 liters/min), and stroke volume (41 ± 7–61 ± 10 ml). Thus, restoration of normal AV synchrony has a marked effect on stroke volume in this setting, and atrial or AV pacing can reverse hypotension and shock in RV AMI complicated by AV dissociation. Therapy for hypotension complicating RV AMI should include the following: intravenous fluid admin-istration to elevate mean RA pressure; attempts to maintain normal sinus rhythm, such as early cardioversion and antiarrhythmic therapy for AF; atrial or AV sequential pacing for AV dissociated rhythms (which are refrac-tory to intravenous atropine or persist after multiple doses of atropine) while avoiding isolated ventricular pacing whenever possible; and intravenous cat-echolamines or afterload-reducing agents when indicated.

Pericarditis

To examine how often pericardial disease is associated with AMI and how often it is diagnosed by ECG, Krainin and associates[38] from Worcester, Mas-sachusetts, determined the frequency of diagnostic (stage 1 present) ST-seg-ment changes in 423 consecutive patients admitted to the coronary care unit because of AMI. Auscultation and ECG were performed at least once daily in all patients and at least twice daily in those presenting with new chest pain of

TABLE 2-2. *Selected clinical and ECG characteristics in 423 patients with AMI ac-cording to the presence or absence of pericarditis. Reproduced with permission from Krainin et al.*[38]

	# PATIENTS		
	PERICARDITIS	NO PERICARDITIS	
# patients	31	392	
Sex			
Male	25	246	$\chi^2 = 4.1$
Female	6	146	$p < 0.05$
Killip class			
I	13	239	
II	12	103	$\chi^2 = 20.8$
III	2	44	$p < 0.001$
IV	4	6	
Infarct			
Q wave	27	206	$\chi^2 = 15.7$
Non-Q wave	3	186	$p < 0.001$
Left BBB	1	0	
Infarct zone (Q wave, n = 233)			
Anterior	13	83	$\chi^2 = 3.2$
Inferior	12	123	NS
Combined	2	0	
Mortality	4	48	$\chi^2 = 2.0$
			NS

any description or a pericardial rub: 31 patients had pericardial rubs, usually detected within the first 4 days after admission (Table 2-2). Only 1 of the 31 had diagnostic ECG changes. The 31 patients with "pericarditis" differed significantly from the 392 patients without pericarditis in several respects: male predominance; Killip classes II, III, and IV; and Q-wave infarcts. However, differences in the location of the infarct and in mortality were not significant. The investigators concluded that during AMI-associated pericarditis, the pericardial rub is the most frequent clinical sign and that ST-segment changes diagnostic of pericarditis are rare. These findings are consistent with confinement of the pericardial involvement to the infarct zone.

IDENTIFYING THE HIGH RISK PATIENT

Familial aggregation of CAD is a well-known phenomenon. Among first-degree relatives of patients with AMI, CAD is at least twice as common as among relatives of control subjects. Spouses of affected patients, however, also have twice the risk of controls. Significant spouse concordance has been found for several risk factors, including BP, lipids, blood glucose, body weight, and cigarette smoking. In general, such spouse concordance has been interpreted as the result of a common marital environment. Under such a hypothesis, concordance should increase over time as marital couples continue to share the same environment. Ten Kate and associates[39] from Seattle, Washington, studied the frequency of AMI and CAD among the first-degree relatives of 126 spouses of male survivors of AMI and compared them with the frequency of AMI in CAD among relatives of 126 age-matched control subjects. Both AMI and CAD were as frequent among the relatives of the wives as among the relatives of their husbands with AMI, but were less frequent among the relatives of control subjects. Familial aggregation of CAD therefore is not limited to patients' relatives, but also affects the wives' families. This finding can be explained by assortative mating, i.e., marriage partners choose mates with similar lifestyles and risk factors that lead to CAD.

Approximately 15% of patients who survive the acute phase of AMI die in the first year after hospital discharge. To identify patients at high and low risk for cardiac death at 1-year follow-up, Olson and colleagues[40] from Long Beach, California, obtained RNA and 24-hour Holter monitor recordings in 115 AMI patients at hospital discharge. The VPC were graded as complicated or uncomplicated. Complicated VPC included unifocal VPC $\geq$ 10/1000 beats for 24 hours, multiform VPC, VPC in pairs, and VT. At hospital discharge, 38 of the 115 patients (33%) had complicated VPC. The LV EF at hospital discharge was 45 $\pm$ 15% (range, 12–74%). During the 1-year follow-up period, there were 12 cardiac deaths. Eight patients died suddenly (death within 2 hours after onset of symptoms) and 4 patients died of AMI. Of the 38 patients with complicated VPC, 8 (21%) had cardiac death at follow-up compared with 4 of 77 patients (5%) with uncomplicated or no VPC (p < 0.01). The LV EF was 29 $\pm$ 13% in cardiac death patients compared with 48 $\pm$ 13% in the survivors (p < 0.001). Sudden death patients had an LV EF of 24 $\pm$ 9% compared with 40 $\pm$ 5% in patients who died of AMI (p < 0.01). High risk patients (patients with complicated VPC and LV EF < 40%) had a 40% mortality rate at 1 year, whereas low risk patients (patients with uncomplicated or

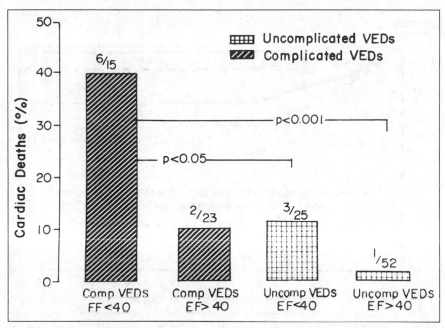

Fig. 2-6. Incidence of cardiac death at follow-up in four subgroups. Subgroup 1 includes patients with complicated VPC and LV EF < 40%, subgroup 2 includes patients with complicated VPC and LV EF > 40%, subgroup 3 includes patients with uncomplicated or no VPC and LV EF < 40%, and subgroup 4 includes patients with uncomplicated or no VPC and LV EF > 40%. VED = VPC. Reproduced with permission from Olson et al.[40]

no VPC and LV EF > 40%) had a 2% mortality rate (p < 0.001) (Fig. 2-6). It was concluded that RNA and 24-hour Holter monitoring at hospital discharge are useful for identifying high and low risk AMI patients at follow-up, and patients with sudden death at follow-up have evidence at hospital discharge of profound impairment of LV function.

Hung and associates[41] from Stanford, Redwood City, and Santa Clara, California, compared the prognostic value of symptom-limited treadmill exercise ECG, exercise thallium myocardial perfusion scintigraphy and rest, and exercise radionuclide ventriculography in 117 men aged 54 ± 9 years, tested 3 weeks after a clinically uncomplicated AMI. During a mean follow-up of 12 months, 8 men had hard medical events (cardiac death, nonfatal VF, or recurrent AMI) and 14 were hospitalized for unstable angina pectoris, CHF, or CABG (total of 22 combined events) (Fig. 2-7). By multivariate analysis (Cox proportional hazards model), peak treadmill work load and the change in LV EF during exercise were significant (p < 0.01) predictors of hard medical events; these 2 risk factors and recurrent ischemic chest pain in the coronary care unit were also significantly predictive (p < 0.001) for combined events. A peak treadmill work load of 4 METs or less or a decrease in EF of 5% or more below the value at rest during submaximal effort distinguished 22 high risk patients (20% of the study population) from 89 low risk patients. The rate of hard medical events within 12 months was 23% (5 of 22 patients), -vs- 2% (2 of 89 patients) in the high and low risk patient subsets, respectively (p < 0.001). Thus, in patients who underwent evaluation 3

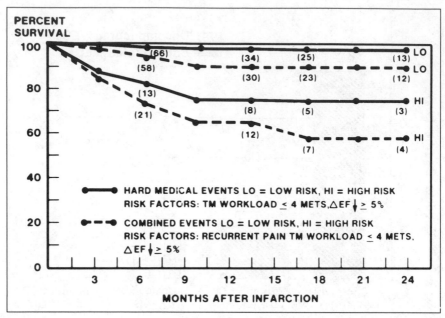

Fig. 2-7. Survival without cardiac events. $\Delta EF\downarrow$ = decrease in ejection fraction during submaximal exercise to below the value at rest; METs = multiples of resting energy expenditure; TM = treadmill.

weeks after a clinically uncomplicated AMI, exercise radionuclide ventriculography contributed independent prognostic information to that provided by symptom-limited treadmill testing and was superior to exercise thallium scintigraphy for this purpose.

Mukharji and associates[42] in a multicenter investigation assessed the risk of sudden coronary death after AMI in 533 patients who survived 10 days after onset of AMI and were followed up to 24 months (mean, 18) in the Multicenter Investigation of the Limitation of Infarct Size. Analysis of multiple clinical and laboratory variables determined before hospital discharge revealed that frequent VPC ($\geq$10/hour) on ambulatory ECG monitoring and LV dysfunction (radionuclide LV EF $\leq$0.40) were independently significant markers of risk for subsequent sudden death believed to be the result of a primary ventricular arrhythmia (Fig. 2-8). The incidence of sudden death was 18% in patients with both LV dysfunction and frequent VPC (11 times that of patients with neither of these findings). Seventy-nine percent of all sudden deaths occurred within 7 months after the index AMI. In 280 survivors reclassified 6 months after AMI with regard to the presence or absence of frequent VPC and LV dysfunction, these risk factors could not be associated with sudden coronary death over a further follow-up period of up to 18 months; the overall incidence of sudden cardiac death was low (1.4%) after 6 months. Thus, the presence of frequent VPC in association with LV dysfunction early after AMI identifies patients at high risk for sudden death over the next 7 months.

To assess alternative criteria for the prediction of multivessel CAD after AMI, Morris and colleagues[43] from Los Angeles, California, compared the

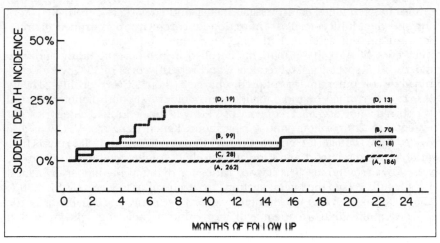

Fig. 2-8.   Incidence of sudden cardiac death (life-table analysis) in each risk group. Group A (314 patients initially at risk) with LV EF >40 and <10/hour VPC; Group B (141 patients) with LV EF of ≤0.40 and <10/hour VPC; Group C (38 patients) with LV EF >0.40 and ≥10/hour VPC; Group D (40 patients) with LV EF of <0.40 and >10/hour VPC. Letters and numbers in parentheses indicate risk group and numbers of patients at risk at 1 and 2 years.

clinical, bicycle ECG, and radionuclide ventriculographic (EF and wall motion) responses in 110 patients undergoing coronary angiography after AMI. Of the 110 patients, 97 had multivessel (≥2) CAD. Clinical or ECG abnormalities were observed in 41 of 97 (sensitivity, 43%) patients with multivessel CAD, and in 2 of 13 (specificity, 85%) patients without multivessel CAD. Among the scintigraphic parameters, the conventional criterion for EF abnormality, an increase of <5%, had a sensitivity of 72% and a specificity of 62% for multivessel CAD, whereas a decrease in EF of ≥5% had a sensitivity of 39% and a specificity of 92% for multivessel CAD. The presence of an exercise wall motion abnormality in the nonadjacent noninfarcted region had a sensitivity of 82% and specificity of 55% for multivessel CAD. A more stringent criterion, worsening of remote wall motion with exercise, had a sensitivity of 52% and specificity of 75%. When this latter criterion was combined with a decrease in EF, the sensitivity for multivessel CAD increased to 62%, specificity remained 75%. The investigators concluded that conventional diagnostic criteria for abnormal clinical, bicycle ECG, or scintigraphic results do not identify patients with additional CAD after AMI with high accuracy. Two alternative ventriculographic parameters—a decrease in EF and wall motion worsening—are similar to clinical parameters in specificity, but have a high sensitivity and information content.

PROGNOSTIC INDEXES

Arrhythmia

Although ventricular arrhythmias and LV dysfunction are 2 major risks for mortality in patients having had an AMI, the relation between these entities has remained controversial. Bigger and coworkers[44] from New York City and the Multicenter Post-Infarction Research Group examined the relations among ventricular arrhythmias, LV dysfunction, and mortality after the occurrence of AMI in 766 patients enrolled in a 9-hospital study and who underwent 2 special tests. Frequency and repetitiveness of VPC were determined by computer analysis of predischarge 24-hour ECG recordings. The LV EF was determined by radionuclide ventriculography and dichotomized at its optimal value of 30%. Frequency of VPC was divided into 3 categories: <1 per hour, 1–2.9 per hour, and ≥3 per hour. Repetitiveness of VPC was also divided into 3 categories: no repetitive VPC, paired VPC, and VPC runs. These variables were related 1 at a time and jointly to total mortality and to deaths caused by arrhythmias. The hazard ratios for dying in the higher or highest risk stratum versus the lowest stratum for each variable were: LV EF <30%, 3.5; VPC runs, 1.9; and VPC frequency of ≥3 per hour, 2.0. The hazard ratio is a probability that a patient will die within a short interval, given that he/she has survived to the beginning of that interval. There were no significant interactions among the 3 variables with respect to effects on the risk of mortality. The LV EF <30% was a better predictor of early mortality (<6 months) and the presence of ventricular arrhythmias was a better predictor of late mortality (after 6 months). The results of this large, multicenter study support the conclusion that ventricular arrhythmias and LV dysfunction are independently related to mortality risk.

Sinus tachycardia often accompanies other indicators of poor prognosis in AMI. Crimm and associates[45] from Durham, North Carolina, evaluated the prognostic significance of in-hospital isolated sinus tachycardia occurring days 1–3 in the absence of other common indicators of poor prognosis in patients with AMI. All patients consecutively admitted directly to the coronary care unit during a 6-year period were evaluated. Patients who had confirmed AMI and no urgent complications during days 1–3 with isolated sinus tachycardia (99 patients) or without isolated sinus tachycardia (159 patients) were included in the study. Both groups were followed for subsequent in-hospital outcome and long-term survival. Univariable and multivariable analysis of historical and demographic characteristics showed no significant differences between the 2 groups (Fig. 2-9). When clinical descriptors of the infarct were evaluated, the group with isolated sinus tachycardia had a significantly higher mean peak creatine kinase level, a larger proportion of anterior infarcts and multiple infarct sites by ECG, a higher incidence of peri-infarction pericarditis, and a higher incidence of recurrent chest pain. Twenty-five patients (25%) in the group with isolated sinus tachycardia had subsequent urgent complications during the hospitalization compared with 11 patients (7%) in the control group. In multivariable analysis, isolated sinus tachycardia was an independent predictor of subsequent urgent complications and mortality.

To assess the prevalence and prognostic implications of complicated VPC after hospital discharge in patients with AMI, Olson and colleagues[46] from Long Beach, California, obtained serial 24-hour Holter recordings in 85 patients during the first 6 weeks after AMI. Recordings were obtained during 2 coronary care unit time intervals, 2 hospital ward time intervals, and 4 weekly time intervals after discharge. Complicated VPC were defined as unifocal VPC ≥10/1000 beats for 24 hours, multiform VPC, pairs, or VT. At 1-year follow-up, there were 9 cardiac deaths (6 sudden and 3 from recurrent

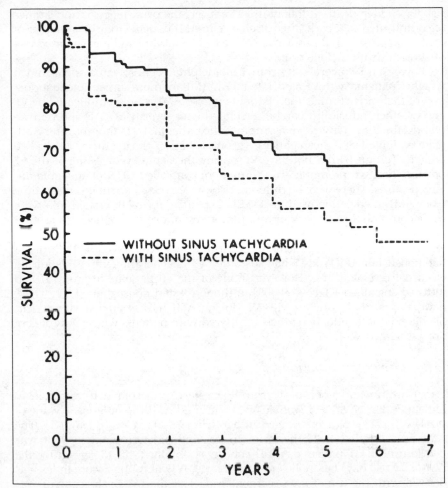

Fig. 2-9.   Survival in 158 admissions without isolated sinus tachycardia and 99 admissions with isolated tachycardia in patients with AMI.

AMI). The mean LV EF at discharge in the cardiac death patients was 29 ± 12% (sudden death patients, 24 ± 11%; AMI death patients, 40 ± 6%) compared with 49 ± 13% in the survivors (p < 0.001). Patients with complicated VPC at discharge (2 weeks after AMI) or during the first 4 weeks after discharge (3–6 weeks after AMI) were significantly more likely to have died suddenly at follow-up compared with patients without complicated VPC. Of the 6 sudden death patients, 4 (66%) had had complicated VPC at discharge compared with 18 of 68 survivors (26%) (p < 0.05). One of 3 patients who died of recurrent AMI had complicated VPC. No Holter data were obtained at hospital discharge in 8 of the survivors. Of the 6 patients with sudden death at follow-up, all had had complicated VPC on ≥3 24-hour Holter recordings during the first 4 weeks after discharge compared with 21 of 76 survivors (28%) (p < 0.001). It was concluded that AMI patients with complicated VPC at discharge or during the first 4 weeks after discharge are at increased risk for sudden death at follow-up. Moreover, the persistence or appearance of complicated VPC early after discharge in AMI patients may be a marker of continued or acquired myocardial electrical instability and for increased risk of sudden death at follow-up.

Kowey and coworkers[47] from Philadelphia, Pennsylvania, determined whether patients with VF associated with AMI are more susceptible to induction of tachyarrhythmias than patients whose AMI is not complicated by VF and whether inducibility can be correlated with severity of CAD and ventricular dysfunction. Fifty-seven asymptomatic patients, 1–24 months after AMI, were evaluated. Seventeen patients (group I) had VF during their AMI and 40 patients (group II) did not have VF during the acute event. None of the 57 patients had symptomatic arrhythmias, uncontrolled CHF, or unstable angina pectoris. There were no differences between the 2 patient groups in time from AMI, medication used, or LV EF. Repetitive forms of arrhythmia were more common during 24-hour ambulatory monitoring in patients in group I (VF group). Programmed extrastimulation was performed and demonstrated that among 17 patients in group I, 8 had no induced arrhythmia, 4 had nonsustained VT, and 5 had sustained VT degenerating into VF requiring electrical reversion in 4. However, none of the 40 patients in group II had induced sustained VT (p < 0.005), although 9 had nonsustained VT. These data suggest that patients with VF during AMI have a greater subsequent likelihood of VT induction when compared with patients whose infarcts are not associated with VF.

Left ventricular function

Nishimura and associates[48] from Rochester, Minnesota, determined in 46 patients (32 men and 14 women) who survived AMI the prognostic value of a 2-D echo. The patients ranged in age from 36–92 years (mean, 61). The AMI was anterior in 21, posterior in 22, and indeterminant in 3; it was transmural in 31 patients. A 2-D echo was obtained 10–15 days after the AMI, i.e., 1–3 days before hospital discharge. A wall motion score index was derived with the use of a 14-segment model of the LV. Each segment was assigned a number corresponding to its wall motion (0 = hyperkinetic, 1 = normal, 2 = hypokinetic, 3 = akinetic, 4 = dyskinetic, and 5 = aneurysm) and the wall motion score index was calculated by dividing the sum of these numbers by the number of segments visualized (1.0 = normal wall motion). During a mean follow-up of 21 months (range, 15–28), 17 patients had a complication: death, recurrence of AMI, CHF of New York Heart Association class III or IV, or angina graded New York Heart Association class III or IV. Patients with complications compared with those without had a significantly higher wall motion score index (2.2 ± 0.4 and 1.7 ± 0.5, p < 0.005). The difference in wall motion score index between those who died and those who survived was not significant because of the small number of deaths. Of 22 patients with a wall motion score index of ≤2, 20 (91%) had no cardiac complication; 15 (88%) of 17 patients with a complication had a wall motion score index of ≥2.0. Thus, a predischarge 2-D echo is useful in identifying a subset of patients at increased risk of complications after AMI.

Norris and associates[49] from Auckland, New Zealand, studied factors associated with cardiac mortality and re-AMI in 325 male survivors <60 years of age (mean, 50) of a first AMI. All patients had undergone exercise

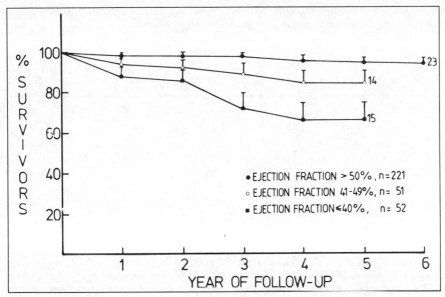

Fig. 2-10. Actuarial survival curves according to the EF for the 324 patients in whom EF could be measured. Numbers after the last data point show numbers of patients at risk during the last year of follow-up. Bars indicate the SE of the estimates. The 3 curves are significantly different $(\chi^2 = 34.0, p < 0.001)$.

testing and cineangiography 4 weeks after AMI, 24% underwent CABG, and 30% received beta blocking drugs. Patients were followed 1–6 years (mean, 3.5). Total cardiac mortality was best predicted by LV EF and by a coronary prognostic index (Fig. 2-10). In contrast, neither the severity of coronary arterial lesions measured with a scoring system nor the results of the exercise test gave significant prediction of mortality. Of the 2 major late sequelae of AMI, reinfarction could not be predicted by any clinical or cineangiocardiographic variable. However, sudden death not associated with reinfarction was significantly more common (p < 0.001) when EF was ≤40% than when it was >40%. Comparison of patients with an EF ≤40% who did or did not die suddenly showed that LV dilation (high volumes at ventriculography) was an added risk factor, but the extent of coronary occlusions and stenoses was not. It is concluded that, at least for groups of patients treated with standard modern methods after MI, the main determinant of medium-term survival is the extent of LV damage. The state of the coronary arteries and the presence of ischemic myocardium during exercise are only of secondary importance for survival.

Greenberg and associates[50] from New York City studied 866 patients surviving the coronary care unit phase of an AMI to identify the variables of prognostic importance in follow-up of 2 years. Data obtained indicate that the single variables reflecting LV dysfunction before AMI and in the acute and recovery phases were history of AMI, rales in the coronary care unit, and predischarge RNA EF <0.40. Patients without these 3 risk characteristics had a 2-year 4.2% mortality rate, whereas patients having all 3 characteristics had a 45% mortality rate (Table 2-3). The data also indicate that rales in the

TABLE 2-3.   *Mortality rates for patients cross-classified by 3 LV dysfunction variables.* *Reproduced with permission from Greenberg et al.*[50]

RALES: NOT ADVANCED/ ADVANCED	EF: ≥0.40/ <0.40	PRIOR AMI: NO/YES	# DEAD	MORTALITY RATE (%)
	488	402	17	4.2
		85	8	9.4
743				
	207	133	21	15.8
		73	10	13.7
	52	42	8	19.0
		10	3	30.0
123				
	63	41	13	31.7
		20	9	45.0

* RNA EF dichotomized at 0.40 and history of prior AMI are added stepwise to rales that are dichotomized at greater than bibasilar. The eight subgroups display a nearly linear increase in mortality rate from 4.2% when all variables are favorable to 45% when all are unfavorable. The number of patients in each clinical subgroup differs because of missing data.

coronary care unit and the predischarge EF are independent predictors of prognosis and each contributes to mortality.

Defects on thallium scanning

To evaluate the safety and usefulness of serial thallium scanning immediately after intravenous dipyridamole, Leppo and associates[51] from Boston and Worcester, Massachusetts, studied 51 patients recovering from AMI. Eight had angina during the procedure, but there were no serious complications. Patients were followed for a mean period of 19 months after hospital discharge. Eleven of 12 patients who died during follow-up or had another AMI had shown transient defects (redistribution) on their predischarge scan, as had 22 of the 24 patients who needed readmission for management of angina. Among all the other clinical or scintigraphic criteria tested, the presence of redistribution on the dipyridamole-thallium scan was the only significant predictor of these serious cardiac events. Twenty-six patients were also given a submaximal exercise test before discharge, of whom 13 subsequently had serious cardiac events. The exercise test had been positive in only 6 of these 13 patients, whereas the dipyridamole-thallium scan had shown a redistribution pattern in 12. The investigators concluded that dipyridamole-thallium scintigraphy after AMI is relatively safe and is a more sensitive predictor of subsequent cardiac events than a submaximal exercise test.

Hung and associates[52] from Stanford, California, assessed the affects of exercise training on exercise myocardial perfusion and LV function in the first 6 months after clinically uncomplicated AMI in 53 consecutive men aged 55 ± 9 years. Symptom-limited treadmill exercise with thallium myocardial perfusion scintigraphy and symptom-limited upright bicycle ergometry with equilibrium gated radionuclide ventriculography were performed 3, 11, and

26 weeks after AMI by 23 men randomized to training and 30 randomized to no training. Peak cycle capacity increased in both groups between 3 and 26 weeks (p < 0.01), but reached higher levels in trained than in untrained patients (803 ± 149 -vs- 648 ± 182 kg-m/min, p < 0.01). Reversible thallium perfusion defects were significantly more frequent at 3 than at 26 weeks: 59 and 36% of patients, respectively (p < 0.05), without significant intergroup differences. Values of LV EF at rest and at submaximal and peak exercise did not change significantly in either group. The increase in functional capacity, i.e., peak treadmill or bicycle workload, that occurred 3–26 weeks after infarction was significantly correlated with the increase in peak exercise heart rate (p < 0.001), but not with changes in myocardial perfusion or LV function determined by radionuclide techniques. Changes in myocardial perfusion or LV function do not appear to account for the improvement in peak functional capacity that occurs within the first 6 months after clinically uncomplicated AMI.

Exercise-induced ST segment elevation

Sullivan and associates[53] from London, England, performed submaximal exercise testing 7–23 days (mean, 11) after AMI in 74 patients (66 men; mean age, 54 years). Follow-up was a mean of 11 months. When compared with patients with no exercise-induced abnormality, ST-segment elevation, ST shift (depression or elevation or both), ST depression, inability to complete 5 metabolic equivalents, and inadequate BP response to exercise were predictive of subsequent cardiac events (cardiac death, LV failure, recurrent AMI, angina). When the presence or absence of specific variables was assessed, only ST elevation and ST shift predicted subsequent cardiac events. The presence of exercise-induced ST elevation was the only exercise test variable that predicted cardiac death. ST segment elevation was therefore the exercise-induced abnormality that best predicted the risk of future complications.

Diabetes mellitus

Oswald and associates[54] from London, England, assessed the prevalence of undiagnosed diabetes mellitus in patients admitted with AMI and the effect of diabetes and admission hyperglycemia on outcome. In the retrospective study admission levels of plasma glucose were higher in patients dying from cardiogenic shock than in survivors, but they were not related to AMI size. In the prospective study, plasma glucose was related to concurrent levels of glycosylated hemoglobin, which were in turn related to outcome: The mortality rate was 23% for those with normal glycosylated hemoglobin, 33% for those with borderline abnormal hemoglobin, and 63% for those with clearly abnormal glycosylated hemoglobin. Cardiogenic shock was more common in the groups with higher glycosylated hemoglobin levels. In addition, admission hyperglycemia was associated with the incidence of cardiogenic shock even after correcting for the effects of glycosylated hemoglobin. All survivors from the clearly abnormal hemoglobin group but none of those from other groups were diabetic at follow-up, suggesting an overall prevalence of undiagnosed diabetes of 5%. The contribution of undiagnosed diabetes mellitus to total mortality after AMI appears at present to be underestimated.

To elucidate the factors involved in the reduced survival rate of diabetic patients after AMI, Jaffe and associates[55] from St. Louis, Missouri, prospectively evaluated 100 patients with well-documented diabetes mellitus and 426 control patients. Infarct size was characterized and the incidence and severity of CHF and subsequent death was analyzed with respect to infarct size. The extent of the index infarct was less in diabetic compared with nondiabetic patients, 16 ± 2 CK-g-eq/m^2 compared with 19 ± 1 ($p < 0.02$). However, CHF was more prevalent in diabetic patients (31% of diabetic patients compared with 16%) (Fig. 2-11). The difference was most prominent in diabetic patients who had sustained prior AMI (50% compared with 16%), but was evident also in diabetic patients with initial AMI (26% compared with 16%). The mortality rate was greater in diabetic patients ($p < 0.04$). When diabetic and nondiabetic patients were stratified with respect to the presence or absence of CHF, survival curves were comparable. The increased incidence of CHF despite a smaller infarct size suggests that additional factors (such as systemic hypertension, autonomic dysfunction, different nature of CAD, and diabetic myopathy) must contribute to myocardial dysfunction and the resultant excess in mortality.

The prognosis of patients with diabetes mellitus surviving hospitalization for AMI has been considered grave. Smith and associates[56] from Tucson, Arizona, compared prognosis of 60 diabetic patients with that of 719 nondiabetic patients who survived the coronary care unit phase of AMI and were

Fig. 2-11. Kaplan-Meier survival curves in diabetic and nondiabetic populations. Diabetic patients had a greater mortality after AMI. Actuarial survival rate was 58% in the diabetic patients and 68% in the nondiabetic patients after 2½ years. The actuarial curves were significantly different ($p < 0.04$). Reproduced with permission from Jaffe et al.[55]

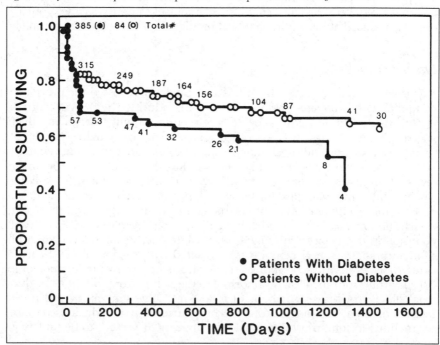

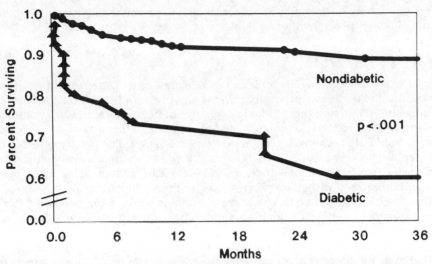

Fig. 2-12.   Kaplan-Meier survivorship curve of diabetic -vs- nondiabetic patients after AMI.

followed an average of 19 months. The mortality rate was 25% in diabetic patients and 8% in nondiabetic patients. These patients had been entered in a multicenter postinfraction program where analysis of the total data base showed 4 significant prognostic factors: cardiac symptoms before AMI, pulmonary rales when the patient was in the coronary care unit, >10 VPC per hour recorded on Holter monitor just before discharge, and a radionuclide EF of >40%. Of these 4 factors, only cardiac symptoms before AMI was significantly more common in diabetic patients (57% in diabetic -vs- 36% in nondiabetic patients). When each of these 4 factors was stratified for severity, the mortality rate was always higher in diabetic patients (Fig. 2-12). The data were examined to determine other factors in diabetic patients who died. Pulmonary rales was significantly more common in diabetic patients who died (6% in survivors -vs- 42% in patients who died). In a multivariate analysis of both diabetic and nondiabetic patients, 5 factors were significant determinants of prognosis. They were, in order of entry into the model, rales, EF <40%, diabetes, symptoms before AMI, and >10 VPC per hour. Either the diabetic state contributes a unique characteristic to the poor prognosis of patients with CAD or coronary atherosclerosis is accelerated in these patients.

Preceding angina pectoris

Matsuda and colleagues[57] from Ube, Japan, evaluated LV function in 31 patients who had total occlusion of the LAD coronary artery and <70% stenosis of the other 2 major coronary arteries or any branch. Of the 31 patients, 15 had a history of angina pectoris before AMI. The patients with angina pectoris before AMI had a significantly better EF, percentage of abnormally contracting segments, and regional wall motion than those without angina pectoris before AMI. These data suggest that the symptom of angina pectoris before AMI could be a favorable sign in preserving LV function when the patients subsequently had AMI.

Psychosocial influences

Crisp and Queenan[58] from London, England, investigated aspects of personality and emotional status that might identify middle-aged men at risk of impending AMI, and they studied the change in these characteristics in survivors of AMI. The study group consisted of alternate patients aged 40–65 years registered with a group in general practice in London. The participants were extensively screened in 1969, 1971, and 1973. Most subjects completed the Crown-Crisp Experimental Index (CCEI) on each occasion. This index is a standardized self-rating inventory of 48 questions allowing scores of 0–16 on 6 scales measuring free-floating anxiety, phobic anxiety, obsessionality and obsessional neurosis, functional somatic complaint, depression, and hysteria. The present report concerns the 26 men admitted to the hospital with a confirmed AMI between screenings or after the final screening: 7 died and 8 had their infarct after the final screening. The remaining 11 were screened after their AMI. Scores on the CCEI before and after AMI were compared with those for the remainder of the male study population (n, 235), from whom the infarct population did not differ significantly in age. The prevalence of ECG evidence of previous AMI was similar in the 2 populations (2 of 26 coronary patients and 18 of 232 controls). Before AMI, the coronary patients had significantly more symptomatic experiences (especially with sweating, heart fluttering, and loss of libido) and were significantly more depressed (especially in respect of feeling sad): 62% had experienced chest pain before the event, compared with 37% who did not have an AMI during the period of study. Those destined for AMI and with chest pain at the time of the previous screening scored no higher on the depression scale than did the remainder, but they did score higher on the anxiety scale at that stage (Fig. 2-13). A striking finding is the change in psychologic status after AMI. The survivors were significantly more anxious, depressed, obsessional, and socially phobic and withdrawn than the general population. They also complained a great deal more of somatic symptoms, some doubtlessly related to the direct physical consequence of their AMI. Noteworthy also are the pre-AMI personality characteristics of obsessionality and of being a worrier but without fear of serious illness, coupled with a raised mean depression score that could not be readily accounted for by the presence of angina or other signals of imminent cardiac catastrophe. The CCEI scoring system in the present study allowed a two thirds correct identification of those persons due for imminent AMI and an overall 82% correct classification of AMI/non-AMI cases.

Ruberman and associates[59] from New York City conducted psychosocial interviews with 2,320 male survivors of AMI, participants in the β-Blocker Heart Attack Trial, and found 2 variables strongly associated with an increased 3-year mortality risk. With other important prognostic factors controlled for, the patients classified as being socially isolated and having a high degree of life stress had more than 4 times the risk of death of the men with low levels of both stress and isolation. An inverse association of education with mortality in this population reflected the gradient in the prevalence of the defined psychosocial characteristics. High levels of stress and social isola-

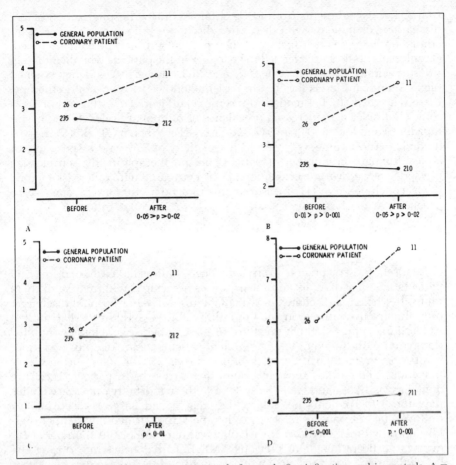

Fig. 2-13.   CCEI scores in coronary patients before and after infarction and in controls. A = anxiety; B = depression; C = social avoidance behavior; D = somatic complaints. Reproduced with permission from Crisp and Queenan.[58]

tion were most prevalent among the least educated men and least prevalent among the best educated. The increase in risk associated with stress and social isolation applied both to total deaths and to sudden cardiac deaths and was noted among men with both high and low levels of ventricular ectopic activity during hospitalization for the AMI. This article was followed by an editorial by Graboys.[60]

Q-T interval

Ahnve and associates[61] from San Diego, California, and Vancouver, Canada, evaluated whether the QT interval, corrected for heart rate, had prognostic importance after AMI. All patients (n, 865) were discharged from the hospital and followed ≥30 days after admission. Because of medication or pacemaker therapy, which influences QT_c, no conclusions could be drawn from QT_c measurements from ECGs obtained during hospitalization before discharge. All patients who died after discharge but within 30 days after admission were on such therapy. When patients on therapy were excluded, QT intervals at discharge tended to be longer in the patients who died than in the survivors, followed for 90, 180, and 365 days. This tendency reached highly significant levels for QT_c. In patients followed 1 year, not on therapy, those who died (n, 13) tended to resemble survivors (n, 201), except for a somewhat older age, increased prevalence of pulmonary rales during hospitalization, and longer QT_c intervals at discharge. When a QT_c of 440 ms was used as a cutoff value, QT_c yielded a sensitivity of 77% and a specificity of 84%. Although the number of patients not on therapy in this sample size precluded a multivariate evaluation of QT_c compared with other risk factors, it was concluded that QT_c measurements may be useful for assessing 1-year prognosis at discharge after AMI.

Digitalis

Madsen and coworkers[62] from San Diego, California, evaluated in 1,599 patients whether digitalis administration is associated with increased mortality after hospital discharge in patients with AMI. After hospital discharge, mortality for the entire group at 4 months was 7.7% and after 1 year, 14.2%. At discharge, approximately one third of these patients were taking digitalis. Compared with those not taking digitalis, patients taking digitalis had more risk factors and a higher incidence of poor prognosis variables during hospitalization. The cardiac mortality rate after 4 months in patients receiving digitalis was 12.5% and after 1 year, 22.4%; these mortality rates were higher than those for patients not taking digitalis (5 and 9.6%, respectively). A multivariate Cox analysis for 1-year outcome demonstrated that neither digitalis nor any other medication variable was more important than age, CHF during the hospitalization, previous AMI, maximal heart rate during the hospitalization, and previous angina as predictors of mortality risk. These data suggest that digitalis therapy at discharge after AMI is not an independent predictor of late mortality.

First nontransmural AMI

Hollander and associates[63] from New York City studied 38 patients with first nontransmural AMI to determine prognosis and clinical markers of a high risk subgroup. A high incidence of reinfarction (18%) was found at a median time of 16 days after nontransmural AMI (7 patients). Reinfarction was uniformly associated with death within 24 hours. A total of 14 patients (37%) either died (8 patients) or required urgent CABG (6 patients). Predominant ST-segment depression with presenting nontransmural AMI and a history of prior angina were associated with increased mortality ($p < 0.05$ and $p = 0.05$, respectively). It was concluded that patients with nontransmural AMI are at high risk for early recurrent AMI. Patients with history of prior angina and predominant ST-segment depression may be at particularly high risk. Reinfarction in these patients is frequently extensive. It is recommended that these patients be considered for early coronary angiography.

Other variables

Madsen and associates[64] in a multicenter study examined long-term prognostic importance of sets of variables from different times in the hospital course after AMI in 818 patients discharged from the hospital. Cardiac mortality during the first year after discharge was 11%. For the end point of death within 1 year after admission, 5 important factors from the history in the first 24 hours of hospitalization were identified by discriminate function analysis: Maximal level of blood urea nitrogen, previous AMI, age, displaced LV apex on physical examination, and sinus bradycardia (negative correlation). When data from the entire hospital period were included, extension of AMI and maximal heart rate also were important. When variables obtained at discharge were included, only the presence of an S_3 gallop and abnormal apex were selected. In subgroups of patients, neither the LV EF nor the presence of complex ventricular arrhythmias during a 24-hour ambulatory monitoring were independent variables. Correct prediction was similar for each analysis, with 55–60% of the deaths and 79–81% of survivors correctly identified. The high risk group consisted of 25% of the patients with 28–30% predictive value for death in the first year. In conclusion, outcome up to 1 year after AMI can be predicted early after admission. Addition of more information later during the hospitalization and at discharge did not improve correct prediction and may be redundant for prognostic evaluation.

TREATMENT

Nitrates

Bussmann and colleagues[65] from Frankfurt, West Germany, recorded VPC continuously in 21 consecutive patients with AMI on magnetic tape by means of an automatic arrhythmia monitor and counted manually. The patients were sequentially assigned to either a control (n, 11) or nitroglycerin group (n, 10). Both groups were comparable for age, onset, localization, and extension of AMI. Recording in the control group was begun at a mean of 9.3 hours after onset of AMI. This interval was 12 hours in the nitroglycerin group. At the start of therapy, the number of VPC was identical in both groups. Ten patients received a mean of 2.1 mg of nitroglycerin per hour intravenously for 48 hours, whereas the control group received no specific therapy. The number of VPC in the control group increased progressively until the sixth hour of registration and reached a maximum of 165% of the baseline value before subsequently declining. Nitroglycerin administration was associated with a significantly more rapid reduction in ventricular arrhythmias: 6 hours after onset of recording the number of VPC had declined to 39% of the baseline value ($p < 0.05$ compared with the control group). This study demonstrates that nitroglycerin reduces VPC during AMI.

Beta blockers

Although long-term control clinical trials of beta blockers in survivors of AMI have demonstrated benefit with respect to mortality from all causes, coronary mortality and sudden cardiac death, several pertinent questions have been raised. First, what is the mechanism of action of the beta blockers; second, should all patients with AMI be treated with beta blockers; and third, can beta blockers be used safely in patients who have been in CHF? A simple classification for patients based on the presence or absence of findings indicative of electrical or mechanical complications early during short-term hospitalization was applied by Furberg and colleagues[66] from Bethesda, Maryland, to the data from the Beta-Blocker Heart Attack Trial (BHAT). In the largest subgroup of BHAT patients who had not reported complications, the 25-month mortality was low and the observed benefit of propranolol therapy small. Patients with electrical complications only had intermittent mortality and a pronounced effect of treatment was observed. Those with mechanical complications had the highest morality and had an intermediate relative benefit of beta blocker treatment. They also reported the most adverse effects. On the basis of these analyses, the investigators suggest that the present practice of prescribing beta blockers in post-AMI patients should not be altered.

A multicenter randomized single-blind study was performed by Roberts and colleagues[67] to evaluate the effects of propranolol administered during the evolution of AMI. Five centers enrolled 269 patients, with 134 receiving propranolol and 135, placebo. Propranolol or placebo was given intravenously on randomization (0.1 mg/kg body weight) and then orally for 9 days to keep the heart rate between 45 and 60 beats/minute. Less than 2% of patients were treated within 4 hours after the onset of symptoms, but 50% received therapy within 8 hours of onset of chest pain, and the remainder between 8 and 18 hours. The heart rates in the propranolol-treated group were significantly lower than those in the placebo group. Baseline characteristics, including the mean heart rate (80 -vs- 81) and the LV EF (49 -vs- 50), were similar in the 2 groups. The primary end point evaluated—infarct size as estimated from plasma creatine kinase MB activity—was virtually identical in the 2 groups, averaging 13 and 14 g-eq of creatine kinase MB per M^2 of body surface area. Peak plasma levels of the enzyme were also similar in the 2 groups. No significant difference was observed between the propranolol and placebo groups in the change in LV EF, extent of area involved in pyrophosphate uptake, R-wave loss on ECGs, or mortality (after 3 years). These results do not support the use of propranolol administered ≥4 hours after the onset of symptoms to limit infarct size.

Gold and associates[68] from Boston, Massachusetts, studied the effect of propranolol on precordial ST-segment elevation in 24 patients with anterior AMI. The ECG response to the drug was correlated with the early angiographic appearance of the LAD coronary artery. After a 30-minute observation period, intravenous propranolol (average dose, 3.5 ± 2.2 mg) was given a mean of 2.8 ± 1.9 hours after the onset of persistent chest pain. Coronary angiography was performed 3.6 ± 2.0 hours after the onset of symptoms. Patients were classified into 2 groups according to the angiographic findings. Group A consisted of 7 patients with a stenotic but patent LAD and 1 patient with excellent collateral blood flow to that area. Group B consisted of 16 patients with a completely occluded LAD and poor or absent collateral blood flow. Patients in group A showed a mean reduction in precordial ST-segment elevation of 77 ± 18% and patients in group B showed a mean reduction of 13 ± 14% (p < 0.005). The LV EF at discharge was 0.6 ± 0.07 in group A and 0.37 ± 0.08 in group B ($p < 0.001$). Thus, the ECG response to intravenous propranolol given early in the course of acute AMI predicts the presence of blood flow in the infarcting zone. The combination of residual blood flow and reduction of ST-segment elevation secondary to propranolol is associated with preservation of ventricular function.

The International Collaborative Study Group[69] randomly assigned 144 patients admitted to the hospital within 4 hours after onset of symptoms of AMI to either intravenous timolol treatment or to placebo. Timolol was given intravenously for the first 24 hours and orally thereafter for the duration of hospitalization. Infarct evolution was assessed by continuous vectorcardiography and creatine kinase release. The timolol group had reduced myocardial ischemia and infarct size as measured by an accelerated reduction of ST-vector magnitude, a significant reduction of maximal cumulative creatine kinase release (30%), and significantly smaller changes in QRS-vector variables (20–25%) (Fig. 2-14). Furthermore, the predicted creatine kinase release and maximal QRS-vector change for a given initial ST-vector magnitude was significantly reduced in the timolol group. Timolol was also associated with significant reductions in pain and need for analgesics and was well tolerated overall. This study supports the use of intravenous timolol in the early phase of suspected AMI to limit infarct size. Timolol has previously been shown to be of long-term benefit to survivors of AMI in terms of prevention of sudden

Fig. 2-14. Mean cumulative release of creatine kinase during the evolution of AMI. Time zero denotes onset of symptoms. Significant differences between the two groups are indicated by vertical dashed lines. Reproduced with permission from the International Collaborative Study Group.[69]

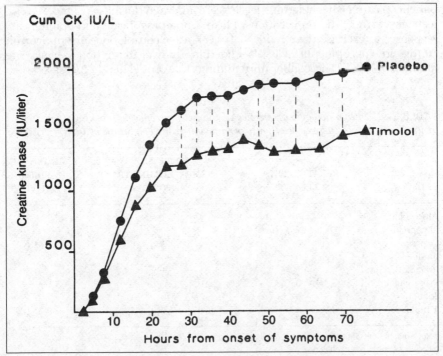

coronary death and reinfarction. Taken together, these studies support the use of timolol for the early and late treatment of patients with AMI.

Three hundred and one patients who had been hospitalized for AMI were <70 years old, in sinus rhythm, and did not have complete BBB were stratified by Olsson and Rehnqvist[70] from Danderyd, Sweden, before discharge according to age, size of AMI, and type of ventricular arrhythmias as determined on a 6-hour ECG. The patients were thereafter randomly assigned to double-run blind treatment with 100 mg metoprolol twice daily or placebo. Repeat 6-hour ECGs were recorded 3 days and 1, 6, and 12 months after treatment had begun. In the placebo group there was a significant increase in the proportion of patients with complex VPC and increased numbers of VPC in the patients during follow-up. In contrast, an initial decrease in the number of PVC was found in the metoprolol group, whereas the complexity of PVC was constant in those patients who continued on metoprolol therapy throughout the follow-up period. The investigators concluded that the increase in complexity and number of PVC after AMI is counteracted but not abolished by long-term treatment with metoprolol.

Metoprolol or placebo was gradually withdrawn during 1 week in 115 coronary disease patients participating in a 3-year, double-blind, post-AMI study performed by Olsson and colleagues[71] from Stockholm, Sweden. During the first month after withdrawal, mental symptoms and increased cardiac symptoms occurred significantly more frequently in the metoprolol group. Disabling symptoms requiring reinstitution of treatment were seen in 14 of 58 in the metoprolol group -vs- 4 of 57 in the placebo group ($p < 0.05$). In the metoprolol group, there was a rebound increase of basal heart rate and of the heart rate response to orthostatic testing during 3 weeks after withdrawal, when compared with values obtained 6 months later. In 27 patients plasma catecholamine levels were analyzed during repeated exercise tests and orthostatic provocations. Plasma norepinephrine and epinephrine responses to exercise were reduced 1 week after completion of withdrawal. At this time norepinephrine levels tended to be lower in relation to heart rate at all work loads. These laboratory findings may be related to increased beta

TABLE 2-4. *Pharmacologic properties of the beta adrenergic blocking drugs tested in long-term trials. Reproduced with permission from Frishman et al.[72]*

DRUG	RELATIVE BETA$_1$ SELECTIVITY	INTRINSIC SYMPATHOMIMETIC ACTIVITY	MEMBRANE-STABILIZING ACTIVITY
Alprenolol*	0	+	+
Metoprolol†	+	0	0
Oxprenolol*	0	+	+
Pindolol	0	++	0
Practolol*	+	+	0
Propranolol	0	0	++
Sotalol*	0	0	0
Timolol	0	0	0

* Not available for clinical use in the United States.
† Results of study not available.

adrenoceptor responsiveness, but unmasking of ischemic symptoms probably contributed to the clinical findings.

Frishman and associates[72] from New York City reviewed the usefulness of beta blocking agents for survivors of AMI. They described the usefulness of 8 different beta blockers for this purpose (Table 2-4).

Ahumada[73] from St. Louis, Missouri, reviewed recent results obtained from large clinical trials demonstrating that long-term administration of beta adrenergic blocking agents to patients after AMI reduced the incidence of death for as long as 2 years. It has been recommended that in the absence of contraindications, all patients be given beta blocking agents after AMI. Ahumada's review of published reports regarding prognosis after AMI demonstrated that patients who have had only 1 AMI and who have good ventricular function thereafter, no complex ventricular ectopic activity, no angina, and negative results of stress testing have a mortality rate no greater than 0.6% per year. For a person in this category, the probability that beta blockade will preclude death is exceedingly low (approximately 1 in 700). Both the commonly described side effects and the recent observation that beta adrenergic blocking agents lower the concentration of serum HDL, potentially reducing the protection against atherosclerosis thought to be conferred by HDL, suggest that it may be unwise to use beta blocking agents in patients who have a very low probability of benefit.

Calcium channel blockers

Heikkilä and Nieminen[74] from Helsinki, Finland, evaluated the effects of intravenous verapamil on hemodynamics and regional LV performance in patients with AMI. Twenty patients having uncomplicated AMI or moderate CHF were randomized to receive either verapamil or placebo and were studied a mean of 12 hours after onset of symptoms. Verapamil, 7.5 mg intravenously, acutely reduced systolic arterial pressure (p < 0.0005), systemic vascular resistance and LV stroke work (p < 0.005) and rate-pressure product (p < 0.05); the heart rate did not alter. The Frank-Starling relation did not change for 1 hour. Segmental wall motion amplitudes were recorded from 8 standardized segments around the left ventricle by a multidirectional M-mode echo technique. The systolic wall motion of the uninvolved LV segments and LV cavity size did not change after verapamil. Verapamil improved mechanical performance in the ischemic segments (p < 0.005). Therefore the overall LV regional contractile function improved (by 11–13%, p < 0.05). This improvement on echo continued after the acute vasodilator response of intravenous verapamil subsided and was preserved for 1 week, the patients having had oral verapamil, 240 mg daily. Chest pain was relieved in 5 of the 6 patients having ongoing angina before verapamil injection. No sequential hemodynamic or echo changes occurred in the placebo-treated patients. Thus, in patients with uncomplicated AMI or AMI with moderate LV dysfunction, verapamil improved contractile function of the acutely ischemic LV segments by hemodynamic unloading or by direct myocardial effect, without manifest depression of the uninvolved myocardium.

Clinical and laboratory observations suggest that nifedipine might prevent progression of threatened AMI by reversing coronary spasm or might limit necrosis during the course of AMI. Muller and collaborators[75] from Boston, Massachusetts, screened 3,143 patients with ischemic pain of >45 minutes duration and randomly assigned 105 eligible patients with threatened AMI and 66 with AMI to receive nifedipine (20 mg orally every 4 hours for 14 days) or placebo plus standard care. Treatment was started 4.6 ± 0.1 hour after the onset of pain. Infarct size was calculated by the creatine kinase (CK) MB method. The incidence of progression to AMI among patients with threatened AMI was not significantly altered by nifedipine (36 of 48 [75%] for placebo-treated and 43 of 57 [75%] for nifedipine-treated patients). Infarct size was similar among placebo and nifedipine-treated patients with threatened AMI who had AMI and for those with AMI. Among 171 eligible patients randomly assigned to drug or placebo, 6-month mortality did not differ significantly, but mortality in the 2 weeks after randomization was significantly higher for nifedipine-treated patients (0% for placebo compared with 8% for nifedipine). There were no significant differences in 2- and 26-week mortality in the group of all participating patients, which included 10 patients randomly assigned therapy but retrospectively determined to be ineligible. Thus, nifedipine therapy did not prevent progression of threatened AMI to the acute event or limit infarct size in patients who sustained an AMI. There was a statistically significant increase in 2-week mortality with nifedipine in the group of eligible patients randomly assigned to a regimen, but mortality was balanced when results were analyzed for all patients taking part in the randomized protocol. The drug should not be used routinely in patients with threatened AMI or AMI when treatment cannot be implemented early within approximately 5 hours after the apparent onset of the AMI.

Gordon and associates[76] from Cape Town, South Africa, randomized 26 patients with AMI (mean delay time, 6 hours after onset of symptoms) to control or nifedipine treatment (10 mg sublingually, followed by 10 mg every 6 hours for 24 hours). Nifedipine reduced arterial BP from 127/78–115/70 mmHg at 30 minutes and continued to reduce the BP significantly for 12–18 hours. Nifedipine also reduced systemic vascular resistance and the rate-pressure product. Cardiac output increased from 4.9 liters/minute before nifedipine to 5.4 liters/minute at 60 minutes. In patients with high initial PA wedge pressures, sublingual nifedipine decreased the wedge pressure more effectively than did 80 mg of furosemide given intravenously. Thus, nifedipine may be useful in patients with early AMI and LV failure.

Factors affecting drug effectiveness

Potential changes in antiarrhythmic drug binding during the early and late hospital phases of AMI could be influenced by α_1-glycoprotein and free fatty acid concentrations, which are the major metabolic parameters modulating serum protein binding. Decreased binding (increased free drug fractions) might occur early in the course of AMI due to competitive influence of increased concentrations of free fatty acids. An increased binding (decreased free drug fractions) mediated by increased binding sites on α_1-glycoprotein might be present for sometime thereafter. Kessler and coworkers[77] from Miami, Florida, tested the hypothesis that the changes in free fatty acid and α_1-glycoprotein concentrations exert asynchronous and opposing influences on the serum protein binding of selected drugs during AMI. Free drug fractions of 2 antiarrhythmic agents with contrasting binding characteristics, quinidine and procainamide, were related to free fatty acid and

α_1-glycoprotein concentrations on days 1–5 and 10 in 20 patients with AMI. The mean free quinidine fraction was elevated on day 1 in patients with stable heart disease and decreased progressively to day 10 as fatty acid concentrations decreased and α_1-glycoprotein concentrations increased. Multiple stepwise regression showed a major influence of changing α_1-glycoprotein concentration on the observed sequential changes in the free quinidine fraction. In contrast, no serial changes in procainamide binding were noted. The investigators concluded that metabolic changes during AMI sequentially alter free quinidine fraction and, consequently, may influence pharmacodynamics.

Coronary artery bypass grafting

Evidence of ischemia after AMI is a serious complication. The precise timing of CABG may be of critical importance. From 1978–1982, 174 patients treated by Hochberg and coworkers[78] from New Jersey underwent CABG within 7 weeks of AMI: 44 (25%) patients required preoperative intraaortic balloon pump support and an additional 18 (10%) required intraaortic balloon pumping to be separated from cardiopulmonary bypass. An average of 2.9 ± 0.1 arteries per patient were bypassed. The hospital mortality was 16%. When mortalities were categorized according to the postinfarction week, hospital mortality fell from 46% for those patients operated on within 1 week of AMI to 6% for those patients operated on 7 weeks after AMI. Of those patients operated on within the first week after AMI, 23% were in cardiogenic shock and 62% required preoperative balloon pumping. However, there was a marked difference in survival when patients in each of

Fig. 2-15. Actuarial survival curves for all 174 patients (divided into EF groupings) after CABG, within 7 weeks of AMI. Reproduced with permission from Hochberg et al.[78]

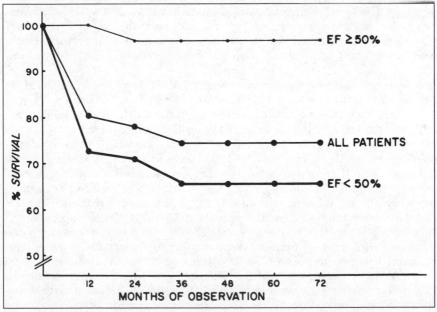

the 7 weekly groups were classified according to EF (Fig. 2-15). All patients with an EF >50% (50 patients) operated on at any time after AMI survived the hospital course with only 1 late death. Conversely, among the 124 patients with an EF <50% operated on within the 7-week interval, there were 27 (22%) hospital deaths. In this latter group, survival rates steadily improved if CABG was performed at a time more remote from the AMI. The difference in early and late survival rates of patients operated on with an EF >50% compared with patients with an EF <50% is highly significant (p < 0.001). The investigators concluded that CABG was safe at any time after AMI for those patients with an EF >50%. If the EF was <50%, operation after AMI should be delayed at least 4 weeks, if possible.

Left ventricular aneurysmectomy

Sir Brian Barratt-Boyes and colleagues[79] from Auckland, New Zealand, reported the surgical results of LV aneurysmectomy in 145 patients treated during a 13-year period. In 113 patients CABG also was undertaken. There were 22 hospital deaths for a 15% mortality and 44 late deaths. The chances of hospital death were increased by worsening New York Heart Association Class, severe CHF, and extensive CAD. Age, LV end-diastolic pressure and volume, and EF had little or no statistical relation to the prediction of operative death. Late results were importantly affected by the presence of angina alone or CHF alone (Fig. 2-16). Thus, if CHF was present, the late mortality was significantly greater than if there was angina as the indication for operation. The presence or absence of the use of furosemide was a predictor of early and late mortality. The investigators identified several incremental risk factors for early and late death after aneurysm resection. Presently other centers are reporting a diminished mortality for aneurysm resection. The definition of LV aneurysm varies among groups. The type of patients submitted to aneurysm resection also may differ among groups and finally the degree of CAD and segmental wall dysfunction may differ. The Auckland experience suggests that angina patients have a better surgical prognosis than those with CHF and that patients on a high dose of furosemide had a worse early and late prognosis than those who do not have need for a diuretic.

Olearchyk and associates[80] from Browns Mills, New Jersey, reported on 244 patients with post-AMI LV aneurysm operated on between 1971 and 1980. Indications for operation were angina in 61%, CHF in 10%, and intractable ventricular arrhythmias in 8%, or a combination of these in 21%. Of the 218 patients who survived the perioperative period (mean, 57 months follow-up) 85% were relieved of angina and 71% were in New York Heart Association class I or II compared with 16% before operation. Cardiac index increased from 2.4 ± 0.7 liters/minute body surface area before LV aneurysmectomy to 3 ± 0.5 liters/minute 1–12 weeks postoperatively. The LV end-diastolic volume decreased from 111 ± 55 ml/M^2 before operation to 73 ± 22 ml/M^2 ($p < 0.001$) ≥ 1 year later. The LV aneurysmectomy alone was performed in 11% of patients with an operative mortality of 8% and an actuarial 10-year survival of $57 \pm 11\%$ (Fig. 2-17). An LV aneurysmectomy with CABG was done in 89% of the patients, with an operative mortality of 11% and an actuarial 10-year survival of $69 \pm 4\%$. An LV aneurysmectomy combined with procedures on the mitral, aortic, or tricuspid valves was done

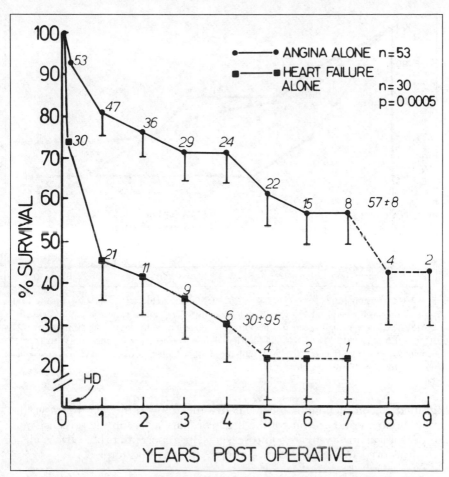

Fig. 2-16. Actuarial survival curves for surgically treated patients with LV aneurysmectomy, comparing those with CHF as their only symptom with those complaining only of angina. The number of patients at risk are noted. Bars indicate ± 1 SE. Reproduced with permission from Barratt-Boyes et al.[79]

in 8% and had a less satisfactory operative result, with an operative mortality of 20% and an actuarial 10-year survival rate of 60 ± 11%. The investigators noted the highest operative mortality when the indication for LV aneurysmectomy was intractable ventricular arrhythmias alone (16%), combined with CHF failure (20%) or combined with angina and CHF (33%), in those in New York Heart Association class IV (16%), and those supported by the intraaortic balloon (44%). Asymptomatic patients had a better 10-year survival rate (90%) than did symptomatic patients (46%). They concluded that functional results are encouraging. The number of patients in New York Heart Association classes I and II increased by 55% and the number of patients in classes III and IV decreased by 70%. Of all the parameters examined, LV aneurysmectomy with grafting of the LAD coronary artery and its diagonal branch yielded the best 10-year survival rate. This series suggests that in the absence of anteroseptal aneurysm the LAD coronary artery should be

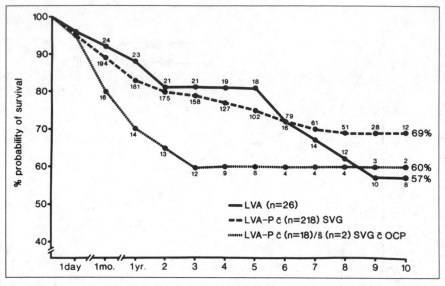

Fig. 2-17. Postoperative survival rates, calculated by the actuarial method, according to the procedure performed. *LVA* (n = 26) = left ventricular aneurysmectomy. *LVA-Pc̄* (n = 218)SVG = left ventricular aneurysmectomy or plication with saphenous vein graft. *LVA-Pc̄* (n = 18)/s̄ (n = 2)SVG c̄ OCP = left ventricular aneurysmectomy or plication with (n = 18) or without (n = 2) saphenous vein graft with and without other cardiac procedures. Reproduced with permission from Olearchyk et al.[80]

grafted. Recommendation for LV aneurysmectomy in the relatively asymptomatic patient and grafting of the LAD coronary artery in the presence of an anteroapical aneurysm are controversial. This report offers objective evidence for improved LV hemodynamics after LV aneurysmectomy.

Heparin

Mombelli and coworkers[81] from Bern, Switzerland, used the plasma level of fibrinopeptide A (FPA) as an index of thrombin action on fibrinogen to investigate the rates of fibrin formation and the effect of the heparin on thrombin in patients with AMI. The FPA levels measured on admission in 19 patients with AMI ranged from 1.7–12.4 ng/ml and were elevated >2.5 ng/ml in 16 patients. A loading dose of 5,000 IU of heparin resulted in a significant decrease within 20 minutes of the mean FPA level and in an FPA normalization on 5 of 16 patients. During the following continuous infusion of 20,000 IU of heparin per day, the mean FPA levels measured on day 0, 1, and 2 were 3.0, 3.2, and 3.4 ng/ml, respectively, with 16 of 46 FPA values within the normal range. In 10 additional patients, the effect of higher concentrations of heparin and the consequences of stopping heparin infusion were studied. An additional 5,000 IU of heparin injected intravenously during continuous infusion of 20,000 IU of heparin per day resulted in a substantial decrease of the plasma FPA level in 3 of 10 measurements. The stopping of heparin infusion led to an impressive increase of the mean FPA level within 2 hours. These data demonstrate increased fibrin formation in patients with

AMI and neutralization of thrombin in vivo by heparin. The observations also suggest that heparin doses higher than those conventionally used may be required to inhibit fibrin formation fully and that additional thrombin may be generated after cessation of heparin infusion.

Thrombolysis

To determine whether subsequent improvement in LV EF can be predicted from preintervention coronary arteriograms, Rogers and coworkers[82] from Birmingham, Alabama, divided 63 patients with AMI into 2 groups based on findings at emergency coronary arteriography at a mean of 7 hours after onset of symptoms. The "no-flow" group demonstrated an occluded infarct-related artery and no easily visible collaterals. The "limited-flow" group revealed either subtotal stenosis or total occlusion of the infarct-related vessel with intact collaterals. At follow-up angiography (contrast or radionuclide) performed 12 ± 7 days after AMI, global LF had increased significantly in patients with limited flow to the infarct zone and successful early reperfusion intervention due primarily to a significant increase in the regional EF in the infarct zone. Global EF decreased significantly below baseline and follow-up in patients with no flow to the infarct zone and unsuccessful early reperfusion intervention due primarily to a decrease in the regional EF of the noninfarct zone. Global and regional EF did not change significantly in patients with no flow to the infarct zone and successful early reperfusion or in patients with limited flow to the infarct zone and unsuccessful early reperfusion intervention. The elapsed time before reperfusion did not relate significantly to the change in either regional or global EF. The magnitude of improvement in both global and regional EF at follow-up was greater among patients with anterior AMI than among those with inferior AMI, possibly because baseline EF was lower in patients with anterior AMI. These data indicate that improvement in global EF is unlikely to occur even after a successful early reperfusion intervention in the absence of preserved flow to the infarct zone. Among patients with subtotally occluded infarct-related arteries or significant collateral flow to the infarct zone, subsequent improvement in global and regional EF in the zone of the AMI frequently occurs. Improvement in both global and regional EF may be more readily demonstrated in patients initially having more severe depression of these parameters. These investigators have identified an important mechanism for improved global and regional EF after reperfusion in AMI.

Leiboff and associates[83] from Washington, D.C., evaluated 55 patients with AMI within 4 hours of onset of symptoms. Each entered into an angiographically controlled trial of intracoronary (IC) streptokinase (STK): 43 patients with total occlusion of the infarct artery were randomized to either IC STK or IC nitroglycerin (NTG), and 12 patients with less-than-complete occlusion received only IC NTG. Reperfusion of a totally occluded vessel was achieved in 69% of STK patients and 17% of IC NTG patients. Time from onset of symptoms to peak creatine kinase (CK) activity was significantly shorter in reperfused patients and patients with subtotal occlusion on initial angiography than in patients with total occlusion who were not reperfused (p < 0.0001). Comparison of radionuclide EF determined acutely and 10–14 days after AMI failed to show improvement in either the STK or IC NTG group (mean decrease, 2.8 and 0.4%, respectively). In contrast, patients with subtotal occlusion on baseline angiography demonstrated a significant (p = 0.05) spontaneous improvement in EF over 2 weeks (7.3% increase).

Blanke and coworkers[84] from New York City have described the kinetics of CK release in patients who had successful reperfusion after receiving IC STK therapy during AMI. Coronary arteriography and biplane ventriculography were performed in 51 patients during the acute (mean, 6.6 hours after the onset of symptoms) and chronic (1–3 months after admission) phase of AMI. Twenty-four patients were treated conventionally and 27 patients had reperfusion achieved with IC STK after 24 ± 20 minutes of infusion. Peak CK and cumulative CK release were derived from serial CK measurements. The LV EF and the length of the akinetic or dyskinetic segments were calculated in the chronic study. The time interval between onset of symptoms and peak CK were shorter for the STK-treated patients compared with those treated conventionally (14 ± 5 compared with 23 ± 7 hours, p = 0.0001). Furthermore, patients receiving STK had a relatively greater release of enzyme for a given infarct size compared with those treated conventionally. These data may be explained by improved washout of CK from the infarct zone secondary to reperfusion after IC STK therapy. The variation in CK release occurring with reperfusion compared with conventional therapy suggests that prediction of infarct size from CK release should be made with great caution when reperfusion has occurred.

Whether administration is IC or intravenous (IV) STK and urokinase activate the fibrinolytic system in the general circulation, inducing what has been called a "systemic lytic state." The lytic state increases the risk of bleeding and is reflected by conversion of plasminogen to plasmin in the circulation, proteolytic depletion of circulating fibrinogen, accumulation of fibrinogen degradation products, and consumption of circulating α_2-antiplasmin. Tissue-type plasminogen activator is a naturally occurring serine protease that activates the fibrinolytic system under physiologic conditions by converting plasminogen to plasmin. It does not bind avidly to circulating plasminogen but has a high affinity for fibrin. Circulating plasminogen binds avidly to the tissue-type plasminogen activator-fibrin complex through the plasminogen-lysine binding sites. Thus, plasminogen is not readily converted to plasmin in the circulation but is converted to plasmin at the fibrin surface of clot while still in association with fibrin. Any plasmin that escapes into the circulation is rapidly inactivated by α_2-antiplasmin. Van de Werf and associates[85] from St. Louis, Missouri, and Leuven, Belgium, induced coronary thrombolysis, confirmed angiographically, within 19–50 minutes with IV or IC tissue-type plasminogen activator in 6 of 7 patients with evolving AMI. Circulating fibrinogen, plasminogen, and α_2-antiplasmin were not depleted by this agent, in contrast to the case in the 2 patients subsequently given STK. In the 1 patient in whom lysis was not inducible with tissue-type plasminogen activator, it was also not inducible with STK. These observations indicate that clot-selective coronary thrombolysis can be induced in patients with AMI by means of tissue-type plasminogen activator, without concomitant induction of a systemic lytic state.

The efficacy of IC urokinase and STK were compared by Tennant and colleagues[86] from Nashville, Tennessee, in 80 patients with AMI in a prospective, randomized, double-blind study. Urokinase was infused into the occluded coronary artery at 6,000 U/minute, and STK was infused at 2,000 U/minute. Maximal duration of infusion was 2 hours. The frequency of successfully opening the artery was similar for patients receiving urokinase (27 of 45, 60%) and those receiving STK (20 of 35, 57%). Fibrinogen levels after infusion were measured in 63 patients. Nineteen of 29 STK patients had fibrinogen levels <100 mg/dl compared with levels of 2 of 34 urokinase patients. Five of 45 (11%) patients receiving urokinase and 10 of 35 receiving STK (29%) had bleeding complications. Major bleeding after early CABG was more frequent in the STK group (4 of 5 compared with a similar group of patients receiving urokinase [0 of 5]). This study demonstrates that although urokinase and STK have equal IC thrombolytic efficacy, patients receiving urokinase have less systemic fibrinolysis and less perioperative bleeding with early CABG than do patients receiving STK. However, IC thrombolysis is still associated with bleeding, and this will continue with IV administration of these agents until the tissue of plasminogen activator becomes available.

To assess the effects on the heart itself of coronary thrombolysis induced with either tissue-type plasminogen activator or STK Sobel and coworkers[87] from St. Louis, Missouri, and Leuven, Belgium, performed positron emission tomography with ^{11}C-palmitate in 19 patients with initial transmural AMI immediately after admission and again within 48–72 hours after IC administration of tissue-type plasminogen activator (n, 2) or STK (n, 17). Clots were persistent in 8 patients treated with STK despite an average dose of 336,000 IU, sufficient to deplete fibrinogen markedly. In the absence of lysis, favorable tomographic changes did not occur. In contrast, in each of the 11 patients in whom lysis was induced (2 with tissue-type plasminogen activator and 9 with STK) myocardial accumulation of ^{11}C-palmitate improved by an average of 29% in late compared with early studies. Results were comparable in patients with anterior and those with inferior AMI. Thus, clot lysis induced with either tissue-type plasminogen activator or STK led to improved regional myocardial metabolism.

Since residual high grade stenoses are frequently present at the site of the previous instruction after reperfusion with STK, Harrison and coworkers[88] from Iowa City, Iowa, tested the hypothesis that lesion rethrombosis after STK infusion is related to luminal size of the residual stenosis. Two independent techniques of analyzing coronary angiogram, quantitative coronary angiography and computer-based videodensitometry, were used to estimate the size of the residual lumen immediately after discontinuation of STK. These techniques were selected because they provided independent estimates of cross-sectional area of a lesion with high degrees of reproducibility and minimal observer variability. Twenty-four patients who had undergone successful reperfusion with STK were studied. Seven patients had lesion rethrombosis documented. Vessel patency was documented by repeat coronary angiography 8–14 days after the initial STK infusion in the other 17 patients. As assessed by quantitative coronary angiography, 7 of 13 patients with minimal luminal cross-sectional areas of <0.4 mm^2 had rethrombosis. None of 11 patients with lumens >0.4 mm^2 had rethrombosis. In the 17 patients with vessels that remained patent, the size of the residual lesion at repeat catheterization was compared with its size immediately after reperfusion with STK. Over the intervening 8–14 days, an average percentage increase in minimal cross-sectional area of 116 ± 34% was observed. In 7 patients minimal luminal cross-sectional area more than doubled. Integrated optical density, an index of the severity of CAD derived from computer-based videodensitometry, was also useful in identifying a subgroup of patients at high risk for rethrombosis of lesion. Sixteen patients were identified as having integrated optical densities <2.5, and 7 of these had rethrombosis of their lesion. Among the 8 patients with integrated optical densities >2.5, none had rethrombosis. These results show that rethrombosis of the artery is in part related to the size of the residual lesion immediately after reperfusion with STK. Arteries with residual stenotic cross-sectional areas <0.4 mm² are at high risk for rethrombosis, whereas vessels with minimal cross-sectional areas of >0.4 mm² are unlikely to develop rethrombosis. Residual size of the lumen may change significantly during the 8–14 days after reperfusion. Thus, these changes may be due to remodeling of a ruptured atherosclerotic plaque, resolution of persistent coronary spasm, or lysis of persistent thrombi.

Ganz and associates[89] from Los Angeles, California, administered to 81 consecutive patients presenting within 3 hours of AMI and without contraindications to thrombolytic or anticoagulant therapy a 15- to 30-minute intravenous infusion of 750,000 or 1.5 million U of STK followed by anticoagulation. Treatment was instituted 130 ± 41 minutes after the onset of symptoms and reperfusion was achieved 36 ± 26 minutes later. Reperfusion of the "infarct artery" was recognized by indirect clinical criteria in 78 patients (96%). In all 66 patients who underwent coronary angiography 3–7 days later, there was complete concordance between indirect and angiographic evidence of reperfusion. In 6 patients there was early reocclusion within 24 hours of treatment; in 4 of these patients, the artery was reopened with an additional dose of STK. Two elderly patients had an intracranial hemorrhage and there were 8 other major hemorrhagic complications, of which 7 were related to procedural trauma. Five patients (6%) died in the hospital.

Yasuno and associates[90] from Hamamatsu City, Japan, performed coronary angioplasty and PTCA in 32 patients with AMI and IC infusion of urokinase in the 25 patients with complete occlusion of an infarct-related coronary artery. Of the latter 25, in 18 the occluded vessel was successfully opened by urokinase. With a small dose of urokinase, the successful opening was achieved in 25% and with a larger dose, in 94%. After PTCA, all patients received glucose-insulin-potassium solution for 76 hours. Repeat angiography 42 days later showed a patent coronary artery in 12 (group A) of 18 patients with successful PTCA. In group A, LV EF increased from 51 ± 13–72 ± 10% and regional wall shortening from 4.5 ± 9.5–29 ± 19%. In contrast, these variables did not change significantly in patients with unsuccessful PTCA or late reocclusion of an infarct-related vessel (group B). These data suggest that successful PTCA with sustained patency of an infarct-related coronary artery has a beneficial effect on the salvage of the jeopardized myocardium, and glucose-insulin-potassium therapy may enhance the beneficial effect of PTCA.

Bleeding continues to be a problem during treatment with both STK and heparin in patients undergoing fibrinolysis for AMI and this may be particularly troublesome during the transition to anticoagulant therapy at the end of the infusion of STK. Hemorrhage was prospectively identified in 26 of 116 consecutive patients (23%) by Timmis and coworkers[91] from Royal Oak, Michigan, who were receiving IC STK for occlusive coronary thrombi producing AMI. Bleeding was not influenced by the dose of STK or the method of cardiac catheterization. Before treatment, prothrombin time and partial thromboplastin time were normal in both bleeders and nonbleeders. Fibrinogen levels measured by bioassay after STK were not significantly lower in patients with major bleeding than in patients with minor bleeding or in nonbleeders. Mean fibrinogen concentrations calculated at sequential 5-hour intervals revealed no net regeneration for the first 20 hours after thrombolysis. The apparent fibrinogen regeneration rate was less than normal for >10 hours but subsequently increased by the second day. The initial apparent latency of fibrinogen regeneration paralleled the sharp rise in fibrinogen degradation products, which began to decline after 20 hours of treatment but remained elevated well into the second day. Because of their anticoagulant effects, these products may interfere with the fibrinogen assay, causing spuriously low results. Thus, whether the early delay in fibrinogen regeneration is real or simply a reflection of the effects of fibrinogen degradation products on the bioassay, it signals the time for caution in initiating systemic heparin therapy. The observations of these investigators should be extended to both IV and IC STK, since heparin therapy appears to reduce the instance of rethrombosis but contributes to further bleeding complications.

Schwarz and associates[92] from Heidelberg, West Germany, assessed retrospectively in 55 consecutive patients with transmural AMI the effect of pretreatment of IV infusion of STK (16,700 U/minute for 90 minutes), started after diagnosis and followed by IC infusion (2,000 U/minute; protocol 1). Another 46 patients with AMI treated previously with IC thrombolysis served as control subjects. Reperfusion at first coronary injection was observed after pretreatment in 25 patients (45%) but in no control patient. Fifteen patients with successful pretreatment (group A), 20 patients with successful treatment according to protocol 2 (group B), and 9 patients with unsuccessful thrombolysis (group C) were restudied after 4 weeks. Data from patients with reinfarction, CABG, or PTCA before restudy were excluded. Thallium-201 scintigraphy was performed before and 24 hours after treatment, serum CK activity was measured every 8 hours for 3 days, and regional EF of AMI was determined before and 4 weeks after treatment. The scintigraphic, enzymatic, and hemodynamic data before treatment indicated severe and comparable ischemia among the 3 groups. The thallium-201 perfusion defect decreased in group A (from 41–21%, p < 0.01) and in group B (from 38–26%, p < 0.01), but did not change in group C (from 37–31%, NS). Peak serum CK levels normalized by the perfusion area of AMI was 20, 33, and 58 U/liter in groups A, B, and C. The mean values of groups A and C were significantly different (p < 0.01). The regional EF of AMI recovered after 4 weeks in group A (from 24–42%, p < 0.001), but not in groups B or C. Time to catheterization from onset of symptoms was similar among the 3 groups; however, start of treatment and angiographic proof of reperfusion (3.5 -vs- 4.5 hours, p < 0.05) was achieved earlier in group A than in group B. Pretreatment with intravenous infusion of STK was followed by reperfusion of AMI in 45% of patients. After 4 weeks, successfully pretreated patients revealed less severe ischemic damage than that in patients treated successfully by IC infusion of STK alone.

Alderman and associates[93] from Stanford, California, in a randomized trial of 28 patients who underwent angiography before and during IV and IC administration of STK achieved recanalization in 73% of the patients who received the drug by the IC route and in 62% of the patients who received the drug by the IV route (NS). Reopening took 28 minutes for IC STK and 39 minutes for IV STK. Patients in whom recanalization was successful using either route of administration had shorter euglobulin lysis times and lower fibrinogen levels than did patients in whom it was not successful (p < 0.05). Bleeding complications were closely correlated with heparinization after thrombolysis rather than with STK itself. These results suggest that early administration of IV STK in the emergency department may yield recanalization rates similar to those for the IC route and may benefit myocardial preservation by restoring flow much earlier.

In 184 consecutive patients with AMI, Taylor and associates[94] from Springfield, Illinois, administered STK. The first 63 patients were treated with IC STK and 44 (70%) had successful thrombolysis. The remaining 121 patients received IV STK immediately after diagnosis of AMI and 99 (82%) were found to have an open infarct artery. Only 58% of patients (14 of 24) who required transfer from out-of-town hospitals for IC STK treatment had successful thrombolysis; in contrast, IV STK given in the local hospital resulted in an 85% (72 of 85) rate of thrombolysis (p = 0.005). Thus, IV STK appears to be at least as effective as IC STK for AMI and is more effective for patients treated in hospitals without catheterization facilities.

To determine the effects of IV thrombolytic therapy on the development of LV thrombi after anterior AMI, Eigler and associates[95] from Los Angeles, California, prospectively studied 22 consecutive patients with RNA and serial 2-D echo: 12 patients who presented within 3 hours after AMI received IV STK followed by IV heparin as thrombolytic treatment and 10 patients who were seen later than 3 hours after the onset of symptoms served as controls. The LV EF was <0.40 in 3 of 12 patients who received STK and in 7 of 19 who did not (control subjects) (p < 0.05). Apical dyssynergy occurred in all 12 patients treated with STK and in 9 of 10 control subjects. In 5 control subjects LV thrombi were present within 36 hours of AMI. Thrombi were detected by 2-D echo in 7 of 10 control subjects and in 1 of 12 patients who received IV STK (p < 0.005). Early thrombolytic therapy with IV STK and heparin appears to reduce significantly the frequency of LV thrombus formation despite persistence of apical dyssynergy.

Kasper and coworkers[96] from Mainz, West Germany, evaluated the fibrinolytic ability and systemic effects on coagulation variables after the IC administration of an acylated STK plasminogen complex (BRL 26921) in 23 patients with AMI. In 22 patients, the infarct artery was totally occluded. Reperfusion occurred in 17 patients (74%), in 2 patients with the use of a guide wire. Reperfusion time in patients receiving BRL 26921 alone was 42 ± 37 minutes; reocclusion occurred in 2 patients subsequently. In patients receiving BRL 26921, fibrinogen levels decreased from 280 ± 65–126 ± 76 mg/dl, factor V decreased from 96 ± 11–53 ± 26%, and factor VIII from 99 ± 1–55 ± 36% (p < 0.001). Reductions in fibrinogen to values <100 mg/dl and a reduction of factor V and factor VIII by >75% occurred in 8 patients; 6 of these demonstrated reperfusion. Nine patients without such severe reductions in fibrinogen and factors V and VIII were also successfully reperfused. Thus, these data indicate that effective IC thrombolysis may be achieved with only moderate effects on peripheral coagulation variables after the IC administration of an acylated STK plasminogen activator.

Ferguson and associates[97] from Iowa City, Iowa, prospectively evaluated the efficacy of STK thrombolytic therapy in 77 consecutive patients presenting within 9 hours of onset of AMI. Serial LV EF was assessed by radionuclide ventriculography, initially (acute) and at 1 month (late). The role of initial

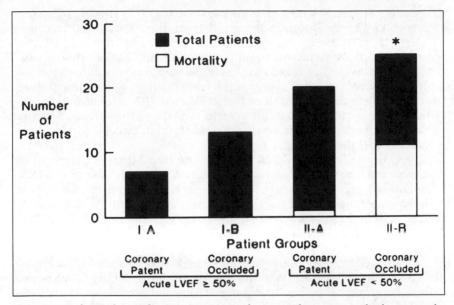

Fig. 2-18. In-hospital mortality rate in patient subgroups. There were no deaths among the patients with a LV EF ≥50% (groups I-A and I-B). There was a significant reduction in mortality in group II-A (mortality 5%) patients who had successful and persistent reperfusion compared with group II-B patients (mortality 44%), who had initial failure of reperfusion or in-hospital coronary reocclusion. *p < 0.01 for mortality in group II-B vs other groups.

LV EF was examined by comparing patients with an acute LV EF >50% (type 1) with those with <50% (type II) (Fig. 2-18). Sixty-five patients (84%) had total coronary occlusion and received STK. Initial successful reperfusion was achieved in 34 patients (52%), but repeat angiograms at 10–14 days revealed persistent patency in only 27 patients. Within the type I and type II classification, 2 patient subgroups were compared: Group A had successful and persistent thrombolysis and group B had initial failure of thrombolysis or in-hospital reocclusion. There was no significant change in global LV EF in any group from acute to 1 month follow-up: group IA: acute EF, 56 ± 2% (mean ± SEM), and late EF, 55 ± 2%; group IB: acute EF, 58 ± 1%, and late EF, 55 ± 2%; group IIA: acute EF, 35 ± 2%, and late EF, 4 + 4%; group IIB: acute EF, 36 ± 2%, and late EF, 41 ± 3%. No patient with an acute EF < 50% died, i.e., group IA patients (n, 7) or group IB patients (n, 13). However, there was a significant difference in the mortality rate between patients with an acute EF <50% who had successful persistent thrombolysis and those in whom thrombolysis failed (groups IIA and IIB: mortality group IIA, 1 of 20 [5%], and mortality group IIB, 11 of 25 [44%]: p = 0.003 group IIA -vs- IIB), with 92% of all deaths occurring in patients with anterior AMI. Thus, the primary demonstrable benefit of STK thrombolysis is a lower mortality rate among patients with an initial LV EF <50%.

White and associates[98] from Iowa City, Iowa, examined reasons for the failure of IC STK to result in coronary thrombolysis in 45 patients with AMI presenting with angiographic evidence of total coronary occlusion. In 25 patients (group A) clot lysis was initially successful; in 20 (group B), reperfusion was unsuccessful. The STK dosage in reperfusion was unsuccessful. The

STK dosage in group A ranged from 84,000–310,000 U (mean, 188,000 ± 12,000); STK dosage in group B ranged from 160,000–360,000 U (mean 267,000 ± 11,000). Before therapy, levels of fibrin degradation products and serum fibrinogen were normal in all patients. After IC STK, fibrin degradation products and serum fibrinogen levels changed similarly in both groups. Eighty-five percent of patients in group B had evidence of a systemic fibrinolytic state. These data suggest that higher doses of STK administered in the same manner are unlikely to result in an increased reperfusion rate. Systemic hematologic markers of fibrinolysis are not helpful in explaining the success or failure of IC thrombolysis.

The clinical effects of IV STK in patients with AMI were compared by Anderson and coworkers[99] from Salt Lake City, Utah, with those of IC STK in a randomized, prospective study. Fifty patients were entered into the study at 2.4 hours after the onset of pain, and 27 were assigned to IV and 23 to IC therapy. The average IC dose of STK was 212,000 U and IV dose, 845,000 U. The STK was administered at 2.8 hours after onset of pain in the IV and at 4.3 hours in the IC groups. Radionuclide EF on day 10 were 54% for the IV and 50% for the IC drug group. Change in EF from days 1–10 tended to be greater after the IV drug: 5 -vs- 1%. Wall motion indexes in the infarct zone showed similar improvement by day 10 in both groups and accelerated enzyme-release kinetics were also noted after both therapies. The ECG summed ST segments diminished rapidly after therapy in both groups and Q wave development was similar with overall R wave loss equivalent and less extensive compared with the historical control subjects. The incidence of early arrhythmias and CHF did not differ in both groups. Post-therapy ischemic events and early CABG tended to be more common in the IC group and bleeding was more common in the IV group. The IV drugs did not decrease early hospital mortality (IV drug, 5 deaths; historical control, 4, and IC drug, 1). At convalescent angiographic evaluation, antegrade perfusion was present in 73% of those receiving IV and 76% of those receiving IC drug. Thus, favorable effects were noted on cardiac function and hospital course after IV STK and early survivors of AMI. However, the early mortality in the IV group could not be ascribed to the drug.

Urban and colleagues[100] from Philadelphia, Pennsylvania, and Richmond, Virginia, evaluated the course of 73 patients who had attempted IC thrombolysis. Fifty-nine patients (81%) had coronary reflow sufficient to control pain and injury current: 52 received thrombolysis alone and 7 had thrombolysis combined with acute coronary angioplasty. Recurrent ischemic events in the hospital were frequent and occurred in 17 patients (29%). These included silent reocclusion (4 patients), recurrent angina (8 patients), and recurrent infarction in the same myocardial zone (5 patients). Late ischemic events occurred in 11 patients (19%) and included silent reocclusion (2 patients) and angina (9 patients). Although acute coronary angioplasty resulted in a high rate of successful myocardial reperfusion, long-term vessel patency was infrequent. The results of CABG, performed in the hospital for severe residual coronary stenosis and angina and later for recurrent angina, were uniformly good. At follow-up of 6–36 months (mean, 19 ± 8) total mortality was 5 patients (8%). Only 16 reperfused patients (27%) were alive and well without recurrent ischemia or interventions. It was concluded that reopening an acutely occluded coronary artery by thrombolysis or angioplasty can be performed in most patients but must be regarded as initial therapy in view of the high incidence of recurrent ischemic events.

Schuler and associates[101] from Heidelberg, West Germany, studied 19 patients undergoing IC fibrinolytic therapy for AMI in whom the site of coronary obstruction was the proximal right coronary artery. The time between the onset of symptoms and hospitalization was <4 hours. These patients were studied prospectively by radionuclide techniques immediately after admission, at 48 hours, and at 4 weeks after AMI. Right and LV EF were calculated from gated blood pool scintigrams and the size of the LV perfusion defect was assessed by thallium-201 scintigraphy. Before the intervention, RV performance was significantly lower (RV EF, 29 ± 8%) than normal (53 ± 7%). The size of the LV perfusion defect was relatively small (less than 25% of LV circumference), and as a consequence, LV pump function was only marginally impaired (LV EF 54 ± 11%). Recanalization of the infarct artery was achieved in 12 patients (group A); in 7 patients the infarct artery remained occluded (group B). Early after the intervention (48 hours), RV performance in group A recovered significantly (RV EF: 30 ± 9% -vs- 39 ± 7%, p < 0.01), and further improvement was noted at 4 weeks (RV EF 43 ± 5%, p < 0.01). In group B, however, RV performance remained depressed early and late after the intervention (RV EF 33 ± 5% -vs- 33 ± 4% at 48 hours, and 32 ± 6% at 4 weeks, NS), and 3 patients with severely impaired RV EF died in the early postinfarction period. In both groups average LV performance remained essentially unchanged within the first weeks after AMI. In conclusion, in most patients with proximal occlusion of the right coronary artery, early recanalization results in swift improvement of initially depressed RV performance; often, recovery of myocardial function is not reflected by changes in LV EF. In contrast, in patients with persistent occlusion, RV AMI may occasionally result in irreversible cardiogenic shock and early death despite adequate LV performance.

Although therapeutic thrombolysis in patients with AMI is becoming a widespread form of therapy, there are few control data comparing this form of treatment with conventional management. The Western Washington Intracoronary Streptokinase In Myocardial Infarction Trial has enrolled 250 patients with AMI. After the coronary angiographic diagnosis of thrombosis, Ritchie and coworkers[102] from Seattle, Washington, randomly assigned patients to receive either conventional therapy with heparin or IC STK followed by heparin. Of the 232 patients who survived at least 60 days, 207 (89%) underwent radionuclide ventriculographic determination of global and regional EF at a single institution at 62 days after AMI. In the first 100 patients, infarct size was also determined by quantitative single-photon emission tomographic imaging with thallium-201 and expressed as a percent of the left ventricle with a perfusion defect. Overall, global EF did not differ between patients treated with STK (46%) and control patients (46%). Similarly, the regional posterolateral, inferior, and anteroseptal EF did not differ between the 2 groups. Infarct size as measured by thallium-201 tomography was 19% of the left ventricle for the STK group and 20% for the control group. When patients were compared within groups by ECG location of AMI, time to treatment, or the presence or absence of artery opening, there were no significant differences between STK and control patients. These investigators concluded that global and regional LV pump function and infarct size determined by thallium-201 tomography did not differ substantially between patients receiving STK and those receiving conventional treatment when measured 8 weeks after AMI.

Hodgson and associates[103] from Ann Arbor, Michigan, performed interventional contrast ventriculography using programmed atrial stimulation in 23 patients with evolving AMI undergoing catheterization for thrombolytic therapy. Postextrasystolic (PES) potentiation was present in 67% of infarct-related segments up to 9 hours after the onset of AMI. The presence of segmental potentiation was not related to time from onset of pain to ventriculography, initial EF, presence of collaterals, LV end-diastolic pressure, or the PES delay. In 18 patients reperfusion was successful using IC STK an average of 6.2 hours after the onset of AMI; in these patients repeat contrast ventriculography was performed an average of 11 days after AMI. Improved chronic segmental ventricular function was predicted by the presence of collaterals in the infarct-related artery at the time of acute catheterization, but was best predicted by analysis of acute PES potentiation. The predictive value of PES analysis was highest in segments without collaterals. Thus, atrial stimulation is safe during AMI and analysis of segmental LV function shows potentially viable myocardium up to 9 hours after the onset of AMI. In addition, analysis of PES segmental function can predict chronic function if reperfusion is successful, especially in segments without collaterals. The PES ventriculographic analysis may allow prospective determination of which patients during AMI are most likely to benefit from acute thrombolytic therapy.

Anderson and colleagues[104] from Salt Lake City, Utah, evaluated the outpatient course of 50 AMI patients, randomly treated with either STK (n, 24) or standard therapy (n, 26), who presented within 2.7 ± 0.7 hours of symptoms. Coronary reperfusion occurred in 19 (79%) of STK patients. Survivors were followed for a mean of 19 months (range, 11–29); information was current in 48 patients (96%). Both groups received antiplatelet therapy for 3 months. Five deaths occurred in the control group and 2 in the STK group. Nonfatal AMI totaled 5 in control patients and 3 in STK patients. Differences in major events (death or nonfatal AMI) favoring STK did not quite reach statistical significance (10 control -vs- 5 STK). A CABG was performed in 7 STK and 4 control patients (NS). Angina occurred in more control than STK patients (p < 0.01), and more control patients used long-acting nitrates (14 control, 3 STK; p < 0.01). Palpitations were noted by 9 control and 1 STK patients (p < 0.01), and documented late arrhythmias were present in 4 control patients and no STK survivors (p < 0.05). Symptoms suggestive of CHF were present in 7 control and 1 STK patients (p < 0.01); 2 control patients were hospitalized for CHF. Use of beta blockers, calcium-channel blockers, and other cardiac medications did not differ. Activity status also was similar. The ECGs in surviving patients at 6 weeks revealed an average of 4.2 ± 2.4 Q waves in control -vs- 3.1 ± 1.5 STK patients (trend NS). Early catheterization with application of STK within about 4 hours of AMI was associated with continued favorable clinical trends after 1.5 years.

Collen and coworkers[105] in a collaborative study from Baltimore, Maryland, Boston, Massachusetts, and St. Louis, Missouri, randomized 45 patients with AMI and angiographically confirmed complete coronary occlusion to treatment of acute coronary thrombosis with IV recombinant human tissue-type plasminogen activator (rt-PA) or placebo. Each of 5 additional consecutive patients was treated with a high dose of rt-PA for 2 hours. Of 33 patients

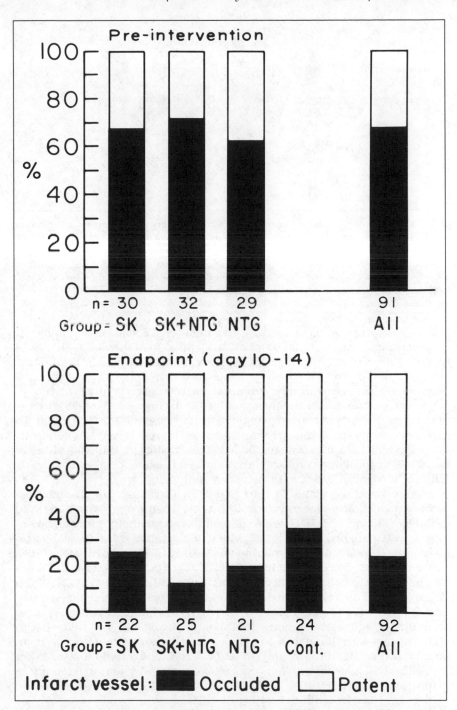

Fig. 2-19. Patency rates for infarct-related coronary arteries before intervention (upper panel) and at days 10–14 (lower panel) in groups of patients with AMI treated with intracoronary STK, STK and NTG, NTG, or conventional therapy. Reproduced with permission from Rentrop et al.[106]

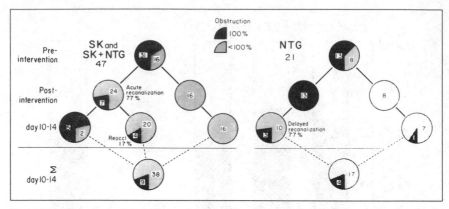

Fig. 2-20. Frequency of complete and incomplete obstruction of the infarct-related coronary artery before intervention, immediately after intervention, and at days 10–14 in 68 patients with paired data. The numbers on the pie graphs correspond to the numbers of patients with the indicated degree of obstruction. The left panel shows pooled data for patients who received an IC infusion of STK (SK) or STK plus NTG; the right panel shows data for those who received IC NTG alone. Reproduced with permission from Rentrop et al.[106]

(75%) receiving the agent over 30–120 minutes, 25 had angiographically proved recanalization within 90 minutes of initiation of therapy. Only 1 of 14 patients given placebo had spontaneous recanalization within 45 minutes. Thirteen placebo-treated patients were crossed over to the IC rt-PA group: 9 had subsequent recanalization within 45 minutes. Levels of circulating fibrinogen decreased after treatment with rt-PA by an average of 8% of baseline values. No patient had a depletion of fibrinogen levels to <100 mg/dl. Six patients who were completely unresponsive to rt-PA were subsequently treated with IC STK and none responded. These results indicate that either IV or IC rt-PA can induce coronary thrombolysis without eliciting clinically significant fibrinogenolysis in patients with AMI.

Rentrop and associates[106] from New York City randomly assigned patients with a clinical diagnosis of AMI to 1 of 4 treatment groups: IC STK, IC NTG, IC STK and IC NTG, or conventional therapy without initial angiography. Of 124 patients, 122 had AMI. Initial angiography revealed total occlusion of the coronary artery responsible for AMI in 67% (61 of 91) (Fig. 2-19). Acute recanalization occurred in 74% (32 of 43) of patients receiving STK but in only 6% (1 of 18) of patients treated with NTG alone (Fig. 2-20). At angiography of all 4 groups on days 10–14 the artery responsible for AMI was patent in 77% (71 of 92) of patients; there was no difference among groups, indicating gradual, endogenous thrombolysis in patients not treated with STK. Patients with subtotal obstruction initially had significant improvement in LV function, significantly lower peak CK levels, and a trend toward lower mortality than patients with total occlusion initially. Mortality at 6 months in patients receiving STK (21%, 13 of 62) did not differ significantly from that in patients not treated with STK (10%, 6 of 61).

Skinner and associates[107] from Des Moines, Iowa, reported their experience with CABG after failed STK infusion for AMI. One hundred and eighty-four patients with AMI underwent immediate catheterization followed by IC STK therapy total (dose 200,000–250,000 U) with or without PTCA: 57 were considered treatment failures based on failure of thrombolysis of a major coronary vessel, failure of PTCA to relieve critical stenosis after successful thrombolysis, occlusion of a coronary artery at attempted PTCA, or continuing profound cardiac decompensation. Twenty-four of 57 treatment failures (42%) underwent immediate CABG: 9 were in profound cardiogenic shock with 8 requiring intraaortic balloon support. Six died (25%) in the hospital; 5 were in the subgroup of those with profound cardiac decompensation preoperatively. The hematologic consequences in this group of 25 patients were an average postoperative blood loss of 1,457 ml per patient and average blood transfusions of 8.2 U per patient. All patients required blood transfusions during and after operation. In 13 patients coagulation profiles were normal. Four patients required reexploration and all patients had some abnormality of clotting activity immediately after heparin reversal characterized by diffuse oozing and requirements for fresh frozen plasma and platelets while in the operating room. Average hospital stay was 15 days.

Laffel and Braunwald[108] from Boston, Massachusetts, reviewed the usefulness and complications of thrombolytic therapy during AMI. This is a superb review on this subject.

Alteration in type A behavior

Friedman and associates[109] from San Francisco, California, enrolled 862 post-AMI patients volunteered to be randomly selected into: a control section of 270 patients, who received group cardiologic counseling, and an experimental section of 592 patients, who received group type A behavior counseling in addition to group cardiologic counseling. Reduction in type A behavior at the end of 3 years was observed in 44% of the 592 participants, who initially were enrolled to receive group cardiologic and type A behavioral counseling. This degree of behavioral reduction was significantly greater than that observed in participants who initially were enrolled to receive only group cardiologic counseling. The 3-year cumulative cardiac recurrence rate was 7% in participants who initially were enrolled to receive group cardiologic and type A behavioral counseling. This was significantly less (p < 0.005) than that (13%) observed in participants who initially were enrolled to receive only cardiologic counseling. This difference in recurrence rates was due to a lower incidence of nonfatal AMI in the patients who had been enrolled in the section receiving type A behavioral as well as cardiologic counseling.

RELATED TOPICS

Serum total cholesterol level within 24 hours of AMI

The relation of the serum total cholesterol (TC) level obtained during AMI to the patient's usual baseline level is unclear. Many physicians tend to ignore TC levels measured during AMI and wait several months before obtaining a repeat TC measurement; in many instances this delays interven-

TABLE 2-5. *Changes in total serum cholesterol levels in patients with recognized and unrecognized AMI: Framingham Heart Study*

	RECOGNIZED AMI (N = 83)	UNRECOGNIZED AMI (N = 175)
Cholesterol level (mg/dl) before AMI (mean)	253 ± 47	244 ± 42
First day of hospital admission cholesterol level (mg/dl; mean)	248 ± 43	
Cholesterol level (mg/dl) after AMI (mean)	245 ± 46	234 ± 42

tional programs. Using the Framingham study cohort of patients, Gore and associates[110] from Framingham, Massachusetts, reviewed the records of all persons sustaining AMI: 83 were identified who had TC levels recorded within 2 years of AMI, within 24 hours of hospitalization for AMI, and within 2 years after hospital discharge. In these patients, there was no statistically significant difference in the TC values measured at these 3 times (Table 2-5). Thus, TC levels drawn within the first 24 hours of AMI accurately reflect a baseline level and can be used in instituting intervention programs.

Usefulness and cost effectiveness of coronary care units

McGregor[111] from Montreal, Canada, summarized studies attempting to evaluate the usefulness of the coronary care unit (CCU). Historically, the CCU has been considered an indispensable component of any acute care hospital. In the early 1960s it was a product of the development of the electric defibrillator and the cardiac monitor. Since patients with AMI were particularly susceptible to malignant arrhythmias, it was logical to concentrate them in special areas where the pieces of equipment could be located. The resulting units became staffed by specialized personnel and spread rapidly throughout the hospital system. Their introduction coincided with a remarkable reduction in case fatality from AMI in North America. Whether or not the reduction in case fatality was the result of the patients being hospitalized in CCU remains uncertain. At the present time therefore there is no direct evidence that management in the CCU favorably influences AMI fatality rates. Furthermore, the difficulties, ethical and otherwise, of carrying out a good trial to establish this are so great that it is unlikely that it will ever be achieved. What policy, then, should be adopted in relation to the use of these expensive facilities? Should all patients with AMI be admitted to the CCU? And for how long after the completion of AMI should they remain therein? McGregor contends that the CCU is an appropriate environment for the management of dangerous arrhythmias and the major complications of AMI, for the management of resting angina until asymptomatic for 24 hours, and for the management of uncomplicated AMI in the absence of all predictors of risk for a period of 24 hours after the last episode of ischemic pain. Longer observation may be desirable only for patients of certain predictors of short-term risk.

Fineberg and associates[112] from Boston, Massachusetts, conducted a cost effectiveness analysis to examine the clinical and economic consequences of alternatives to admission to a CCU for patients who have a relatively low probability of AMI. This analysis showed that admission to an intermediate care unit providing resuscitative facilities and prophylactic lidocaine is highly cost effective. For patients with about a 5% probability of AMI, admission to a CCU would cost $2.04 million per life saved and $139,000 per year of life saved compared with intermediate care. For the expected number of such patients annually in the USA, the cost would be $297 million to save 145 lives. At probabilities of AMI up to about 20%, the incremental cost to save a year of life by choosing a CCU over an intermediate care unit would be higher than the estimated cost of saving a year of life by treating a 40 year old man with mild systemic hypertension. The results suggest that many patients who have a low risk of AMI would be appropriate candidates for admission to an intermediate care unit.

Each year 1.5 million patients are admitted to a CCU for suspected acute CAD; for half of these patients, the diagnosis is ultimately "ruled out." Pozen and associates,[113] in a Prospective Multicenter Clinical Trial involving the emergency rooms of 6 New England hospitals ranging in type from urban teaching centers to rural nonteaching hospitals, developed a scheme to help emergency room physicians reduce the number of CCU admissions of patients without acute cardiac ischemia. From data on 2,801 patients, a predictive instrument was developed for use in a hand-held programmable calculator, which requires only 20 seconds to compute a patient's probability of having acute cardiac ischemia. In a prospective trial that included 2,320 patients in the 6 hospitals, physicians' diagnostic specificity for acute ischemia increased when the probability value determined by the instrument was made available to them. Rates of false positive diagnosis decreased without any increase in rates of false negative diagnosis. Among study patients with a final diagnosis of "not acute ischemia," the number of CCU admissions decreased 30%, without any increase in missed diagnoses of ischemia. The proportion of CCU admissions that represented patients without acute ischemia dropped from 44–33%. Widespread use of this predictive instrument could reduce the number of CCU admissions in this country by more than 250,000 per year.

Transtelephonic coronary intervention

Capone and associates[114] from Providence, Rhode Island, and Buffalo, New York, evaluated 284 patients in a pilot study of the effects of subsequent mortality and morbidity of a prehospital program for post-AMI patients experiencing recurrent chest pain: 161 in a program incorporating patient education, routine transtelephonic follow-up, and emergency prehospital CCU-controlled intervention; 124 in a control group receiving usual medical care. Cardiac mortality over a median of 13-months follow-up was significantly reduced in the treatment group (6%) -vs- control (13%, p = 0.036), although the incidence of acute events (nonfatal AMI plus cardiac death) was similar in both groups. This suggests that the program does not affect the acute incident, but rather the mortality subsequent to it. Prehospital ventricular arrhythmias, present in 7 of 54 treatment patients with recurrent chest pain, did not recur after self-injection by a prefilled lidocaine syringe; only 1 patient who was initially arrhythmia-free had VPC after lidocaine injection. Delay from onset of symptoms to hospital arrival was 1.9 hours. Routine telephone follow-up uncovered ventricular arrhythmias in 30% of treatment patients and, despite the program's patient educational efforts, unreported angina in 20% of the treatment group. In the treatment group there were 99 emergency calls placed by 62 patients, 50% within 12 weeks after discharge and 80% by 35 weeks, resulting in 74 Emergency Department evaluations and 57 hospital admissions. Overuse of the emergency system occurred with only 1 patient, and physician acceptance was high. This approach to the care of the patient discharged after an AMI is practical and results in a significant reduction of 1-year post-AMI mortality.

References

1. KANNEL WB, ABBOTT RD: Incidence and prognosis of unrecognized myocardial infarction: an update on the Framingham Study. N Engl J Med 311:1144–1147, Nov 1, 1984.
2. SPODICK DH, FLESSAS AP, JOHNSON MM: Association of acute respiratory symptoms with onset of acute myocardial infarction: perspective investigation of 150 consecutive patients and matched control patients. Am J Cardiol 53:481–482, Feb 1, 1984.
3. MUKHARJI J, MURRAY S, LEWIS SE, CROFT CH, CORBETT JR, WILLERSON JT, RUDE RE: Is anterior ST depression with acute transmural inferior infarction due to posterior infarction? A vectorcardiographic and scintigraphic study. J Am Coll Cardiol 4:28–34, July 1984.
4. ROUBIN GS, SHEN WF, NICHOLSON M, DUNN RF, KELLY DT, HARRIS PJ: Anterolateral ST segment depression in acute inferior myocardial infarction: angiographic and clinical implications. Am Heart J 107:1177–1182, June 1984.
5. BLANKE H, COHEN M, SCHLUETER GU, KARSCH KR, RENTROP KP: Electrocardiographic and coronary arteriographic correlations during acute myocardial infarction. Am J Cardiol 54:249–255, Aug 1, 1984.
6. BRAAT SH, BRUGADA P, DULK K, OMMEN V, WELLENS HJJ: Value of lead V₄R for recognition of the infarct coronary artery in acute inferior myocardial infarction. Am J Cardiol 53:1538–1541, June 1, 1984.
7. NADOR F, DE MARTINI M, BINDA A, RADRIZZANI D, CIRO E, LOTTO A: Hemodynamic evaluation by M-mode echocardiography in acute myocardial infarction. Am Heart J 108:38–43, July 1984.
8. KAN G, VISSER CA, LIE KI, DURRER D: Measurement of left ventricular ejection fraction after acute myocardial infarction: a serial cross sectional echocardiographic study. Br Heart J 51:631–636, June 1984.
9. ARVAN S, VARAT MA: Persistent ST-segment elevation and left ventricular wall abnormalities: a 2-dimensional echocardiographic study. Am J Cardiol 53:1542–1546, June 1, 1984.
10. ERLEBACHER JA, WEISS JL, WEISFELDT ML, BULKLEY BH: Early dilation of the infarcted segment in acute transmural myocardial infarction: role of infarct expansion in acute left ventricular enlargement. J Am Coll Cardiol 4:201–208, Aug 1984.
11. VAN REET RE, QUINONES MA, POLINER LR, NELSON JG, WAGGONER AD, KANON D, LUBETKIN SJ, PRATT CM, WINTERS WL: Comparison of two-dimensional echocardiography with gated radionuclide ventriculography in the evaluation of global and regional left ventricular function in acute myocardial infarction, J Am Coll Cardiol 2:243–252, Feb 1984.

12. HIRSOWITZ GS, LAKIER JB, GOLDSTEIN S: Right ventricular function evaluated by radionuclide angiography in acute myocardial infarction. Am Heart J 108:949–954, Oct 1984.

13. FOX KAA, BERGMANN SR, MATHIAS CJ, POWERS WJ, SIEGEL BA, WELCH MJ, SOBEL BE: Scintigraphic detection of coronary artery thrombi in patients with acute myocardial infarction. J Am Coll Cardiol 4:975–986, Nov 1984.

14. MASUDA Y, YOSHIDA H, MOROOKA N, WATANABE S, INAGAKI Y: The usefulness of x-ray computed tomography for the diagnosis of myocardial infarction. Circulation 70:217–225, Aug 1984.

15. WALINSKY P, SMITH JB, LEFER AM, LEBENTHAL M, URBAN P, GREENSPON A, GOLDBERG S: Thromboxane A$_2$ in acute myocardial infarction. Am Heart J 108:868–872, Oct 1984.

16. DePACE NL, HAKKI A-H, ISKANDRIAN AS: Effects of resting ischemia assessed by thallium scintigraphy on QRS scoring system for estimating left ventricular function quantified by radionuclide angiography in acute myocardial infarction patients. Am Heart J 107:1210–1214, June 1984.

17. HACKEL DB, REIMER KA, IDEKER RE, MIKAT EM, HARTWELL TD, PARKER CB, BRAUNWALD EB, BUJA M, GOLD HK, JAFFE AS, MULLER JE, RAABE DS, RUDE RE, SOBEL BE, STONE PH, ROBERTS R, THE MILIS STUDY GROUP: Comparison of enzymatic and anatomic estimates of myocardial infarct size in man. Circulation 70:824–835, Nov 1984.

18. SINUSAS AJ, HARDIN NJ, CLEMENTS JP, WACKERS FJ: Pathoanatomic correlates of regional left ventricular wall motion assessed by equilibrium radionuclide angiocardiography: a postmortem correlation. Am J Cardiol 54:975–981, Nov 1, 1984.

19. BUSSMANN WD, SEHER W, GRUENGRAS M: Reduction of creatine kinase and creatine kinase-MB indexes of infarct size by intravenous verapamil. Am J Cardiol 54:1224–1230, Dec 1, 1984.

20. FEIGL D, ASHKENAZY J, KISHON Y: Early and late atrioventricular block in acute inferior myocardial infarction. J Am Coll Cardiol 4:35–38, July 1984.

21. SCLAROVSKY S, STRASBERG B, HIRSHBERG A, ARDITI A, LEWIN RF, AGMON J: Advanced early and late atrioventricular block in acute inferior wall myocardial infarction. Am Heart J 108:19–24, July 1984.

22. STRASBERG B, PINCHAS A, ARDITTI A, LEWIN RF, SCLAROVSKY S, HELLMAN C, ZAFRIR N, AGMON J: Left and right ventricular function in inferior acute myocardial infarction and significance of advanced atrioventricular block. Am J Cardiol 54:985–987, Nov 1, 1984.

23. GRENADIER E, ALPAN G, MAOR N, KEIDAR S, BINENBOIL C, MARGULIES T, PALANT A: Polymorphous ventricular tachycardia in acute myocardial infarction. Am J Cardiol 53:1280–1283, May 1, 1984.

24. STRATTON JR, RITCHIE JL: The effects of antithrombotic drugs in patients with left ventricular thrombi: assessment with indium-111 platelet imaging and two-dimensional echocardiography. Circulation 69:561–568, March 1984.

25. JOHANNESSEN K, NORDREHAUG JE, LIPPE G: Left ventricular thrombosis and cerebrovascular accident in acute myocardial infarction. Br Heart J 51:553–556, May 1984.

26. MELTZER RS, VISSER CA, KAN G, ROELANDT J: Two-dimensional echocardiographic appearance of left ventricular thrombi with systemic emboli after myocardial infarction. Am J Cardiol 53:1511–1513, June 1, 1984.

27. NORTHCOTE RJ, HUTCHISON SJ, McGUINNESS JB: Evidence for the continued existence of the postmyocardial infarction (Dressler's) syndrome. Am J Cardiol 53:1201–1202, Apr 1, 1984.

28. MEIZLISH JL, BERGER HJ, PLANKEY M, ERRICO D, LEVY W, ZARET BL: Functional left ventricular aneurysm formation after acute anterior transmural myocardial infarction. N Engl J Med 311:1001–1006, Oct 18, 1984.

29. FOSTER CJ, SEKIYA T, BROWNLEE WC, GRIFFIN JF, ISHERWOOD I: Computed tomographic assessment of left ventricular aneurysms. Br Heart J 52:332–338, Sept 1984.

30. HOCHMAN JS, PLATIA EB, BULKLEY BH: Endocardial abnormalities in left ventricular aneurysms. Ann Intern Med 100:29–35, Jan 1984.

31. EDWARDS BS, EDWARDS WD, EDWARDS JE: Ventricular septal rupture complicating acute myocardial infarction: identification of simple and complex types in 53 autopsied hearts. Am J Cardiol 54:1201–1205, Dec 1, 1984.

32. GEFT IL, SHAH PK, RODRIGUEZ L, HULSE S, MADDAHI J, BERMAN DS, GANZ W: ST elevations in leads V_1 to V_5 may be caused by right coronary artery occlusion and acute right ventricular infarction. Am J Cardiol 53:991–996, Apr 1, 1984.

33. MORGERA T, ALBERTI E, SILVESTRI F, PANDULLO C, DELLA MEA MT, CAMERINI F: Right precordial ST and QRS changes in the diagnosis of right ventricular infarction. Am Heart J 108:13–18, July 1984.

34. BRAAT SH, DE ZWAAN C, BRUGADA P, COENEGRACHT JM, WELLENS HJJ: Right ventricular involvement with acute inferior wall myocardial infarction identifies high risk of developing atrioventricular nodal conduction disturbances. Am Heart J 107:1183–1187, June 1984.

35. JUGDUTT BI, HARAPHONGSE M, BASUALDO CA, ROSSALL RE: Evaluation of biventricular involvement in hypotensive patients with transmural inferior infarction by two-dimensional echocardiography. Am Heart J 108:1417–1426, Dec 1984.

36. JUGDUTT BI, SUSSEX BA, SIVARAM CA, ROSSALL RE: Right ventricular infarction: two-dimensional echocardiographic evaluation. Am Heart J 107:505–518, March 1984.

37. LOVE JC, HAFFAJEE CI, GORE JM, ALPERT JS: Reversibility of hypotension and shock by atrial or atrioventricular sequential pacing in patients with right ventricular infarction. Am Heart J 108:5–13, July 1984.

38. KRAININ FM, FLESSAS AP, SPODICK DH: Infarction-associated pericarditis: rarity of diagnostic electrocardiogram. N Engl J Med 311:1211–1214, Nov 8, 1984.

39. TEN KATE LP, BOMAN H, DAIGER SP, MOTULSKY AG: Increased frequency of coronary heart disease in relatives of wives of myocardial infarct survivors: assortative mating for lifestyle and risk factors? Am J Cardiol 53:399–403, Feb 1, 1984.

40. OLSON HG, LYONS KP, TROOP P, BUTMAN S, PITERS KM: The high-risk acute myocardial infarction patient at 1-year follow-up: identification at hospital discharge by ambulatory electrocardiography and radionuclide ventriculography. Am Heart J 107:358–366, Feb 1984.

41. HUNG J, GORIS ML, NASH E, KRAEMER HC, DEBUSK RF, BERGER WE, LEW H: Comparative value of maximal treadmill testing, exercise thallium myocardial perfusion scintigraphy and exercise radionuclide ventriculography for distinguishing high- and low-risk patients soon after acute myocardial infarction. Am J Cardiol 53:1221–1227, May 1, 1984.

42. MUKHARJI J, RUDE RE, POOLE WK, GUSTAFSON N, THOMAS LJ, STRAUSS HW, JAFFE AS, MULLER JE, ROBERTS R, RAABE DS, CROFT CH, PASSAMANI E, BRAUNWALD E, WILLERSON JT, MILIS STUDY GROUP: Risk factors for sudden death after acute myocardial infarction: two-year follow-up. Am J Cardiol 54:31–36, July 1, 1984.

43. MORRIS DD, ROZANSKI A, BERMAN DS, DIAMOND GA, SWAN HJC: Noninvasive prediction of the angiographic extent of coronary artery disease after myocardial infarction: comparison of clinical, bicycle exercise electrocardiographic, and ventriculographic parameters. Circulation 70:192–201, Aug 1984.

44. BIGGER JT, FLEISS JL, KLEIGER R, MILLER JP, ROLNITZKY LM, THE MULTICENTER POST-INFARCTION RESEARCH GROUP: The relationships among ventricular arrhythmias, left ventricular dysfunction, and mortality in the 2 years after myocardial infarction. Circulation 69:250–258, Feb 1984.

45. CRIMM A, SEVERANCE HW, COFFEY K, MCKINNIS R, WAGNER GS, CALIFF RM: Prognostic significance of isolated sinus tachycardia during the first three days of acute myocardial infarction. Am J Med 76:983–988, June 1984.

46. OLSON HG, LYONS KP, TROOP P, BUTMAN SM, PITERS KM: Prognostic implications of complicated ventricular arrhythmias early after hospital discharge in acute myocardial infarction: a serial ambulatory electrocardiography study. Am Heart J 108:1221–1229, Nov 1984.

47. KOWEY PR, FRIEHLING T, MEISTER SG, ENGEL TR: Late induction of tachycardia in patients with ventricular fibrillation associated with acute myocardial infarction. J Am Coll Cardiol 3:690–695, March 1984.

48. NISHIMURA RA, REEDER GS, MILLER FA, ILSTRUP DM, SHUB C, SEWARD JB, TAJIK AJ: Prognostic value of predischarge 2-dimensional echocardiogram after acute myocardial infarction. Am J Cardiol 53:429–432, Feb 1, 1984.

49. NORRIS RM, BARNABY PF, BRANDT PWT, GEARY GG, WHITLOCK RML, WILD CJ, BARRATT-BOYES BG: Prognosis after recovery from first acute myocardial infarction: determinants of rein-

farction and sudden death. Am J Cardiol 53:408–413, Feb 1, 1984.

50. GREENBERG H, McMASTER P, DWYER EM JR: Left ventricular dysfunction after acute myocardial infarction: results of a prospective multicenter study. J Am Coll Cardiol 4:867–874, Nov 1984.

51. LEPPO JA, O'BRIEN J, ROTHENDLER JA, GETCHELL JD, LEE VW: Dipyridamole-thallium-201 scintigraphy in the prediction of future cardiac events after acute myocardial infarction. N Engl J Med 310:1014–1018, Apr 19, 1984.

52. HUNG J, GORDON EP, HOUSTON N, HASKELL WL, GORIS ML, DEBUSK RF: Changes in rest and exercise myocardial perfusion and left ventricular function 3 to 26 weeks after clinically uncomplicated acute myocardial infarction: effects of exercise training. Am J Cardiol 54:943–950, Nov 1, 1984.

53. SULLIVAN ID, DAVIES DW, SOWTON E: Submaximal exercise testing early after myocardial infarction: prognostic importance of exercise induced ST segment elevation. Br Heart J 52:147–153, Aug 1984.

54. OSWALD GA, CORCORAN S, YUDKIN JS: Prevalence and risks of hyperglycemia and undiagnosed diabetes in patients with acute myocardial infarction. Lancet 1:1264–1267, June 9, 1984.

55. JAFFE AS, SPADARO JJ, SCHECHTMAN K, ROBERTS R, GELTMAN EM, SOBEL BE: Increased congestive heart failure after myocardial infarction of modest extent in patients with diabetes mellitus. Am Heart J 108:31–37, July 1984.

56. SMITH JW, MARCUS FI, SEROKMAN R, MULTICENTER POSTINFARCTION RESEARCH GROUP: Prognosis of patients with diabetes mellitus after acute myocardial infarction. Am J Cardiol 54:718–721, Oct 1, 1984.

57. MATEUDA Y, OGAWA H, MORITANI K, MATSUDA M, NAITO H, MATSUZAKI M, IKEE Y, KUSUKAWA R: Effects of the presence or absence of preceding angina pectoris on left ventricular function after acute myocardial infarction. Am Heart J 108:955–958, Oct 1984.

58. CRISP AH, QUEENAN M: Myocardial infarction and the emotional climate. Lancet 1:616–619, March 17, 1984.

59. RUBERMAN W, WEINBLATT E, GOLDBERG JD, CHAUDHARY BS: Psychosocial influences on mortality after myocardial infarction. N Engl J Med 311:552–559, Aug 30, 1984.

60. GRABOYS TB: Stress and the aching heart. N Engl J Med 311:594–595, Aug 30, 1984.

61. AHNVE S, GILPIN E, MADSEN EB, FROELICHER V, HENNING H, ROSS J JR: Prognostic importance of QTc interval at discharge after acute myocardial infarction: A multicenter study of 865 patients. Am Heart J 108:395–400, Aug 1984.

62. MADSEN EB, GILPIN E, HENNING H, AHNVE S, LEWINTER M, MAZUR J, SHABETAI R, COLLINS D, ROSS J JR: Prognostic importance of digitalis after acute myocardial infarction. J Am Coll Cardiol 3:681–689, March 1984.

63. HOLLANDER G, OZICK H, GREENGART A, SHANI J, LICHSTEIN E: High mortality early reinfarction with first nontransmural myocardial infarction. Am Heart J 108:1412–1416, Dec 1984.

64. MADSEN EB, GILPIN E, HENNING H, AHNVE S, LEWINTER M, CERETTO W, JOSWIG W, COLLINS D, PITT W, ROSS J: Prediction of late mortality after myocardial infarction from variables measured at different times during hospitalization. Am J Cardiol 53:47–54, Jan 1, 1984.

65. BUSSMANN W-D, NEUMANN K, KALTENBACH M: Effects of intravenous nitroglycerin on ventricular ectopic beats in acute myocardial infarction. Am Heart J 107:940–944, May 1984.

66. FURBERG CD, HAWKINS CM, LICHSTEIN E, FOR THE BETA-BLOCKER HEART ATTACK TRIAL STUDY GROUP: Effect of propranolol in postinfarction patients with mechanical or electrical complications. Circulation 69:761–765, Apr 1984.

67. ROBERTS R, CROFT C, GOLD HK, TYLER MD, HARTWELL TD, JAFFE AS, MULLER JE, MULLIN SM, PARKER C, PASSAMANI ER, POOLE WK, RAABE DS, RUDE RE, STONE PH, TURI ZG, SOBEL BE, WILLERSON JT, BRAUNWALD E, MILIS STUDY GROUP: Effect of propranolol on myocardial-infarct size in a randomized blinded multicenter trial. N Engl J Med 311:218–225, July 26, 1984.

68. GOLD HK, LEINBACH RC, HARPER RW: Usefulness of intravenous propranolol in predicting left anterior descending blood flow during anterior myocardial infarction. Am J Cardiol 54:264–268, Aug 1, 1984.

69. INTERNATIONAL COLLABORATIVE STUDY GROUP: Reduction of infarct size with the early use of timolol in acute myocardial infarction. N Engl J Med 310:9–15, Jan 1, 1984.

70. Olsson G, Rehnqvist N: Ventricular arrhythmias during the first year after acute myocardial infarction: influence of long-term treatment with metoprolol. Circulation 69:1129–1134, June 1984.

71. Olsson G, Hjemdahl P, Rehnqvist N: Rebound phenomena following gradual withdrawal of chronic metoprolol treatment in patients with ischemic heart disease. Am Heart J 108:454–462, Sept 1984.

72. Frishman WH, Furberg CD, Friedewald WT: β-Adrenergic blockade for survivors of acute myocardial infarction. N Engl J Med 310:830–837, March 29, 1984.

73. Ahumada GG: Identification of patients who do not require beta antagonists after myocardial infarction. Am J Med 76:900–904, May 1984.

74. Heikkilä J, Nieminen MS: Effects of verapamil in patients with acute myocardial infarction: hemodynamics and function of normal and ischemic left ventricular myocardium. Am Heart J 107:241–247, Feb 1984.

75. Muller JE, Morrison J, Stone PH, Rude RE, Rosner B, Roberts R, Pearle DL, Turi ZG, Schneider JF, Serfas DH, Tate C, Scheiner E, Sobel BE, Hennekens CH, Braunwald E: Nifedipine therapy for patients with threatened and acute myocardial infarction: a randomized, double-blind, placebo-controlled comparison. Circulation 69:740–747, Apr 1984.

76. Gordon GD, Mabin TA, Isaacs S, Lloyd EA, Eichler HG, Opie LH: Hemodynamic effects of sublingual nifedipine in acute myocardial infarction. Am J Cardiol 53:1228–1232, May 1, 1984.

77. Kessler KM, Kissane B, Cassidy J, Pefkaros KC, Kozlovskis P, Hamburg C, Myerburg RJ: Dynamic variability of binding of antiarrhythmic drugs during the evolution of acute myocardial infarction. Circulation 70:472–478, Sept 1984.

78. Hochberg MS, Parsonnet V, Gielchinsky I, Hussain SM, Fisch DA, Norman JC: Timing of coronary revascularization after acute myocardial infarction: early and late results in patients revascularized within seven weeks. J Thorac Cardiovasc Surg, 88:914–921, Dec 1984.

79. Barratt-Boyes BG, White HD, Agnew TM, Pemberton JR, Wild CJ: The results of surgical treatment of left ventricular aneurysms: an assessment of the risk factors affecting early and late mortality. J Thorac Cardiovasc Surg 87:87–98, Jan 1984.

80. Olearchyk AS, Lemole GM, Spagna PM: Left ventricular aneurysm: ten years' experience in surgical treatment of 244 cases. Improved clinical status, hemodynamics, and long-term longevity. J Thorac Cardiovasc Surg 88:544–553, Oct 1984.

81. Mombelli G, Imhof V, Haeberli A, Straub PW: Effect of heparin on plasma fibrinopeptide A in patients with acute myocardial infarction. Circulation 69:684–689, Apr 1984.

82. Rogers WJ, Hood WP, Mantle JA, Baxley WA, Kirklin JK, Zorn GL, Nath HP: Return of left ventricular function after reperfusion in patients with myocardial infarction: importance of subtotal stenoses or intact collaterals. Circulation 69:338–349, Feb 1984.

83. Leiboff RH, Katz RJ, Wasserman AG, Bren GB, Schwartz H, Varghese PJ, Ross AM: A randomized, angiographically controlled trial of intracoronary streptokinase in acute myocardial infarction. Am J Cardiol 53:404–407, Feb 1, 1984.

84. Blanke H, von Hardenberg D, Cohen M, Kaiser H, Karsch K, Holt J, Smith H Jr, Rentrop P: Patterns of creatine kinase release during acute myocardial infarction after nonsurgical reperfusion: comparison with conventional treatment and correlation with infarct size. J Am Coll Cardiol 3:675–680, March 1984.

85. Van de Werf F, Ludbrook PA, Bergmann SR, Tiefenbrunn AJ, Fox KA, De Geest H, Verstraete M, Collen D, Sobel BE: Coronary thrombolysis with tissue-type plasminogen activator in patients with evolving myocardial infarction. N Engl J Med 310:609–613, March 8, 1984.

86. Tennant SN, Dixon J, Venable TC, Page HL, Roach A, Kaiser AB, Frederiksen R, Tacogue L, Kaplan P, Babu NS, Anderson EE, Wooten E, Jennings HS, Breinig J, Campbell WB: Intracoronary thrombolysis in patients with acute myocardial infarction: comparison of the efficacy of urokinase with streptokinase. Circulation 69:756–760, Apr 1984.

87. Sobel BE, Geltman EM, Tiefenbrunn AJ, Jaffe AS, Spadaro JJ, Ter-Pogossian MM, Collen D, Ludbrook PA: Improvement of regional myocardial metabolism after coronary thrombolysis induced with tissue-type plasminogen activator or streptokinase. Circulation 69:983–990, May 1984.

88. HARRISON DG, FERGUSON DW, COLLINS SM, SKORTON DJ, ERICKSEN EE, KIOSCHOS JM, MARCUS ML, WHITE CW: Rethrombosis after reperfusion with streptokinase: importance of geometry of residual lesions. Circulation 69:991–999, May 1984.

89. GANZ W, GEFT I, SHAH PK, LEW AS, RODRIGUEZ L, WEISS T, MADDAHI J, BERMAN DS, CHARUZI Y, SWAN HJC: Intravenous streptokinase in evolving acute myocardial infarction. Am J Cardiol 53:1209–1216, May 1, 1984.

90. YASUNO M, SAITO Y, ISHIDA M, SUZUKI K, ENDO S, TAKAHASHI M: Effects of percutaneous transluminal coronary angioplasty: intracoronary thrombolysis with urokinase in acute myocardial infarction. Am J Cardiol 53:1217–1220, May 1, 1984.

91. TIMMIS GC, GANGADHARAN V, RAMOS RG, HAUSER AM, WESTVEER DC, STEWART J, GOODFLIESH R, GORDON S: Hemorrhage and the products of fibrinogen digestion after intracoronary administration of streptokinase. Circulation 69:1146–1152, June 1984.

92. SCHWARZ F, HOFMANN M, SCHULER G, OLSHAUSEN K, ZIMMERMANN R, KUBLER W: Thrombolysis in acute myocardial infarction: effect of intravenous followed by intracoronary streptokinase application on estimates of infarct size. Am J Cardiol 53:1505–1510, June 1, 1984.

93. ALDERMAN EL, JUTZY KR, BERTE LE, MILLER RG, FRIEDMAN JP, CREGER WP, ELIASTAM M: Randomized comparison of intravenous versus intracoronary streptokinase for myocardial infarction. Am J Cardiol 54:14–19, July 1, 1984.

94. TAYLOR GJ, MIKELL FL, MOSES HW, DOVE JT, BATCHELDER JE, THULL A, HANSEN S, WELLONS HA, SCHNEIDER JA: Intravenous versus intracoronary streptokinase therapy for acute myocardial infarction in community hospitals. Am J Cardiol 54:256–260, Aug 1, 1984.

95. EIGLER N, MAURER G, SHAH PK: Effect of early systemic thrombolytic therapy on left ventricular mural thrombus formation in acute anterior or myocardial infarction. Am J Cardiol 54:261–263, Aug 1, 1984.

96. KASPER W, ERBEL R, MEINERTZ T, DREXLER M, RÜCKEL A, POP T, PRELLWITZ W, MEYER J: Intracoronary thrombolysis with an acylated streptokinase plasminogen activator (BRL 26921) in patients with acute myocardial infarction. J Am Coll Cardiol 4:357–363, Aug 1984.

97. FERGUSON DW, WHITE CW, SCHWARTZ JL, BRAYDEN GP, KELLY KJ, KIOSCHOS, M, KIRCHNER PT, MARCUS ML: Influence of baseline ejection fraction and success of thrombolysis on mortality and ventricular function after acute myocardial infarction. Am J Cardiol 54:705–711, Oct 1, 1984.

98. WHITE CW, SCHWARTZ JL, FERGUSON DW, BRAYDEN GP, KELLY KJ, KIOSCHOS JM, MARCUS ML: Systemic markers of fibrinolysis after unsuccessful intracoronary streptokinase thrombolysis for acute myocardial infarction. Am J Cardiol 54:712–717, Oct 1, 1984.

99. ANDERSON JL, MARSHALL HW, ASKINS JC, LUTZ JR, SORENSEN SG, MENLOVE RL, YANOWITZ FG, HAGAN AD: A randomized trial of intravenous and intracoronary streptokinase in patients with acute myocardial infarction. Circulation 70:606–618, Oct 1984.

100. URBAN PL, COWLEY M, GOLDBERG S, VETROVEC G, HASTILLO A, GREENSPON AJ, KUSIAK V, GREENBERG R, WALINSKY P, CAMMARATO J, MAROKO P: Intracoronary thrombolysis in acute myocardial infarction: clinical course following successful myocardial reperfusion. Am Heart J 108:873–878, Oct 1984.

101. SCHULER G, HOFMANN M, SCHWARZ F, MEHMEL H, MANTHEY J, TILLMANNS H, HARTMANN S, KUBLER W: Effect of successful thrombolytic therapy on right ventricular function in acute inferior wall myocardial infarction. Am J Cardiol 54:951–957, Nov 1, 1984.

102. RITCHIE J, DAVIS KB, WILLIAMS DL, CALDWELL J, KENNEDY JW: Global and regional left ventricular function and tomographic radionuclide perfusion: the Western Washington Intracoronary Streptokinase Myocardial Infarction Trial. Circulation 70:867–875, Nov 1984.

103. HODGSON JM, O'NEILL WW, LAUFER N, BOURDILLON PDV, WALTON JA, PITT B: Assessment of potentially salvageable myocardium during acute myocardial infarction: use of postextrasystolic potentiation. Am J Cardiol 54:1237–1244, Dec 1, 1984.

104. ANDERSON JL, McILVAINE PM, MARSHALL HW, BRAY BE, YANOWITZ FG, LUTZ JR, MENLOVE RL, HAGAN AD: Long-term follow-up after intracoronary streptokinase for myocardial infarction: a randomized, controlled study. Am Heart J 108:1402–1408, Dec 1984.

105. COLLEN D, TOPOL EJ, TIEFENBRUNN AJ, GOLD HK, WEISFELDT ML, SOBEL BE, LEINBACH RC, BRINKER JA, LUDBROOK PA, YASUDA I, BULKLEY BH, ROBISON AK, HUTTER AM, BELL WR, SPADARO JJ, KHAW BA, GROSSBARD EB: Coronary thrombolysis with recombinant human tissue-type

plasminogen activator: a prospective, randomized, placebo-controlled trial. Circulation 70:1012–1017, Dec 1984.

106. Rentrop KP, Feit F, Blanke H, Stecy P, Schneider R, Rey M, Horowitz S, Goldman M, Karsch K, Meilman H, Cohen M, Siegel S, Sanger J, Slater J, Gorlin R, Fox A, Fagerstrom R, Calhoun WF: Effects of intracoronary streptokinase and intracoronary nitroglycerin infusion on coronary angiographic patterns and mortality in patients with acute myocardial infarction. N Engl J Med 311:1457–1463, Dec 6, 1984.

107. Skinner JR, Phillips SJ, Zeff RH, Kongtahworn C: Immediate coronary bypass following failed streptokinase infusion in evolving myocardial infarction. J Thorac Cardiovasc Surg 87:567–570, Apr 1984.

108. Laffel GL, Braunwald E: Thrombolytic therapy: a new strategy for the treatment of acute myocardial infarction (second of two parts). N Engl J Med 311:770–776, Sept 20, 1984.

109. Friedman M, Thoresen CE, Gill JJ, Powell LH, Ulmer D, Thompson L, Price VA, Rabin DD, Breal WS, Dixon T, Levy R, Bourg E: Alteration of type A behavior and reduction in cardiac recurrences in postmyocardial infarction patients. Am Heart J 108:237–248, Aug 1984.

110. Gore JM, Goldberg RJ, Matsumoto AS, Castelli WP, McNamara PM, Dalen JE: Validity of serum total cholesterol level obtained within 24 hours of acute myocardial infarction. Am J Cardiol 54:722–725, Oct 1, 1984.

111. McGregor M: Myocardial ischemia: towards better use of the coronary care unit. Am J Med 76:887–890, May 1984.

112. Fineberg HV, Scadden D, Goldman L: Care of patients with a low probability of acute myocardial infarction: cost effectiveness of alternatives to coronary-care-unit admissions. N Engl J Med 310:1301–1307, May 17, 1984.

113. Pozen MW, D'Agostino RB, Selker HP, Sytkowski PA, Hood WB: A predictive instrument to improve coronary-care-unit admission practices in acute ischemic heart disease: a prospective multicenter clinical trial. N Engl J Med 310:1273–1278, May 1, 1984.

114. Capone RJ, Visco J, Curwen E, VanEvery S: The effect of early prehospital transtelephonic coronary intervention on morbidity and mortality: experience with 284 postmyocardial infarction patients in a pilot program. Am Heart J 107:1153–1160, June 1984.

3

Arrhythmias, Conduction Disturbances, and Cardiac Arrest

ARRHYTHMIAS IN HEALTHY INDIVIDUALS

Dickinson and Scott[1] from Leeds, England, performed ambulatory 24-hour monitoring for 2 consecutive periods of 24 hours in 100 boys aged 14–16 years. Heart rates during monitoring ranged from 45–200 beats/minute during the day and from 23–95 beats/minute during sleep. Sinus arrhythmia was present in all boys and was the only variation in 17. Sudden variations in the PP interval occurred in 41 boys, but a precise diagnosis of the mechanism was usually impossible; 15 had changes compatible with sinus arrest or temporary complete sinoatrial block and 1 boy had a pattern compatible with type II second-degree sinoatrial block. Escape rhythms were noted in 26, first-degree AV block in 12, and second-degree AV block in 11. Mobitz type I second-degree AV block occurred in 1 boy. In 41 boys VPC occurred and in 75% of them it was uniform and in 25% it was multiform. Short episodes of VT were recorded in 3 boys.

ATRIAL FIBRILLATION/FLUTTER

Approximately a third of hyperthyroid patients have AF. The prevalence of coexistent AF and thyroid dysfunction in institutionalized older patients is uncertain. To fill this void Cobler and associates[2] from Rochester, New York, determined the cardiac rhythm and thyroid status of 316 patients >65 years of age residing in a nursing home. One of the 9 elderly men and 5 of the 16 women with AF had laboratory evidence or a history of hyperthyroidism. The elderly patients with cardiac rhythms other than AF (n, 291) had only a 1.7% prevalence of hyperthyroidism. The analysis for elderly women demonstrated a statistically significant association between AF and hyperthyroidism, but the association was not statistically significant for men. These findings indicate that hyperthyroidism is common in institutionalized elderly women with AF.

The effect of Corwin, a new oral beta$_1$ partial agonist, on the ventricular response to AF was studied by Molajo and associates[3] from Manchester, England, in 10 digitalized patients during 24-hour ambulatory ECG and during exercise on a treadmill and a double-blind placebo control crossover trial. Of the 10 patients, 8 had MS, 1 had "lone AF," and 1 had CAD. Corwin reduced maximum heart rate during exercise from 162–120 beats/minute and reduced the peak heart rate during ambulatory ECG from 113–90 beats/minute, consistent with a beta adrenoreceptor antagonist action at higher levels of sympathetic nervous system activity. Minimum heart rate during ambulatory ECG increased from 62–70 beats/minute, indicating that at lower levels of sympathetic activity the drug acts as a beta antagonist. The drug increased exercise tolerance significantly. Serum digoxin concentrations were not affected by Corwin. Thus, Corwin appears to be effective in stabilizing heart rate during AF both at rest and during exercise in digitalized patients.

Buxton and associates[4] from Philadelphia, Pennsylvania, evaluated the effects of cycle length and stimulation site on intraatrial conduction and refractoriness in 19 patients with and without atrial flutter (AFL) or AF using the extrastimulus technique. Nineteen patients with spontaneous sustained AFl or AF were compared with 19 control patients. Programmed stimulation was performed at the right atrium and coronary sinus at drive cycle lengths of 600 and 450 ms. The atrial effective refractory period was similar in the patients with atrial arrhythmias and the control group. The RA effective refractory period at a drive cycle length of 700 ms was significantly shorter in patients with AF (211 ms) than in patients with AFl (235 ms, p = 0.05). The conduction time of late (coupling intervals more than 50% of the drive cycle length) premature impulses was similar in the patients with atrial arrhythmias and the control group. However, early extrastimuli (coupling intervals less than 50% of the drive cycle length) at a drive cycle length of 600 ms produced significantly more intraatrial conduction delay in the patients with atrial arrhythmias than in the control patients. At a drive cycle length of 450 ms, similar delays in intraatrial conduction occurred in the patients with and without atrial arrhythmias because of an increase in the maximal observed intraatrial conduction delay in the control patients. This study shows that delay in conduction of early premature atrial stimuli at a drive cycle length of 700 ms is a marker of patients with spontaneous AFl and AF. At a drive cycle length of 450 ms, increase in intraatrial conduction delay in response to early extrastimuli appears to be a physiologic response of the normal atrium.

SUPRAVENTRICULAR TACHYCARDIA WITH OR WITHOUT SHORT P-R INTERVAL SYNDROMES

Electrophysiologic studies

Bar and associates[5] from Maastricht, The Netherlands, studied 187 patients with clinically documented SVT with a narrow (<0.12 seconds) QRS complex admitted for electrophysiologic study. The diagnoses were circus movement tachycardia using an accessory pathway in 50 patients, AV nodal tachycardia in 50 patients, atrial flutter in 50 patients, atrial tachycardia in 27, and an accessory tachycardia retrogradely using a slowly conducting accessory pathway in 10 patients. On retrospective analysis, 5 criteria on the 12-lead ECG during tachycardia were analyzed for their value in making the diagnosis of site of origin. These criteria were P-wave location, axis of the P wave, atrial rate, alternation of the QRS complex, and AV relation. Fifty-seven patients with a narrow QRS tachycardia were prospectively studied using the 5 criteria. A correct diagnosis was made in 48 of the 57 patients (84%). Thus, in most patients with a narrow QRS tachycardia, information from the 12-lead ECG is adequate for diagnosis.

Brugada and colleagues[6] from Maastricht, The Netherlands, assessed factors playing a role in initiation of AV nodal reentrant SVT utilizing antegradely a slow and retrogradely a fast conducting AV nodal pathway in 38 patients having no accessory pathways and showing discontinuous antegrade AV nodal conduction curves during atrial stimulation. Twenty-two patients (group A) underwent an electrophysiologic investigation because of recurrent paroxysmal SVT that had been documented by ECG before the study Sixteen patients (group B) underwent the study because of a history of palpitations (15 patients) or recurrent VT (1 patient); in none of them had SVT ever been documented by ECG before the investigation. Of the 22 patients, 21 of group A demonstrated continuous retrograde conduction curves during ventricular stimulation. In 20, tachycardia was initiated by either a single atrial premature beat (18 patients) or by 2 atrial premature beats. Fifteen of the 16 patients of group B had discontinuous retrograde conduction curves during ventricular stimulation, with a long refractory period of their retrograde fast pathway. Tachycardia was initiated by multiple atrial premature complexes in 1 patient. Thirteen of the remaining 15 patients received atropine. Thereafter, tachycardia could be initiated in 3 patients by a single atrial premature beat, by 2 atrial premature beats in 1 patient, and by incremental atrial pacing in another patient. In the remaining 8 patients tachycardia could not be initiated. These observations indicate that the pattern of ventriculoatrial conduction found during ventricular stimulation is a marker for ease of initiation of AV nodal tachycardia in patients with discontinuous antegrade AV nodal conduction curves.

Since the normal AV conduction system constitutes the antegrade limb of the reentry circuit in patients with SVT due to unidirectional retrograde accessory pathway (URAP), the antegrade properties are important in determining the rate of tachycardia. Thus, Henglein and associates[7] from Houston, Texas, determined if there was abnormal antegrade conduction in URAP patients having a concealed anomalous conduction pathway without preexcitation. In 26 patients (aged 1–18 years) with URAP, antegrade conduction properties were evaluated. During electrophysiologic study, the interval from the low septal RA potential to the His bundle potential (LSRA-H) in sinus rhythm (SR) was found to be <60 ms in 7 of the 18 patients with left-sided URAP and in 1 of 2 patients with septal URAP. Each of the 6 patients with right-sided URAP had an LSRA-H ≥70 ms. During atrial extrastimulus testing, LSRA-H failed to prolong >100 ms in 4 of 6 patients with left-sided URAP and LSRA-H of <60 ms in SR as well as in the 1 of 2 patients with septal URAP in whom the LSRA-H in SR was <60 ms. During rapid atrial pacing, 1:1 AV node conduction was found at a pacing rate of >200 beats/minute in the 1 patient with septal URAP and in 7 of 14 patients with left-sided URAP who could be assessed. Three of these patients had progression from 1:1 AV conduction to 2:1 AV block without intervening Wenckebach. Therefore accelerated AV node conduction in SR and reduced AV node function during rapid atrial pacing or extrastimulus testing was found in 44% of patients with left-sided or septal URAP. Since these patients are at higher risk for faster ventricular response to atrial flutter and AF and for high frequency during SVT, these findings are of clinical relevance. Each patient with right-sided URAP had normal antegrade conduction times but the occurrence of right-sided URAP was less common. This difference in AV nodal conduction between patients with right-sided versus left-sided URAP suggests that a developmental abnormality might be responsible for both the left URAP and the enhanced AV nodal conduction.

Factors determining tachycardia induction using ventricular stimulation in AV nodal reentrant SVT utilizing the slow pathway for antegrade and the fast pathway for retrograde conduction were analyzed in 53 patients by Wu and associates[8] from Taipei, Taiwan, and Los Angeles, California. Sixteen patients had tachycardia induced by ventricular stimulation. In 15, tachycardia was inducible with incremental ventricular pacing. In 4 of these 15 patients, the tachycardia was also induced with V_1V_2 testing, whereas in 11 patients, the tachycardia was not induced with V_1V_2 testing. In 9 of the latter 11 patients, tachycardia could be induced with $V_1V_2V_3$ testing, suggesting that the retrograde effective refractory period (ERP) of the right bundle or the relative refractory period of the His-Purkinje system (HPS) was the limiting factor for tachycardia induction during V_1V_2 testing. In 1 remaining patient, tachycardia was induced with $V_1V_2V_3$ testing, which provoked a premature ventricular beat, leading to tachycardia induction. Tachycardia was not induced by ventricular stimulation in 37 patients. Factors deterring tachycardia induction in these patients may be related to the retrograde ERP or functional refractory period (FRP) of the HPS, the retrograde ERP of the fast pathway, and an insufficient conduction delay of the circuit (retrograde fast and antegrade slow pathways) to allow antegrade conduction of the slow pathway. It was concluded that AV nodal reentrant SVT can be induced by ventricular stimulation in approximately 30% of patients with incremental ventricular pacing and/or ventricular extrastimulus testing. Induction of tachycardia with ventricular stimulation, nevertheless, is frequently limited by the retrograde FRP or ERP of the HPS, the retrograde ERP of the fast pathway, and possibly by an insufficient conduction delay of the circuit.

Orthodromic reciprocating tachycardia and AF are the predominant clinical arrhythmias in patients with the WPW syndrome. During electrophysiologic study of 435 patients referred for evaluation of WPW syndrome, Bardy and colleagues[9] from Durham, North Carolina, observed 42 (10%) with preexcited reciprocating tachycardia defined as a macro-reentrant tachycardia that used an accessory AV pathway for antegrade conduction. Ages of the patients ranged from 9–67 years; 33 were males, 9 female, and 8 had Ebstein's anomaly. Preexcited reciprocating tachycardia cycle length was 220–430 ms. Significant hemodynamic compromise in the laboratory directly related to preexcited reciprocating tachycardia occurred in only 1 patient. In 10 patients, a transformation to AF was seen after a spontaneously occurring premature atrial contraction. Only 17 of the 42 patients with preexcited reciprocating tachycardia during electrophysiologic study had the same tachycardia documented clinically. These 17 patients were more often younger with multiple accessory pathways and with no history of orthodromic reciprocating tachycardia when compared with 25 patients in whom preexcited reciprocating tachycardia could be induced only in the laboratory. Preexcited reciprocating tachycardia was induced in 6% of the patients with single accessory pathways and 33% of those with multiple pathways. In the 20 patients with multiple accessory pathways, the spectrum of reentrant circuits included fusion over 2 or more accessory pathways or fusion over both an accessory pathway and the AV node. No patient with true antidromic reciprocating tachycardia had a posterior septal accessory AV pathway and only in patients with multiple accessory pathways was the posterior septal accessory AV pathway used as the antegrade limb.

Ajmaline

Ajmaline is an alkaloid derived from the Indian plant Rauwolfia serpentina and has been found useful in experimental and clinical atrial and ventricular arrhythmias. Although the drug has been successful in management of arrhythmias associated with the WPW syndrome, no information is available concerning the efficacy in patients with paroxysmal SVT that is mediated by dual AV nodal pathways. Sethi and colleagues[10] from New Delhi, India, evaluated electrophysiologic effects of 50 mg intravenous (IV) ajmaline in 10 patients with AV nodal reentrant paroxysmal SVT utilizing the slow pathway for antegrade and the fast pathway for retrograde conduction. Ajmaline terminated the SVT in all 10 patients in 17–165 seconds: by ventriculoatrial block in 8, AH block in 1, and intraatrial reentry in 1. The predrug SVT cycle length increased significantly before the SVT was terminated from 289–374 ms. The increase in cycle length was a function of both AH and HA prolongation. In all 10 patients ajmaline depressed conduction through the retrograde fast pathway, as was evident from the increase in mean ventricular-paced cycle length producing ventriculoatrial block from <280–438 ms and the increase in the effective refractory period of the ventriculoatrial conduction system from <241–<298 ms. The drug abolished ventriculoatrial conduction in 4 cases. The effective refractory period of the antegrade fast pathway was unchanged after ajmaline, but conduction through the antegrade slow pathway was depressed. The SVT could not be reinduced in 8 subjects, predominantly because of inhibition of the retrograde pathway. The investigators concluded that ajmaline terminates AV nodal reentrant SVT by blockade of the retrograde fast pathway, although effects on the antegrade slow pathway also were observed.

Amiodarone

Alboni and associates[11] from Ferrara, Italy, and New York City evaluated whether the electrophysiologic effects of intravenous (IV) amiodarone in patients with reentrant SVT could predict the efficacy of long-term oral therapy with this drug. The effects of oral and IV amiodarone were studied in 27 patients with SVT. In 14 the SVT circuit involved a concealed AV bypass for retrograde conduction (group I), and in 13 a concealed atrio-His bypass (group II). Intravenous amiodarone induced significant prolongation of the AH interval, the refractory periods of the atrium, AV node, His-Purkinje system, and ventricular myocardium. The ventriculoatrial interval was slightly prolonged in group I patients and did not change in group II patients after administration of the drug. In both groups, the effective refractory period of the concealed bypass was prolonged by IV amiodarone. During control state, SVT could be induced in all patients; after IV administration of the drug, SVT was present in 6 patients in group I and in 8 patients in group II. In all cases in which IV amiodarone prolonged the effective refractory period of the concealed bypass to >350 ms, the drug always prevented SVT even when given orally. All but 2 patients, 1 from each group, remained asymptomatic after oral amiodarone. In the patient from group I, SVT had been prevented by IV amiodarone, whereas in the patient from group II SVT could not be induced by ventricular stimulation during the control state, but appeared after IV administration of the drug. These data indicate that: (1) therapy with oral amiodarone is effective in most patients with SVT irrespective of the type of bypass fibers, i.e., atrio-His or Kent's bundle; (2) effective suppression of induction of SVT with IV amiodarone is a predictor of efficacy of amiodarone in 93% of the cases. However, a lack of response to IV amiodarone is not a predictor of lack of efficacy of oral amiodarone; (3) prolongation of the effective refractory period of the concealed bypass tract to >350 ms appears to have a favorable predictive value in oral administration; (4) a change in the inducibility of SVT after IV amiodarone appears to have a negative predictive value in controlling SVT with the oral drug.

Wellens and colleagues[12] from Maastricht, The Netherlands, studied the electrophysiologic effects of intravenous and oral amiodarone in 12 patients (9 with WPW syndrome and 3 with VT) with programmed stimulation. Intravenous and oral amiodarone had a similar effect of lengthening on the effective refractory period of the AV node. Only intravenous amiodarone prolonged the AH interval. Oral amiodarone was more effective than intravenous amiodarone in lengthening the antegrade effective refractory period of the accessory AV pathway. Only oral amiodarone prolonged the effective refractory period of atrium and ventricle and the HV interval. Intravenous amiodarone slowed the rate of circus movement tachycardia in patients with WPW syndrome, and further slowing was observed after oral amiodarone. Termination of tachycardia by intravenous amiodarone predicted prevention of reinitiation of tachycardia during oral therapy. These data indicate that intravenous and oral amiodarone do not have the same electrophysiologic effects, but it is not clear whether cumulative effects, active metabolites, or both are responsible for these differences. It is difficult, if not impossible, to predict the individual antiarrhythmic effects of amiodarone from the outcome of electrophysiologic studies.

Gomes and colleagues[13] from New York City conducted electrophysiologic studies in 9 patients with reentrant paroxysmal SVT during a control period and after 5 mg/kg body weight of intravenous amiodarone administered as a slow continuous infusion over 15–20 minutes. All 9 patients had induction of sustained SVT during control studies. In 7 of 9 patients (group 1) the SVT was due to AV nodal reentry, and in 2 of 9 patients (group 2) a concealed retrograde bypass tract was incorporated in the reentrant process. In group 1, after amiodarone, all 7 patients lost the ability to sustain SVT with either absence of atrial echoes (1 patient) or induction of ≤3 echo beats (6 patients) with termination of SVT in the antegrade pathway (3 patients) or retrograde pathway (2 patients) or both (1 patient). In group 2, after amiodarone, both patients lost the ability to sustain SVT with absence of atrial echoes (1 patient) on induction of a single echo beat (1 patient) with block in the retrograde pathway (the concealed retrograde bypass tract). Amiodarone significantly increased atrial cycle length for AV nodal Wenckebach block, antegrade functional refractory period of the AV node, antegrade effective refractory period of the AV node, ventricular paced cycle length for ventriculoatrial block, and the retrograde functional refractory period of the ventriculoatrial conducting system. Thus, intravenous amiodarone inhibited induction of sustained reentrant SVT by inducing block in the antegrade or retrograde or both limbs of the reentrant circuit and was shown to have significant depressant effects on both antegrade and retrograde AV nodal conduction and refractory periods.

Kappenberger and associates[14] from Zurich, Switzerland, studied the effect of oral amiodarone in 12 patients with the WPW syndrome and life-threatening rapid ventricular response via an accessory pathway during spontaneous AF. The effective refractory period of the accessory pathway in the antegrade direction was ≤280 ms during control study in all patients. After amiodarone therapy, the effective refractory period remained ≤280 ms in 7 of the 12 patients. During incremental atrial pacing, the longest atrial pacing cycle length that produced block over an accessory pathway ranged from 200–310 ms (mean, 261 ± 42) during the control period and 240–980 ms (mean, 377 ± 198) after amiodarone therapy. During AF, the shortest ventricular response via the accessory pathway could be measured in 10 of 12 of the patients both before and after amiodarone treatment and ranged from 200–290 ms (234 ± 30) and 250–500 (mean, 302 ± 75), respectively. The average RR interval during AF before and after the drug ranged from 200–390 ms (mean, 280 ± 55) and 280–650 ms (mean, 396 ± 116), respectively. Thus, the safety of amiodarone in the WPW syndrome should be established by electrophysiologic studies and induction of AF, because amiodarone is not protective in all patients with WPW.

Diltiazem

Hung and associates[15] from Taipei, Taiwan, gave diltiazem, 0.25 mg/kg, intravenously during induced tachycardia in 6 patients with AV nodal reentrant tachycardia (group 1) and in 24 patients with AV reentrant tachycardia incorporating a retrogradely conducting accessory pathway (group II). In all

6 group I and in 15 of 24 group II patients, tachycardias terminated within 1 minute after diltiazem administration, with a weak link in the antegrade direction. In 3 other patients in group II, tachycardias were terminated by a VPC within 1 minute. In the remaining 6 patients in group II, in whom tachycardia failed to terminate, rates of tachycardia decreased as a result of suppression of antegrade AV nodal conduction by diltiazem. Electrophysiologic studies were performed subsequently 2 hours after the third dose of 90 mg of diltiazem, which was given orally at 8-hour intervals. In 18 responders to intravenous diltiazem who were subjected to oral diltiazem testing, sustained SVT could be induced in only 2. Of the 6 nonresponders, sustained tachycardias could not be induced in 3. Twelve patients, including 11 responders and 1 nonresponder to intravenous diltiazem who responded to oral diltiazem testing, were discharged with oral diltiazem therapy, 90 mg every 8 hours, with follow-up periods of 2–13 months (mean, 7 ± 4). The frequency of recurrent SVT decreased significantly; 8 patients were free of tachycardias and 4 had occasional recurrences of SVT that required no hospital visit. In conclusion, intravenous diltiazem is effective in terminating SVT. Termination of SVT by intravenous diltiazem predicts subsequent electrophysiologic and clinical responses to oral diltiazem.

Disopyramide

Brugada and Wellens[16] from Maastricht, The Netherlands, studied the effect of intravenous and oral disopyramide on the mechanisms of the arrhythmia in 11 patients with the common type of AV nodal paroxysmal reentrant tachycardia. Programmed electrical stimulation of the heart was used to initiate and terminate tachycardia and to evaluate the effect of disopyramide on mode of initiation and termination of tachycardia. Disopyramide was given intravenously to all patients during tachycardia. This resulted in termination of tachycardia, by block in the antegrade slow pathway in 1 and in the retrograde fast pathway in 3 patients. In these 4 patients, reinitiation of tachycardia was no longer possible. In these 4 patients, oral disopyramide prevented spontaneous and pacing-induced AV nodal tachycardia. In 4 of the remaining 7 patients in whom tachycardia was not terminated by intravenous disopyramide, reinitiation of the arrhythmia during programmed stimulation was prevented by the drug. In these 4 patients, oral disopyramide was also effective in preventing spontaneous occurrence of tachycardia. In 3 patients, tachycardia was not terminated and its reinitiation was not prevented by intravenous disopyramide. Only 1 of these 3 patients received disopyramide by mouth, and it failed to prevent reinitiation and spontaneous tachycardia. In conclusion, disopyramide by mouth failed to prevent reinitiation and spontaneous tachycardia. It is an effective drug in patients with AV nodal paroxysmal reentrant tachycardia. A good correlation was found between intravenous and oral effect of disopyramide on the mechanisms of the arrhythmia. The study of the effect of intravenous disopyramide predicted the outcome of oral disopyramide therapy.

Encainide

Kunze and associates[17] from Hamburg, West Germany, studied the effect of intravenous and oral encainide in 12 patients with an accessory AV pathway: 8 had WPW syndrome and 4 had a concealed accessory pathway. Electrophysiologic studies were performed before and after intravenous encainide, 1.0–1.5 mg/kg, and 4 weeks after oral encainide, 75–200 mg/day. Mean follow-up was 19 ± 6 months. During sinus rhythm, intravenous and oral encainide significantly prolonged the AH and HV intervals. In patients with WPW syndrome, after intravenous encainide, antegrade conduction over the accessory pathway was blocked in 3 patients, and the antegrade effective refractory period of the accessory pathway was markedly increased in 3. Five of these 6 patients had a control value of the antegrade accessory pathway ERP of less than 270 ms. Antegrade accessory pathway block was maintained in 2 patients after oral encainide therapy. Retrograde accessory pathway block or marked increase of retrograde accessory pathway ERP was seen in 4 of 9 patients after intravenous encainide and in 2 of 7 after oral therapy. Encainide either prevented induction of circus movement tachycardia (intravenous, 4 of 11 patients; oral, 2 of 7 patients) or significantly prolonged tachycardia cycle length (intravenous, 7 of 11 patients; oral, 5 of 7 patients). During long-term follow-up of 9 patients, 6 patients had no recurrences of tachyarrhythmia after individual adjustment of encainide dosage. One patient had worsening of SVT after intravenous encainide therapy and 4 patients complained of visual blurring; in 1 patient it was so severe that it required withdrawal of the drug. No correlation was found between plasma concentration of encainide or its metabolites and changes of electrophysiologic or clinical variables. Thus, in most patients with an accessory pathway, encainide blocks or prolongs antegrade conduction over the accessory pathway and has a beneficial effect on circus movement tachycardia, either by preventing induction of tachycardia or by prolonging tachycardia cycle length.

Abdollah and associates[18] from Maastricht, The Netherlands, studied the electrophysiologic effects and clinical efficacy of intravenous (IV) and oral encainide in 13 patients with accessory AV pathways (7 overt, 1 intermittent, and 5 concealed) and drug resistant supraventricular arrhythmias (5 paroxysmal AF, 1 atrial tachycardia, and 7 with orthodromic circus movement tachycardia). Previously, therapy had failed with a mean of 3 conventional antiarrhythmic agents. In 5 patients, amiodarone administration had also been unsuccessful. All patients underwent programmed electrical stimulation of the heart before and after 1.5 mg/kg of IV encainide. Seven patients were restudied during oral encainide therapy (mean, 156 ± 54 mg/day) 3 days to 6 weeks (mean, 21 days) later. Antegrade conduction over the accessory AV pathway blocked in 4 of 7 patients after IV encainide. Oral encainide blocked antegrade conduction over the accessory pathway in 3 of 4 patients. This change in antegrade conduction was independent of the predrug value for the antegrade refractory period of the accessory AV pathway. Intravenous and oral encainide had minimal effects on retrograde conduction over the accessory AV pathway. The clinical effect of oral encainide was studied in 12 patients. Four patients responded to oral encainide and have been free of arrhythmia or side effects for 2–20 months (average, 10). Encainide failed to prevent the clinical arrhythmia in 2 patients. In 4 patients with atrial arrhythmias, circus movement tachycardia developed during oral encainide therapy. In 1 patient the frequency of circus movement tachycardia increased with oral encainide treatment. Five of the previous 7 patients also had central nervous system side effects. In conclusion, encainide has a marked effect on antegrade conduction and a minimal effect on retrograde conduction over the accessory AV pathway. Oral encainide was effective in controlling supraventricular arrhythmia in 4 of 12 of this selected group of patients with accessory AV pathways. Failure to control the initial arrhythmia, facilitation of circus movement tachycardia, and central nervous system side effects led to discontinuation of oral encainide in the other patients.

Ethmozine

Chazov and colleagues[19] from Moscow, USSR, performed electrophysiologic studies in 11 patients with AV nodal reentrant SVT before and after intravenous administration of 1.5–2 mg/kg ethmozine. Initially, 9 of 11 patients had induction of sustained SVT, and 2 remaining patients had nonsustained SVT and atrial echoes, respectively. Ethmozine terminated induced SVT in 6 of 9 patients. In 6 of 9 patients ethmozine prevented the development of sustained SVT, indicating that ethmozine depressed retrograde fast pathway AV nodal conduction. In 4 patients atrial echoes were abolished. In the 2 remaining cases ethmozine prevented the induction of nonsustained SVT. In only 3 of these 9 patients was sustained SVT induced. Antegrade fast and slow pathway properties did not significantly change with ethmozine administration. Effective refractory period (ERP) of the ventriculoatrial (VA) conduction system and ventricular paced cycle length producing VA block was 305 ± 40 (mean ± SEM) and 347 ± 38 ms before and 424 ± 105 and 475 ± 71 ms after ethmozine administration, respectively (p < 0.01; n, 8), suggesting depression of retrograde pathway with ethmozine administration. Ethmozine significantly (p < 0.05) lengthened PA, AH, HV, and PR intervals (36 ± 11–45 ± 14 ms, 84 ± 21–93 ± 17 ms, 42 ± 8–50 ± 7 ms, and 163 ± 23–190 ± 31 ms, respectively). No significant change was observed in sinus rate, QRS and QT intervals, or ERP of atrium and ventricle. Thus, a single intravenous dose of ethmozine terminated induced SVT and prevented induction of sustained SVT in most patients, reflecting depression of retrograde fast pathway conduction.

Catheter ablation

In patients with supraventricular arrhythmias in whom drug therapy is ineffective or poorly tolerated, any tachycardia pacing or specific localized ablative surgical or catheter techniques may be indicated. In others the interruption of AV nodal conduction may be considered. Originally this was achieved at open heart surgery, but a catheter technique has been developed. Nathan and associates[20] from London, England, described the catheter technique used from 3 English centers; 45 patients with refractory supraventricular arrhythmias were treated by high energy shocks delivered to the AV conduction system from a conventional transvenous pacing catheter. In a mean interval of 10 months, 26 patients (74%) had persistent complete heart block, 2 (6%) had intermittent complete heart block, and 3 (9%) had first-degree heart block. Three patients continued to have conducted AF, but with slower ventricular rates than previously, and 1 had normalization of dual atrio-His conduction. In 1 patient a septal accessory pathway was ablated. Thirty patients (86%) are completely symptom-free without additional therapy. There were no important long-term complications. Transvenous ablation of atrioventricular conduction is a safe and effective technique for treating a wide range of refractory atrial and junctional arrhythmias.

Fisher and coworkers[21] from New York City tested the possibility that electrical ablation of accessory pathways in 8 patients with symptomatic WPW syndrome could be provided from the coronary sinus. Shocks were limited to 40–80 J, except in 1 patient who received shocks of 100 and 150 J. From 2–26 shocks were administered to each accessory pathway. Immediately after the shocks, all accessory pathways were blocked. However, evidence of accessory pathway conduction recurred in each patient. The only significant complication occurred in the patient receiving shocks of 100 and 150 J who had rupture of the coronary sinus requiring pericardial drainage. These data are encouraging in suggesting this possible approach for altering accessory pathway conduction in patients with the symptomatic arrhythmias coexistent with the WPW syndrome.

Surgical ablation

The permanent or recurring form of junctional reciprocating tachycardia (PJRT) is so named because of its characteristic incessant nature and refractoriness to medical therapy. Guarnieri and colleagues[22] from Durham, North Carolina, reported 9 patients with PJRT refractory to medical therapy who were referred for evaluation and electrophysiologic study. All 9 patients had the characteristic clinical and electrophysiologic features of PJRT. Each patient demonstrated near incessant reciprocating tachycardia with a 1:1 AV relation and with a retrograde P wave (P') occurring closer to the succeeding QRS complexes (long RP'). With initiation of the tachycardia, there was no prolongation of the PR or AH interval. All patients had evidence of early retrograde atrial activation in their posterior atrial septa and this retrograde limb had properties of decremental conduction. Eight of the 9 patients underwent elective surgical ablation of the retrograde limb tachycardia, and in 7 patients it was successful. Epicardial and endocardial atrial maps recorded during PJRT demonstrated that the site of earliest retrograde activation was in the posterior atrial septum near the coronary sinus orifice. The 7 patients in whom surgery was successful left the hospital in sinus rhythm with antegrade conduction, and all were free of tachycardia during the mean followup period of 31 months. In the 2 remaining patients PJRT was controlled by interruption of the antegrade limb of the tachycardia, the AV node-His bundle. In 1 patient this was done under direct vision at surgery after an unsuccessful attempt at pathway dissection. The other underwent closed chest ablation of the AV node with a catheter. Both remained well and left the hospital free of tachycardia. This study demonstrates that PJRT, which is characteristically refractory to medical therapy, can be successfully managed by surgical ablation of the retrograde limb of the tachycardia.

VENTRICULAR ARRHYTHMIAS

Holter Monitoring and/or electrophysiologic study for guiding management

The ability to assess prognosis in patients with serious ventricular arrhythmias treated with antiarrhythmic drugs by the degree of complexity of the 24-hour ambulatory ECG was evaluated in 59 survivors of VT and VF by Vlay and associates[23] from Baltimore, Maryland, and Stony Brook, New York. After conventional therapy had failed, patients were treated with investigational drugs until symptomatic VT was abolished. A Holter monitor recording, obtained once the therapeutic regimen was established, was graded for the presence or absence of asymptomatic VT. Fifty-two patients were asymptomatic at discharge and were followed for 700 days. Of 44 patients followed for 1 year, none had recurrent syncope or died if asymptomatic VT was absent at 1 month (p < 0.002). After 700 days, 27 patients (82%) without asymptomatic VT at 1 month were doing well, compared with 11 patients (58%) with asymptomatic VT at 1 month (p < 0.002). In patients at risk for sudden cardiac arrest, early abolition of asymptomatic VT on ambulatory monitoring can be used to predict a good long-term clinical response.

Platia and Reid[24] from Baltimore, Maryland, evaluated 44 patients with primary VF or recurrent VT who had been stabilized on an antiarrhythmic regimen before electrophysiologic study and in whom 24–72 hours of ambulatory ECG monitoring were performed. The long-term predictive value of these 2 tests was compared retrospectively for a 12–32 month (mean, 18) follow-up period during which all patients continued receiving the same antiarrhythmic drug regimen. Data obtained indicate that electrophysiologic testing induced VT in 26 patients; 23 had a poor clinical outcome for a positive predictive value of electrophysiologic testing of 88%. In 18 patients with a negative electrophysiologic test, only 1 died suddenly or sustained VT; thus, the negative predictive value of this test was 94%. Ambulatory ECG monitoring predicted outcome in 7 of 10 patients with a positive recording for a positive predictive value of 70% and in 17 of 34 patients with negative ambulatory monitor recordings for a negative predictive value of 50%. However, predictive accuracy of the electrophysiologic study was significantly higher than that of the ambulatory ECG monitoring (p < 0.001). These data indicate that electrophysiologic testing has certain advantages over ambulatory ECG monitoring in a high risk patient group for predicting risks of sudden death and recurrent sustained VT.

Ezri and associates[25] from Chicago, Illinois, studied 19 patients with sustained VT with 24-hour Holter recordings before control electrophysiologic studies (EPS) and before each drug trial. Successful drug or surgical treatment (with the exception of amiodarone) was based on noninducibility of VT. Among the 8 noninducible and nonamiodarone medically treated patients, 2 had significant VPC reduction and/or Lown class improvement. The remaining 6 had no change or worsening of Holter findings, despite noninducibility of sustained VT. Among the 6 amiodarone-treated patients, 5 of whom were persistently inducible before discharge, 4 had improved and 2 had worsened Holter findings compared with controls. None of the 5 surgically managed patients were inducible postoperatively, and 3 of the 5 had no change or worsening of Holter findings. It was concluded that EPS are superior to Holter findings in assessing successful management, and Holter findings may be concordant or discordant during EPS serial drug trials or after surgery and therefore cannot predict the success or failure of the intervention.

Electrophysiologic induction

To analyze the significance of the different types of ventricular arrhythmias, Brugada and coworkers[26] from Maastricht, The Netherlands, evaluated in a prospective study the effect of from 1–4 ventricular premature stimuli in 52 patients without (non-VT group) and 50 patients with (prior-VT group) documented VT or VF. More than half of the patients in the prior-VT group had CAD. In most patients of the non-VT group the heart was normal. In 44 of the 50 patients in the prior-VT group, the clinically documented ventricular arrhythmia was initiated by programmed ventricular stimulation of the heart. In 88% of these 44 patients, 1 or 2 VPC were required to initiate the clinical arrhythmia. A ventricular arrhythmia could be initiated in 31 of the 52 patients in the non-VT group. The ventricular arrhythmias included nonsustained monomorphic VT (2 patients), 6–25 complexes of sustained polymorphic VT (24 patients), and VF (5 patients). In 70% of the patients in the non-VT group 3 or 4 VPC were required to initiate the ventricular arrhythmia. These results indicate that not only the number of extrastimuli required to initiate ventricular arrhythmias but also the type of ventricular arrhythmia initiated differed between patients with and without history and clinical documentation of ventricular arrhythmia.

Buxton and associates[27] from Philadelphia, Pennsylvania, performed electrophysiologic studies in 83 consecutive patients with spontaneous nonsustained VT. The VT was inducible in 52 patients (nonsustained VT only in 37 patients, nonsustained and sustained VT in 13, and sustained VT only in 2). During a follow-up of 3–111 months (mean, 33), 10 patients died suddenly, 5 with CAD and 5 with dilated cardiomyopathy. All patients dying suddenly had an EF ≤0.40. Sudden death occurred in 4 of 15 patients with inducible sustained VT, 2 of 37 patients with only nonsustained VT and 4 of 31 patients without inducible VT (Fig. 3-1). One patient with dilated cardiomyopathy and VT inducible only by isoproterenol died suddenly. Three of 5 patients with CAD who had sudden death had had inducible sustained VT, but 3 of 5 patients with cardiomyopathy who had sudden death had no inducible VT. Multivariate analysis revealed that patients with inducible sustained VT or an EF ≤0.40 had a 3-fold increased risk of sudden death, and patients with both factors had a 7-fold increased risk of sudden death (Fig. 3-2). This study demonstrates that patients with nonsustained VT with an EF >0.40 have an uncomplicated course; however, noninducibility does not predict such a course, particularly in patients with cardiomyopathy. The most powerful predictor of risk for sudden cardiac death is a LV EF ≤0.40, but the presence of inducible sustained VT is an independent risk factor for sudden death.

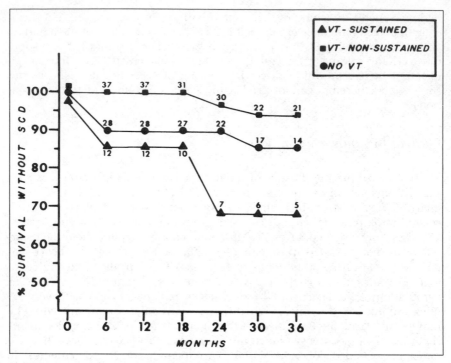

Fig. 3-1. Actuarial survival curves of patients with spontaneous nonsustained VT relating risk of sudden cardiac death (SCD) to arrhythmias induced at electrophysiologic study. Numbers accompanying each symbol denote patients in each group at risk for sudden death at the beginning of each period.

Programmed ventricular stimulation has been demonstrated to be useful both diagnostically and in the evaluation of drug therapy in patients with recurrent VT, out-of-hospital cardiac arrest, and syncope of unknown cause. A basic premise of this technique is that VT is provocable rarely, if ever, in patients who have never had spontaneous episodes of VT. There have as yet been no reports on the specificity of stimulation protocols that use a current intensity greater than twice diastolic threshold. Accordingly, Morady and associates[28] from San Francisco, California, studied the effects of programmed RV and LV stimulation with up to 3 extrastimuli at an intensity level of 5 mA in 52 patients who had never had a documented or suspected episode of spontaneous VT or VF. A maximum response of 1–5 intraventricular reentry beats was induced in 52% of patients. Nonsustained VT (≥6 repetitive beats terminating spontaneously within 30 seconds) was never induced in the 16 patients without structural heart disease but was induced (usually with triple extrastimuli) in 4 of 9 patients with MVP and in 37% of 27 patients with other types of heart disease. Sustained VT was never induced; however, sustained VF was induced in 2 patients. Therefore, during programmed RV and LV stimulation with up to 3 extrastimuli (with 2 ms pulses, 5 mA in intensity): a maximum response of 1–5 repetitive beats is a nonspecific finding of no predictive value; nonsustained VT was not induced in patients without structural heart disease who had not had spontaneous VT; nonsustained VT was frequently induced in patients with structural

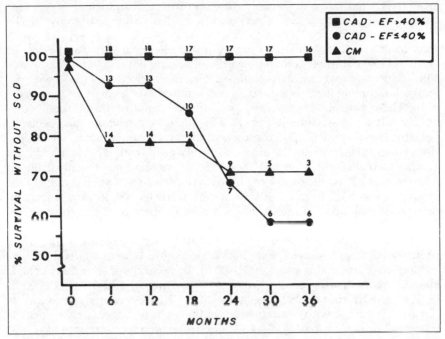

Fig. 3-2.   Actuarial survival curves of patients with spontaneous nonsustained VT relating risk of sudden cardiac death (SCD) to underlying heart disease. The numbers next to each symbol represent number of patients in each group at risk of sudden cardiac death at the beginning of each period depicted. CM = cardiomyopathy.

heart disease who had not previously been known to have had VT; the induction of sustained VT appears to be a response specific to patients who have had spontaneous VT or VF; and sustained VF can be induced infrequently in patients who have never had spontaneous VT or VF.

Gomes and colleagues[29] from New York City undertook a prospective study of programmed electrical stimulation with up to 2 extrastimuli and burst pacing in 73 patients with high grade VPC who had no evidence of sustained VT, sudden death, or syncope as determined by 48 hours of monitoring in the coronary care unit and 48 hours of Holter monitoring. Fifty-six patients (77%) had CAD, 10 (14%) had cardiomyopathy or valvular heart disease, and 7 (10%) had no evident heart disease. Thirty-seven patients (51%) had Lown grade IVB VPC. Yet, 30 (41%) had Lown grade IVA VPC, and 6 (8%) had Lown grade III VPC. Programmed electrical stimulation identified 2 groups of subjects: group 1 comprised 20 patients in whom VT or VF was induced, group 2 comprised 53 patients in whom no ventricular arrhythmia or only 2–4 repetitive ventricular responses were induced. There was a significant difference between the presence of CAD, healed AMI, and EF <40% in group 1 compared with group 2. There was no significant difference in the grade of VPC between the 2 groups. Of 20 patients from group 1, 17 were placed on antiarrhythmic therapy, whereas group 2 patients were randomly assigned to prophylactic antiarrhythmic therapy. A total of 70 patients were followed up for 30 ± 15 months. The incidence of sustained VT or sudden death or both was significantly higher in group 1 compared with group 2. There was no difference in the occurrence of sudden or nonsudden cardiac death between the treated and untreated patients in group 2. The probability of surviving 12 and 48 months was significantly lower in group 1 than in group 2. In this study, programmed electrical stimulation defines high and low risk subsets for sudden death among patients with high grade VPC. Patients in whom arrhythmias are not inducible and those with EF >40% have a low incidence of sudden death and an excellent 1–2-year survival. These patients did not need prophylactic antiarrhythmic therapy.

Doherty and associates[30] from Philadelphia, Pennsylvania, prospectively performed in 56 patients programmed ventricular stimulation in 56 consecutive patients from both the RV apex and the RV outflow track: 37 patients had documented clinical sustained VT and 19 patients had no clinical sustained spontaneous VT in the absence of antiarrhythmic drugs. The sensitivity of VT induction was 65% from the RV apex, 76% from the RV outflow tract, and 89% with combined stimulation at both RV sites. The specificity from the RV apex, the RV outflow tract, and both sites combined was 100%. When sustained VT was induced from both sites (51%) it was usually of the same morphologic characteristics, axis, and cycle length. When sustained VT was induced at 1 site and nonsustained VT at the second site, the morphologic characteristics or axis usually differed. Of patients who had VT induced at both RV sites during the baseline study, 37% had VT rendered noninducible during treatment with conventional antiarrhythmic agents. No patients whose VT was induced at only 1 RV site responded to conventional drugs. Thus, programmed ventricular stimulation at a second RV site is frequently helpful in evaluating VT. Inducibility at only 1 of 2 RV sites predicts a poor response to conventional antiarrhythmic drugs.

Buxton and associates[31] from Philadelphia, Pennsylvania, compared clinical and electrophysiologic characteristics of 6 patients who had repetitive monomorphic VT after a healed AMI (group A) with those of 22 patients who had this arrhythmia without structural heart disease (group B). The VT had a right BBB morphologic pattern in 5 of 6 group A patients and a left BBB morphologic pattern in all group B patients. Endocardial catheter activation mapping was performed in 4 group A patients and in 9 group B patients during VT. In all group A patients the site of VT origin was on the border of the previous infarction; in all group B patients VT originated at the RV outflow tract. Pacing and programmed stimulation induced VT in 5 of 6 group A patients and 7 of 22 group B patients (p = 0.03). Isoproterenol infusion provoked VT in 4 group A patients and 9 group B patients. Type I antiarrhythmic agents suppressed VT in 4 group A patients and in 14 group B patients, whereas propranolol suppressed VT in 3 of 3 group A patients tested and in 12 of 20 group B patients. Verapamil suppressed spontaneous VT in 1 group A patient and in 4 group B patients. During a mean follow-up of 19 months for group A and 40 months for group B, no patient died suddenly or had cardiac arrest.

To evaluate the timing of the RV apical electrogram in relation to the QRS complex during VT, Almendral and associates[32] from Philadelphia, Pennsylvania, analyzed in 56 patients 94 episodes of sustained uniform VT. The timing of the RV apical electrogram varied and could be recorded from 33 ms before to 180 ms (mean, 77 ± 44 ms) after the onset of the QRS complex. The timing of the RV apical electrogram, expressed both as an absolute value and as a percentage of a QRS width, was significantly different when right BBB morphology VT (95 ± 37 ms) and left BBB morphology VT (40 ± 34) were compared (p < 0.001). The timing of the RV apical electrogram, expressed as a percentage of the QRS width, was significantly different when VT with different axes were compared in the right BBB VT group (p < 0.01). A left BBB VT, compared with a right BBB VT, predicted an RV apical electrogram occurring in the first 35% of the QRS with a sensitivity of 74%, a specificity of 91%, and a positive predictive value of 84%. Right BBB VT with a right and inferior axis were usually associated with the latest occurring RV apical electrogram. A right BBB VT with a right and inferior axis predicted an RV apical electrogram inscribed in the latter half of the QRS with a sensitivity of 65%, a specificity of 84%, and a positive predictive value of 80%. Thus, the timing of the RV apical electrogram relative to the onset of the QRS can have markedly different values in sustained VT, which may be to some predictable from the QRS morphologic pattern. These findings may have important implications in the application of electrical devices that depend on synchronization to the RV apical electrogram for the delivery of their impulses. More appropriate synchronization may improve the efficacy and safety of these devices.

Exercise induced

Weiner and associates[33] from Boston, Massachusetts, investigated the determinants and prognostic significance of ventricular arrhythmias during exercise testing. Such arrhythmias were identified in 86 patients from a consecutive series of 446 patients who underwent treadmill exercise testing during cardiac catheterization. The prevalence of these arrhythmias was 19% of the total group but increased to 30% in the 120 patients with 3-vessel or LM CAD (Fig. 3-3). Patients with exercise-induced arrhythmias were more likely to have 3-vessel or LM CAD, a lower resting EF, ≥2 mm of ischemic ST depression, and more severe segmental wall motion abnormalities than patients without this finding (p < 0.05). Repeat exercise testing in 22 patients with exercise-induced arrhythmias after CABG revealed that persistence of these arrhythmias was associated with either severe wall motion abnormalities preoperatively or residual ischemic ST depression during the postoperative exercise testing. At a mean follow-up period of 5.3 years, the presence of exercise-induced ventricular arrhythmias was not associated with increased cardiac mortality in the medically treated patients.

Fleg and Lakatta[34] from Baltimore, Maryland, assessed the prevalence of VT associated with maximal treadmill exercise in 597 men and in 325 women volunteers, aged 21–96 years (mean, 54 ± 16). Ten subjects, 7 men and 3 women, with exercise-induced VT were identified, representing 1.1% of those tested; only 1 was less than age 65 years. All episodes of VT were asymptomatic and nonsustained. In 9 of 10 subjects, VT developed at or near peak exercise. The longest run of VT was 6 beats; multiple runs of VT were present in 4 subjects. Two subjects had exercise-induced ST-segment depression, but subsequent exercise thallium scintigraphic results were negative in each. Compared with a group of age- and sex-matched control subjects, those with asymptomatic, nonsustained VT displayed no difference in exercise duration, maximal heart rate, or the prevalence of coronary risk factors or exercise-induced ischemia as measured by ECG and thallium scintigraphy. Over a mean follow-up period of 2 years, no subject has developed symptoms

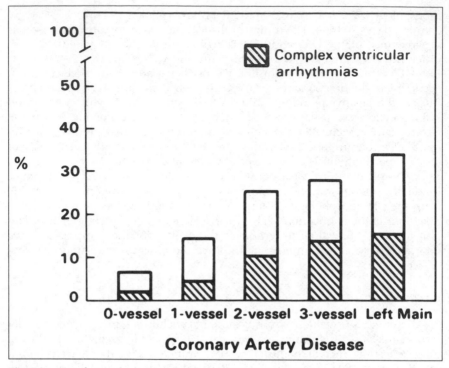

Fig. 3-3. Prevalence of exercise-induced ventricular arrhythmias according to the number of diseased coronary vessels.

of heart disease or experienced syncope or sudden death. Thus, exercise-induced VT in apparently healthy subjects occurs almost exclusively in the elderly, is limited to short, asymptomatic runs of 3–6 beats usually near peak exercise, and does not portend increased cardiovascular morbidity or mortality rates over a 2-year period of observation.

Economics of electrophysiologic testing

Ferguson and associates[35] from Newark, New Jersey, examined clinical and economic results of antiarrhythmic therapy selected on the basis of electrophysiologic (EP) studies in patients with recurrent VT and compared with previously administered empiric therapy. Twenty-nine patients with recurrent VT and organic heart disease, aged 39–78 years (mean, 59) were evaluated. All patients had empiric therapy before EP studies and EP-based therapy after EP evaluation. Hospital records were analyzed from arrhythmia diagnosis 1–39 months (mean, 8) before EP evaluation until completion of follow-up 1–20 months (mean, 13) after EP studies. Clinical efficacy was assessed by comparing actual antiarrhythmic death or occurrences during EP-based therapy with predicted values on empiric therapy. During empiric therapy, 1–7 unsuccessful drug trials (mean, 4) were performed, with arrhythmia recurrences noted in all patients during a mean 7.5-month VT duration. Of 29 patients, 27 required 1–70 electrical terminations. There were 64 hospitalizations (mean, 2) with a total length of hospital stay of 913 days (mean, 31). The EP evaluation required 90 procedures (mean, 3) with a length of stay of 690 days (mean, 24). During a follow-up period of 1–26.5 months (mean, 13) on EP-based therapy, 1 patient died suddenly. There were 5 repeat hospitalizations for adverse effects with a total length of stay of 48 days (mean, 2). There was a significant reduction in arrhythmia recurrences and sudden death (p < 0.05) and hospital charges (p < 0.01) with EP-based therapy compared with empiric therapy. Thus, EP-based therapy has favorable clinical and economic results in patients with recurrent VT.

Relation between premature ventricular complex site of origin and LV function

It has been suggested that the effect of a VPC on LV function depends on the site of origin of the VPC and that the subsequent impairment of LV performance during a VPC may be more pronounced if baseline LV dysfunction is present. To evaluate these concepts, Rolfe and associates[36] from Columbus, Ohio, performed RNA phase image analysis of spontaneous VPC after acquisition of images from VPC alone by a new gating procedure. The sites of VPC were localized to 1 of 3 RV or 5 LV regions by this method. The LV function during VPC was assessed and compared with baseline by noting the LV EF during VPC, the difference between sinus LV EF and VPC EF, and the normalized VPC EF (VPC EF/sinus EF). Twenty-four patients had LV VPC sites and 19 had RV sites. The LV function during a VPC appeared to be independent of either the ventricle of origin of the VPC or a specific site of origin within the ventricles. In addition, no correlation between coupling interval and any of the variables measured was demonstrated. These data suggest that the effects of VPC on ventricular performance seen during ventricular ectopic activity are independent of the site of origin of the VPC, baseline wall motion abnormalities, or VPC coupling interval.

Vulnerability to VF with clinically manifest VT

Ventricular vulnerability may be assessed by measuring the threshold current for the induction of VF. This technique has been widely utilized in animal experimentation and has been safely applied in a small number of clinical studies. Kowey and associates[37] from Boston, Massachusetts, measured the VF threshold, using the single-stimulus technique in 10 patients with CAD just before institution of cardiopulmonary bypass. There were no adverse effects of VF threshold measurement. Three patients had nonsustained VT on 24-hour ambulatory monitoring and had VF thresholds of 10, 14, and 16 mA. In this group VF was induced without any preceding repetitive ventricular responses. Seven patients had no repetitive forms on ambulatory monitoring. Their VF thresholds ranged from 30–>40 mA (mean, >37). Repetitive VPC were regularly observed in this group at current intensities, which ranged from 53–80% of the VF threshold. Thus, patients with manifest VT appear to have an enhanced vulnerability to VF.

Factors predicting syncope during VT

Hamer and associates[38] from Los Angeles, California, performed programmed electrical stimulation (PES) in 40 patients who had a history of
recurrent ventricular arrhythmias. The PES initiated sustained VT in each
patient. Twenty patients remained alert and oriented during arrhythmia, but
syncope occurred in the remaining 20 patients. The only factor that could be
known before PES that was associated with the occurrence of syncope during
the study was a clinical history of syncope (p < 0.01). In particular, impaired
resting ventricular function was not an important determinant of syncope.
During PES, syncope was related to the rapidity of VT (syncope, 253 ± 37
beats/min; nonsyncope, 193 ± 24 beats/min; p < 0.001) and was a consequence of the degree of hypotension induced (<50 mmHg mean arterial
pressure). Antiarrhythmic drugs prevented syncope if they reduced the rate
of VT to <200 beats/minute in patients prone to syncope. It was concluded
that reduced ventricular function is not related to syncope from VT, but that
syncope during PES can often be predicted from a clinical history and is
predominantly determined by the rate of induced VT. Antiarrhythmic drugs
may be lifesaving if they reduce the rate of VT even if they cannot prevent its
occurrence.

VT of left BBB configuration
in RV dilation

Rowland and associates[39] from London, England, performed electrophysiologic studies in 5 patients with isolated RV dilation of undetermined cause.
All had been asymptomatic before onset of palpitations or cardiac arrest,
both of which occurred in adolescents or early adult life. The VT had been
associated with syncope in 4 patients and 3 had been resuscitated from VF.
The ECG during VT showed a left BBB pattern and endocardial mapping,
and electrophysiologic study confirmed the RV origin. The presenting VT
could be induced in all patients by programmed stimulation and in 3 patients VT of differing configuration could be induced, but the RV origin and
left BBB pattern were maintained. Cineangiography, cross-sectional echo,
and multigated RNA confirmed the dilated right ventricle. On a resting ECG,
T-wave inversion over the right precordial leads was the sole abnormality.
There were no signs of right-sided CHF and exercise tolerance was normal.
Thus, VT complicating RV dilation may be associated with serious symptoms
and ventricular electrical instability, and in adults it may be suspected on
clinical grounds by inverted T waves in the right precordial leads.

Postoperative ventricular arrhythmias

Development of VT or VF during the postoperative period is a dreaded but
poorly understood complication of cardiac operations. In a series from Virginia Medical Center, Kron and associates[40] reported on 18 (1.4%) of 1,251
patients who underwent cardiac operations during a 3-year period who had
new sustained VT (12 patients) or VF (6 patients) not caused by but resulting
in hemodynamic compromise. Lidocaine was being administered to 10 patients for suppression of previously noted ventricular ectopic activity, but it
did not prevent the occurrence of the arrhythmia. The initial episode was

fatal in 5 patients. Nine of the remainder had repeat episodes with 3 deaths. Five of 10 survivors underwent electrophysiologic studies after initial resuscitation. In all 5, programmed ventricular stimulation reproduced the clinical arrhythmia. The investigators suggested that a cardiac operation may unmask or induce potentially lethal arrhythmias that previously had not been apparent. They also noted that pharmacologic suppression of ventricular ectopic activity does not necessarily prevent VT or VF in the early postoperative period.

Amiodarone

The collaborative Group for Amiodarone Evaluation[41] from Milan, Italy, tested the clinical efficacy of a low dosage schedule of amiodarone in 58 patients with severe ventricular arrhythmias refractory to other drug treatments. The initially chosen regimen of 400 mg was effective at the end of the first controlled trial period (after 4 weeks) in 73% of the patients. The responsiveness was maintained with the smaller dosage of 200 mg in 68% of this group. The response was reestablished also in the patients who became nonresponders during the low dose regimen when they returned to the initial (400 mg) dosage. No relation was found between clinical response and blood levels of amiodarone and of its deethylated metabolite. Adverse effects more often associated with amiodarone therapy were rare. However, careful monitoring of thyroid function allowed the detection in 10% of the patients of biochemically and functionally documented, but clinically silent, hypo- or hyperthyroidism.

McGovern and associates[42] from Boston, Massachusetts, and Charlottesville, Virginia, studied the determinants of long-term clinical outcome in 45 patients with recurrent VT or VF who were treated with amiodarone as a sole antiarrhythmic agent. Of the 42 patients, 11 (26%) either died suddenly or had recurrent, symptomatic, sustained VT during a mean follow-up period of 10 months (range, 0.3–45). Of the 19 patients without inducible VT/VF during electrophysiologic study while receiving amiodarone, 1 patient died suddenly but no patient had recurrent VT/VF. Ten of the 23 patients (43%) with persistently inducible arrhythmia have died suddenly or have had recurrent VT/VF (Fig. 3-4). Using survival and stepwise logistic regression analyses, 2 significant independent predictors of recurrent arrhythmia were identified: persistently inducible VT during electrophysiologic testing in patients receiving amiodarone therapy (p < 0.002) and the LV EF at rest (p < 0.05). The predictive accuracy of the response to serial electrophysiologic testing during amiodarone therapy was 67%, the sensitivity was 58%, and the specificity was 91%. Thus, serial electrophysiologic testing is useful for determining the prognosis in patients with inducible VT/VF treated with amiodarone.

Saal and associates[43] from Seattle, Washington, measured serum levels of quinidine or procainamide in patients who had amiodarone added to their antiarrhythmic regimen. Doses of quinidine or procainamide were held constant. All 11 patients had an increase in the serum quinidine level, and 11 of 12 other patients had an increase in the serum procainamide level. The dose requirement to maintain a stable plasma level of quinidine or procainamide decreased by 37 and 20%, respectively. Clinical toxicity occasionally occurred with the increase in serum levels of quinidine and procainamide, and the doses of these drugs should be decreased when amiodarone is administered concurrently.

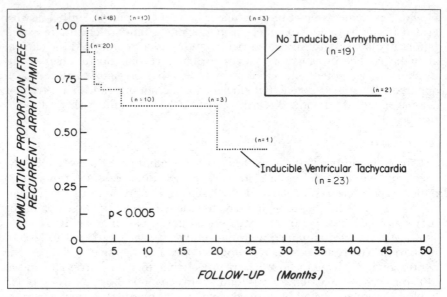

Fig. 3-4. Life-table curves for 42 patients classified according to the results of electrophysiologic testing during amiodarone therapy. Recurrent arrhythmia is defined as recurrent symptomatic VT or sudden death. Numbers in parentheses indicate the number of patients still being treated with amiodarone at that time.

Nademanee and coworkers[44] from Los Angeles, California, evaluated the interaction of amiodarone and digoxin in 28 patients receiving long-term digoxin therapy. The administration of amiodarone (600–1,600 mg/day) increased serum digoxin levels from 0.97 ± 0.45–1.98 ± 0.84 ng/ml (p < 0.001) (Fig. 3-5). Nine patients had gastrointestinal side effects, central nervous system reactions occurred in 5, and cardiovascular reactions occurred in 4 patients. Amiodarone resulted in a 31% prolongation of digoxin elimination half-life from 49 ± 9–65 ± 29 hours. Total body clearance was reduced significantly by 29% and nonrenal clearance mechanisms showed a similar decrease. Thus, these data indicate that caution should be observed when digoxin and amiodarone are given to the same patient and such an individual should be monitored closely for evidence of digoxin toxicity.

Mostow and coworkers[45] from Cleveland, Ohio, determined whether intravenous loading with amiodarone might provide more rapid suppression of complex ventricular arrhythmias than occurs with chronic oral loading. Eleven patients were studied. Each patient received a single intravenous dose kinetic study, followed by a 2-stage infusion of amiodarone that resulted in a serum concentration of 2–3 μg/ml. In 7 patients, arrhythmias during hours 24–48 after the infusion were compared with arrhythmias without therapy. Amiodarone therapy reduced episodes of VT by 85% (p < 0.01), paired VPC by 74% (p < 0.01), and VPC by 60% (p < 0.05). In 4 patients, the control period was associated with symptomatic arrhythmias precluding further evaluation. In 3 patients, symptomatic arrhythmias were abolished during the 24-hour evaluation period. Two of 11 patients with severe LV dysfunction developed significant hypotension during amiodarone loading. Thus, these

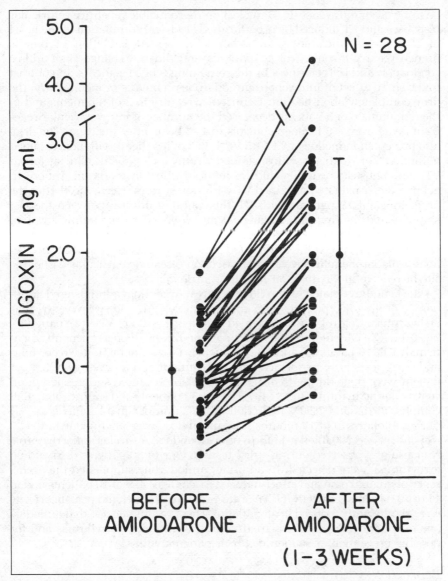

Fig. 3-5. Changes in steady state serum digoxin concentrations induced by the concomitant administration of amiodarone (600–1,600 mg/day; mean, 1,251 ± 335) for 7–21 days (mean, 13.3 ± 5.3). Each closed circle represents a value from 1 patient. The vertical bars indicate standard deviations from the mean values. Amiodarone increased digoxin levels in all patients. Reproduced with permission from Nademanee et al.[44]

data indicate that intravenous loading with amiodarone may result in a therapeutic serum concentration that is effective in the suppression of life-threatening ventricular arrhythmias, and caution should be utilized with administering large intravenous doses of amiodarone to patients with markedly impaired LV function.

Hariman and associates[46] from New York City studied the effects of amiodarone given intravenously (5 mg/kg) on reproducible repetitive ventricular responses and VT induced by programmed electrical stimulation of the heart in 32 patients. Intravenous amiodarone prevented induction of bundle branch reentry in only 2 of 11 patients and did not change His-Purkinje conduction and refractoriness in the remaining 9 of 11 patients. In contrast to the small effect of intravenous amiodarone on bundle branch reentry, the drug completely abolished intraventricular reentry in 3 of 9 patients and in the remaining 6 of 9 patients decreased the number of intraventricular reentrant beats from ≤5 beats in controls to 1–2 beats after the drug. The drug also prevented induction of VT (≥5 VPC) in 3 of 5 patients with nonsustained VT and in 3 of 7 patients with sustained VT. In 2 of 7 patients with sustained VT, only nonsustained VT could be induced after drug administration. In another 2 of 7 patients, sustained VT with slower rates was induced after the drug. In 11 of 12 patients with VT the coupling interval between the last stimulus and the first ventricular beat increased after drug administration. These effects of intravenous amiodarone occurred in the absence of effect on ventricular effective refractory period. These findings suggest that intravenous amiodarone may have greater effect on diseased ventricular tissue, the site of reentry in VT, than on healthy ventricular tissue.

Kaski and associates[47] from Buenos Aires, Argentina, administered amiodarone orally to 30 patients with chronic stable CAD and severe ventricular arrhythmias. Control studies revealed frequent (>30/hr) VPC (27 patients), bigeminy (21 patients), couplets (29 patients), R-on-T phenomenon (14 patients), VT (16 patients), and VF (1 patient). Two 24-hour Holter recordings and stress tests were performed before treatment and an average of 3.6 per patient were done during treatment. Amiodarone caused suppression of all ventricular arrhythmias in 13 (43%) of the 30 patients and suppression of all complex forms and >90% reduction of VPC number in 14 patients (47%) during a follow-up of 12 months. The mean dose was 590 mg/day in the 27 responders and 300 mg/day in the 3 nonresponders. A similar antiarrhythmic response was observed during stress testing. One of 30 patients died and no arrhythmias were detected. In addition, amiodarone suppressed the occurrence of anginal pain and effort-induced ST changes in 9 of 10 patients and in 11 of 13 patients, respectively. The rate-pressure product and peak heart rate were significantly reduced in all patients. These results suggest that amiodarone may be ideally suited for treatment of ventricular arrhythmias and for possible prevention of sudden death in patients with CAD.

Bepridil

Levy and associates[48] from Marseille, France, evaluated intravenous and oral bepridil using serial electrophysiologic studies in 9 patients with recurrent sustained VT unresponsive to usual therapy. Intravenous bepridil treatment terminated sustained, well tolerated, pacing-induced VT in 3 of 6 patients and prevented the initiation of VT in 2 and in a patient in whom the drug failed to restore sinus rhythm. Oral bepridil was administered at a loading dose of 800 mg on day 1, and 500–600 mg the following days, and programmed electrical stimulation was repeated 2–6 days after initial study. Oral bepridil therapy prevented VT initiation in 6 patients. The tachycardia cycle length was prolonged (30–105 ms) in patients in whom VT remained inducible. In 1 patient the tachycardia cycle length significantly shortened after bepridil and prompt cardioversion was required. Five of the 6 patients with successful results underwent long-term oral treatment with bepridil. The VT recurred in 1 patient during the hospitalization period and an adverse effect (paralytic ileus) in another patient required drug discontinuation. Three patients remained symptom-free over a follow-up of 4–13 months. These data suggest that bepridil may be useful in patients with recurrent, sustained VT.

Bethanidine

Benditt and associates[49] from Minneapolis, Minnesota, studied antiarrhythmic and electrophysiologic actions of bethanidine sulfate, a chemical analog of bretylium tosylate, using programmed cardiac electrical stimulation in 14 survivors of out-of-hospital cardiac arrest unassociated with AMI. Before bethanidine sulfate was administered, sustained VT was inducible in 11 patients and reproducible nonsustained VT in 3 patients. Bethanidine sulfate shortened sinus cycle length and absolute and relative ventricular refractory periods measured during sinus rhythm, but did not alter ventricular effective refractory period measured during ventricular pacing. Bethanidine sulfate prevented inducible VT in 8 patients (57%), increased the number of extrastimuli needed to induce VT in 2 patients, and was ineffective in 4 patients. In contrast, in only 1 of 26 trials with other conventional and investigational antiarrhythmic drugs in these patients was VT prevented. Orthostatic hypotension was a prominent side effect of bethanidine sulfate therapy, but could be reversed in most patients by concomitant administration of protriptyline. Five patients in whom bethanidine sulfate was effective in the laboratory have been treated chronically (400–600 mg 4 times daily), and all were alive at 3–40 months. In the remaining 9 patients, 8 were treated empirically because no drug was effective in the laboratory and 1 was treated with quinidine, which appeared to be protective during testing. Four of these 9 patients, including the patient treated with quinidine, died suddenly during follow-up. Thus, although bethanidine sulfate therapy is difficult to initiate because of orthostatic hypotensive side effects, it may be useful in treating patients at high risk of recurrent cardiac arrest.

Somberg and associates[50] from New York City performed studies in 20 patients with symptomatic VT to determine the efficacy of bethanidine compared with procainamide in preventing VT induced by programmed electrical stimulation. Before administering bethanidine, 5–10 mg/kg, the patients received 15 mg of protriptyline orally 24 and 2 hours before electrophysiologic studies to prevent the orthostatic hypotensive effects of bethanidine. Sustained VT was induced in 8 and nonsustained VT (≥10 beats terminating spontaneously) was induced in 4 patients. Bethanidine, 5 mg/kg, protected 7 patients, and 10 mg/kg protected 1 additional patient. Procainamide, 1,000 and 1,500 mg intravenously, protected 8 of 16 patients. Bethanidine prevented VT induction in 50% of the patients not protected by procainamide. Bethanidine facilitated VT induction in 3 patients, and procainamide facilitated VT induction in 1 patient. Four patients with symptomatic VT have received bethanidine therapy for an average of 11 ± 1 months, without clinical recurrence of the VT. Concomitant administration of protriptyline attenuated the acute hemodynamic changes caused by bethanidine and chronic combined therapy of protriptyline and bethanidine abolished the severe orthostatic changes in BP caused by bethanidine. These studies show that bethanidine is effective in preventing VT induction and, thus, its use may not be restricted only to cases of primary VF.

Flecainide

Meinertz and associates[51] from Mainz, West Germany, assessed the antiarrhythmic efficacy and safety of oral flecainide during a controlled 2-week and a subsequent 48-week long-term trial. Fifteen patients with frequent (>30 per hour) and complex ventricular arrhythmias (Lown grade IVA or IVB) who had been resistant or intolerant to 2 or more antiarrhythmic agents, were studied. Antiarrhythmic efficacy was controlled by 24-hour Holter monitoring at 2, 12, 24, and 48 weeks. The administration of 100–200 mg flecainide twice daily resulted in >90% suppression of VPCs and of complex ventricular arrhythmias in 14 of 15 patients. The minimum effective therapeutic dose could be titrated in 9 of 14 patients to 100 mg twice daily, in 3 of 14 patients to 150 mg twice daily, and in 2 of 14 patients to 200 mg twice daily. During this therapy and a mean plasma concentration of 886 ± 103 ng/ml, PQ and QRS duration and QTc time and JTc interval were not significantly changed. Side effects (gastrointestinal complaints, nausea, obstipation, dizziness, visual disturbances, headache, and impaired potency) occurred in 5 of 14 patients after 12 weeks, in 3 of 4 patients after 24 weeks, and in only 2 of 14 patients after 48 weeks. Side effects were described as mild and tolerable and did not limit flecainide therapy except in 1 patient, who discontinued therapy after 3 days because of intense gastrointestinal symptoms. Thus, flecainide is highly effective and well tolerated in the long-term treatment of serious ventricular arrhythmias.

Lorcainide

Somani and colleagues[52] from Toledo, Ohio, examined the effects of lorcainide on serum electrolytes and osmolality in 33 patients with organic heart disease and complex ventricular arrhythmias. In 8 patients, a mean decrease in serum Na^+ of 8.2 ± 3.2 mEq/liter was observed after a single 200 mg intravenous dose of lorcainide. Sixteen of 33 patients developed significant hyponatremia and hypoosmolality during oral treatment with lorcainide. In all except 2 patients, serum Na^+ returned to normal values within 3–12 months of continued lorcainide therapy. Low serum Na^+ and hypoosmolality in the absence of volume depletion, clinically manifested edema, and unaltered renal, adrenal, cardiac, or thyroid function suggest that this antiarrhythmic drug produced the syndrome of inappropriate antidiuretic hormone secretion (SIADH), which appeared to be transient and asymptomatic. These findings suggest that SIADH is an important side effect of lorcainide therapy. It is recommended that serum Na^+ be carefully monitored in patients started on lorcainide therapy, and extreme caution should be exercised in prescribing diuretics to patients with persistent hyponatremia.

Magnesium

Tzivoni and associates[53] from Jerusalem and Tiqva, Israel, described the successful use of magnesium sulfate ($MgSO_4$) in 3 patients with torsade de pointes (TDP). The QT intervals before TDP were 0.70, 0.64, and 0.56 seconds. A bolus of 1.0–2.0 g MgSO$_4$ 25% abolished the TDP in all 3 patients. There was no immediate shortening in the QT interval in any patient after MgSO$_4$. Thus, magnesium can be given safely even in patients with AMI, angina pectoris, or systemic hypertension, conditions in which isoproterenol is contraindicated.

Mexiletine

Singh and associates[54] from Worcester, Massachusetts, evaluated the efficacy and safety of oral mexiletine compared with oral quinidine in suppressing VPC in a single-blind randomized study of 51 patients in ≤12 weeks: 26 patients were randomized to the mexiletine group and 25 to the quinidine group. The drugs were administered in an increasing dose regimen to suppress the VPC by 70% from the baseline value in both groups. Mexiletine reduced the average number of VPC by 70% of the baseline number in a comparable fashion to quinidine, 69% in the mexiletine group -vs- 70% in the quinidine group (p > 0.05). There was a comparable reduction (≥50%) of ventricular couplets from the baseline value in the 2 groups, 78% in the mexiletine group -vs- 86% in the quinidine group. The effect of mexiletine on suppression of VT was also similar, 72% in the mexiletine group -vs- 71% in the quinidine group. There was no significant difference in the 2 groups in side effects. This study shows the comparable efficacy and tolerance of mexiletine and quinidine for the control of ventricular arrhythmias in a large number of patients with diverse forms of heart diseases.

Stein and colleagues[55] from Boston, Massachusetts, evaluated mexiletine in 313 patients with VT refractory to conventional antiarrhythmic drugs. Therapy with mexiletine was continued long-term in 107 patients who responded to the drug and were free of side effects during a short-term evaluation in the hospital. During an average follow-up of 23 months (range, 0.1–70 months), 19 patients died (18%). Eleven patients had sudden death (3.6% per year), and 6 patients died of progressive CHF and 2 of noncardiac causes. Nonfatal ventricular arrhythmia recurred in 14 patients (5% per year). Overall, 25 patients had recurrent arrhythmia (incidence of 6% per year). Side effects occurred in 13 patients after an average of 5 months and were primarily gastrointestinal and neurologic. Sixty-one patients (57%) were continued on mexiletine therapy for an average of 32 months (range, 1–70 months). Outcome during long-term therapy was not related to drug dose, blood level, or presenting arrhythmia. Thus, this drug is effective and well tolerated during long-term use.

Schoenfeld and associates[56] from Boston, Massachusetts, described their experience in >300 patients and indicated that suppression of inducible ventricular arrhythmias by mexiletine either alone or in combination with another antiarrhythmic agent was achieved in approximately 30% of patients. Furthermore, suppression was sometimes achieved when mexiletine was tested in combination with a type IA antiarrhythmic or beta adrenergic blocking agent in patients for whom neither agent alone had been effective. The likelihood of suppressing inducible VT with mexiletine therapy alone or in combination varied as a function of the spontaneous ventricular arrhythmia with which a patient presented at the time of electrophysiologic study; patients presenting with sustained VT appeared to have inducible arrhythmias that were more difficult to suppress. A significant incidence of adverse effects attributable to mexiletine was observed, particularly gastrointestinal and neurologic effects. These side effects, although common, were frequently eliminated by reducing the dosage of the drug and administering the drug with food. Facilitation of arrhythmia induction also was observed in a small percentage of patients. This experience suggests that selected patients with ventricular arrhythmias that are refractory to conventional antiarrhythmic agents may derive long-term benefit from chronic therapy with oral mexiletine.

Nadolol

Nademanee and associates[57] from Los Angeles, California, evaluated the antiarrhythmic effect of nadolol, a long-acting, nonselective beta antagonist without intrinsic sympathomimetic or membrane-stabilizing properties, in 36 patients with ventricular arrhythmias as determined by 3 baseline 24-hour Holter recordings at a time when subjects were receiving placebo. Nadolol was administered once daily at a dose of 40–80 mg and increased at weekly intervals to a maximum daily dose of 640 mg. Thereafter, the drug was stopped gradually and placebo was given again for 2 weeks. Nadolol was effective in reducing VPC in 17 of 36 patients (48%), in reducing ventricular couplets in 24 of 27 patients (89%), and in reducing nonsustained runs of VT in all 13 subjects. Serum nadolol levels obtained at dosages resulting in a 75% reduction in VPC varied from 58–853 ng/ml. In most subjects studied, a nadolol dosage of 160 mg/day or less was effective for arrhythmia suppression.

Pirmenol

Anderson and associates[58] from Salt Lake City, Utah, assessed the antiarrhythmic efficacy and safety of oral pirmenol during a controlled, dose-ranging, and short-term maintenance study in 12 patients with frequent (>480/8 hours) VPC. Eleven patients responded favorably (>70% VPC suppression) to a trial of different doses. Mean interval (8 hours) suppression of VPC frequency was 95% in these 11 and 86% in the entire group. Suppression for 24 hours was similar in responders (88%). Repetitive VPC were essentially eliminated. The mean effective dose was 316 mg/day (105 mg/8 hours). The average predose (trough) plasma concentration at the end of dose ranging was 1.4 μg/ml and the drug elimination half-life was 7.3 hours (n, 12). Of 11 responding patients, 10 completed a 2-week outpatient trial. Pirmenol continued to be effective and tolerated in 8 patients, maintaining an overall average outpatient VPC suppression of 80%. The ECG intervals were mildly prolonged after multiple dosing (PR, +7%; QRS, +12%; QTc, +8%; all p < 0.01). The BP and heart rate did not change during treatment. The echo EF was maintained. Thus, oral pirmenol appears to be effective, conveniently administered, and well tolerated as an antiarrhythmic agent for control of VPC.

Procainamide

Marchlinski and coworkers[59] from Philadelphia, Pennsylvania, evaluated 33 patients with sustained ventricular arrhythmias undergoing electrophysiologic testing after intravenous and again after oral procainamide administration. These patients were subsequently divided into 2 groups: group 1 with 15 patients with concordant serum procainamide concentrations with less than a 3 μg/ml difference after intravenous and oral procainamide therapy and group 2 with 18 patients with discordant serum procainamide concentrations after intravenous and oral therapy. In these studies, patients in group 1 responded to programmed stimulation in a similar manner after intravenous and oral procainamide therapy with no inducible ventricular arrhythmias in 5 of 15 patients. However, in patients in group 2, three of 18 patients had no inducible arrhythmia after intravenous compared with 7 of 18 patients after oral procainamide therapy. There was a different response to programmed stimulation after oral compared with intravenous procainamide in 6 of 18 patients in group 2 but in none of 15 patients in group 1 (p = 0.02). These data indicate that intravenous procainamide closely predicts the electrophysiologic effects of oral procainamide when similar serum procainamide concentrations are achieved.

Propafenone

Salerno and associates[60] from Minneapolis, Minnesota, evaluated the effectiveness of oral propafenone for treatment of VPC in 12 patients, using a single-blind, double-ranging trial followed by double-blind comparison with placebo and then an open label, long-term protocol. During dose ranging, 8 of 12 patients achieved ≥80% suppression of total VPC (mean, 83%) (p < 0.01 -vs- single-blind placebo). Paired VPC were suppressed ≥90% and ventricular tachycardia was eliminated in 11 of the 12 patients (p < 0.01). The effectiveness of propafenone for treatment of VPC was confirmed during the double-blind trial (p < 0.05 -vs- double-blind placebo) and during treatment for 6 months (p < 0.05 -vs- initial single-blind placebo). Propafenone prolonged the PR interval by 16% (p < 0.01 -vs- single-blind placebo) and the QRS interval by 18% (p < 0.001). The LV systolic performance decreased as assessed by 2-D echo (p < 0.01 -vs- single-blind placebo). Propafenone increased serum digoxin levels in 5 of 5 patients (mean increase, 83%). Side effects included exacerbation of CHF (1 patient) and conduction abnormalities (2 patients). Thus, propafenone is effective for treatment of total and repetitive VPC. Although generally well tolerated, the drug reduces LV systolic function and AV conduction and increases serum digoxin levels.

Shen and coworkers[61] from San Francisco, California, studied 28 patients with recurrent VT to determine the efficacy of a new antiarrhythmic agent, propafenone. Propafenone was given at a loading dose of 2 mg/kg in all patients. Subsequently, in the first 14 patients (group A) 1 mg/minute was administered and in the second 14 patients (group B) 2 mg/minute by continuous infusion was administered. Propafenone significantly prolonged AV nodal and His-Purkinje conduction time and the QRS duration (p < 0.001). However, it did not change sinus node recovery time or mean arterial BP. The administration of propafenone slightly increased RA, PA, and PA wedge pressure and caused a reduction in cardiac index (2.6 ± 0.8 liters/min/M^2 before propafenone and 2.3 ± 0.7 liters/min/M^2 afterward, p < 0.001). Propafenone did not influence the inducibility of VT in patients in group A, but it did prevent inducibility of sustained VT in 3 patients in group B. These data suggest that propafenone may be a useful addition to currently available antiarrhythmic agents when given intravenously as a 2 mg/kg loading dose followed by 2 mg/minute of sustained infusion.

De Soyza and colleagues[62] from Little Rock, Arkansas, treated 30 patients with clinically significant ventricular ectopic activity with propafenone. Patients had a minimum mean of >30 VPC/hour documented by continuous 48-hour ambulatory ECG recording. Twenty-five patients qualified as responders, defined as >85% reduction of ventricular ectopic activity compared with baseline, and completed a double-blind placebo crossover phase. Significant reduction in single ventricular ectopic activity per hour, paired VPC per hour, and VT beats per hour were observed. Almost total abolition of VT and paired VPC was achieved. Side effects were minimal and well tolerated. A significant prolongation of the PR interval occurred. QRS prolongation and prolongation of the corrected QT interval were observed in some patients, with new left BBB developing in 2 patients. These initial results are encouraging.

Naccarella and associates[63] from Bologna, Italy, studied the efficacy of propafenone in 21 patients with ventricular arrhythmias refractory to previous antiarrhythmic medications. Group A included 10 patients with chronic VPC, 6 of whom had nonsustained VT and 4 of whom had recurrent, sustained VT; all received propafenone, 900 mg/day. Group B included 11 patients, all with chronic VPC, 9 of whom had nonsustained VT and 5 of whom had sustained VT; all received propafenone, 450 mg/day. Drug efficacy was evaluated as a $\geq 70\%$ reduction in VPC frequency with complex VPC abolition in ambulatory monitoring and suppression of nonsustained VT and sustained VT during a follow-up period $\leq 154 \pm 58$ days in group A and 96 ± 42 days in group B. Drug plasma levels were measured during chronic therapy in pharmacologic steady state. In group A, propafenone reduced the frequency of chronic VPC in 9 patients and abolished nonsustained VT in 4 of 6 and sustained VT in 3 of 4; in group B, propafenone reduced the frequency of chronic VPC in 6 patients and abolished nonsustained VT in 6 of 9 and sustained VT in 3 of 5. Two patients with recurrences of sustained VT in this group were later successfully treated with propafenone, 900 mg/day; overall, 8 of 9 patients with recurrences of sustained VT were successfully treated with 900 mg/day. The lowest mean plasma level in pharmacologic steady state was 1.16 ± 0.83 µg/ml in group A and 0.54 ± 0.67 µg/ml in group B ($p \leq 0.05$). Plasma levels were generally higher in patients who received 900 mg/day compared with those who received 450 mg/day and were higher in responders to different therapeutic end points than in nonresponders. Side effects, including hypotension and PR and QRS prolongation, were observed in 5 patients, but required a dose reduction in only 1 patient. Thus, propafenone is an effective antiarrhythmic drug in the treatment of refractory chronic VPC of nonsustained VT and of recurrences of sustained VT. The dose of 900 mg/day is more effective in controlling recurrences of VT.

Quinidine

Torres and associates[64] from New York City evaluated the safety and efficacy of intravenous quinidine gluconate, using intermittent boluses of 80 mg/ml every 5 minutes for a total dose of 800 mg in 61 patients. Patients were referred because of out-of-hospital cardiac arrest (12), symptomatic VT (24), asymptomatic VT (18), syncope of unknown origin (6), and supraventricular arrhythmias (1). Clinical CHF was present in 74% of patients, with a mean EF of 45 ± 3 for all patients. Quinidine prevented VT induction in 78% of patients at a mean dose of 9.6 mg/kg and facilitated VT induction in 7% of patients. Quinidine failed to decrease mean arterial pressure in 14 patients, and in the remaining 47 patients arterial pressure decreased by 16%. Six patients had hemodynamically significant hypotension. Two patients had hypotension severe enough to require saline administration, and 4 had hypotension not needing fluid replacement; 16% of patients had other side effects. Quinidine can be administered safely by intermittent infusion and is effective in preventing programmed stimulation induction of VT.

Tocainide -vs- lidocaine

In a double-blind parallel study, Morganroth and associates[65] from Philadelphia, Pennsylvania, gave either tocainide (50 patients) or lidocaine (49 patients) intravenously as 2 bolus injections 15 minutes apart, plus a fixed-rate infusion that started at the first bolus, to 99 patients with acute ventricular tachyarrhythmias after open heart surgery. If needed, a third bolus was administered and simultaneously the infusion rate was doubled. The boluses and initial infusion rate for tocainide treatment were, respectively, 250, 250, and 125 mg and 1.04 mg/minute, and for lidocaine treatment, 100, 50, and 50 mg and 2.08 mg/minute. When efficacy was defined as 80% or greater reduction in single VPC or complete abolition of ventricular couplets or VT, no difference in efficacy between the 2 treatments was found by bedside ECG monitoring. By computer analysis of 24-hour taped ECGs and a regression analysis of the proportion of patients responding favorably to treatment, it was estimated that ≥80% reduction of single VPC occurred in 55% of patients during tocainide treatment and in 48% of patients during lidocaine treatment; abolition of couplets occurred in 74 and 68% of patients, respectively; and abolition of VT in 87 and 73% of patients, respectively. These treatment-related differences were different. Adverse reactions occurred in 5 patients (10%) given tocainide and led to discontinuation of treatment in 3 patients. Adverse reactions were reported in 9 patients (18%) given lidocaine and led to discontinuation of treatment in 4 patients. Thus, tocainide was at least as effective, if not more effective than lidocaine when administered intravenously for the treatment of acute ventricular arrhythmias occurring immediately after cardiac surgery.

Complications of drugs

To obtain information germane to identifying patients at increased risk for developing torsade de pointes (TDP) resulting from quinidine, Bauman and associates[66] from Chicago, Illinois, performed a mail solicitation and obtained the records of 31 patients with documented TDP due to quinidine. All 31 patients had heart disease: CAD, 11 patients (36%); rheumatic, 5 patients (16%); hypertensive, 4 patients (13%); cardiomyopathic, 4 patients (13%); other, 7 patients (22%). Quinidine was administered for the following reasons: AF or atrial flutter, 22 patients (71%); VPC, 6 patients (19%); VT or SVT, 3 patients (10%). The 31 patients were receiving quinidine, 650–2,400 mg/day (mean, 1,097), and 14 patients had serum quinidine levels of 1.4–10.6 μg/ml (mean, 3.7). The TDP occurred within 1 week of initiation of quinidine therapy in 23 (74%) of the patients. Twenty-eight (90%) patients were receiving digoxin, and 5 (24%) of 21 patients had hypokalemia at the time of TDP. Off of quinidine therapy, corrected QT (QTc) intervals in 24 patients ranged from 390–580 ms (mean, 470) and were prolonged in 17 patients (71%). On quinidine therapy, QTc intervals in 23 patients ranged from 390–630 ms (mean, 510) and were prolonged in 21 patients (91%). Therefore patients with TDP due to quinidine usually had heart disease complicated by AF, were receiving digoxin, and were receiving moderate dosages of quinidine for <1 week before TDP. Approximately two thirds of patients with TDP due to quinidine had long QT intervals while off of quinidine.

Sudden death has occurred in monkeys fed large doses of probucol, a cholesterol-lowering drug, given in combination with an atherogenic diet. These monkeys develop prolonged QT intervals and high serum levels of probucol. Browne and associates[67] from Indianapolis, Indiana, investigated the effect of probucol on QT interval and the incidence of ventricular ectopic activity during a double-blind placebo-controlled study in 16 patients with <600 VPC/day and a corrected QT interval of <0.44 second. Seven patients received probucol and 9 patients received placebo. Three 24-hour continuous ECG recordings were obtained before entry into the study and 3 additional recordings were obtained after 6 months of drug or placebo therapy. A 15-second ECG tracing was sampled from the continuous ECG recording every 30 minutes and, for the group, 15,000 QT intervals were measured, permitting construction of QT versus R-R regression lines for each patient before and during therapy. Comparison of the regression lines revealed that the measured QT interval prolonged 20 ± 18 ms during the awake state and 24 ± 20 ms during sleep (mean ± SD) at matched heart rates in the 7 patients receiving probucol (p < 0.01). Using Bazett's formula to correct for rate, corrected QT interval prolonged 22 ± 23 ms in the awake state and 20 ± 18 ms in the asleep state (p < 0.01). In probucol-treated patients QT interval prolongation was directly related to increasing probucol plasma levels (p < 0.05). The VPC did not increase in either group. Therefore, probucol prolongs QT interval in humans but does not increase the number of VPC in patients with normal QT intervals before probucol treatment. Although the magnitude of QT prolongation in these patients is small, monitoring of the QT interval while administering probucol may be indicated in certain patients.

Subendocardial resection

Paramount to the success of surgery in the management of VT has been the ability to localize the site of origin of VT by endocardial mapping procedures. Cassidy and coworkers[68] from Philadelphia, Pennsylvania, assessed the value of endocardial catheter mapping in 52 patients in sinus rhythm and with 102 morphologically distinct VT. The local bipolar electrograms from various LV regions were assessed and quantitatively classified with respect to the characteristics of amplitude and duration. With the use of this assessment, the investigators found that electrograms from the site of origin were of significantly lower amplitude and longer duration; however, because such an overlap occurred with electrograms that were not from sites of origin, this did not serve as a useful clinical marker. Various types of electrograms, including normal, abnormal, fractionated, abnormal late, fractionated late, and longest, were evaluated with respect to sensitivity, specificity, and positive predictive value. No type possessed the ability to localize reliably the site of origin of VT. These workers therefore concluded that endocardial catheter mapping during sinus rhythm is not useful as a guide in localized surgical therapy for VT. Surgery guided only by the results of mapping during sinus rhythm would result in a more extensive excision than that directed by maps obtained during VT and some cases would result in the exclusion of the area considered to be the site of origin of the VT.

In patients with LV aneurysm the percentage of the endocardial border zone demonstrating fragmented electrical activity correlates with the occurrence of recurrent VT. Wiener and colleagues[69] from New York City presented results achieved by excising these areas of fragmentation in addition to resecting the aneurysm. Eight patients with LV aneurysm and VT refractory to drugs were studied. Each patient underwent intraoperative epicardial and endocardial mapping during stable sinus rhythm. After aneurysmectomy, areas of the endocardial border zone which demonstrated fragmented activity were excised. Mapping was then repeated to ensure that major areas of fragmentation did not remain. Mapping was completed in <20 minutes in each patient. One patient died of pump failure before hospital discharge and a second patient, who was arrhythmia-free, died of pump failure 12 months postoperatively. Six patients are alive and free of areas of VT 5–25 months (mean, 12) postoperatively. It was concluded that excision of areas of fragmented electrical activity in the endocardial border zone of LV aneurysm is useful to surgical therapy for VT. This approach allows an excision directed to arrhythmogenic areas without the need for tachycardia induction in the operating room.

Ostermeyer and associates[70] described 40 consecutive patients who underwent electrophysiologically guided encircling endocardial ventriculotomy (EEV) for treatment for recurrent sustained VT. Twelve patients had a complete EEV (group I) and 28 had a partial EEV (group II). The partial EEV was done at the site of earliest electrical activation during VT. There were no significant differences between the 2 groups in age, New York Heart Association functional class, CAD, LV aneurysm location, concomitant CABG, and LV function preoperatively. One patient of the complete and 2 patients of the partial EEV did not survive the postoperative period. Eight patients of group I and 19 of group II were free of VT (no spontaneous or inducible VT 3 weeks postoperatively, both 73%). Five patients of the complete and 5 patients in the partial EEV groups developed severe LV dysfunction (46 -vs- 8%; p = 0.025). In addition three of the 11 survivors of complete EEV died late due to CHF compared to 1 of 26 survivors of partial EEV. The investigators contend that map-directed partial EEV is superior to complete EEV because of a decreased incidence of LV dysfunction postoperatively. The number of patients free of inducible VT is similar to that reported for endocardial resection (Harken procedure) from other institutions.

Miller and coworkers[71] from Philadelphia, Pennsylvania, retrospectively evaluated the first 100 patients who underwent mapping-guided subendocardial resection (SER) at their hospital for drug-refractory sustained VT caused by CAD. There were 91 survivors of surgery with 200 morphologically distinct types of VT. Eighty-three patients (91%) were cured of VT by SER alone (60 patients, 66%) or by SER in combination with antiarrhythmic drug therapy (23 patients, 25%). There were 4 late sudden deaths and 4 patients continued to have rare episodes of spontaneous VT after surgery despite receiving antiarrhythmic drugs. A model of multivariate analysis identified disparate sites of origin of VT and the absence of a discrete LV aneurysm as the only independent variables associated with failure of surgery alone. Inferior wall site of origin and right BBB morphology of VT were also significantly associated with failure of surgery to cure VT. Mapping-guided SER is a highly effective mode of treatment for drug-refractory VT, despite the existence of groups of patients with higher-than-average surgical failure rates.

CARDIAC ARREST

Epidemiology

Data from the Framingham Heart Study were used to investigate the frequency of and risk factors for sudden coronary death (SCD) in men and women in a report by Schatzkin and colleagues[72] from Boston, Massachusetts. The original Framingham cohort comprised 2,336 men and 2,873 women who were followed with biennial examinations: 69 men and 34 women in the cohort died suddenly and unexpectedly in 26 years of observation. This represented 22 and 23%, respectively, of all CAD deaths. The incidence rates of SCD for men and women were, respectively, 151 and 53 deaths per 100,000 person-years. Predictors of SCD in men that emerged from multiple logistic regression analysis were LV hypertrophy by ECG, age, serum cholesterol, number of cigarettes smoked daily, relative weight, and systolic BP. An interaction term reflecting the product of age and serum cholesterol was negatively correlated with SCD, indicating that cholesterol was a more potent predictor of SCD in younger as opposed to older men. The risk profile for SCD in women differed, with significant factors being age, vital capacity, hematocrit, serum cholesterol (marginal), and serum glucose (marginal). Classic CAD risk factors for men appear to be operative for SCD in men. In women the picture is less clear, but limitations in data may partially account for some of the sex differences in predictors of SCD.

During exercise

To examine the risk of primary cardiac arrest during vigorous exercise, Siscovick and associates[73] from Chapel Hill, North Carolina, interviewed the wives of 133 men without known prior heart disease who had primary cardiac arrest during vigorous exercise. The patients were classified according to their activity at the time of cardiac arrest and the amount of their habitual vigorous activity. From interviews with wives of a random sample of healthy men, the investigators estimated the amount of time members of the community spent in vigorous activity. Among men with low levels of habitual activity, the relative risk of cardiac arrest during exercise compared with that at other times was 56. The risk during exercise among men at the highest level of habitual activity also was elevated, but only by a factor of 5. Among the habitually vigorous men, the overall risk of cardiac arrest, i.e., during and not during vigorous activity, was only 40% that of the sedentary men. Although the risk of primary cardiac arrest is transiently increased during vigorous exercise, habitual vigorous exercise is associated with an overall decreased risk of primary cardiac arrest.

During ambulatory ECG recording

To characterize the events that precede and precipitate sudden cardiac death, Kempf and Josephson[74] from Philadelphia, Pennsylvania, analyzed long-term ECGs of 27 patients who died suddenly while being monitored. In 20 patients sudden death was associated with ventricular tachyarrhythmias (VT/VF) and in 7 it was associated with bradyarrhythmias. Seventeen of the patients were men and 10 were women. Twenty-one patients had CAD, 2 had idiopathic dilated cardiomyopathy, 2 had MS and 1 patient had MVP. Four patients with VT/VF had a previous nonfatal cardiac arrest. In the 20 patients with tachyarrhythmia-related sudden death, ⩾3 VT beats always preceded degeneration to VF. In 5 patients, the frequency or complexity of ventricular arrhythmias increased in the hour before death. In 11 of 20, there was a ⩾20% increase in underlying heart rate in the hour before sudden death. The R-on-T phenomenon was observed in 4 patients. The long-short phenomenon was observed in 4 patients. The long-short phenomenon initiated VT/VF in 2 patients. Only 2 patients with VT/VF were resuscitated. No patient with bradyarrhythmia-related sudden death had manifest AV block or BBB. Two of 7 patients had an episode of nonsustained bradycardia in the hour before arrest. No patient was resuscitated. In conclusion, VT that degenerates into VF is the most common arrhythmia associated with sudden cardiac death, and VT/VF is frequently preceded by an increase in heart rate and complex ectopic activity. The VT is most often initiated by late VPC. Twenty-five percent of patients who had sudden cardiac death had associated bradyarrhythmias that may occur without premonitory events.

Out-of-hospital management

Survival after out-of-hospital cardiac arrest is poor in communities served only by basic ambulance services, but conventional advanced prehospital care is not an option for most rural communities. Stults and associates[75] from Iowa City, Iowa, trained ambulance technicians in 18 small communities (average population, 10,400) to recognize and defibrillate VF. Neither endotracheal intubation nor medication was used. Twelve additional communities of similar size where such early defibrillation was not attempted provided control data. In the communities where early defibrillation was available, 12 of 64 patients (19%) who were found in VF were resuscitated and discharged alive from the hospital; this was true of only 1 of 31 such patients (3%) in the control communities, where only basic life support was available. Ten (83%) of the long-term survivors received electrical shocks administered solely by the technicians. Early defibrillation by minimally trained ambulance technicians is an effective approach to emergency cardiac care in rural communities.

Wilson and associates[76] from Durham, North Carolina, analyzed the outcome in 126 consecutive patients with nontraumatic out-of-hospital cardiac arrest to determine the effectiveness of a standard ambulance system over 22 months. Therapy was limited to basic life support (administration of oxygen by mask, intravenous fluids, closed-chest massage, and artificial respiration) by emergency medical technicians. Of the 126 patients, 28 (22%) survived to hospital admission and 11 (9%) to hospital discharge. Two patient subgroups had a higher discharge rate: those with an initial rhythm of VT or VF (7 of 50, 14%) and those with an initial BP ≥ 90 mmHg and a heart rate of >50 beats/minute (3 of 6). For patients in cardiac arrest before ambulance arrival, there was no difference in outcome between those who did and those who did not receive prior cardiopulmonary recessitation.

Prognosis after successful resuscitation

Morady and coworkers[77] from San Francisco, California, evaluated 19 patients surviving a cardiac arrest unassociated with an AMI and with a normal electrophysiologic study, including no inducible VT despite programmed stimulation. Fourteen patients with CAD had cardiac arrest during exertion or an episode of angina in 11. Twenty-four ambulatory ECG recordings demonstrated infrequent or no VPC in 10 and an ischemic response during exercise in 6 of 9 patients. Eight of these patients underwent CABG and 6 were treated with antianginal medication. Only 3 patients received an antiarrhythmic drug. With a follow-up period of 26 ± 15 months (mean ± SD), only 1 patient died suddenly. Two patients had coronary artery spasm and were treated with appropriate medication and had no recurrence of cardiac arrest during 7 and 36 months of follow-up, respectively. Three patients had cardiomyopathy or no identifiable heart disease and were treated with nadolol or amiodarone, and they have had no recurrence of cardiac arrest over 3–27 months of follow-up. Thus, these data indicate that in patients surviving a cardiac arrest and with a normal electrophysiologic study, those with CAD or coronary artery spasm have a good prognosis with treatment directed primarily at the underlying heart disease. Natural history of recurrent arrhythmia in patients with cardiomyopathy or no identifiable heart disease surviving a cardiac arrest and with a normal electrophysiologic study remains to be determined.

Tresch and colleagues[78] from Milwaukee, Wisconsin, followed 139 survivors of prehospital cardiac arrest after their hospital discharge. Eighty patients were studied with coronary angiography and cardiac catheterization; 34 underwent CABG. After a maximum follow-up of 105 months, 89 patients were still alive. The probability of survival at 0.5, 1, 2, 3, 4, and 5 years was 88, 86, 78, 70, 63, and 59%, respectively. Of the 43 cardiac deaths, 37 (86%) were secondary to documented recurrent VF or occurred suddenly. Twelve percent of the total population had recurrent VF in the first year after the initial cardiac arrest, 16% within 2 years, and 22% within 3 years. Of the 37 survivors dying from recurrent VF, 32% died within the first 3 months after hospital discharge, 46% in the first year, 64% within 2 years, and 78% within the first 3 years. Most survivors were capable of resuming normal activities after hospital discharge. Only 7% had permanent neurologic impairment. Sixty-eight percent of the patients who were employed at the time of their prehospital cardiac arrest returned to full-time employment. In 34 surgically treated patients, there were 6 (18%) cardiac deaths. Four deaths were related to recurrent VF, with 1 occurring in the immediate postoperative period; the other 3 were related to recurrent VF and occurred 36 months (2 deaths) and 49 months after the initial prehospital cardiac arrest.

Vlay and associates[79] from Baltimore, Maryland, and Stony Brook, New York, prospectively evaluated the relation of specific coronary arterial and LV segments to subsequent clinical outcome in 80 persons who were survivors of sudden coronary death and had failed conventional antiarrhythmic therapy. There were 68 men and 12 women with an average age of 51 years who were treated with investigational antiarrhythmic agents, rendered asymptomatic, and followed for 16 ± 14 (SD) months. At the end of the study 48 patients (60%) were alive and asymptomatic, and 32 (40%) had experienced either recurrent syncope (5) or sudden cardiac death (27). The independent relation of clinical and angiographic variables was performed in a univariate fashion using a Kaplan-Meier survival analysis and then multivariate logistic analysis was used to consider all clinical and arteriographic variables simultaneously. The results reconfirmed the importance of EF and LV filling pressure on outcome. Coronary arterial and LV segmental analyses provided additional predictive power. The survival outcome was found to be inversely related to the degree of proximal LAD coronary arterial narrowing: at 1 year, 90% of patients with minimal LAD narrowing were alive and asymptomatic in contrast with 70% who had partial and 40% who had complete proximal LAD obstruction ($p < 0.005$). Analysis of the posterobasal LV segment wall motion demonstrated that 100% of patients with minimal dysfunction were alive and asymptomatic at 1 year, whereas only 52% of patients with severe dysfunction were alive ($p < 0.001$). A multivariate analysis using both LAD narrowing and posterobasal dysfunction correctly predicted 39 of 43 patients (91%) who were alive and 11 of 15 patients (73%) who were dead or syncopal, for a predictive accuracy of 86%. These results suggest that specific segmental cardiac lesions may accurately identify subsets of sudden cardiac death survivors who are at either exceptionally high or low risk for subsequent arrhythmic events.

Findings at necropsy

Warnes and Roberts[80] from Bethesda, Maryland, described the amount and distribution of coronary arterial narrowing by atherosclerotic plaque at necropsy in 70 persons with sudden coronary death. They ranged in age from 22–81 years (mean, 50). Of 3,484 5 mm segments examined (mean, 50 per patient) from the major (LM, LAD, LC, and right) coronary arteries, 950 (27%) were narrowed 76–100% in cross-sectional area (XSA), 1,127 (32%), 51–75%; 689 (20%), 26–50%; and 718 (21%), 0–25% (Figs. 3-6, 3-7). More extensive severe narrowing occurred in the proximal than in the distal halves of the LAD, LC, and right coronary arteries. Comparison between the 31 previously symptomatic patients (angina pectoris or a clinical AMI or both) with the 39 who had previously been asymptomatic disclosed a significantly higher mean percent of severely narrowed (76–100% XSA) 5 mm segments (30 -vs- 25%, $p < 0.005$) and lower mean percent of minimally narrowed (0–25% XSA) segments in the symptomatic group (15 -vs- 25%, $p < 0.001$). Comparison of the 31 patients who had a healed myocardial infarction at necropsy with the 39 patients who did not discloses a higher mean percent of 5 mm segments narrowed 76–100% in XSA (33 -vs- 24%, $p < 0.001$) and a lower mean percent of segments narrowed minimally in those with a LV scar (13 -vs- 26%, $p < 0.001$). Comparison between patients whose hearts weighed >450 g with those whose hearts weighed ≤450 g disclosed a higher

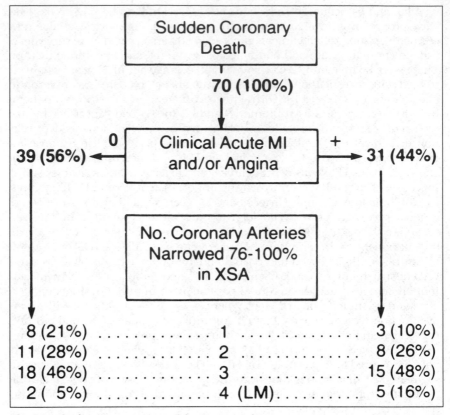

Fig. 3-6. Qualitative comparison of the 39 previously asymptomatic patients with the 31 who had clinical AMI or angina pectoris or both before sudden coronary death. XSA = cross-sectional area.

mean percent of severely narrowed segments (19 -vs- 23%, p < 0.01) and a lower mean percent of minimally narrowed segments (29 -vs- 24%, p < 0.005) in the group with enlarged hearts.

Warnes and Roberts[81] from Bethesda, Maryland, analyzed clinical and morphologic findings among 70 persons with sudden coronary death (SCD), comparing the 13 with a coronary thrombus to the 57 without a coronary thrombus. The 13 with a thrombus were younger than those without (mean age, 43 -vs- 51 years), had a lower mean percent of cross-sectional area (XSA) narrowing by plaque at the site of maximal coronary stenosis (89 -vs- 95%) (Fig. 3-8), and had a higher mean percent of 5 mm segments of the 4 major epicardial coronary arteries minimally narrowed (0–25% in XSA) by plaque (27 -vs- 19%) (Fig. 3-9). No differences occurred in the 2 groups with regard to sex, previous angina pectoris or clinical AMI, healed myocardial infarction at necropsy, mean heart weight, number of major coronary arteries narrowed 76–100% in XSA by atherosclerotic plaque, or the mean percent of 5 mm segments of the 4 major epicardial coronary arteries narrowed 76–100% in XSA by atherosclerotic plaque. Thus, coronary thrombi are infrequent in patients with SCD, and when observed, their significance is uncertain be-

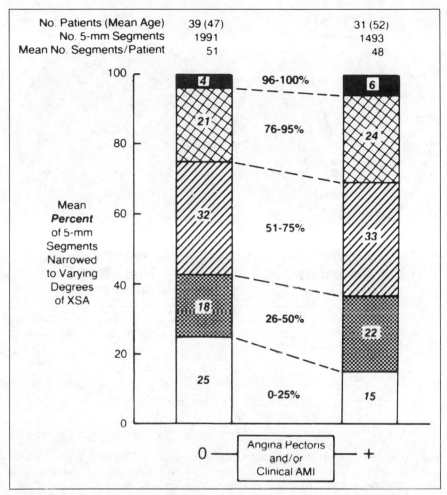

Fig. 3-7. Mean percents of 5 mm segments of the sum of the 4 major coronary arteries narrowed to varying degrees in cross-sectional area (XSA) in 70 patients with sudden coronary death: comparison of 39 patients without and 31 patients with a clinical AMI or angina or both.

cause persons with SCD without coronary thrombi have similar amounts of severe coronary narrowing.

Davies and Thomas[82] from London, England, studied at necropsy 100 subjects who died of CAD in <6 hours and found coronary thrombus in 74. There was no difference in incidence between those who died in <15 minutes, those who died 15–60 minutes, and those who died >60 minutes. Among 26 cases without an intraluminal thrombus, plaque fissuring was found in 21; thus, in only 5 cases was no acute arterial lesion demonstrated. No intraluminal thrombi were found in age-matched controls. Of the 74 thrombi, 48 were found at sites of preexisting high grade stenosis; 14 were found at points of previous stenosis of <50% of the diameter of the lumen. Forty-seven percent of the thrombi were found in the right coronary artery; only 30% were found in the LAD coronary artery.

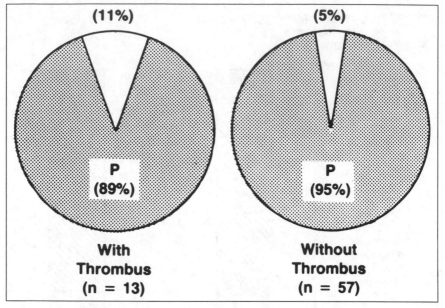

Fig. 3-8. Mean amount of cross-sectional area coronary arterial narrowing at site of maximal narrowing by atherosclerotic plaque (P) alone in 70 subjects with sudden coronary death, 13 with and 57 without coronary thrombus.

SUDDEN INFANT DEATH SYNDROME

Using 24-hour ambulatory ECG recordings and 120-lead body surface potential maps, Montague and associates[83] from Halifax, Canada, compared the prevailing cardiac rate and rhythm, instance and frequency of arrhythmia, and rate and pattern of ventricular repolarization at the body surface in 17 infants at risk of sudden infant death syndrome (SIDS) and in 17 age- and sex-matched control subjects. Sinus rhythm was the prevailing rhythm in both study groups and there were no intergroup differences in average overall awake or asleep sinus rates, nor in temporal variability of sinus rate. Atrial and ventricular ectopic activity were equally uncommon in both study groups. Although there were smooth and bipolar body surface distributions of ST-T and QRST time integrals in both study groups, the average rate of ventricular repolarization (QTc), measured from the 12-lead ECG, 120-lead body surface potential maps, and 24-hour ECG, was consistently shorter in the at-risk group than in the control group. However, temporal variability of QTc was not different between the 2 groups. Thus, significant cardiac arrhythm and QT prolongation are not found in infants at increased risk for SIDS. Rather, there is an abbreviated ventricular repolarization interval in at-risk infants. In combination with the findings of intergroup similarity of average sinus rate and temporal variability of sinus rate and ventricular repolarization rate, the data suggest a subtle, constant difference in cardiac autonomic activity, most likely an increase in sympathetic tone, in at-risk sub-

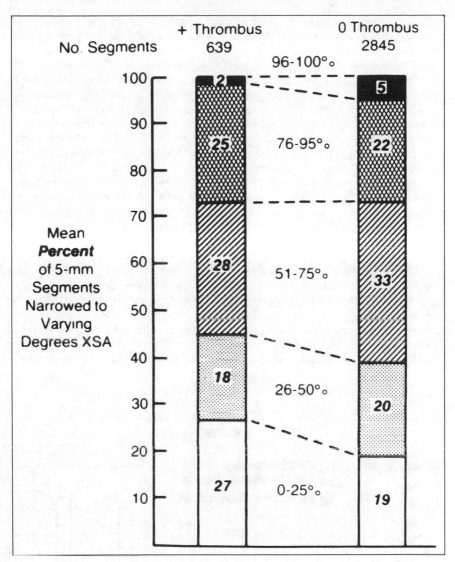

Fig. 3-9. Mean percents of 5 mm segments of the 4 major coronary arteries narrowed to varying degrees in cross-sectional area (XSA) in the 13 patients with and in the 57 patients without coronary artery thrombus.

jects. The role of this altered cardiac autonomic activity in the causation of SIDS remains undetermined.

SYNCOPE

Almost all patients who present with syncope have 24-hour ambulatory ECG monitoring primarily to exclude an arrhythmogenic cause. The usefulness of 24-hour ambulatory ECG monitoring in patients with syncope has not been well defined, although several studies of small numbers of selective patients have indicated that it might be helpful. Gibson and Heitzman[84] from Burlington, Vermont, evaluated the effectiveness of an open referral ECG monitoring service in identifying an arrhythmogenic cause for syncope. During a 5-year period, 7,364 patients of all ages underwent ambulatory 24-hour ECT (Holter) monitoring using a 2-channel recorder. Of these, 1,512 patients (21%) were referred because of syncope. During monitoring, 15 patients had syncope and 7 of the episodes were related to an arrhythmia, usually VT (Fig. 3-10). Presyncope was reported in 241 patients, with a related arrhythmia in 24. Thus, an arrhythmia-related symptom that could be diagnostic was present in only 2% of the patients monitored. However, syncope or presyncope without an associated arrhythmia might be considered a negative diagnostic clue and occurred in 225 (15%). High grade AV block was present in 15 and VT in 116; only 6 (5%) reported associated symptoms. An age-related incremental increase in AV arrhythmias was found. In 415 of the 1,004 patients (41%) aged 60 years or more, arrhythmias that are conventionally associated with sinoatrial disease were recorded. Using stringent diagnostic criteria, the sick sinus or tachybradycardia syndrome was present in 33 (3%). Many older patients (70%) were taking drugs that could be arrhythmogenic, hypotensive, or both. It was concluded that an open referral 24-hour ambulatory monitoring service rarely results in identifying relevant symptom-related arrhythmias in patients with syncope. It records many asymptomatic arrhythmias that can compound rather than resolve the diag-

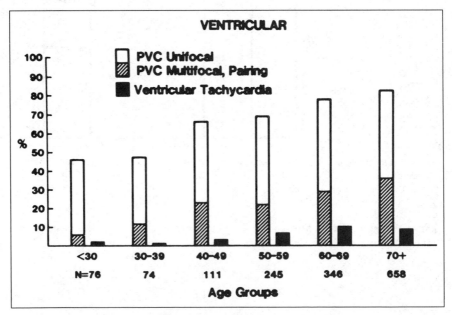

Fig. 3-10. The percentage incidence of ventricular arrhythmias by age groups. PVC = ventricular premature contractions.

nostic problem in older patients, because the data obtained could lead to unnecessary therapy. An iatrogenic cause for syncope should always be considered.

SLEEP-APNEA SYNDROME

In the sleep apnea syndrome in which the usual complaints are daytime sleepiness, loud snoring, and restless sleep, the daytime breathing pattern is normal. During sleep, however, monitoring reveals that multiple apneic episodes lead to nocturnal pulmonary and systemic hypertension and cor pulmonale. Most but not all patients with sleep apnea are overweight. Various cardiac arrhythmias arise, and during the period of apnea there may be systemic arterial oxygen desaturation. Sleep apnea is classified as central when there is a lack of inspiratory effort, obstructive when respiratory effort is made against an upper airway obstruction, or mixed. A pattern of sinus arrhythmia—bradycardia during apnea, followed by abrupt tachycardia—has been observed in a small number of patients with a sleep apnea syndrome. The cyclical variation of heart rate can be identified by computer analysis that provides plots of the R-R interval between QRS complexes over 24 hours. In the present study, Guilleminault and associates[85] from Stanford, California, recorded an ECG in 400 sleep apnea patients with an intact autonomic nervous system for 24 hours with simultaneous polygraph recording at night to evaluate factors resulting in cyclical variation of heart rate. At onset of sleep apnea all showed progressive bradycardia, followed by abrupt tachycardia on resumption of breathing. The ECG pattern, which was identifiable by computer analysis, was used as a screening tool for sleep apnea. It was not seen in controls without the sleep apnea syndrome. A subgroup of patients with sleep apnea and impairment of autonomic nervous system of the heart (heart transplants, autonomic neuropathy, Shy-Drager syndrome) did not show the cyclical heart rate pattern. In obstructive sleep apneic patients with normal autonomic nervous function, atropine sulfate blocked the pattern by eliminating the bradycardia component, whereas 100% oxygen, even at high rates of administration, caused only moderate blunting of the heart rate variation. The ECG changes observed in sleep apnea syndrome therefore are mediated by the autonomic nervous system; hypoxia is not the only factor involved.

BUNDLE BRANCH BLOCK

Ventricular activation in the human heart with left BBB has been limited by experimental preparations, effects of general anesthesia, and such conditions as AMI, LV hypertrophy, fibrosis, and ischemia. Vassallo and coworkers[86] from Philadelphia, Pennsylvania, performed endocardial catheter mapping in 18 patients with left BBB. Four patients had no organic heart disease (group I), 6 had cardiomyopathy (group II), and 8 had CAD and previous

AMI (group III). Twelve patients had 1 septal site of LV endocardial break-through, and 6 had 2 LV endocardial breakthrough sites with 1 site always being septal. There was no significant difference among the groups with respect to time of LV breakthrough. Total LV endocardial activation time was significantly longer in group III (119 ms) than group I (81 ms) and group II (61 ms). Duration of total RV endocardial activation was 36 ms. The final site of RV activation was at 44 ms after the onset of the QRS complex. The investigators conclude that (1) RV activation occurs before initiation of LV activation in patients with left BBB, (2) LV endocardial activation in patients with left BBB most likely occurs as a result of right-to-left transseptal activation, (3) LV endocardial activation sequence in patients with left BBB is heterogenous, and (4) patients with CAD and left BBB have significantly longer total LV endocardial activation times than patients with no organic heart disease or those with cardiomyopathy.

Faster heart rates shorten refractoriness more in some tissues than in others. Chilson and associates[87] from Indianapolis, Indiana, investigated whether faster heart rates shorten relative refractoriness more in the right than left bundle branch. Premature atrial stimulation at <2 basic cycle lengths was performed in 314 patients with no evidence of AV conduction system disease. In 10 patients, both functional and left BBB developed with premature atrial stimulation. Functional right BBB occurred at the longer basal cycling, and functional left BBB at the shorter cycle length in 8 patients. In 2 patients functional right and functional left BBB were present at the same cycle length, but functional left BBB occurred at a shorter premature atrial coupling interval. For all patients, the mean functional right bundle branch relative refractoriness was 438 ms at a basic cycle length of 847 ms, and functional left bundle branch relative refractoriness was 357 ms at a cycle length of 622 ms. The HV interval was 45 ± 15 ms at control and increased with functional left BBB to 77 ± 19 ms, but not with functional right BBB. Thus, relative refractoriness of the right and left bundle branches are rate dependent and discordant. At longer cycle lengths, relative refractoriness of the right bundle branch is greater than that of the left, and at shorter cycle lengths relative refractoriness of the left bundle branch is greater than that of the right. The relative refractory period curves "cross over" and can explain the presence of both functional right and left BBB in the same patient.

Morady and associates[88] from San Francisco, California, performed electrophysiologic testing in 32 patients with BBB and unexplained syncope. The testing included programmed ventricular stimulation with up to triple extrastimuli. The infranodal conduction time (HV) was 70 ms in ≤70 patients. Pathologic infranodal block during atrial pacing occurred in 2 patients. Unimorphic VT was induced in 9 patients (28%) and polymorphic VT in 5 (16%). A permanent pacemaker was implanted in patients with infranodal block during atrial pacing and, generally, in patients with an HV of ≥70 ms. Patients with inducible unimorphic or sustained polymorphic VT were treated with an antiarrhythmic drug. The mean follow-up period was 19 ± 14 months ($\pm$SD). Three patients died suddenly: a noncompliant patient with inducible sustained VT; a patient with a normal electrophysiologic study treated empirically with quinidine for VPC; and a patient with an HV of 70 ms and no inducible VT treated with a permanent pacemaker. The actuarial incidence of sudden death was 10% at 45 months of follow-up.

Only 2 patients had recurrent syncope; both had a normal electrophysiologic study. Approximately 50% of patients with BBB and unexplained syncope who undergo electrophysiologic testing are found to have a clinically significant abnormality (HV of ⩾70 ms, infranodal block during atrial pacing and inducible unimorphic VT), and some patients have >1 abnormality. Long-term management guided by the results of electrophysiologic testing generally is successful in preventing recurrent syncope. Patients who have a normal electrophysiologic study or who have inducible nonsustained polymorphic VT usually have a benign prognosis when left untreated.

The presence of left BBB on 12-lead ECG may obscure the diagnosis of other ECG abnormalities, including LV hypertrophy. Klein and colleagues[89] from Sacramento, California, retrospectively reviewed ECGs of patients with left BBB and LV hypertrophy as determined by echo to evaluate several ECG parameters as predictors of LV hypertrophy. The ECG evaluation included precordial voltage as measured by the sum of the S wave in leads V_1 or V_2 plus R wave in lead V_6, QRS duration, mean frontal plane QRS axis, R wave amplitude in lead aV_L, intrinsicoid deflection, and the presence or absence of criteria for LA enlargement. In the presence of left BBB and LV hypertrophy, precordial voltage was greater, QRS duration more prolonged ($p < 0.001$), and LA enlargement more frequently present than when LV hypertrophy was not present. There was no difference in limb lead voltage, intrinsicoid deflection, or mean frontal plane QRS axis. Furthermore, the criterion of SV_2 + RV_6 > 4.5 mV demonstrated a sensitivity of 86% and a specificity of 100%. It was concluded that a voltage criterion of SV_2 + RV_6 > 4.5 mV is diagnostic of LV hypertrophy in the presence of left BBB; furthermore, QRS duration of >160 ms plus LA enlargement strongly supports the diagnosis of LV hypertrophy.

PACEMAKERS AND CARDIOVERTERS

Hanley and associates[90] from Rochester, Minnesota, analyzed reasons for pacemaker insertion and other factors at the Mayo Clinic for the years 1961, 1971, and 1981. As indicated by the accompanying tables (Tables 3-1, 3-2, 3-3, and 3-4), major changes in trends and practices occurred. In addition to numerical growth, the indications for permanent pacing and the technologic alternatives available expanded considerably. Of interest, at least to me (WCR), the surgeons did all of the pacemaker implantations in 1971, whereas the cardiologists did 96% of the pacemaker implantations in 1981.

Three types of carotid sinus (CS) syndrome have been described: cardio-inhibitory, vasodepressor, and mixed. For the treatment of symptomatic patients with associated significant cardioinhibition, permanent ventricular demand pacing systems usually are implanted. Even with this pacing modality, some patients remain symptomatic because of continued (and at times aggravated) vasodepression. Madigan and associates[91] from Columbia, Missouri, assessed the effects of loss of atrial preloading and orthostasis after carotid massage in patients with carotid sinus hypersensitivity. Eleven patients were studied using constant intraarterial pressure measurements during either ventricular (VVI) or atrioventricular sequential (DVI) pacing in both supine and upright positions. The measurements performed included the

TABLE 3-1. *Summary of data and analysis by patient and procedure subgroups. Reproduced with permission from Hanley et al.*[90]

	1961	1971	1981	ABSOLUTE CHANGE (%), 1971–1981
Patient groups				
All patients*	12	138	262	Increased 90
No previous pacemaker	10	72	210	Increased 192
Previous pacemaker(s)	2	66	52	Decreased 21
Pacemaker placement	10	134	253	Increased 89
Postinfarction	0	0	7	
Surgical bradycardia	1	4	11	Increased 175
Pacemaker syndrome†	0	0	5	
Procedures: 1 only	11	116	234	Increased 102
2	1	22	28	Increased 27
3	0	9	5	Decreased 44
4	0	3	0	Decreased 100
Procedure groups				
All procedures*	13	172	295	Increased 72
No previous pacemaker	11	92	236	Increased 157
Previous pacemaker(s)	2	80	59	Decreased 26
No pacemaker implant	0	4	9	Increased 125
Pacemaker placement	11	141	258	Increased 83
Operator				
Surgeon	13	172	13	Decreased 92
Cardiologist	0	0	282	
Procedure duration (min)	...	92	78	Decreased 15
Male patients (%)	67	63	66	Increased 5
Mean age (yr)	49.8	66.7	66.2	Decreased 0.7

* Excludes 6 in 1971 and 18 in 1981 in whom epicardial leads only were inserted during a cardiac operation (that is, prophylactic lead placement). All patients in 1961 had epicardial leads inserted at thoracotomy (three during a cardiac operation).
† Not recognized in 1961 or 1971.

TABLE 3-2. *Indications for pacing (no previous pacemaker group). Reproduced with permission from Hanley et al.*[90]

INDICATION	1961 (%)	1971 (%)	1981* (%)	RELATIVE CHANGE (%), 1971–1981
Sinus node disease	0	11	41	Increased 30
High grade heart block	100	85	60	Decreased 25
Conduction system disease	0	0	11	Increased 11
Carotid sinus hypersensitivity	0	0	5	Increased 5
Vasovagal syncope	0	1	4	Increased 3
Supraventricular tachycardia	0	0	1	Increased 1
VT	0	1	1	0
Cardiogenic (unspecified)†	0	2	2	Increased 0

* Figures for 1981 total more than 100% because more than one indication for pacing was identified in certain patients.
† Patients thought to have a cardiogenic cause for syncope (mechanism not defined).

TABLE 3-3. *Pacing mode used (no previous pacemaker group). Reproduced with permission from Hanley et al.*[90]

MODE*	1961 (%)	1971 (%)	1981 (%)
VOO	100	0	0
VVI	0	100	75
AAI	0	0	1
DVI	0	0	21
DDD	0	0	2
VDD	0	0	1

* Three-letter code established by the Inter-Society Commission for Heart Disease Resources. The first letter designates the chamber paced (A = atrium, V = ventricle, D = dual); the second, the chamber sensed (A = atrium, V = ventricle, D = dual, O = none); and the third, the response to sensing (I = inhibited, T = triggered, D = dual [atrial triggered and ventricular inhibited], 0 = none). VOO = ventricular fixed-rate pacing; VVI = ventricular demand pacing; AAI = atrial demand pacing; DVI = atrioventricular sequential pacing; DDD = atrioventricular sequential, atrioventricular sensing pacing; and VDD = atrial synchronous, ventricular inhibited pacing.

TABLE 3-4. *Information about leads used (no previous pacemaker group).* *Reproduced with permission from Hanley et al.*[90]

	1961 (%)	1971 (%)	1981 (%)
Lead location			
Endocardial	0	92	94
Epicardial	100	8	6
Site of pacemaker			
Ventricle	100	100	77
Atrium	0	0	22
Coronary sinus	0	0	1
Lead polarity			
Unipolar	0	18	40
Bipolar	100	82	60
Sheath material			
Silicone	100	100	56
Urethane	0	0	44

* Total number of leads used was 75 in 1971 and 269 in 1981.

magnitude of decrease in arterial BP, the rate of decrease of BP, and the percent change in BP from baseline values. After carotid massage, all 11 patients had greater hemodynamic change with the VVI than DVI pacing mode, whether in the supine or upright position. The decreases in systolic BP were: DVI (supine), 29 mmHg; VVI (supine), 48 mmHg; DVI (upright), 27 mmHg; and VVI (upright), 59 mmHg (mean group values, p < 0.001). The rates of decrease of systolic BP were: DVI (supine), 2.9 mmHg/s; VVI (supine), 5.7 mmHg/s; DVI (upright), 4.1 mmHg/s; and VVI (upright), 8.3 mmHg/s (mean group values, p < 0.001). VVI pacing, particularly in the upright position, resulted in a significant increase in the incidence of patient symptoms (p = 0.03). Thus, in CS hypersensitivity, VVI pacing results in significant hemodynamic deterioration compared with the DVI mode. This aggravation of the vasodepressor component results in increased patient symptoms, and therefore DVI is the optimal pacing mode.

In an investigation performed by Nitsch and colleagues[92] from Bonn, West Germany, LV performance was studied by gated RNA during pacing (60 or 70–120 beats/min) in 55 patients (37 with CAD, 12 with cardiomyopathy, and 6 with myocarditis) having programmable ventricular or dual-chamber AV demand pacemakers. Twenty-three patients were followed 4–6 months. In 16 patients the findings in ventricular (VVI) and dual-chamber AV (DDD) pacing were compared. In all patients end-diastolic volume (EDV) decreased and cardiac output increased when the pacing rate was changed from 60–70–120 beats/minute. In the patient group with VVI pacemakers, EDV decreased by 7.5% ± 3.5% (p < 0.01) and cardiac output increased by 54% ± 19% (p < 0.01). The results were independent of the underlying heart disease. After 4–6 months, a reduction of both cardiac output and EF was found in 6 of the 23 patients. Compared with VVI pacing, a significantly higher cardiac output (2–16%) was derived from DDD pacing. The results indicate the dependence of LV performance on the pacing rate and the benefit of DDD pacing. Since gated RNA provides the means to determine the effect of different pacing modes on LV performance, an optimal pacing mode may be found for each individual.

Mahmud and coworkers[93] from Milwaukee, Wisconsin, evaluated patients undergoing ventricular pacemaker insertion to identify those at risk for developing endless loop tachycardia. A pacing protocol was designed to assess the effects of AV sequential pacing on ventriculoatrial (VA) conduction in 13 subjects without evidence of VA conduction during routine electrophysiologic testing. The absence of VA conduction was indicated by pacing the ventricle at several cycle lengths without obtaining a retrograde atrial capture. Using the AV sequential method, the presence or absence of VA conduction was tested utilizing a premature ventricular stimulus superimposed over a wide range of coupling intervals. With AV sequential pacing, a premature ventricular stimulus was propagated to the atria in 5 of 13 patients, with VA intervals ranging from 200–460 ms (mean, 304 ± 97). These data suggest that in patients with absent VA conduction during routine testing, the ability of a paced ventricular impulse to propagate retrogradely may be demonstrated by AV sequential pacing. Thus, patients at risk for endless loop tachycardia after insertion of dual chamber (DDD) pacemakers may be identified using these methods.

Development of a permanent transvenous cardioversion system to obviate the need for thoracotomy and permit implantation under local anesthesia, just as permanent transvenous pacing systems are implanted, is obvious. Zipes and associates[94] from Indianapolis, Indiana, tested the efficacy and safety of a fully programmable cardioverter weighing 95 g, in terminating sustained VT. The device was implanted transvenously under local anesthesia in 7 patients. On command from a programmer or automatically, the cardioverter delivered shocks through a lead inserted at the apex of the right ventricle. It also served as a demand ventricular pacemaker and could perform programmed ventricular stimulation or overdrive pacing. Cardioversion of VT required <0.5 J (mean) and was well tolerated by the patients, who were awake and not sedated. In 1 patient, a shock terminated VT with the device in the automatic mode but produced AF with a rapid ventricular response that was intermittently recognized as VT, triggering additional shocks. One such shock in the ST segment produced VF that was terminated transthoracically in the emergency room, without residual impairment. The investigators concluded that cardioversion of sustained VT by means of an implantable catheter device is feasible, but for the present its use in the automatic mode must be cautious and selective. The unit's small size, ease of implantation, usefulness for noninvasive electrophysiologic studies, programmability, and bradycardia-pacing functions are advantages.

By the mid-1970s prototype external and internal devices for the automatic detection of VF had been developed. By 1982 the use of an automatic external defibrilator to deliver electric countershocks to patients in out-of-hospital cardiac arrest was reported for the first time. Cummins and associates[95] from Seattle, Washington, described the use of an automatic external defibrillator by paramedics to detect VF and to deliver cardia countershocks in 39 persons with out-of-hospital cardiac arrest. The automatic external defibrillator identified and delivered ⩾1 countershock to 13 of the 16 patients in VF (81% sensitivity). The automatic external defibrillator responded correctly to all 21 of the non-VF rhythms (8 other electrical rhythms, 13 asystole) with no countershocks (100% specificity). In 2 patients the rhythm could not be assessed. The device caused no injuries to patients or personnel. The performance of the automatic external defibrillator also was analyzed by considering each 15 s segment of VF as a separate challenge; the device delivered a countershock in 19 of 29 such segments (66%). What should be the minimum acceptable performance for a device that automatically detects and countershocks VF? Since the device was being evaluated in anticipation of placing it in the homes of high risk patients, where relatives would be responsible for its application, the standards may differ from those required when a device is used in such a setting as a coronary care unit, where its performance should be at least equal to that of the personnel for whom it substitutes. In the home setting, however, the device does not substitute for another method, but acts where no method of defibrillating previously existed.

The previous decade has witnessed a rapid increase in the use of pacemakers. In 1981, an estimated 118,000 pacemakers were implanted in patients in the USA. There is concern that the use of pacemakers may be "excessive." Accordingly, Phibbs and associates[96]—a self-appointed committee—outlined criteria for permanent cardiac pacing in the treatment of bradyarrhythmias. This report is timely and merits careful reading. This committee designated the following as indications for pacemaker implantation: (1) Complete heart block; (2) second-degree AV block; (3) second-degree AV block in the bundle branch system; (4) incomplete AV block within the bundle of His; (5) incomplete AV block in the AV node; (6) sinoatrial disease (sick sinus syndrome). Findings or measurements not constituting indications for pacemaker implantation included the following: (1) Isolated prolongation of HV interval or other intra-His abnormality without evidence of failure of AV conduction; (2) prolonged PR interval or first-degree AV block; (3) electrophysiologic prolongation of the refractory period of the AV node without documentation of failure of AV conduction; (4) AV nodal block evoked only by atrial pacing; (5) anticipation of sinus node slowing for the "tachy" state of a bradycardia-tachycardia type of sick sinus syndrome; (6) vasodepressor syncope; (7) asymptomatic sinus node slowing; (8) abnormalmalities of conduction or electrophysiologic findings in a patient taking cardioactive drugs that may affect such findings; (9) chronotropic incompetence. Borderline indications for pacemaker implantation included: (1) Transient AV block with complicating bifascicular or BBB appearing acutely during AMI; (2) infra-His block produced only by pacing without clinical or ECG evidence of spontaneous failure of AV conduction; (3) bradyarrhythmia caused by an essential drug. In most cases, decrease in dosage or change of medication is all that is needed.

This article was followed by an editorial by Bhandari and Rahimtoola[97] who pointed out that the report does not evaluate: (1) the role of cardiac pacing in the treatment of tachyarrhythmias; (2) the role of temporary pacing, or (3) the special problems of bradyarrhythmias in patients with AMI.

Fully automatic pacing systems rely on accurate identification of spontaneous atrial signals for physiologically responsive pacing. These signals must be discriminated from far-field ventricular activity, which might otherwise be sensed in the atrium. To amplify on the previously reported superiority of bipolar signals and high impedance circuitry for atrial sensing, Timmis and associates[98] from Royal Oak, Michigan, studied the effects of various intraatrial electrode positions on the atrial and ventricular contribution to electrograms recorded in this chamber. Compared with other intraatrial endocardial sites, RA signals were greatest in amplitude and slew rate in the RA appendage, averaging 3.3 ± 0.41 mV and 1.15 ± 0.16 V/s (mean $\pm$ SEM), respectively. These values were substantially higher than in the low right atrium ($p < 0.001$ and 0.0005 for amplitude and slew rate, respectively) and the high RA lateral wall ($p < 0.05$ for slew rate). The RA appendage electrograms also had significantly higher amplitude and slew rate than far-field R waves recorded here ($p < 0.0001$ for both). Additionally, the greatest difference in spectral content between atrial and far-field ventricular signals was also observed in the RA appendage. Thus, parameters in the domain of both time and frequency identified the RA appendage as the superior location for atrial sensing. Except for phrenic nerve problems with pacing, the high right atrium also appears to be a suitable electrode location for sensing. These considerations are germane in light of a growing number of atrial active and passive fixation leads now being employed for physiologic pacing.

RELATED TOPICS

Diagnostic electrophysiologic stimulation— policy statement

This article is a position paper put together by the Health and Public Policy Committee of the American College of Physicians.[99] Endocardial electrical stimulation, of course, is a diagnostic technique for evaluating sinus node function, the AV conduction system, and tachyarrhythmias. Electrode catheters inserted into the heart detect and stimulate cardiac electrical activity to provide information about the heart's electrical conduction system. Because activity is measured in several sites, several catheters must be placed in the right side of the heart and at times in the left ventricle as well. When severe or life-threatening arrhythmias are induced during stimulation, the efficacy of pharmacologic agents in preventing or suppressing the initiation of these arrhythmias may be evaluated. Electrophysiologic studies generally require that the patient be on the cardiac catheterization table for 2–5 hours. Extensive analysis of records by the examiner is required. When the studies show that the arrhythmia being evaluated is resistant to standard pharmacologic agents, sequential studies done 1–14 (usually 2–3) days apart to permit clearance of each drug may be needed. These procedures are done in the hospital and the length of hospital stay may range from 5–40 days. The indications for electrophysiologic testing are listed in Table 3-5. The estimated cost of a single electrophysiologic study is >$2,000, not including hospital costs. This committee concluded that endocardial electrical stimulation was an expensive invasive diagnostic technique that is the state of the art method for evaluating and guiding therapy for some patients with complex arrhythmias. The procedure was indicated in patients with VF or recurrent sustained VT who have not recently had an AMI. The procedure is also useful in patients with symptomatic arrhythmias in whom noninvasive findings are inconclusive. The procedures may be useful in subsets of patients with severe symptomatic arrhythmias, preexcitation syndromes, SVT, or unexplained syncope. The procedure entails significant risk, expense, and psychologic strain to the patient. It should be done in institutions in which emergency cardiovascular surgical backup is available and only by physicians who have had special training in clinical electrophysiology.

Drug levels in long-term antiarrhythmic therapy

Maintenance of adequate serum blood levels is crucial to successful antiarrhythmic therapy. Squire and associates[100] from New York City determined serum levels of 4 antiarrhythmic agents (long-acting procainamide, quinidine sulfate, quinidine gluconate, and disopyramide) in 98 consecutive ambulatory patients receiving long-term oral therapy (Fig. 3-11). Medication dosages, dosing intervals, and time elapsed from last dosage until blood sampling were determined. Seventy-five patients (77%) had subtherapeutic blood levels (with mean levels less than 50% of the suggested minimum), and only 22 patients (23% of the suggested minimum), and only 22 patients (23%) had therapeutic levels. Even among the 61 patients who claimed to have taken their medications within the 6 hours before blood sampling, 43 (70%) had subtherapeutic levels. These ratios held among all subgroups studied. Physicians should be aware of the high proportion of patients receiving long-term oral antiarrhythmic therapy with inadequate serum blood levels when planning therapeutic regimens.

Sotalol, hypokalemia, syncope, and torsade de pointes

McKibbin and associates[101] from Johannesburg, South Africa, described 13 patients who developed syncope and a prolonged QT interval while taking therapeutic doses of sotalol. Polymorphous VT was observed in 12 of the 13 patients and criteria typical of torsade de pointes were present in 10. In 12 patients sotalol had been given with hydrocholorothiazide in a combined preparation but with inadequate or no potassium supplementation. Serum potassium concentrates were reduced in 8 patients. Four patients were tak-

TABLE 3-5. *Clinical indications for electrophysiologic testing. Reproduced with permission from the Health and Policy Committee, American College of Physicians.*[99]

INDICATED	POSSIBLY INDICATED	NOT INDICATED
Sinus node dysfunction		
Significant symptoms (syncope, presyncope) and bradyarrhythmic sick sinus syndrome diagnosed by ambulatory ECG monitoring or atropine stimulation	Asymptomatic sinus node dysfunction	Symptoms clearly related to a sinus bradyarrhythmia; asymptomatic sinus bradycardia
AV conduction block		
Suspected AV that cannot be diagnosed by scalar ECG (type I AV block with BBB, and apparent type II AV block with normal QRS complex)	Asymptomatic AV block and inability to determine noninvasively the level of block; concealed junctional extrasystole suspected	Symptoms clearly related to high grade AV block; asymptomatic patients with AV block in whom the level of the block can be determined from scalar ECG and various diagnostic maneuvers
VT		
Sustained VT; selection of electropharmacologic therapy for this disorder		Asymptomatic, nonsustained VT, particularly without structural heart disease; VT in the setting of AMI
Syncope/cardiac arrest		
Recurrent syncope with no identifiable cause after thorough noninvasive and neurologic evaluation, particularly if organic heart disease is present; cardiac arrest without a documented cause (AMI, respiratory failure, severe aortic stenosis, pulmonary embolus, cardiac tamponade); before cardiac electrosurgery or implantable defibrillator therapy	Syncope and BBB	Cardiac arrest secondary to known causes
Intraventricular conduction delay		
Tachycardia (general)		
Severe tachycardia-related symptoms (angina, hypotension, pulmonary edema, syncope); recurrent tachycardia resistant to empiric antiarrhythmic therapy; differentiate supraventricular tachycardia with aberrant conduction from VT; before initiation of nonpharmacologic therapy (overdrive pacing, catheter ablation, implanted defibrillator) or cardiac electrosurgery		Asymptomatic patient
Supraventricular tachycardia		
WPW syndrome and AF or atrial flutter; WPW syndrome suspected but not documented by noninvasive tests	Asymptomatic WPW syndrome with an apparent short refractory period; symptomatic WPW when prescription of digitalis or verapamil is considered	Slow, well-tolerated tachycardia with accessory pathway excluded; asymptomatic patient with accessory pathway included and apparent long refractory period

* Under "Indicated", electrophysiologic testing is usually useful; under "Possibly Indicated," sometimes useful; and under "Not Indicated," rarely useful.

ing other drugs known to prolong the QT interval, including disopyramide (3 patients) and tricyclic antidepressants (2 patients). The QT returned to normal in all patients after withdrawal of the drugs and correction of the hypokalemia. Thus, even in low dosages, sotalol may be hazardous in the presence of hypokalemia or when combined with drugs that also prolong the QT interval. The use of sotalol concurrently with potassium-losing diuretics may expose the patient to unnecessary risk and should be avoided unless class III antiarrhythmic actions of this unique beta adrenoreceptor blocking agent also is required.

Antiglobulin tests and immune hemolytic anemia after procainamide therapy

To characterize the autoimmune phenomena in patients receiving procainamide, Kleinman and associates[102] from Los Angeles, California, studied the prevalence of positive direct antiglobulin (Coombs') tests and immune hemolytic anemia in 100 such patients and compared them with 100 age- and sex-matched controls. There was a significant increase in the frequency of positive direct antiglobulin tests in patients receiving procainamide (21 -vs- 10%). The mechanism of red cell sensitization in patients receiving procainamide was the production of red cell autoantibody, which was serologically indistinguishable from that seen in warm autoimmune hemolytic anemia. In contrast, positive direct antiglobulin tests in control patients were due to the presence of complement components. Red cell autoantibody production secondary to procainamide was not correlated with a higher-than-expected frequency of antinuclear antibodies of the clinical syndrome of drug-induced lupus erythematosus. In the 100 patients receiving procainamide, 3 cases of immune hemolytic anemia were identified. In 2 of the 3 cases, the anemia resolved after the medication was discontinued and did not require steroid therapy. Thus, procainamide often results in the production of red cell autoimmune phenomena.

Abdominal computerized tomography with amiodarone

Although amiodarone is known to cause elevation of hepatic function tests, the effect of this drug on abdominal computerized tomography (CT) scans in patients on amiodarone therapy is unknown. Since iodine is in its molecular structure, the presence of amiodarone or its metabolites might be expected to produce higher CT numbers similar to the effect of contrast agents. Shenasa and associates[103] from Milwaukee, Wisconsin, tested this hypothesis. The CT scans were performed in 25 patients receiving amiodarone, 14 receiving short-term (mean, 2.5 ± 1.3 days) and 19 receiving long-term therapy (mean, 130 ± 75 days) and in a control group not receiving amiodarone. Gastrointestinal symptoms (if any) and liver function tests (LFT) before instituting amiodarone and at the time of CT scan also were documented. The CT scans showed a modestly increased density in multiple organs in the short-term group, but a markedly increased hepatic density in all but 1 patient in the long-term group. Presence of gastrointestinal symptoms or abnormal LFT did not appear to correlate with the CT number. Such findings suggest that increased hepatic density on CT scan is to be expected in patients receiving long-term amiodarone therapy, and although the exact

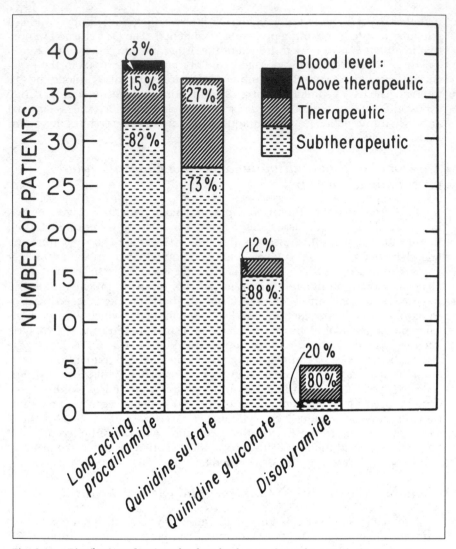

Fig. 3-11. Distribution of patients by drug level range for each antiarrhythmic drug.

biologic pathways of amiodarone metabolism are uncertain, the liver appears to be a major site of drug storage and metabolism.

Effects on ventricular function of disopyramide, procainamide, and quinidine

To evaluate the effects of 3 commonly used antiarrhythmic agents, disopyramide, procainamide, and quinidine on LV function, Wisenberg and associates[104] from London, Canada, administered these 3 agents in random sequence after control RNA performed at rest and during exercise in 17 patients. Drug dosages were tailored to achieve therapeutic blood levels 5 minutes before and 2–3 hours after drug administration. The mean dose of disopyramide was 141 ± 26 mg every 6 hours, procainamide, 441 ± 100 mg every 4 hours, and quinidine, 401 ± 101 mg of the gluconate preparation every 6 hours. The patients received the appropriate dosage for ≥7 days before repeat RNA was performed. The EF at rest was: control, 60 ± 13%; disopyramide, 55 ± 11%; procainamide, 58 ± 11%; and quinidine, 59 ± 12%. The exercise EF was: control, 61 ± 14%; disopyramide, 58 ± 13%; procainamide, 58 ± 12%; and quinidine, 61 ± 13%. In neither case, at rest nor during exercise, was there any significant difference observed between any of the agents or between any individual agent and control. However, at rest 8 subjects had a ≥5% decrease from the control value with disopyramide, 5 had a ≥5% decrease with procainamide, and 6 had a ≥5% decrease with quinidine, whereas during exercise the decreases were 8, 6, and 5%, respectively. These values were not statistically significant but suggest that caution should be taken in administering all 3 agents, particularly to patients with impaired LV function, because individual sensitivity to a given agent may precipitate a significant decline in LV function.

Chronic tachycardia and LV dysfunction

Kugler and associates[105] from Omaha, Nebraska, studied 5 children aged 3 weeks to 14 years who had chronic tachycardia and LV dysfunction as manifested by decreased LV shortening fraction on echo. In addition, 3 of 5 had cardiomegaly on radiography, 3 of 5 had ventricular or atrial enlargement or both on ECG, and 3 of 5 had symptoms of CHF. In 4 patients SVT was present, and irregular VT occurred in 1. Rates varied from 150–214. After effective drug therapy, fractional shortening improved to normal (20 ± 2–36 ± 2), cardiomegaly resolved on radiography and hypertrophy resolved on ECG. This is an intriguing study about the effects of chronic tachycardia at rates that were not fast enough to cause rapid clinical deterioration. In the 3 oldest patients the rates were 150–160 beats/minute, and in the infant age group 190 and 214 beats/minute. Various combinations of drugs were required to achieve adequate control of rate. In all patients, echo indices of ventricular function returned to normal. The exact mechanism for the LV dysfunction is unclear. It certainly behooves the clinician to prove the absence of an ectopic focus in patients whose heart rate persistently appears above normal.

Ambulatory ECG monitoring in women without heart disease

Romhilt and associates[106] from Richmond, Virginia, evaluated cardiac arrhythmias in apparently normal women by randomly selecting within the age decades of 20–60, 200 of the 788 women employees of a company. After exclusions for cardiac and medical reasons and refusals to participate, 101 subjects underwent 24-hour ambulatory ECG monitoring. The mean heart rate was 82 beats/minute, but was higher in smokers (p < 0.05). Supraventricular premature complexes were present in 28 of 101 subjects (28%); the prevalence increased with age (p < 0.001), but the frequency was <1 per hour in 24 of 28. In 34 of 101 subjects (34%) VPC occurred; the frequency was <1 an hour in 25 of 34. The VPC were complex (Lown grade ≥3) in 10 (10%) and multifocal in 9 of 10; there was 1 couplet each in 3 and 1 run of 4 VPC in

1 subject. The VPC were present in 20 of 42 subjects (48%) taking any medication (primarily oral contraceptives, estrogenic hormones, and maintenance thyroid), compared with 14 of 59 subjects (24%) not taking medication (p < 0.01). In women <40 years of age, VPC were present in 8 of 15 women (53%) taking contraceptives, compared with 4 of 33 (12%) not taking contraceptives (p < 0.001). The VPC occurred in 7 of 12 subjects (58%) taking thyroid medication, compared with 27 of 89 (30%) not taking thyroid medication (p < 0.03). In the 59 subjects not taking medication only 1 subject averaged >1 VPC/hour and 1 had 1 couplet. Thus, the prevalence and frequency of cardiac arrhythmias were low in randomly sampled, apparently normal women; however, the prevalence of VPC was significantly lower in subjects not taking medication.

Atrioventricular dissociation detected by suprasternal M-mode echo

Ruckel and associates[107] from Mainz, West Germany, studied 22 patients by suprasternal M-mode echo during VT. Adequate echoes were obtained from 19 patients. Thirteen patients showed AV dissociation and 6 patients a ventriculoatrial contraction obtained from the suprasternal notch. In 1 of these 6 patients, a 2:1 block retrograde was found by echo. In another patient, an intermittent block occurred in the retrograde direction. In 4 patients, a constant relation between the QRS complex and LA contraction soon after the beginning of the QRS complex was seen, demonstrating a 1:1 ventriculoatrial conduction. According to the LA contraction obtained from the suprasternal echo, 13 patients showed AV dissociation and 6 patients a retrograde conduction to the LA. From the analysis of the 12-lead standard ECG obtained simultaneously during VT, AV dissociation could be recognized in only 3 patients. Thus, AV dissociation during VT is more easily diagnosed with suprasternal M-mode echo than with the standard ECG.

References

1. DICKINSON DF, SCOTT O: Ambulatory electrocardiographic monitoring in 100 healthy teenage boys. Br Heart J 51:179–183, Feb 1984.
2. COBLER JL, WILLIAMS ME, GREENLAND P: Thyrotoxicosis in institutionalized elderly patients with atrial fibrillation. Arch Intern Med 144:1758–1760, Sept 1984.
3. MOLAJO A, COUPE MO, BENNETT DH: Effect of Corwin (ICI 118587) on resting and exercise heart rate and exercise tolerance in digitalized patients with chronic atrial fibrillation. Br Heart J 52:392–395, Oct 1984.
4. BUXTON AE, WAXMAN HL, MARCHLINSKI FE, JOSEPHSON ME: Atrial conduction: effects of extrastimuli with and without atrial dysrhythmias. Am J Cardiol 54:755–761, Oct 1, 1984.
5. BAR FW, BRUGADA P, DASSEN WRM, WELLENS HJJ: Differential diagnosis of tachycardia with narrow QRS complex (shorter than 0.12 second). Am J Cardiol 54:555–560, Sept 1, 1984.
6. BRUGADA P, HEDDLE B, GREEN M, WELLENS HJJ: Initiation of atrioventricular nodal reentrant tachycardia in patients with discontinuous anterograde atrioventricular nodal conduction curves with and without documented supraventricular tachycardia: observations on the role of a discontinuous retrograde conduction curve. Am Heart J 107:685–697, Apr 1984.

7. HENGLEIN D, GILLETTE PC, GARSON A JR, PORTER CJ: Antegrade conduction and AV node function in patients with unidirectional retrograde accessory pathways. Am Heart J 107:411–417, March 1984.

8. WU D, KOU H-C, YEH S-J, LIN F-C, HUNG J-S: Determinants of tachycardia induction using ventricular stimulation in dual pathway atrioventricular nodal reentrant tachycardia. Am Heart J 108:44–55, July 1984.

9. BARDY GH, PACKER DL, GERMAN LD, GALLAGHER JJ: Preexcited reciprocating tachycardia in patients with Wolff-Parkinson-White syndrome: incidence and mechanisms. Circulation 70:377–391, Sept 1984.

10. SETHI KK, JAISHANKAR S, GUPTA MP: Salutary effects of intravenous ajmaline in patients with paroxysmal supraventricular tachycardia mediated by dual atrioventricular nodal pathways: blockade of the retrograde fast pathway. Circulation 70:876–883, Nov 1984.

11. ALBONI P, SHANTHA N, PIRANI R, BAGGIONI F, SCARFO S, TOMASI AM, MASONI A: Effects of amiodarone on supraventricular tachycardia involving bypass tracts. Am J Cardiol 53:93–98, Jan 1, 1984.

12. WELLENS HJJ, BRUGADA P, ABDOLLAH H, DASSEN WR: A comparison of the electrophysiologic effects of intravenous and oral amiodarone in the same patient. Circulation 69:120–124, Jan 1984.

13. GOMES JAC, KANG PS, HARIMAN RJ, EL-SHERIF N, LYONS J: Electrophysiologic effects and mechanisms of termination of supraventricular tachycardia by intravenous amiodarone. Am Heart J 107:214–221, Feb 1984.

14. KAPPENBERGER LJ, FROMER MA, STEINBRUNN W, SHENASA M: Efficacy of amiodarone in the Wolff-Parkinson-White Syndrome with rapid ventricular response via accessory pathway during atrial fibrillation. Am J Cardiol 54:330–335, Aug 1, 1984.

15. HUNG J, YEH S, LIN F, FU M, LEE Y, WU D: Usefulness of intravenous diltiazem in predicting subsequent electrophysiologic and clinical responses to oral diltiazem. Am J Cardiol 54:1259–1269, Dec 1, 1984.

16. BRUGADA P, WELLENS HJJ: Effects of intravenous and oral disopyramide on paroxysmal atrioventricular nodal tachycardia. Am J Cardiol 53:88–92, Jan 1, 1984.

17. KUNZE KP, KUCK KH, SCHLUTER M, KUCH B, BLEIFELD W: Electrophysiologic and clinical effects of intravenous and oral encainide in accessory atrioventricular pathway. Am J Cardiol 54:323–329, Aug 1, 1984.

18. ABDOLLAH H, BRUGADA P, GREEN M, WEHR M, WELLENS HJJ, PAULUSSEN G: Clinical efficacy and electrophysiologic effects of intravenous and oral encainide in patients with accessory atrioventricular pathways and supraventricular arrhythmias. Am J Cardiol 54:544–549, Sept 1, 1984.

19. CHAZOV EI, ROSENSHTRAUKH LV, SHUGUSHEV KK: Ethmozin. II. Effects of intravenous drug administration on atrioventricular nodal reentrant tachycardia. Am Heart J 108:483–489, Sept 1984.

20. NATHAN AW, WARD DE, BENNETT DH, BEXTON RS, CAMM AJ: Catheter ablation of atrioventricular conduction. Lancet 1:1280–1284, June 9, 1984.

21. FISHER JD, BRODMAN R, KIM SG, MATOS JA, BRODMAN LE, WALLERSON D, WASPE LE: Attempted nonsurgical electrical ablation of accessory pathways via the coronary sinus in the Wolff-Parkinson-White syndrome. J Am Coll Cardiol 4:685–694, Oct 1984.

22. GUARNIERI T, SEALY WC, KASELL JH, GERMAN LD, GALLAGHER JJ: The nonpharmacologic management of the permanent form of junctional reciprocating tachycardia. Circulation 69:269–277, Feb 1984.

23. VLAY SC, KALLMAN CH, REID PR: Prognostic assessment of survivors of ventricular tachycardia and ventricular fibrillation with ambulatory monitoring. Am J Cardiol 54:87–90, July 1, 1984.

24. PLATIA EV, REID PR: Comparison of programmed electrical stimulation and ambulatory electrocardiographic (Holter) monitoring in the management of ventricular tachycardia and ventricular fibrillation. J Am Coll Cardiol 4:493–500, Sept 1984.

25. EZRI MD, HUANG SK, DENES P: The role of Holter monitoring in patients with recurrent sustained ventricular tachycardia: an electrophysiologic correlation. Am Heart J 108:1229–1236, Nov 1984.

26. BRUGADA P, GREEN M, ABDOLLAH H, WELLENS HJJ: Significance of ventricular arrhythmias initiated by programmed ventricular stimulation: the importance of the type of ventricular arrhythmia induced and the number of premature stimuli required. Circulation 69:87–92, Jan 1984.

27. BUXTON AE, MARCHLINSKI FE, WAXMAN HL, FLORES BT, CASSIDY DM, JOSEPHSON ME: Prognostic factors in nonsustained ventricular tachycardia. Am J Cardiol 53:1275–1279, May 1, 1984.

28. MORADY F, SHAPIRO W, SHEN E, SUNG RJ, SCHEINMAN MM: Programmed ventricular stimulation in patients without spontaneous ventricular tachycardia. Am Heart J 107:875–882, May 1984.

29. GOMES JAC, HARIMAN RI, KANG PS, EL-SHERIF N, CHOWDHRY I, LYONS J: Programmed electrical stimulation in patients with high-grade ventricular ectopy: electrophysiologic findings and prognosis for survival. Circulation 70:43–51, July 1984.

30. DOHERTY JU, KIENZLE MG, BUXTON AE, MARCHLINSKI FE, WAXMAN HL, JOSEPHSON ME: Discordant results of programmed ventricular stimulation at different right ventricular sites in patients with and without spontaneous sustained ventricular tachycardia: a prospective study of 56 patients. Am J Cardiol 54:336–342, Aug 1, 1984.

31. BUXTON AE, MARCHLINSKI FE, DOHERTY JU, CASSIDY DM, VASSALLO JA, FLORES BT, JOSEPHSON ME: Repetitive, monomorphic ventricular tachycardia: clinical and electrophysiologic characteristics in patients with and patients without organic heart disease. Am J Cardiol 54:997–1002, Nov 1, 1984.

32. ALMENDRAL JM, GROGAN W, CASSIDY DM, VASSALLO JA, MARCHLINSKI FE, BUXTON AE, DOHERTY MU, JOSEPHSON ME: Timing of the right ventricular apical electrogram during sustained ventricular tachycardia: relation to surface QRS morphology and potential clinical implications. Am J Cardiol 54:1003–1007, Nov 1, 1984.

33. WEINER DA, LEVINE SR, KLEIN MD, RYAN TJ: Ventricular arrhythmias during exercise testing: mechanism, response to coronary bypass surgery and prognostic significance. Am J Cardiol 53:1553–1557, June 1, 1984.

34. FLEG JL, LAKATTA EG: Prevalence and prognosis of exercise-induced nonsustained ventricular tachycardia in apparently healthy volunteers. Am J Cardiol 54:762–764, Oct 1, 1984.

35. FERGUSON D, SAKSENA S, GREENBERG E, CRAELIUS W: Management of recurrent ventricular tachycardia: economic impact of therapeutic alternatives. Am J Cardiol 53:531–536, Feb 1, 1984.

36. ROLFE SJ, RASOR T, SHAFFER PA, SANITATE PA, BASHORE TM: Relation between premature ventricular contraction site of origin (defined by radionuclide phase analysis) and subsequent left ventricular function. Am J Cardiol 53:1028–1033, Apr 1, 1984.

37. KOWEY PR, KHURI S, JOSA M, VERRIER RL, SHARMA S, KIELY JP, FOLLAND ED, PARISI AF: Vulnerability to ventricular fibrillation in patients with clinically manifest ventricular tachycardia. Am Heart J 108:884–889, Oct 1984.

38. HAMER AWF, RUBIN SA, PETER T, MANDEL WJ: Factors that predict syncope during ventricular tachycardia in patients. Am Heart J 107:997–1005, May 1984.

39. ROWLAND E, McKENNA WJ, SUGRUE D, BARCLAY R, FOALE RA, KRIKLER DM: Ventricular tachycardia of left bundle branch block configuration in patients with isolated right ventricular dilatation. Br Heart J 51:15–24, Jan 1984.

40. KRON IL, DIMARCO JP, HARMAN PK, CROSBY IK, MENTZER RM JR, NOLAN SP, WELLONS HA JR: Unanticipated postoperative ventricular tachyarrhythmias. Ann Thorac Surg 38:317–322, Oct 1984.

41. COLLABORATIVE GROUP FOR AMIODARONE EVALUATION: Multicenter controlled observation of a low-dose regimen of amiodarone for treatment of severe ventricular arrhythmias. Am J Cardiol 53:1564–1569, June 1, 1984.

42. McGOVERN B, GARAN H, MALACOFF RF, DIMARCO JP, GRANT G, SELLERS D, RUSKIN JN: Long-term clinical outcome of ventricular tachycardia or fibrillation treated with amiodarone. Am J Cardiol 53:1558–1563, June 1, 1984.

43. SAAL AK, WERNER JA, GREENE L, SEARS GK, GRAHAM EL: Effect of amiodarone on serum quinidine and procainamide levels. Am J Cardiol 53:1264–1267, May 1, 1984.

44. NADEMANEE K, KANNAN R, HENDRICKSON J, OOKHTENS M, KAY I, SINGH BN: Amiodarone-digoxin

interaction: clinical significance, time course of development, potential pharmacokinetic mechanisms and therapeutic implications. J Am Coll Cardiol 4:111–116, July 1984.

45. Mostow ND, Rakita L, Vrobel TR, Noon D, Blumer J: Amiodarone: intravenous loading for rapid suppression of complex ventricular arrhythmias. J Am Coll Cardiol 4:97–104, July 1984.

46. Hariman RJ, Gomes JAC, Kang PS, El-Sherif N: Effects of intravenous amiodarone in patients with inducible repetitive ventricular responses and VT. Am Heart J 107:1109–1117, June 1984.

47. Kaski JC , Girotti LA, Elizari MV, Lázzari JO, Goldbarg A, Tambussi A, Rosenbaum MB: Efficacy of amiodarone during long-term treatment of potentially dangerous arrhythmias in patients with chronic stable ischemic heart disease. Am Heart J 107:648–655, Apr 1984.

48. Levy S, Cointe R, Metge M, Faugere G, Valeix B, Gerard R: Bepridil for recurrent sustained ventricular tachycardias: assessment using electrophysiologic testing. Am J Cardiol 54:579–581, Sept 1, 1984.

49. Benditt DG, Benson DW, Dunnigan A, Kriett JM, Pritzker MR, Bacaner MB: Antiarrhythmic and electrophysiologic actions of bethanidine sulfate in primary ventricular fibrillation or life-threatening ventricular tachycardia. Am J Cardiol 53:1268–1274, May 1, 1984.

50. Somberg JC, Butler B, Torres V, Flowers D, Tepper D, Wynn J, Keren G, Miura DS: Antiarrhythmic action of bethanidine. Am J Cardiol 54:343–346, Aug 1, 1984.

51. Meinertz T, Zehender MK, Geibel A, Treese N, Hofmann T, Kasper W, Pop T: Long-term antiarrhythmic therapy with flecainide. Am J Cardiol 54:91–96, July 1, 1984.

52. Somani P, Temesy Armos PN, Leighton RF, Goodenday LS, Fraker TD Jr: Hyponatremia in patients treated with lorcainide, a new antiarrhythmic drug. Am Heart J 108:1443–1448, Dec 1984.

53. Tzivoni D, Keren A, Cohen AM, Loebel H, Zahavi I, Chenzbraun A, Stern S: Magnesium therapy for torsades de pointes. Am J Cardiol 53:528–530, Feb 1, 1984.

54. Singh JB, Rasul AM, Shah A, Adams E, Flessas A, Kocot SL: Efficacy of mexiletine in chronic ventricular arrhythmias compared with quinidine: a single-blind, randomized trial. Am J Cardiol 53:84–87, Jan 1, 1984.

55. Stein J, Podrid PJ, Lampert S, Hirsowitz G, Lown B: Long-term mexiletine for ventricular arrhythmia. Am Heart J 107:1091–1098, May 1984.

56. Schoenfeld MH, Whitford E, McGovern B, Garan H, Ruskin JN: Oral mexiletine in the treatment of refractory ventricular arrhythmias: the role of electrophysiologic techniques. Am Heart J 107:1071–1078, May 1984.

57. Nademanee K, Schleman MM, Singh BN, Morganroth J, Reid PR, Stritar JA: Beta-adrenergic blockade by nadolol in control of ventricular tachyarrhythmias. Am Heart J 108:1109–1115, Oct 1984.

58. Anderson JL, Lutz JR, Nappi JM: Pirmenol for control of ventricular arrhythmias: oral dose-ranging and short-term maintenance study. Am J Cardiol 53:522–527, Feb 1, 1984.

59. Marchlinski FE, Buxton AE, Vassallo JA, Waxman HL, Cassidy DM, Doherty JU, Josephson ME: Comparative electrophysiologic effects of intravenous and oral procainamide in patients with sustained ventricular arrhythmias. J Am Coll Cardiol 4:1247–1254, Dec 1984.

60. Salerno DM, Granrud G, Sharkey P, Asinger R, Hodges M: A controlled trial of propafenone for treatment of frequent and repetitive ventricular premature complexes. Am J Cardiol 53:77–83, Jan 1, 1984.

61. Shen EN, Sung RJ, Morady F, Schwartz AB, Scheinman MM, DiCarlo L, Shapiro W: Electrophysiologic and hemodynamic effects of intravenous propafenone in patients with recurrent ventricular tachycardia. J Am Coll Cardiol 3:1291–1297, May 1984.

62. de Soyza N, Terry L, Murphy ML, Thompson CH, Doherty JE, Sakhaii M, Dinh H: Effect of propafenone in patients with stable ventricular arrhythmias. Am Heart J 108:285–290, Aug 1984.

63. Naccarella F, Bracchetti D, Palmieri M, Marchesini B, Ambrosioni E: Propafenone for refractory ventricular arrhythmias: correlation with drug plasma levels during long-term treatment. Am J Cardiol 54:1008–1014, Nov 1, 1984.

64. Torres V, Flowers D, Miura D, Somberg J: Intravenous quinidine by intermittent bolus for electrophysiologic studies in patients with ventricular tachycardia. Am Heart J 108:1437–1442, Dec 1984.

65. Morganroth J, Panidis IP, Harley S, Johnson J, Smith E, MacVaugh H: Efficacy and safety of intravenous tocainide compared with intravenous lidocaine for acute ventricular arrhythmias immediately after cardiac surgery. Am J Cardiol 54:1253–1258, Dec 1, 1984.

66. Bauman JL, Bauernfeind RA, Hoff JV, Strasberg B, Swiryn S, Rosen KM: Torsade de pointes due to quinidine: observations in 31 patients. Am Heart J 107:425–430, March 1984.

67. Browne KF, Prystowsky EN, Heger JJ, Cerimele BJ, Fineberg N, Zipes DP: Prolongation of the QT interval induced by probucol: demonstration of a method for determining QT interval change induced by a drug. Am Heart J 107:680–684, Apr 1984.

68. Cassidy DM, Vassallo JA, Buxton AE, Doherty JU, Marchlinski FE, Josephson ME: The value of catheter mapping during sinus rhythm to localize site of origin of ventricular tachycardia. Circulation 69:1103–1110, June 1984.

69. Wiener I, Mindich B, Pitchon R: Fragmented endocardial electrical activity in patients with ventricular tachycardia: a new guide to surgical therapy. Am Heart J 107:86–90, Jan 1984.

70. Ostermeyer J, Breithardt G, Borggrefe M, Godehardt E, Seipel L, Bircks W: Surgical treatment of ventricular tachycardias: complete versus partial encircling endocardial ventriculotomy. J Thorac Cardiovasc Surg 87:517–525, April 1984.

71. Miller JM, Kienzle MG, Harken AH, Josephson ME: Subendocardial resection for ventricular tachycardia: predictors of surgical success. Circulation 70:624–631, Oct 1984.

72. Schatzkin A, Cupples LA, Heeren T, Morelock S, Mucatel M, Kannel WB: The epidemiology of sudden unexpected death: risk factors for men and women in the Framingham Heart Study. Am Heart J 107:1300–1306, June 1984.

73. Siscovick DS, Weiss NS, Fletcher RH, Lasky T: The incidence of primary cardiac arrest during vigorous exercise. N Engl J Med 311:874–877, Oct 4, 1984.

74. Kempf FC, Josephson ME: Cardiac arrest recorded on ambulatory electrocardiograms. Am J Cardiol 53:1577–1582, June 1, 1984.

75. Stults KR, Brown DD, Schug VL, Bean JA: Prehospital defibrillation performed by emergency medical technicians in rural communities. N Engl J Med 310:219–223, Jan 26, 1984.

76. Wilson BH, Severance HW, Raney MP, Pressley JC, McKinnis RA, Hindman MC, Smith M, Wagner GS: Out-of-hospital management of cardiac arrest by basic emergency medical technicians. Am J Cardiol 53:68–70, Jan 1, 1984.

77. Morady F, DiCarlo L, Winston S, Davis JC, Scheinman MM: Clinical features and prognosis of patients with out of hospital cardiac arrest and a normal electrophysiologic study. J Am Coll Cardiol 4:39–44, July 1984.

78. Tresch DD, Keelan MH Jr, Siegel R, Troop PJ, Bonchek LI, Olinger GN, Brooks HL: Long-term survival after prehospital sudden cardiac death. Am Heart J 108:1–5, July 1984.

79. Vlay SC, Reid PR, Griffith LSC, Kallman CH: Relationship of specific coronary lesions and regional left ventricular dysfunction to prognosis in survivors of sudden cardiac death. Am Heart J 108:1212–1220, Nov 1984.

80. Warnes CA, Roberts WC: Sudden coronary death: relation of amount and distribution of coronary narrowing at necropsy to previous symptoms of myocardial ischemia, left ventricular scarring and heart weight. Am J Cardiol 54:65–73, July 1984.

81. Warnes CA, Roberts WC: Sudden coronary death: comparison of patients with to those without coronary thrombus at necropsy. Am J Cardiol 54:1206–1211, Dec 1, 1984.

82. Davies MJ, Thomas A: Thrombosis and acute coronary-artery lesions in sudden cardiac ischemic death. N Engl J Med 310:1137–1140, May 3, 1984.

83. Montague TJ, Finley JP, Mukelabai K, Black SA, Rigby SM, Spencer A, Horacek BM: Cardiac rhythm, rate and ventricular repolarization properties in infants at risk for sudden infant death syndrome: comparison with age- and sex-matched control infants. Am J Cardiol 54:301–307, Aug 1, 1984.

84. Gibson TC, Heitzman MR: Diagnostic efficacy of 24-hour electrocardiographic monitoring for syncope. Am J Cardiol 53:1013–1017, Apr 1, 1984.

85. GUILLEMINAULT C, WINKLE R, CONNOLLY S, MELVIN K, TILKIAN A: Cyclical variation of the heart rate in sleep apnea syndrome: mechanisms, and usefulness of 24 h electrocardiography as a screening technique. Lancet 1:126–130, Jan 21, 1984.

86. VASSALLO JA, CASSIDY DM, MARCHLINSKI FE, BUXTON AE, WAXMAN HL, DOHERTY JU, JOSEPHSON ME: Endocardial activation of left bundle branch block. Circulation 69:914–923, May 1984.

87. CHILSON DA, ZIPES DP, HEGER JJ, BROWNE KF, PRYSTOWSKY EN: Functional bundle branch block: discordant response of right and left bundle branches to changes in heart rate. Am J Cardiol 54:313–316, Aug 1, 1984.

88. MORADY F, HIGGINS J, PETERS RW, SCHWARTZ AB, SHEN EN, BHANDARI A, SCHEINMAN MM, SAUVE MJ: Electrophysiologic testing in bundle branch block and unexplained syncope. Am J Cardiol 54:587–591, Sept 1, 1984.

89. KLEIN RC, VERA Z, DeMARIA AN, MASON DT: Electrocardiographic diagnosis of left ventricular hypertrophy in the presence of left bundle branch block. Am Heart J 108:502–506, Sept 1984.

90. HANLEY PC, VLIETSTRA RE, MERIDETH J, HOLMES DR, BROADBENT JC, OSBORN MJ, McGOON DC, CONNOLLY DC: Two decades of cardiac pacing at the Mayo Clinic (1961 through 1981). Mayo Clin Proc 59:268–274, Apr 1984.

91. MADIGAN NP, FLAKER GC, CURTIS JJ, REID J, MUELLER KJ, MURPHY TJ: Carotid sinus hypersensitivity: beneficial effects of dual-chamber pacing. Am J Cardiol 53:1034–1040, Apr 1, 1984.

92. NITSCH J, SEIDERER M, BÜLL U, LÜDERITZ B: Evaluation of left ventricular performance by radionuclide ventriculography in patients with atrioventricular versus ventricular demand pacemakers. Am Heart J 107:906–911, May 1984.

93. MAHMUD R, DENKER S, LEHMANN MH, AKHTAR M: Effect of atrioventricular sequential pacing in patients with no ventriculoatrial conduction. J Am Coll Cardiol 4:273–277, Aug 1984.

94. ZIPES DP, HEGER JJ, MILES WM, MAHOMED Y, BROWN JW, SPIELMAN SR, PRYSTOWSKY EN: Early experience with an implantable cardioverter. N Engl J Med 311:485–490, Aug 23, 1984.

95. CUMMINS RO, BERGNER L, EISENBERG M, MURRAY JA: Sensitivity, accuracy, and safety of an automatic external defibrillator. Lancet 2:318–320, Aug 11, 1984.

96. PHIBBS B, FRIEDMAN HS, GRABOYS TB, LOWN B, MARRIOTT HJL, NELSON WP, PRESTON T: Indications for pacing in the treatment of bradyarrhythmias. JAMA 252:1307–1311, Sept 14, 1984.

97. BHANDARI AK, RAHIMTOOLA SH: Indications for cardiac pacing in patients with bradyarrhythmias: do we know all the answers? JAMA 252:1327–1328, Sept 14, 1984.

98. TIMMIS GC, WESTVEER DC, GADOWSKI G, STEWART JR, GORDON S: The effect of electrode position on atrial sensing for physiologically responsive cardiac pacemakers. Am Heart J 108:909–916, Oct 1984.

99. HEALTH AND PUBLIC POLICY COMMITTEE, AMERICAN COLLEGE OF PHYSICIANS, PHILADELPHIA, PENNSYLVANIA: Diagnostic endocardial electrical recording and stimulation. Ann Intern Med 100:452–454, Mar 1984.

100. SQUIRE A, GOLDMAN ML, KUPERSMITH J, STERN EH, FUSTER V, SCHWEITZER P: Long-term antiarrhythmic therapy: problem of low drug levels and patient noncompliance. Am J Med 77:1035–1038, Dec 1984.

101. McKIBBIN JK, POCOCK WA, BARLOW JB, MILLAR RNS, OBEL IW: Sotalol, hypokalemia, syncope, and torsade de pointes. Br Heart J 51:157–162, Feb 1984.

102. KLEINMAN S, NELSON R, SMITH L, GOLDFINGER D: Positive direct antiglobulin tests and immune hemolytic anemia in patients receiving procainamide. N Engl J Med 311:809–812, Sept 27, 1984.

103. SHENASA M, VAISMAN U, WOJCIECHOWSKI M, DENKER S, MURTHY V, AKHTAR M: Abnormal abdominal computerized tomography with amiodarone therapy and clinical significance. Am Heart J 107:929–933, May 1984.

104. WISENBERG G, ZAWADOWSKI AG, GEBHARDT VA, PRATO FS, GODDARD MD, NICHOL PM, RECHNITZER PA, GRYFE-BECKER B: Effects on ventricular function of disopyramide, procainamide and quinidine as determined by radionuclide angiography. Am J Cardiol 53:1292–1297, May 1, 1984.

105. KUGLER JD, BAISCH SD, CHEATHAM JP, LATSON LA, PINSKY WM, NORBERG W, HOFSCHIRE PJ: Im-

provement of left ventricular dysfunction after control of persistent tachycardia. J Pediatr 105:543–548, Oct 1984.

106. ROMHILT DW, CHAFFIN C, CHOI SC, IRBY EC: Arrhythmias on ambulatory electrocardiographic monitoring in women without apparent heart disease. Am J Cardiol 54:582–586, Sept 1, 1984.

107. RUCKEL A, KASPER W, TREESE N, HENKEL B, POP T, MEINERTZ T: Atrioventricular dissociation detected by suprasternal M-mode echocardiography: a clue to the diagnosis of ventricular tachycardia. Am J Cardiol 54:561–563, Sept 1, 1984.

4

Systemic Hypertension

MISCELLANEOUS TOPICS

National Committee Report

Since publication of the 1980 Report of the Joint National Committee on Detection, Evaluation, and Treatment of High Blood Pressure, several events have occurred that affect successful management of patients with systemic hypertension: Publication of major clinical trial results, introduction of new antihypertensive agents, evidence concerning effectiveness of nonpharmacologic treatment, and further analysis of the epidemiologic data base relating BP with the risk of premature morbidity and mortality. These events led the director of the National Heart, Lung, and Blood Institute, as chairman of the National High Blood Pressure Education Program Coordinating Committee, to establish a new Joint National Committee to revise earlier recommendations. The present report[1] includes recommendations on the following topics: screening and referral procedures, classification according to BP, use of nonpharmacologic therapy, revised stepped-care approach, management of mild systemic hypertension, patient-professional interaction, and management of BP in special groups, including blacks, children, and pregnant women. This, of course, is an important report, since >60 million persons in the USA either have an elevated BP (≥140/90 mmHg) or have reported that a physician has told them that they have systemic hypertension. The stepped care approach to drug therapy and the antihypertensive agents are summarized in (Tables 4-1 and 4-2).

TABLE 4-1. *Stepped-care approach to drug therapy.* Reproduced with permission from The Joint National Committee on Detection, Evaluation, and Treatment of High Blood Pressure.*[1]

STEP	DRUG REGIMENS
1	Begin with less than a full dose of either a thiazide-type diuretic or a beta blocker†; proceed to full dose if necessary and desirable
2	If BP control is not achieved, either add a small dose of an adrenergic-inhibiting agent‡ or a small dose of thiazide-type diuretic; proceed to full dose if necessary and desirable§; additional substitutions may be made at this point‖
3	If BP control is not achieved, add a vasodilator, hydralazine hydrochloride, or minoxidil for resistant cases
4	If BP control is not achieved, add guanethidine monosulfate

* See Table 4-2 for specific dosages.

† Beta blockers include atenolol, metoprolol tartrate, nadolol, oxprenolol hydrochloride, pindolol, propranolol hydrochloride, and timolol maleate.

‡ These include centrally acting adrenergic inhibitors (clonidine hydrochloride, guanabenz acetate, and methyldopa), peripherally acting adrenergic inhibitors (guanadrel sulfate and reserpine), and an alpha$_1$ adrenergic blocker (prazosin hydrochloride).

§ A high percentage (70–80%) of patients with mild hypertension will respond to the above regimen using steps 1 and 2.

‖ An angiotensin-converting enzyme inhibitor (Table 4-2) may be substituted at steps 2 through 4 if side effects limit use of other agents or if other agents are ineffective. Slow channel calcium-entry blockers (diltiazem hydrochloride, nifedipine, and verapamil hydrochloride) have not been approved for therapy in hypertension but may be acceptable as steps 2 or 3 drug.

Circadian Pattern

Weber and associates[2] from Long Beach and Irvine, California, performed ambulatory BP monitoring using a portable noninvasive device capable of automatically measuring and recording BP every 7.5 minutes during a 24-hour study period in 34 normal volunteers on 2 separate occasions, 2–8 weeks apart, to test the consistency of the whole-day BP pattern. The average of all systolic BPs measured during the second study day was within 10 mmHg of that measured during the first study day in 79% of the subjects, and the respective diastolic BP averages were within 5 mmHg of each other in 65% of the subjects; 53% satisfied both of these criteria. The reproducibility of the circadian pattern of the BP was tested by dividing the 24-hour day into 12 consecutive 2-hour BP averages. When the corresponding 2-hour periods on the 2 study days were matched, there were strong correlations (r > 0.70) within most subjects for both the systolic and diastolic BP averages of the 2-hour periods (76 and 68% of subjects) and for the relative rank values of the periods (62 and 56%). Moreover, there were no significant differences between the averages (for all subjects together) on the 2 study days of the highest and lowest systolic and diastolic 2-hour BP values; similarly, the times at which these extreme values occurred on the 2 study days corresponded closely. Thus, in normal subjects there is a strong tendency for the circadian pattern and the actual levels of BP to be consistent between 24-hour study periods.

Sphygmomanometer cuff size and obesity

Most investigators agree that arterial BP increases as body weight and skin-fold thickness increase. Whether this increase is due in part to some measurement artifact caused by a larger arm circumference remains controversial. Although a standard size sphygmomanometer cuff (13 by 26 cm) may give a spuriously elevated reading in obese patients, the magnitude and prevalence of this error has not been emphasized. Despite the importance of correctly assessing BP, authorities do not yet agree on the size of sphygmomanometer cuff that ordinarily should be used. Some continue to recommend a standard cuff for regular use, reserving the large ones for very obese patients. Others advocate that a large cuff (14 by 37 cm) be used for all patients. Because of the several discordant views, Linfors and associates[3] from Durham, North Carolina, used standard, large adult, and thigh-sized cuffs in random order to take BP in 470 patients. The prevalence of definite high BP (≥160/95 mmHg) and borderline high BP (≥140/90–<160/95 mmHg) were the same with all 3 cuffs in patients with an arm circumference <35 cm, a body mass index <34, and a weight of <95 kg. The large adult and thigh cuffs did not underestimate the prevalence of high BP in these nonobese patients. The prevalences of high BP and borderline high BP were 2-fold greater with the standard cuff than with the large adult or thigh cuffs in obese patients (arm circumference ≥35 cm or body mass index ≥34 or weight ≥95 kg). Routine use of the large adult cuff will provide accurate BP measurement and avoid unneeded evaluation and treatment.

Adipose tissue cellularity and hemodynamic indexes

Epidemiologic studies have repeatedly shown a positive relation between BP and body weight. Achimastos and associates[4] from Paris, France, determined fat cell weight, fat cell number, and hemodynamic indexes in 25 obese men with sustained elevation of arterial BP. Fat cell weight (and not fat cell number) was positively correlated with overweight (r = 0.51) and mean arterial BP (r = 0.57) in basal conditions. After body weight reduction, BP decreased significantly through a decrease in cardiac index due to a predominant decrease in heart rate. Simultaneously, fat cell weight decreased significantly. The ratio between the change in BP and the change in body weight, i.e., the ability to decrease pressure per unit weight loss, was positively related to the level of initial BP and reached a plateau >120 mmHg of the initial mean arterial pressure. The investigators suggest that, in patients with obesity and hypertension, high BP is associated with hypertrophic obesity, and after body weight reduction, the simultaneous decrease in BP, heart rate, and fat-cell weight could be mediated by neurogenic mechanisms.

Effect of physical fitness

Blair and associates[5] from Dallas, Texas, measured physical fitness assessed by maximal treadmill testing in 4,820 men and 1,219 women aged 20–65 years. Participants had no history of cardiovascular disease and were normotensive at baseline. We followed up these persons for 1–12 years (median, 4 years) for the development of systemic hypertension. Multiple logistic risk analysis was used to estimate the independent contribution of physical

TABLE 4-2. *Antihypertensive Agents. Reproduced with permission from The Joint National Committee on Detection, Evaluation, and Treatment of High Blood Pressure.*[1]

TYPE OF DRUG	DOSAGE RANGE* (MG/DAY)	
	INITIAL	MAXIMUM†
Diuretics		
Thiazides and related sulfonamide diuretics		
Bendroflumethiazide	2.5	5
Benzthiazide	25.0	50
Chlorothiazide sodium	250.0	500
Chlorthalidone	25.0	50
Cyclothiazide	1.0	2
Hydrochlorothiazide	25.0	50
Hydroflumethiazide	25.0	50
Indapamide	2.5	5
Methyclothiazide	2.5	5
Metolazone	2.5	5
Polythiazide	2.0	4
Quinethazone	50.0	100
Trichlormethiazide	2.0	4
Loop diuretics		
Bumetanide‡	0.5	10§
Ethacrynic acid	50.0	200§
Furosemide	80.0	480§
Potassium-sparing agents		
Amiloride hydrochloride	5.0	10
Spironolactone	50.0	100
Triamterene	50.0	100
Adrenergic Inhibitors		
Beta adrenergic blockers‖		
Atenolol	25.0	100
Metoprolol tartrate	50.0	300
Nadolol	20.0	120
Oxprenolol hydrochloride	160.0	480
Pindolol	20.0	60‖
Propranolol hydrochloride	40.0	480‖
Propranolol, long acting	80.0	480
Timolol maleate	20.0	60‖
Central-acting adrenergic inhibitors		
Clonidine hydrochloride	0.2	1.2‖
Guanabenz acetate	8.0	32‖
Methyldopa	500.0	2,000‖
Peripheral-acting adrenergic antagonists		
Guanadrel sulfate	10.0	150‖
Guanethidine monosulfate	10.0	300
Rauwolfia alkaloids		
Rauwolfia (whole root)	50.0	100
Reserpine	0.05	0.25

TABLE 4-2. *Antihypertensive Agents. Reproduced with permission from The Joint National Committee on Detection, Evaluation, and Treatment of High Blood Pressure.*[1] *(Continued)*

TYPE OF DRUG	DOSAGE RANGE* (MG/DAY)	
	INITIAL	MAXIMUM†
Alpha₁-adrenergic blocker		
Prazosin hydrochloride	1.0	20‖
Combined alpha and beta-adrenergic blockers		
Labetalol¶	200.0	1,200
Vasodilators		
Hydralazine hydrochloride	50.0	300‖
Minoxidil	5.0	100‖
Angiotensin converting enzyme inhibitors		
Captopril	37.5	150‖
Enalapril maleate¶	10.0	40
Slow channel calcium-entry blocking agents§		
Diltiazem hydrochloride	120.0	240**
Nifedipine	30.0	180**
Verapamil hydrochloride	240.0	480**

* The dosage range may differ slightly from manufacturers recommended dosage.
† The maximum suggested dosage may be exceeded in resistant cases.
‡ This drug has not yet been approved by the Food and Drug Administration for the treatment of hypertension.
§ This drug is usually given in divided doses twice daily.
‖ Atenolol and metoprolol are cardioselective; oxprenolol and pindolol have partial agonist activity.
¶ This drug has not yet been approved by the FDA.
** This drug is usually given in divided doses three or four times daily.

fitness to risk of becoming hypertensive. After adjustment for sex, age, follow-up interval, baseline BP, and baseline body-mass index, persons with low levels of physical fitness (72% of the group) had a relative risk of 1.52 for the development of hypertension when compared with highly fit persons. Risk of hypertension developing also increased substantially with increased baseline BP.

Cade and associates[6] from Gainesville, Florida, studied 105 patients with established diastolic systemic hypertension (diastolic BP consistently >90 mmHg) in an exercise program to examine the effect of aerobic conditioning on BP. In 4 patients, the decrease in mean BP was <5 mmHg; in all others, there was a significant decline in arterial BP. In 58 patients who were not taking drug medication in the preexercise period, mean BP decreased by 15 mmHg. Of 47 patients receiving drug therapy during the preexercise period, 24 were able to discontinue all medication. Mean BP in this group decreased from 117 ± 7–97 ± 9 mmHg as a result of exercise. In patients still taking antihypertensive drugs, mean pressure decreased from 121 ± 29–104 ± 18 mmHg after 3 months of exercise. It is concluded that in patients physically and emotionally able to exercise, a significant decline in BP can be achieved.

Effect of nutrient intake

McCarron and associates[7] from Portland, Oregon, used a data base of the National Center for Health Statistics, Health and Nutrition Examination Survey I (HANES I), to perform a computer-assisted comprehensive analysis of the relation of 17 nutrients to the BP profile of adult Americans. Subjects included 10,372 individuals, 18–74 years of age, who denied a history of systemic hypertension and intentional modification of their diet. Significant decreases in the consumption of calcium, potassium, vitamin A, and vitamin C were identified as the nutritional factors that distinguished hypertensive from normotensive subjects (Fig. 4-1). Lower calcium intake was the most consistent factor in hypertensive individuals. Across the population, higher intakes of calcium, potassium, and sodium were associated with lower mean systolic BP and lower absolute risk of hypertension. Increments of dietary calcium were also negatively correlated with body mass. Even though these correlations cannot be accepted as proof of causation, they have implications for future studies of the association of nutritional factors and dietary patterns

Fig. 4-1. Standardized mean differences in nutrient intakes between hypertensive subjects (≥160 mmHg) and normotensive subjects. Reproduced with permission from McCarron et al.[7]

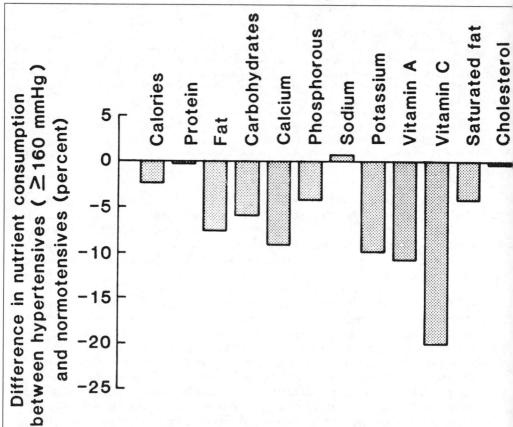

with hypertension in America. These investigators made the following conclusions: (1) predictable nutritional differences existed between individuals with high BP and those with normal BP; (2) deficiencies rather than excesses are the principal nutritional patterns that characterize the hypertensive person in America; (3) reduced consumption of calcium and potassium is the primary nutritional marker of systemic hypertension with reductions in vitamins A and C also being present; (4) dairy products are the food group for which reduced consumption is most closely related to high BP in the USA; (5) these observations are largely independent of age, race, sex, body mass index, and alcohol consumption; (6) diets low in sodium are associated with higher BP and high sodium diets are associated with lowest BP. These observations raise the question of whether sodium restriction is routinely advisable in many hypertensive patients. These observations obviously imply potentially important relations among nutrients and BP regulation in humans. These observations need to be confirmed.

Effect of platelet calcium

Intracellular free calcium has been implicated in vascular smooth muscle contraction and in the pathophysiology of essential systemic hypertension. Erne and associates[8] from Basel, Switzerland, studied free calcium levels in blood platelets, which have many features in common with vascular smooth muscle cells. With use of an intracellularly trapped fluorescent dye, the free-calcium concentration in platelets was found to be elevated in 9 patients with borderline hypertension, who were compared with 38 normotensive subjects. There was a close correlation between the free-calcium level and both systolic and diastolic BP (n, 92). Antihypertensive treatment with calcium-entry blockers (n, 15), beta adrenoceptor blockers (n, 12), or a diuretic (n, 6) resulted in a reduction in free calcium, and this correlated with the decrease in BP. The intracellular free calcium concentration in platelets may be determined by the same humoral or pharmacologic factors that determine the height of BP.

Exercise RNA responses

The effectiveness of exercise treadmill testing in diagnosing CAD in patients with systemic hypertension is limited by a high rate of false positive results. Exercise radionuclide and ventriculography, however, relies on different criteria (EF and wall motion). Wasserman and associates[9] from Washington, D.C., evaluated this procedure in 37 hypertensive and in 109 normotensive patients with chest pain, using coronary arteriography as the indicator of CAD. In the hypertensive cohort there was no difference in the EF at rest between the 17 patients with CAD and the 20 without it. Neither group had a significant mean change in EF from rest to exercise (-1.9 ± 2 and $-1.4 \pm 1\%$, respectively). A wall motion abnormality developed during exercise in 5 of the 17 hypertensive patients with CAD (29%) and in 4 of the 20 without it (20%). In the normotensive cohort, however, the peak exercise EF were significantly different. The 71 patients with CAD had a mean decrease of 3.6 ± 1% in contrast to the patients without CAD, who had an increase of 6 ± 1%. An exercise-induced wall motion abnormality was seen in 35 of the 71 patients with CAD (48%), compared with 3 of the 38 without it (8%). The investigators concluded that exercise radionuclide ventriculography is inadequate as a screening test for coronary atherosclerosis in hypertensive patients with chest pain.

Effect of alcohol

Several population and clinical studies have demonstrated a relation between alcohol intake and BP. During alcohol withdrawal, alcoholic patients have high BP, which settles during recovery, the presser effect being associated with increased plasma cortisol and catecholamine levels. In nonalcoholics, however, evidence on the acute effects of alcohol on BP is conflicting. The presser effects of alcohol in hypertensive patients have not been examined. Potter and Beevers[10] from Birmingham, England, therefore studied the effect of alcohol on BP in 16 men with systemic hypertension who regularly drank up to 80 g of alcohol daily. Antihypertensive treatment was stopped 2 weeks before the men were admitted to hospital for a 7-day study. The BP remained high in 8 patients who continued their regular alcohol consumption up to the 4th day after admission. In the next 4 days no alcohol was taken and diastolic and systolic BP decreased significantly. Eight other patients had no alcohol for the first 3 days after admission, but they resumed alcohol consumption from days 4–7. In these patients, BP decreased slightly after admission. Reintroduction of alcohol produced statistically significant increases in both systolic and diastolic pressures. This study demonstrated a pressor effect of alcohol in patients with hypertension and confirms the link between alcohol and BP reported in population studies. The mechanism of alcohol-induced hypertension is uncertain and is more likely to be due to an effect of alcohol rather than to the pressor response produced by alcohol withdrawal.

Extracellular fluid volume and sodium

Lebel and associates[11] from Quebec, Canada, studied in 38 young patients with borderline systemic hypertension and in 37 age- and sex-matched control subjects interrelations between systemic arterial pressure, extracellular fluid (ECF) volume, exchangeable sodium (Na), and the renin-angiotensin-aldosterone system. The ECF volume and exchangeable sodium were subnormal in borderline hypertensive patients. In normal subjects, volume data did not relate to arterial pressure; in contrast, negative correlations were observed between arterial pressure and ECF volume or exchangeable Na in patients with borderline hypertension (in hypertensive women, $r \geq 0.7$, $p < 0.01$). Plasma renin activity was consistently elevated in borderline hypertension, mainly in the upright posture, and these values were inversely correlated with ECF volume and exchangeable Na. No correlation was observed between arterial pressure and plasma renin activity. These results show that slight elevation of arterial pressure in the early stage of hypertension induces a proportional decrease in ECF volume, suggesting that the phenomenon of pressure-natriuresis is operative in young borderline hypertensive persons. The renin-angiotensin system is activated in these patients, in part to preserve sodium homeostasis.

LEFT VENTRICULAR HYPERTROPHY

Fouad and coworkers[12] from Cleveland, Ohio, evaluated diastolic cardiac function in hypertensive patients to determine whether it is affected before alterations in either EF or cardiac output. Eleven normal subjects (group 1), 5 hypertensive subjects without evidence of LV hypertrophy (group 2), and 18 hypertensive subjects with increased LV mass by echo (group 3) were studied by M-mode echo and radionuclide ventriculography. Systolic function was assessed by measuring EF, maximal rate of ejection, and percent LV shortening. No differences in these variables describing systolic function were found between hypertensive and normotensive subjects. No correlation was found between systolic BP and LV mass. There were, however, differences in diastolic function between normotensive and hypertensive subjects. The maximal rate of LV filling decreased progressively from group 1 to group 3 subjects and reached statistical significance in hypertensive subjects with LV hypertrophy. The LV maximal filling rate correlated inversely with LV mass and LV end-systolic diameter, but positively with LV fractional shortening and EF. These data suggest that impairment of early LV filling develops in relation to LV hypertrophy resulting from systemic arterial hypertension and that it may be detected even before definite evidence of systolic dysfunction is apparent.

Shapiro and McKenna[13] from London, England, used digitized M-mode echo to determine the relation between the degree of LV hypertrophy and abnormalities of isovolumic relaxation and diastolic function in 56 patients with varying degrees of nonmalignant systemic hypertension without evidence of CAD, LV dilation, or clinical CHF. In addition, 10 athletes with hypertrophy and 20 normal subjects were studied. Athletes and patients with moderate (systolic BP, 175–200 mmHg) and severe hypertension (>200 mmHg) had a significant increase in LV mass. Cavity dimensions were normal in hypertensive patients and increased in athletes. Systolic function was normal in all groups. Regardless of the degree of hypertrophy, patients with hypertension had a prolonged isovolumic relaxation period and delayed mitral valve opening. Patients with hypertrophy also had a reduced rate and prolonged duration of rapid early diastolic dimension increase and posterior wall thinning. Athletes, however, who had an equivalent degree of hypertrophy to patients with moderate or severe hypertension had entirely normal function. Measurements of diastolic function were significantly correlated with wall thickness and LV mass. These indices of hypertrophy, particularly posterior wall thickness and the sum of posterior wall and septal thickness, were positively correlated with the duration of isovolumic relaxation and delay in mitral opening and negatively with the peak rate of early diastolic dimension increase and wall thinning. Thus, in hypertensive patients with nondilated LV hypertrophy there appears to be a relation between the degree of wall thickening and abnormalities of diastolic function.

Messerli and associates[14] from New Orleans, Louisiana, designed a study to detect and quantify cardiac arrhythmias in patients with systemic hypertension with LV hypertrophy. Continuous ambulatory ECG tracings and arterial BP were recorded for 24 hours in 14 normotensive subjects, 10 with established essential hypertension without LV hypertrophy, and in 16 hypertensive patients with LV hypertrophy by ECG criteria. Urinary excretion of norepinephrine was simultaneously measured over 4 successive 4-hour and 1 8-hour period. Patients with LV hypertrophy had significantly more ventricular (but not atrial) premature contractions than those without LV hypertrophy or than normotensive subjects. Five patients with LV hypertrophy had episodes of >30 VPC/minute. Higher grade ventricular ectopic activity, such as coupled VPC, was seen in 2, and multifocal VPC were seen in 3 in the group with LV hypertrophy (Table 4-3). No difference in urinary catecholamine excretion rates among the 3 groups was seen. The LV hypertrophy has been shown to be an independent risk factor for sudden death and AMI, and ECG monitoring of patients with LV hypertrophy allows identification of those who have the highest risk and therefore require the most aggressive therapeutic intervention.

Devereux and associates[15] from New York City and Long Beach, California, evaluated relations among BP, blood viscosity and echo LV muscle mass in 24 patients with essential hypertension and in 13 normotensive control subjects. The LV mass was greater in the hypertensive patients than in the control subjects (225 ± 69 -vs- 170 ± 31 g) as was blood viscosity at a shear rate of 104 s^{-1} (4.7 ± 0.1 -vs- 4.3 ± 0.2 cp). Among the hypertensive patients, LV mass was most closely related to viscosity at 104 s^{-1} (r = 0.80), whereas only weak correlations were found between LV mass and systolic or diastolic BP. The 14 hypertensive patients with normal LV mass had viscosity similar to that in control subjects (4.5 ± 0.3 -vs- 4.3 ± 0.2 cp), whereas viscosity was consistently increased (5.0 ± 0.4 cp) in hypertensive patients with LV hypertrophy. Thus, increased blood viscosity may be a determinant of or a response to hypertensive cardiac hypertrophy.

TABLE 4-3. *Prevalence of premature atrial and ventricular contractions (mean ± SD).*

		HYPERTENSIVE	
	NORMOTENSIVE	WITHOUT LVH	WITH LVH
APC per 24 hours	1.08 ± 1.78	1.0 ± 1.5	9.3 ± 25
VPC per 24 hours	8.17 ± 20.1	10.0 ± 22.1	475 ± 852*
Mean heart rate (beats per minute)	77 ± 3.0	75 ± 2.6	74 ± 3.6

* p < 0.01 versus both other groups.
LVH = left ventricular hypertrophy; APC = premature atrial contractions.

The development and regression of cardiac hypertrophy in patients with systemic hypertension do not depend solely on the level of the arterial BP, but seem also to be modulated by various neurohumoral factors. Adrenergic factors play an important role where sympatholytic drugs and beta adrenergic blocking drugs do enduce regression of LV hypertrophy. Other antihypertensive agents, such as vasodilators and diuretic drugs, have been ineffective in that regard. Nakashima and associates[16] from Cleveland, Ohio, studied 7 patients with LV hypertrophy from systemic hypertension to evaluate serial changes of LV mass and function after initiation of the new converting enzyme inhibitor MK-421. The LV mass and function were determined serially at the end of a placebo period and at 5 days, 1, 3, and 7 months after the initiation of MK-421, using both 2-D guided M-mode echo and radionuclide techniques. All patients except 1 had LV hypertrophy and all had normal LV function (EF derived from gated blood pool method >49%). There was an inverse relation between LV fractional shortening (percent FS) and end-systolic stress before medication. The LV mass decreased significantly at 3 and 7 months (−10, and −12%, respectively) accompanied with persistent decrease of mean BP, which occurred as early as 5 days after start of therapy (133 ± 5 mmHg at control to 112 ± 4 mmHg at day 5). During reversal of LV hypertrophy, the inverse correlation between FS and end-systolic stress remained significant, with no difference from the placebo period and from this relation in the normal group. Moreover, percent FS, EF, and stroke index remained unchanged. Thus, LV hypertrophy in patients with systemic hypertension can be reversed without deterioration of LV function. Moreover, overall LV function is likely to be determined by afterload even after reversal of LV hypertrophy.

TREATMENT

Therapeutic motivation—decreased life-insurance premiums

It is well known that elevated BP substantially increases mortality and requires therefore high premium payments for life insurance coverage. Most life insurance companies are willing to reduce the cost of yearly premiums when BP is successfully treated and controlled for several years. Physicians should bring these facts to their patients' attention as a motivating factor to improve adherence to therapy[17] (Fig. 4-2).

Breaking tablets in half

The primary goal of chronic drug therapy is to find a dose that maximizes efficacy and minimizes toxicity. To make it easier to tailor doses individually, manufacturers often score tablets to assist breaking. To find out if such tablets really break evenly, Stimpel and associates[18] from Zurich, Switzerland, took 100 tablets of each of 14 brands of antihypertensive drugs and broke them into 2 halves, using the scoring line. They weighed the whole tablet and the 2 halves separately on precision scales. The theoretical weight

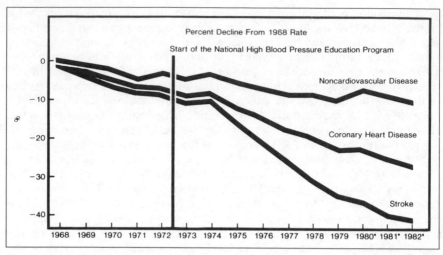

Fig. 4-2. United States age-adjusted mortality rates (ages 35–74 years). Asterisk indicates provisional data. Data from the National Center for Health Statistics and the National Heart, Lung, and Blood Institute. Reproduced with permission from Moser et al.[17]

of each half was 50% of the whole and they grouped weights as within 5% of expected (45–55%), 5–10% off in either direction (40–44% or 56–60%), or more than 10% in error (<40% or >60%). If ≥95% of the half-tablet weights were within 5% of expected, the divisibility of the tablet was classified as "excellent." If ≥95% of the tablet halves were within 10%, divisibility was "moderate." For the remainder, divisibility was "poor." Only 2 brands tested divided well. Most others tested broke easily but deviations in half-tablet weights of up to 10% were frequent and some tablets were unsuitable for breaking, by hand or otherwise. In all cases, the weight loss after breaking was not important. Clearly, any assumption that halving a tablet will lead to accurate doses is invalid. This potential source of inaccuracy could be even more significant in clinical situations (this study was done under ideal conditions) and the pharmaceutical industry should attempt to solve the problem, either by improving divisibility or, even better, by marketing a wider range of unscored tablets to provide all the doses that might be indicated clinically.

Sodium restriction and loading

Since young patients with borderline hypertension are at least 3 times more likely to develop established essential hypertension than are age-matched normotensive controls, Fujita and colleagues[19] from Ibaraki, Japan, evaluated sodium susceptibility in subjects with borderline hypertension while studying the effect of salt loading after salt deprivation with a diuretic in 21 young patients with borderline hypertension and 12 age-matched normal subjects. Treatment with a diuretic caused significant decreases in mean BP in subjects with borderline hypertension but not in normotensive subjects. In borderline hypertensives, the subsequent sodium loads resulted in a significant increase in mean BP, but sodium did not change mean BP in normotensive subjects. There was a good correlation between the increments in mean

BP with sodium loads and the decrements in mean BP with a diuretic for each patient. After diuretics, cardiac index as measured by echo decreased significantly, but calculated total peripheral resistance remained unchanged in subjects with borderline hypertension. After sodium chloride administration each day for 7 days, cardiac index and stroke index increased significantly but resistance remained unchanged. Overall, the increments of mean BP with sodium loads did not correlate with the changes in cardiac index but did correlate with the changes in resistance. In the young patients with borderline hypertension, plasma norepinephrine and epinephrine concentrations and plasma renin activity was significantly higher than in normotensive subjects. These results suggested that young patients with borderline hypertension differed from normal subjects in that they displayed a BP increase due to a disproportionate increase in cardiac index and an inadequate decrease in total peripheral resistance in response to a short-term increase in dietary sodium and that adrenosympathetic overactivity and increased activity of the renin-angiotensin system may be partly involved. These observations suggest that potassium supplementation may prevent the BP increase with the sodium loading by attenuating the increase in cardiac output, possibly as a result of the natriuresis.

To determine whether moderate restriction of dietary sodium content or supplementation of potassium intake reduces BP in patients with mild systemic hypertension (BP between 140/90 and 180/105 mmHg after resting supine for 15 minutes on 2 consecutive outpatient visits ≥10 days apart), Richards and associates[20] from Christ Church, New Zealand, put 12 patients on 3 different diets, a controlled diet (180 mM sodium/day), a sodium restricted diet (80 mM/day), and a potassium supplemented diet (200 mM potassium/day). Each diet was taken for ≥4 weeks and the sequence of the regimens was randomized. At the completion of each regimen, intraarterial pressure was recorded continuously, and vasoactive hormones were measured hourly, for 24 hours, under standardized conditions, in hospital. Compared with the control diet, sodium restriction was associated with lower BP readings in 7 patients, higher levels in 5, and an overall reduction in mean pressures of only 4.0/3.0 mmHg. Individual differences in BP between these 2 diets correlated closely with concomitant differences in plasma renin activity. Potassium supplementation also resulted in variable changes in arterial BP and the mean difference in BP recordings (0.1/0.8 mmHg) was insignificant. The results show that moderate restriction of sodium intake or supplementation of dietary potassium has variable effects on arterial BP in individuals with mild essential hypertension and that overall the BP changes induced are small.

Niarchos and associates[21] from New York City treated 71 patients with diuretics and another 32 with low sodium diets, all of whom had *systolic* BP ≥160 mmHg and diastolic BP ≤90 mmHg). In the 71 who were treated with diuretics, body weight decreased from 69 ± 1–69 ± 1 kg and systolic BP from 178 ± 2–152 ± 2 mmHg. Plasma renin activity increased from 1.78 ± 0.30–7.32 ± 1.78 ng/ml/hour and urinary aldosterone from 10 ± 1–23 ± 4 μg/24 hours. The greatest decrease in systolic BP occurred in patients in the low renin group (−32 ± 2 mmHg), whereas it decreased by 24 ± 2 mmHg in the normal renin group; however, BP did not change significantly in the high renin group. In the 32 patients who were treated with low sodium diet, the 24-hour urinary sodium excretion decreased from 143 ± 10–48 ± 5 mEq, body weight decreased from 71 ± 2.50–70 ± 2.47 kg, systolic BP decreased from 174 ± 2–156 ± 3 mmHg, and diastolic BP decreased from 90 ± 1–87 ± 1 mmHg. Plasma renin activity increased from 2.25 ± 0.33–4.27 ± 0.43 ng/ml/hour and urinary aldosterone from 9 ± 1–15 ± 2 μg/24 hours. The decrease in the systolic BP was related to the pretreatment 24-hour urinary sodium excretion. The smallest decrease in systolic BP occurred in the patients with high renin in values (−1 ± 9 mmHg; n, 5), whereas the decrease in systolic BP in the low renin (n, 12) and normal renin groups (n, 15) was similar, −22 ± 2 mmHg and −21 ± 3 mmHg, respectively. These results indicate that both diuretic therapy and low sodium diet are effective antihypertensive means in most patients with isolated systolic hypertension and low or normal plasma renin activity.

Maxwell and associates[22] from Los Angeles, California, in a controlled prospective study compared 2 groups of obese hypertensive subjects during 12 weeks of hypocaloric protein-supplemented fast containing 40 mEq of sodium daily. One group received additional sodium chloride sufficient to maintain baseline sodium intake measured before the fast (210 mEq/day). Sodium restriction resulted in greater weight loss and slightly greater BP reduction only during the initial week of fasting. Thereafter, despite sodium equilibrium, further substantial weight loss and BP reduction were identical in both groups, the decrement in weight being linear (1.89 kg/week) and the BP reduction asymptotic. Although the initial reduction in BP during the first week of supplemented fast may be attributable to negative salt and water balance, the further reduction in BP during a period of constant sodium balance must be caused by weight loss per se or by the triggering of other antihypertensive mechanisms associated with weight reduction.

To test the utility of a qualitative chloride titrator strip in facilitating compliance with a reduced sodium intake diet, Luft and associates[23] from Indianapolis, Indiana, enrolled 32 patients into a randomized crossover trial comprising 2 study periods of 4 weeks each. The study periods were begun after the patients had undergone extensive instruction in the diet and the use of the strip. A high degree of correlation between the patient's and the laboratory's interpretation of the strip results occurred in 29 subjects. Ability to use the strip was not related to level of education. A total of 12 patients achieved compliance with the diet when using the strips. Of these, 9 were able to achieve compliance without the strips. Ten patients (30%) had significantly lower sodium intake when using the strips than when they did not use them. Thus, the use of the chloride titrator strip can be mastered by most patients and, in conjunction with dietary counseling, can facilitate compliance with a reduced sodium intake diet.

Diuretic-induced hypokalemia

The arrhythmogenic propensity of diuretic-induced hypokalemia is controversial. There is a consensus about the ill effects of hypokalemia in patients receiving digitalis preparations and the advisability of correcting this electrolyte abnormality by administration of potassium supplements. Hypokalemia in patients not receiving digitalis, however, is believed by some to be of benign nature and by others to warrant prompt correction. Madias and associates[24] from New York City investigated the potential arrhythmogenic effects of diuretic-induced hypokalemia. Each patient received hydrochlorothiazide therapy for 1 month. The ambulatory ECG monitoring was done a month after receiving placebo and 2 and 4 weeks after hydrochlorothiazide therapy. Serum potassium level averaged 4.4 ± 0.09 mEq/liter after the placebo trial and 3.4 ± 0.07 and 3.0 ± 0.06 mEq/liter after 2 and 4 weeks of therapy, respectively: 16 patients had no arrhythmias; 4 patients had 329 ± 140 VPC while receiving placebo, and 341 ± 203 and 315 ± 158 VPC/24 hours after 2 and 4 weeks of therapy, respectively. Thus, patients with uncomplicated hypertension and no arrhythmias before diuretic therapy did not experience arrhythmias as a result of diuretic-induced hypokalemia of 1 month's duration. Patients with low grade ventricular ectopic activity before therapy did not progress to higher grades of ventricular ectopic activity after diuretic treatment for 4 weeks.

Diuretic-induced hypokalemia often leads to the routine use of potassium chloride (KCl) supplements in potassium-sparing diuretic therapy. In 1981 >7.5 million prescriptions for KCl and 19 million prescriptions for potassium-sparing diuretic drugs were prescribed for patients with systemic hypertension at a cost >$250 million. Hypokalemia, plasma potassium ≤3.5 mEq/liter, occurs in approximately 20% of patients with essential hypertension who receive diuretic therapy. Severe hypokalemia (<3.0 mEq/liter) occurs less frequently. Whether the hypokalemia reflects a true deficit of total body potassium is controversial. Although numerous studies have shown that diuretic therapy results in a mild decrease of plasma potassium and in an initial increase in urinary potassium excretion, studies assessing the duration and severity of kaliuresis in patients with overt hypokalemia are scarce. Papademetriou and associates[25] from Washington, D.C., studied 2 groups of patients with uncomplicated systemic hypertension. Group 1 included 11 patients who had overt hypokalemia with diuretic drug treatment, and group 2 included 11 patients who remained normokalemic. After baseline studies without treatment were performed, both groups received hydrochlorothiazide, 50 mg twice daily. Plasma potassium was significantly reduced within the first day of treatment and stabilized by day 7 in both groups. The average decrease in plasma potassium was 1.0 ± 0.1 mEq/liter in the first group and 0.6 ± 0.2 mEq/liter in the second group. Cumulative losses of potassium were approximately 200 mEq in the hypokalemic group and were minimal in the normokalemic group, as assessed by 24-hour urinary collections. Patients in the hypokalemic group also had a greater reduction in body weight and BP. Supplementation with KCl, 96 mEq/day, or triamterene, 200 mg/day, in 9 hypokalemic patients resulted in an increase of plasma potassium to approximately 3.5 mEq/liter, leveling off by day 7, and a cumulative potassium retention of approximately 200 mEq. Thus, overt thiazide-induced hypokalemia was associated with small and biologically unimportant losses of potassium from body stores. With replacement therapy, the estimated amount of retained potassium also was small.

Relaxation and biofeedback

Systemic hypertension in pregnancy occurs in about 10% of women and can adversely affect the health of both mother and baby. Although its etiology is unclear, it has been suggested that pregnancy hypertension is particularly likely in patients with a family history of essential hypertension. Emotional factors also are believed to be important. The most commonly used drugs in the management of hypertension during pregnancy are methyldopa, diuretics, and beta blocking agents. There is still some doubt, however, about their safety to the fetus. Because of their possible adverse effects on the fetus, the use of drugs during pregnancy, of course, should be based on clear evidence that they are essential. The safest treatment of hypertension in pregnancy appears to be bed rest accompanied by sedation, but this form of treatment is quite costly and disruptive. Several studies have used biofeedback training to reduce BP in hypertensive patients with varying degrees of success. In a study of the effectiveness of systemic relaxation training alone or combined with feedback in the treatment of systemic hypertension in pregnancy, Little and associates[26] from London, England, studied 60 pregnant women weekly for 6 weeks: 18 were given relaxation therapy alone (group A), 18, relaxation plus biofeedback (group B), and the findings were compared with 24 controls. Whereas two thirds of the control group had to be admitted to the hospital during their pregnancies, less than a third of each experimental group had to be admitted. The experimental groups also had significantly lower systolic and diastolic BP than the control group. There were no significant differences between groups A and B in hospital admission rates or BP measurements. Thus, it appears worthwhile to carry on with this approach to the treatment of hypertension in pregnancy. Biofeedback does not seem to add greatly to the effect achieved and therefore it would be cheap and simple to set up groups for mothers at risk of hypertension to practice just the systematic relaxation. This approach could provide a cost-effective way of reducing hospital admissions and would be a most acceptable form of treatment for pregnant women.

Beta blocking agents

Vincent and associates[27] from Rotterdam, The Netherlands, compared the effects of graded infusions of the beta agonist isoproterenol (nonselective), prenalterol (beta$_1$ selective), and albuterol (beta$_2$ selective) on plasma potassium and on norepinephrine levels in subjects who had borderline hypertension. Potassium levels decreased with all 3 agonists, and norepinephrine levels increased with isoproterenol and albuterol. These effects on potassium and norepinephrine were closely correlated and occurred at the same dose ranges as the cardiovascular responses. The decrease in plasma potassium was probably caused by activation of beta receptors, mainly on skeletal muscle, with subsequent stimulation of active sodium-potassium transport across the cellular membrane. The increase in plasma norepinephrine may have been due to activation of beta receptors on sympathetic nerve endings. Activation of these presynaptic receptors is known to enhance the release of norepinephrine during nerve stimulation. For a given increase in heart rate and cardiac contractility, as measured by the heart rate-corrected duration of total electromechanical systole, which are mainly beta$_1$ responses, the effects on potassium and norepinephrine were in the order: albuterol $>$ isoproterenol $>$ prenalterol. Beta blockade with propranolol (nonselective), 80 mg 4 times a day, or atenolol (beta$_1$ selective), 100 mg once a day, antagonized the hypokalemic effect of isoproterenol and the increase in norepinephrine levels, but when isoproterenol was infused in doses high enough to overcome the blockade of the heart rate response, the effects on norepinephrine and potassium were abolished by propranolol and not by atenolol. Thus, the receptors in question appear to be of the beta$_2$ subtype. Epinephrine, which is known to circulate in high concentrations under stressful conditions, is generally considered to be the endogenous activator of these receptors. Beta blockers may prevent hypokalemia and may suppress sympathetic activity, which could contribute to their so-called cardioprotective action. The evidence presented here and in other studies that beta$_2$-type receptors are involved in stress-induced hypokalemia and in presynaptic facilitation of norepinephrine release warrants further consideration of the clinical significance of beta blocker selectivity.

To assess changes in LV function during antihypertensive treatment using pindolol, a beta adrenocepter blocking drug with potent intrinsic sympathomimetic activity, Plotnick and associates[28] from Baltimore, Maryland, obtained serial echo measurements in 70 hypertensive patients before and during 15 weeks of treatment with pindolol. For analysis, the patients were separated into 3 groups on the basis of their baseline LV fractional shortening (group I, 35 patients with normal fractional shortening of ≥28%; group II, 16 patients with abnormal fractional shortening of 21–27%; and group III, 19 patients with markedly abnormal fractional shortening of ≤20%). More than half of the patients in groups I and II had decreases in mean BP of ≥10% in response to pindolol, but only one fourth of group III patients had similar responses. Patients with normal pretreatment fractional shortening had a mild decrease in fractional shortening during pindolol treatment, whereas patients with either abnormal or markedly abnormal fractional shortening had an increase in fractional shortening. This increase in fractional shortening suggests the possibility that the partial agonist or intrinisic sympathomimetic activity of pindolol may play a role in preserving LV function in patients with borderline or impaired function.

Cressman and associates[29] from Cleveland, Ohio, investigated the intravenous administration of labetalol, a combined alpha and beta adrenergic receptor blocking agent, which reduced diastolic BP by ≥30 mmHg in 15 of 17 patients with severe hypertension (supine diastolic BP ≥125 mmHg). A method of repeated intravenous injection of the drug produced a prompt but gradual reduction of arterial BP without the induction of a reflex tachycardia. Side effects were mild and of brief duration despite the presence of hypertensive complications in many patients. Hypotension, coronary insufficiency, or neurologic deterioration did not occur. Labetalol appears to be a suitable alternative to the direct vasodilating agents in the management of patients with severe hypertension and hypertensive emergencies.

Bucindolol is a newly developed, nonselective beta adrenergic blocking agent with intrinsic sympathomimetic activity and direct vasodilator properties. Rotmensch and associates[30] from Philadelphia, Pennsylvania, compared in 14 patients with mild to moderate essential systemic hypertension the effects of bucindolol, hydrochlorothiazide, and their combination on BP, heart rate, and variables of the renin-aldosterone system with those after placebo. Bucindolol's antihypertensive effect was evident within the first hour after drug administration, maximal at 2–3 hours, and lasted for as long as 12 hours. Compared with placebo values (108 ± 5 mmHg), both bucindolol (97 ± 9 mmHg) and hydrochlorothiazide (99 ± 10 mmHg) alone significantly and comparably reduced the 12-hour averaged standing diastolic BP, with the combination resulting in approximately additive effects (91 ± 9 mmHg). Although bucindolol alone did not affect heart rate, it attenuated the hydrochlorothiazide-induced increase in heart rate. There was a tendency for bucindolol to decrease plasma renin activity. Except for transient postural hypotension in 2 patients, bucindolol was well tolerated.

A series of studies on various therapeutic aspects of beta adrenergic blocking drugs has been carried out by the Veterans Administration Cooperative Study Group on Antihypertensive Agents. In 1 study directed by Freis[31] from Washington, D.C., the diastolic BPs of 49% of 132 men with mild to moderate hypertension were controlled (<90 mmHg) with once-daily nadolol. In a similar group, 85% were controlled with nadolol plus bendroflumethiazide, both given once daily. Nadolol alone was as effective as diuretic alone, although in another study comparing propranolol and hydrochlorothiazide, the latter was somewhat more effective. In both trials black patients tended to respond better to the diuretic, whereas white patients responded better to the beta blocker. Although high renin hypertensive patients tended to respond better to the beta blocker and low renin patients to the diuretic, the relations were not close enough to provide a dependable guide to treatment. Sixty percent of patients whose BP was not controlled on the nadolol-containing regimens reached goal BP (<90 mmHg) with the addition of hydralazine, 25–100 mg twice daily.

Captopril

The manufacturer of captopril, E.R. Squibb and Sons, made available to Frohlich and associates[32] from New Orleans, Louisiana, Philadelphia, Pennsylvania, and Chicago, Illinois, the total data base of clinical studies for determining the safety and efficacy of captopril therapy for systemic hypertension. From review of these data and from review of previous published reports, Frohlich and associates identified a small subgroup of clinically complex patients at a particular risk of side effects and in whom the drug must be used with caution. Evidence was available that demonstrated that lower doses (≤150 mg/day with modest doses of diuretic agents) were effective in both short- and long-term therapy, and the incidence of side effects was substantially reduced. They concluded that the benefit-risk ratio was substantially improved and that the use of captopril as a primary agent in the management of systemic hypertension may be considered. This is a superb article on an important drug.

In a Veterans Administration Cooperative Study Group on Antihypertensive Agents,[33] 495 men with uncomplicated systemic hypertension (diastolic BP, 92–109 mmHg) were randomized to 1 of 5 captopril regimens at the following doses: 12.5 mg 3 times a day, 25 mg 3 times a day, 37.5 mg twice daily, 50 mg 3 times a day, or placebo 3 times a day. After 7 weeks, BP reduction with each captopril dose was greater than in the placebo group, averaging 10.2–14.2/8.6–10.5 mmHg. Captopril, 37.5 mg/day, was as effective as 150 mg/day. Hydrochlorothiazide, 25 mg twice daily, was added for 7 more weeks to all patients receiving placebo and to two thirds of those randomized to captopril therapy. The BP reduction averaged 12.0/8.7 mmHg in those receiving hydrochlorothiazide alone and 24.9–26.4/14.4–17.3 mmHg in those receiving a combination of hydrochlorothiazide and captopril. Added hydrochlorothiazide greatly enhanced the antihypertensive response. The 15 terminations (4.3%) related to captopril were not life threatening.

Thus, captopril treatment of uncomplicated hypertension may be initiated with 37.5 mg/day, half the currently recommended dose.

Chlorthalidone

Previous studies have shown that controlling the diastolic BP for >6 months frequently permits the use of fewer drugs in lower doses in most patients with moderately severe and severe systemic hypertension. Prompted by these observations, Finnerty[34] from Washington, D.C., decreased the dosage of chlorthalidone (monotherapy) in a stepwise fashion and then discontinued the drug entirely after the diastolic BP had been maintained at <85 mmHg for 6 months in 67 patients with mild systemic hypertension (diastolic BP 92–104 mmHg). These patients were followed for 48 months. Initially, a dose of 25 mg/day of chlorthalidone was just as effective as 50 mg in controlling the diastolic BP in all patients, and it was not until the dose was reduced to 12.5 mg/day that the diastolic BP increased in 8 patients. Annoying symptoms and metabolic side effects were decreased or eliminated. Chlorthalidone therapy was discontinued in 36 of the 67 patients. The ability to discontinue therapy in these patients suggests the possibility of intermittent, rather than continuous, lifelong therapy.

Clonidine

The centrally acting agent clonidine has been used as a single agent oral antihypertensive therapy. It was recently incorporated into a skin patch that produces a steady release of the agent through the skin over 7 days. Weber and associates[35] from Long Beach and Irvine, California, used the self-adhesive patches containing a 7-day supply of transdermal clonidine in 20 patients with mild systemic hypertension. The skin patches (3 by 5 cm^2) which were changed by the patients every week, reduced diastolic BP to <90 mmHg in 12 patients. When placebo-containing patches were substituted in these 12 patients after 3 months of treatment, BP increased slowly to its pretreatment level. Side effects appeared to be milder than those experienced during conventional oral antihypertensive treatment. Plasma clonidine concentrations were lower than peak levels after oral administration. Thus, this new method for treating systemic hypertension was convenient and well tolerated and may increase patient compliance.

Clonidine recently became available as a transdermal preparation with a duration of action of ≥1 week. In a multicenter study, Weber and associates[36] evaluated the effectiveness of transdermally administered clonidine hydrochloride in 85 patients with mild essential hypertension. The drug was incorporated into small self-adhesive delivery systems (pliable skin patches, 3.5 cm^2) designed to deliver continuously 0.1 mg/day of clonidine hydrochloride. These devices were changed by the patients themselves at weekly intervals. Diastolic BP decreased by ≥10% in 37 patients and was normalized (<90 mmHg) in 54 patients (64%); 17 of these responding patients required only 1 skin patch, 27 required 2, and the other 10 responders required 3. The antihypertensive action of the transdermal clonidine was sustained for the full 3 months of study. Side effects were similar to those during conventional oral treatment, but appeared to be milder.

Farsang and coworkers[37] examined the effects of clonidine, naloxone, and their combination on arterial BP, heart rate (HR), and hemodynamic and biochemical parameters in 29 patients with essential hypertension. Naloxone is an opiate antagonist and recent reports in experimental animals demonstrated that this agent could inhibit the antihypertensive agent of clonidine. Treatment for 3 days with clonidine reduced BP and HR, and these effects were quickly reversed by a single injection of intravenous (IV) naloxone in 17 patients (responders), but not in the remaining 12 (nonresponders). Responders revealed higher control values for cardiac output, stroke index, and plasma renin activity (PRA), and plasma epinephrine levels than did nonresponders. Basal BP was similar in the 2 groups, but clonidine decreased BP, PRA, and plasma epinephrine more in responders than in nonresponders. Naloxone given during placebo treatment had no significant effects. During clonidine treatment, naloxone increased BP, HR, total peripheral resistance, PRA, and plasma epinephrine and norepinephrine, and decreased stroke volume in responders, whereas in nonresponders its only effect was a small increase in HR. The investigators concluded that in a subset of hyperadrenergic, hypertensive patients the antihypertensive effect of clonidine involves a naloxone reversible inhibition of central sympathetic outflow, probably mediated by the release of an endogenous opioid.

Antihypertensive medications have a variable effect on renal hemodynamics and may contribute to renal insufficiency in some patients. Since clonidine has actually been found to improve renal hemodynamics in patients with essential hypertension, Green and associates[38] from Richmond, Virginia, studied the effects of clonidine therapy in 6 patients with renal transplant systemic hypertension. Baseline measurements of BP and renal hemodynamics were made in 6 patients after 2 weeks of therapy with furosemide. Clonidine was then added and titrated until BP was controlled. Repeated measurements of renal hemodynamics were made 4 and 16 weeks after clonidine therapy was begun. Glomerular filtration and effective renal plasma flow, assessed by inulin and aminohippurate sodium clearances, were preserved during prolonged clonidine therapy.

Prazosin

Prazosin hydrochloride is an alpha$_1$ adrenoceptor antagonist introduced in 1976 primarily as a second-step therapy for treatment of essential systemic hypertension. Recent reports have suggested that prazosin may be used as an effective first-step therapy for systemic hypertension without development of tolerance. No information is available on the effects of prazosin monotherapy for treatment periods in excess of 8 weeks on renal function and body fluid composition. Consequently, Bauer and associates[39] from Columbia, Missouri, studied 14 hypertensive men in whom the BP was normalized with prazosin monotherapy. Each underwent assessment of renal function and body fluid composition after 3–6 weeks and 5–6 months and after 2 weeks of withdrawal of therapy. Neither short- nor long-term prazosin therapy had any adverse effect on the glomerular filtration rate or effective renal plasma flow. Renal vascular resistance was decreased 14% during short-term therapy, but not during long-term therapy. Urine flow rate, urine osmolality, free water clearance, and fractional sodium and potassium excretions were statistically unchanged throughout drug therapy. Plasma volume and extracellular fluid volume were increased after both short- and long-term therapy. Long-term prazosin monotherapy effectively lowers BP without resulting in drug tolerance; however, sodium retention probably limits its antihypertensive effectiveness.

Drug combinations and comparisons

Since calcium-channel blockers reduce arterial smooth muscle tone and lower BP, they may be regarded as LV unloading agents. Guazzi and colleagues[40] from Milan, Italy, examined LV unloading efficacy of nifedipine (15 patients) and verapamil (14 patients) in hypertensive decompensated patients during a 1-month treatment period. Nifedipine persistently reduced systemic vascular resistance (SVR), mean arterial BP, mean PA wedge pressure, and LV diastolic diameter, and improved cardiac index and velocity of circumferential fiber shortening (VCF). All patients had relief from dyspnea and reduction in heart size. The only side effect was ankle edema in 6 patients. Verapamil reduced SVR and mean arterial BP and was not effective on PA wedge pressure, LV diastolic diameter, and VCF. The drug was discontinued in 2 patients who developed severe dyspnea at rest after 3–4 days of treatment. Clinical symptoms and signs did not improve in the remaining patients despite persistent pressure reduction. A less potent vasodilating action of verapamil and a prominent depression in cardiac contractility may account for the differential results with the 2 compounds, despite a shared vasodilating antihypertensive effect. These findings indicate that functional changes in the failing hypertensive heart may differ from one calcium blocker to another as the result of interaction and relative preponderance of influence on afterload and contractility.

Weber and Drayer[41] from Long Beach and Irvine, California, treated patients with mild to moderate essential hypertension with beta blockers and diuretics given separately and in combination. During single-drug therapy, most patients had clearly superior antihypertensive responses to either 1 type of drug or the other; only rarely were the beta blockers and the diuretic equally effective in an individual patient. A poor response to diuretic therapy tended to predict a good response to a beta blocker, and vice versa. Pretreatment renin measurements were not helpful in predicting the differing responses to single-drug treatment in this study population. These findings indicate that when 1 type of drug is ineffective as monotherapy in treating hypertension, the other type should be substituted before considering combination treatment. Combined therapy with the beta blockers and diuretics also gave variable results, although poor antihypertensive responses could be attributed to excessive stimulation of the renin-aldosterone system by the diuretic component of the combination. The effectiveness of this form of treatment might thus be enhanced by the use of low diuretic doses.

Weinstein and associates[42] from Jerusalem, Israel, studied the effect of a single dose of 500 mg of methyldopa with 50 mg of hydrochlorothiazide and 5 mg of amiloride hydrochloride in 21 patients with mild to moderate systemic hypertension (systolic BP >160 and diastolic BP >95 mmHg). It was shown that the average morning BP changed from 182/103 ± 15/9–145/83 ± 16/8 mmHg after 1 day of treatment. Similarly, the average of 7 hourly measurements (7 BP) dropped from 170/99 ± 11/7–145/86 ± 11/8 mmHg. In 12 patients the same therapy lowered the morning BP from

186/104 ± 16/9–144/83 ± 15/8 mmHg and the 7 BP from 168/98 ± 10/7–142/83 ± 12/7 mmHg after 3 weeks. After 8 weeks, normal values were still maintained. The LV mass was elevated in all the patients (330 ± 67) and dropped by an average of 12 and 17% by 3 and 8 weeks after initiation of therapy. Unchanged LV and diastolic volume and decreased muscle thickness indicate true reduction in hypertrophy in addition to the BP-lowering effect of this combined single-dose therapy described.

Hornung and colleagues[43] from Harrow, England, performed an open crossover trial to compare the 24-hour profiles of BP reduction after chronic therapy with propranolol and verapamil. Nineteen patients were studied by continuous ambulatory intraarterial recording and the order of drug administration was decided by random allocation. Drug dosage was twice daily and titrated according to casual clinic pressures (propranolol, 40–240 mg twice a day; verapamil, 120–240 mg twice a day). Mean hourly BP and heart rate values were obtained over a 24-hour cycle, and the responses to isometric and dynamic exercise were also examined. Both drugs were shown to produce a uniform and comparable reduction in BP throughout the whole day, together with a reduction in heart rate, which was greater with propranolol. Comparable effects also were seen on the pressor responses to exercise. Both drugs were equally well tolerated and caused no patient withdrawals. It was concluded that oral verapamil given twice daily showed a similar degree of efficacy to propranolol and provided 24-hour BP control. This slow calcium-channel inhibitor may be useful as initial therapy for hypertension, particularly for those patients in whom beta adrenoreceptor blockers are contraindicated.

Guazzi and coworkers[44] from Milan, Italy, tested nefedipine (10 mg 4 times a day) and captopril (25 mg four times a day) alone and in combination in 14 patients with severe hypertension. Each study period was of 1 week's duration and circulatory response was evaluated through hourly pressure and pulse rate readings. The decrease in BP after oral nifedipine was maximal ≤1 hour and was generally accompanied by palpitation and increase in heart rate. With a 6-hourly dosing regimen, the tendency of BP to recover after each dose was interrupted by the next dose so that values remained significantly reduced throughout the 24 hours, although BP fluctuations were still evident. The antihypertensive action of captopril was similar, but the magnitude and the duration of the decrease in BP were less pronounced. When the converting-enzyme inhibitor was combined with the calcium-channel blocker, pressure fluctuations were not abolished, but the antihypertensive response was definitely enhanced, so that the normal BP was maintained for several hours. Additional positive effects of captopril were mitigation of the heart rate reaction and prevention of the ankle edema elicited by nifedipine. A balance in arteriolar and venular dilation prompted by captopril is the suggested mechanism for these effects. With the 2-drug combination, LV function was not reduced and possibly improved; blood urea nitrogen and serum electrolyte and creatinine concentration were not affected. Plasma renin activity increased with captopril and reverted toward baseline with the addition of nifedipine, suggesting an interference of the calcium-channel blocker with the release of renin. Thus, these investigators showed that the combination of a calcium-blocker and the converting-enzyme inhibitor appears to be more effective and better suited than each drug alone for treating patients with severe hypertension.

Niarchos and Laragh[45] from New York City investigated the role of the renin system in the maintenance of the elevated systolic BP in isolated systolic hypertension in 31 patients who received long-term treatment with propranolol (120 mg daily) and in another group of 22 patients with isolated systolic systemic hypertension who received a test dose of captopril (25 or 50 mg). The greatest systolic BP decrease (35 ± 5 mmHg) by propranolol occurred in the high renin group (n, 9), whereas in the normal renin group (n, 13), systolic BP was decreased by propranolol by 22 ± 5 mmHg. For all the propranolol-treated patients, the decrement in the systolic BP by propranolol was related to the control plasma renin activity and to the concurrent change in plasma renin activity. Captopril decreased the systolic BP by 55 ± 10 mmHg in the high renin group (n, 11) and by 17 ± 5 mmHg in the normal renin group (n, 6), whereas the smallest decrease 12 ± 5 mmHg in systolic BP occurred in the low renin group (n, 5). In all the captopril-tested patients (n, 22), the decrease in systolic BP by captopril was related to the control plasma renin activity. These results indicate that the plasma renin activity value indicates the participation of the renin-angiotensin system in the maintenance of the elevated systolic BP in patients with isolated systolic hypertension.

Effects of therapy on serum glucose, cholesterol, and triglyceride levels

Helgeland and associates[46] from Oslo, Norway, determined serum glucose levels, triglyceride levels, and body weight from a controlled drug trial in men, aged 40–49 years, with uncomplicated mild systemic hypertension (average initial BP, 156/97 mmHg in the treatment group and 155/96 mmHg in the control group). The drug treatment started with hydrochlorothiazide alone, and methyldopa was added when necessary. If side effects occurred, methyldopa was replaced by propranolol. No detailed advice about diet, smoking, or weight reduction was given to any group. The untreated control subjects had a small increase in serum glucose levels during 5 years, from 6.08–6.21 mM/liter. Those treated with hydrochlorothiazide alone and those treated with hydrochlorothiazide plus methyldopa had a small increase in serum glucose levels of the same order as that in the control subjects. However, those receiving the thiazide and propranolol combination had a sizeable increase in glucose levels, from 5.96–6.53 mM/liter. This increase was significantly greater than the increase in the other groups. The thiazide and propranolol group also had a significant increase in serum triglyceride levels. There was no difference in serum potassium levels in the different drug groups. These results indicate that moderate thiazide doses do not have significant effects on serum glucose levels in this age group. Propranolol in combination with thiazide seems to increase the level of serum glucose.

It is now well established that thiazide-type diuretic drugs raise the serum total cholesterol (TC) and LDL cholesterol and sometimes triglyceride. Nondiuretic antihypertensive drugs with the exception of sotalol do not affect serum TC in this way, but beta blocking drugs usually increase triglyceride levels and lower HDL cholesterol. Hydralazine, clonidine, and prazosin hydrochloride appear to have beneficial effects on serum lipids or lipoproteins or both. Ames and Peacock[47] from New York City utilized spironolactone as therapy for systemic hypertension and evaluated the effect of this drug on serum lipid concentrations. They selected 23 men from the multiple risk factor intervention trial (MRFIT) in New York City and all 23 had increase in serum TC levels after the start of antihypertensive treatment with hydrochlorothiazide or chlorthalidone. Eleven of the 23 men were randomly changed to therapy with spironolactone and the remainder continued with thiazide-type diuretic treatment and therefore served as a control group. After receiv-

Fig. 4-3. Serum cholesterol and triglyceride levels (mean ± SEM) during each of 3 periods of drug treatment. In second period, 1 of 2 subgroups of men with hypertension was switched from chlorthalidone to spironolactone therapy (n, 11); other subgroup remained on chlorthalidone therapy (n, 12) and served as control. Decrease in levels of serum total cholesterol and triglyceride was significantly greater ($p < 0.05$ and < 0.01, respectively) in group switched to spironolactone. In period 3, when chlorthalidone therapy was resumed in this group, increase in cholesterol levels was significantly different ($p < 0.01$) from that in control group. Reproduced with permission from Ames and Peacock.[47]

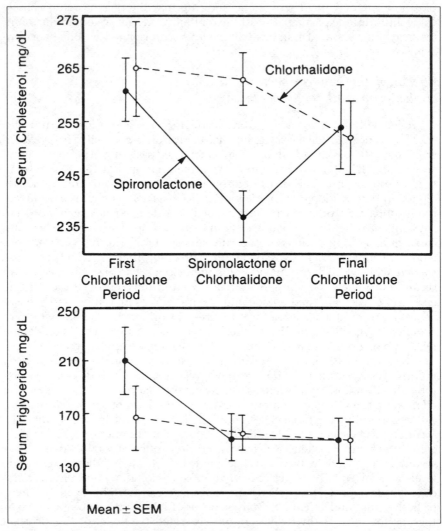

ing spironolactone, TC levels decreased by 24 mg/dl whereas TC levels decreased by only 3 mg/dl in the 12 men still receiving chlorthalidone (Fig. 4-3). The triglyceride levels decreased by 58 mg/dl after the change to spironolactone therapy, whereas it decreased by 10 mg/dl during continued chlorthalidone treatment. When the 11 men again received chlorthalidone, their TC levels increased 16 mg/dl, whereas TC levels decreased by 11 mg/dl in men receiving uninterrupted chlorthalidone treatment. These observations suggest that spironolactone may be a preferable alternative to thiazide-type agents as first-line therapy for hypertension because of the more favorable influence on serum lipid concentrations.

References

1. The Joint National Committee on Detection, Evaluation, and Treatment of High Blood Pressure: The 1984 report of the Joint National Committee on Detection, Evaluation, and Treatment of High Blood Pressure. Arch Intern Med 144:1045–1057, May 1984.
2. Weber MA, Drayer JIM, Nakamura DK, Wyle FA: The circadian blood pressure pattern in ambulatory normal subjects. Am J Cardiol 54:115–119, July 1, 1984.
3. Linfors EW, Blessing CL, Neelon FA: Spurious hypertension in the obese patient: effect of sphygmomanometer cuff size on prevalence of hypertension. Arch Intern Med 144:1482–1485, July 1984.
4. Achimastos A, Raison J, Levenson J, Safar M: Adipose tissue cellularity and hemodynamic indexes in obese patients with hypertension. Arch Intern Med 144:265–268, Feb 1984.
5. Blair SN, Goodyear NN, Gibbons LW, Cooper KH: Physical fitness and incidence of hypertension in healthy normotensive men and women. JAMA 252:487–490, July 27, 1984.
6. Cade R, Mars D, Wagemaker H, Zauner C, Packer D, Privette M, Cade M, Peterson J, Hood-Lewis D: Effect of aerobic exercise training on patients with systemic arterial hypertension. Am J Med 77:785–790, Nov 1984.
7. McCarron DA, Morris CD, Henry HJ, Stanton JL: Blood pressure and nutrient intake in the United States. Science 224:1392–1398, June 29, 1984.
8. Erne E, Bolli P, Burgisser E, Buhler FR: Correlation of platelet calcium with blood pressure: effect of antihypertensive therapy. N Engl J Med 310:1084–1088, Apr 26, 1984.
9. Wasserman AG, Katz RJ, Varghese J, Leiboff RH, Bren GG, Schlesselman S, Varma VM, Reba RC, Ross AM: Exercise radionuclide ventriculographic responses in hypertensive patients with chest pain. N Engl J Med 311:1276–1280, Nov 15, 1984.
10. Potter JF, Beevers DG: Pressor effect of alcohol in hypertension. Lancet 1:119–122, Jan 21, 1984.
11. Lebel M, Grose JH, Blais R: Abnormal relation of extracellular fluid volume and exchangeable sodium with systemic arterial pressure in early borderline essential hypertension. Am J Cardiol 54:1267–1271, Dec 1, 1984.
12. Fouad FM, Slominski JM, Tarazi RC: Left ventricular diastolic function in hypertension: relation to left ventricular mass and systolic function. J Am Coll Cardiol 3:1500–1506, June 1984.
13. Shapiro LM, McKenna WJ: Left ventricular hypertrophy: relation of structure to diastolic function in hypertension. Br Heart J 51:637–642, June 1984.
14. Messerli FH, Ventura HO, Elizardi DJ, Dunn FG, Frohlich ED: Hypertension and sudden death: increased ventricular ectopic activity in left ventricular hypertrophy. Am J Med 77:18–22, July 1984.
15. Devereux RB, Drayer JIM, Chien S, Pickering TG, Letcher RL, DeYoung JL, Sealey JE, Laragh JH: Whole blood viscosity as a determinant of cardiac hypertrophy in systemic hypertension. Am J Cardiol 54:592–595, Sept 1, 1984.

16. Nakashima Y, Fouad FM, Tarazi RC: Regression of left ventricular hypertrophy from systemic hypertension by enalapril. Am J Cardiol 53:1044–1049, Apr 1, 1984.

17. Moser M, Rafter J, Gajewski J: Insurance premium reductions: a motivating factor in long-term hypertensive treatment. JAMA 251:756–757, Feb 10, 1984.

18. Stimpel M, Kuffer B, Groth H, Vetter W: Breaking tablets in half. Lancet 1:1299, June 9, 1984.

19. Fujita T, Noda H, Ando K: Sodium susceptibility and potassium effects in young patients with borderline hypertension. Circulation 69:468–476, March 1984.

20. Richards AM, Espiner EA, Maslowski AH, Nicholls MG, Ikram H, Hamilton EJ, Wells JE: Blood-pressure response to moderate sodium restriction and to potassium supplementation in mild essential hypertension. Lancet 1:757–761, Apr 7, 1984.

21. Niarchos AP, Weinstein DL, Laragh JH: Comparison of the effects of diuretic therapy and low sodium intake in isolated systolic hypertension. Am J Med 77:1061–1068, Dec 1984.

22. Maxwell MH, Kushiro T, Dornfeld LP, Tuck ML, Waks AU: BP changes in obese hypertensive subjects during rapid weight loss: comparison of restricted v unchanged salt intake. Arch Intern Med 144:1581–1584, Aug 1984.

23. Luft FC, Sloan RS, Lang CL, Cohen SJ, Fineberg NS, Miller JZ, Weinberger MH: Influence of home monitoring on compliance with a reduced sodium intake diet. Arch Intern Med 144:1963–1965, Oct 1984.

24. Madias JE, Madias NE, Gavras HP: Nonarrhythmogenicity of diuretic-induced hypokalemia: its evidence in patients with uncomplicated hypertension. Arch Intern Med 144:2171–2176, Nov 1984.

25. Papademetriou V, Price M, Johnson E, Smith M, Freis ED: Early changes in plasma and urinary potassium in diuretic-treated patients with systemic hypertension. Am J Cardiol 54:1015–1019, Nov 1, 1984.

26. Little BC, Benson P, Beard RW, Hayworth J, Hall F, Dewhurst J, Priest RG: Treatment of hypertension in pregnancy by relaxation and biofeedback. Lancet 1:865–867, Apr 21, 1984.

27. Vincent HH, Bocmsma F, Veld AJ, Derkx FHM, Wenting GJ, Schalekamp MADH: Effects of selective and nonselective B-agonists on plasma potassium and norepinephrine. J Cardiovasc Pharmacol 6:107–114, 1984.

28. Plotnick GD, Fisher ML, Wohl B, Hamilton JH, Hamilton BP: Improvement in depressed cardiac function in hypertensive patients during pindolol treatment. Am J Med 76:25–30, Jan 1984.

29. Cressman MD, Vidt DG, Gifford RW Jr, Moore WS, Wilson DJ: Intravenous labetalol in the management of severe hypertension and hypertensive emergencies. Am Heart J 107:980–985, May 1984.

30. Rotmensch HH, Rocci ML, Vlasses PH, Swanson BN, Fedder IL, Soyka L, Ferguson RK: Bucindolol, a beta-adrenoceptor blocker with vasodilatory action: its effect in systemic hypertension. Am J Cardiol 54:353–356, Aug 1, 1984.

31. Freis ED: Veterans Administration cooperative study on nadolol as monotherapy and in combination with a diuretic. Am Heart J 108:1087–1091, Oct 1984.

32. Frohlich ED, Cooper RA, Lewis EJ: Review of the overall experience of captopril in hypertension. Arch Intern Med 144:1441–1444, July 1984.

33. Veterans Administration Cooperative Study Group on Antihypertensive Agents: Low-dose captopril for the treatment of mild to moderate hypertension: I. Results of a 14-week trial. Arch Intern Med 144:1947–1953, Oct 1984.

34. Finnerty FA: Step-down treatment of mild systemic hypertension. Am J Cardiol 53:1304–1307, May 1984.

35. Weber MA, Brewer DD, Drayer JIM, Lipson JL: Transdermal continuous antihypertensive therapy. Lancet 1:9–11, Jan 7, 1984.

36. Weber MA, Drayer JIM, McMahon G, Hamburger R, Shah AR, Kirk LN: Transdermal administration of clonidine for treatment of high BP. Arch Intern Med 144:1211–1213, June 1984.

37. Farsang C, Kapocsi J, Vajda L, Varga K, Malisak Z, Fekete M, Kunos G: Reversal by naloxone of the antihypertensive action of clonidine: involvement of the sympathetic nervous system. Circulation 69:461–467, March 1984.

38. Green S, Zawada ET, Muakkassa W, Johnson M, MacKenzie T, McClanahan M, Graybill A, Goldman M: Effect of clonidine therapy on renal hemodynamics in renal transplant hypertension. Arch Intern Med 144:1205–1208, June 1984.
39. Bauer JH, Jones LB, Gaddy P: Effects of prazosin therapy on BP, renal function, and body fluid composition. Arch Intern Med 144:1196–1200, June 1984.
40. Guazzi MD, Cipolla C, Della Bella P, Fabbiocchi F, Montorsi P, Sganzerla P: Disparate unloading efficacy of the calcium channel blockers, verapamil and nifedipine, on the failing hypertensive left ventricle. Am Heart J 108:116–123, July 1984.
41. Weber MA, Drayer JIM: Single-agent and combination therapy of essential hypertension. Am Heart J 108:311–316, Aug 1984.
42. Weinstein M, Hilewitz H, Rogel S: The effect of single-dose methyldopa and diuretic on BP and left ventricular mass. Arch Intern Med 144:1629–1632, Aug 1984.
43. Hornung RS, Jones RI, Gould BA, Sonecha T, Raftery EB: Propranolol versus verapamil for the treatment of essential hypertension. Am Heart J 108:554–560, Sept 1984.
44. Guazzi MD, De Cesare N, Galli C, Salvioni A, Tramontana C, Tamborini G, Bartorelli A: Calcium-channel blockade with nifedipine and angiotensin converting-enzyme inhibition with captopril in the therapy of patients with severe primary hypertension. Circulation 70:279–284, Aug 1984.
45. Niarchos AP, Laragh JH: Renin dependency of blood pressure in isolated systolic hypertension. Am J Med 77:407–414, Sept 1984.
46. Helgeland A, Leren P, Foss O, Hjermann I, Holme I, Lund-Larsen PG: Serum glucose level during long-term observation of treated and untreated men with mild hypertension: the Oslo Study. Am J Med 76:802–805, May 1984.
47. Ames RP, Peacock PB: Serum cholesterol during treatment of hypertension with diuretic drugs. Arch Intern Med 144:719–724, Apr 1984.

5

Valvular Heart Disease

MITRAL REGURGITATION

Value of pulmonary arterial V wave

Although V waves recorded in the PA wedge and LA positions have been hemodynamic indicators of MR, the physiologic significance and clinical implications of an early diastolic V wave in the PA have not been adequately defined. Grose and colleagues[1] from New York City investigated the PA early diastolic V wave in patients and experimental animals with MR. V waves exceeding systolic pressure in the PA were recorded in the pulmonary trunk with micromanometer catheters both in patients and in animals, eliminating the possibility of catheter artifact. In experimental preparations, aortic closure preceded pulmonic closure by 33 ± 12 ms at baseline. With the creation of acute MR, a PA V wave occurred in 6 of 8 animals. Early pulmonic valve closure occurred only in 6 animals with a PA V wave, and pulmonic closure preceded aortic closure by 28 ± 7 ms during MR. Of 70 patients with severe MR at cardiac catheterization, 14 had a PA V wave. In 5 patients recordings with micromanometer catheters were made and early pulmonic closure also was observed in 4 of those patients who had PA V waves at rest or on provocation. The patients with PA V waves had a more acute onset of symptoms, shorter duration of MR, higher PA wedge V waves, and lower PA resistances than patients without them and were more likely to have nonrheumatic MR. Thus, the recording of PA V waves provides hemodynamic and diagnostic information in patients with MR.

Reconstruction operation

Recently several investigators have reopened the question as to the role of the mitral chordae papillary muscle tethering apparatus as it affects postoperative LV performance after mitral valve surgery. Bonchek and associates[2] from Milwaukee, Wisconsin, analyzed preoperative and postoperative catheterization data in 10 of 18 patients who underwent mitral reconstruction with preservation of the native valves. They found a significant decrease in LV end-diastolic volume index (from $143 \pm 39-84 \pm 21$ ml/M^2) and end-systolic volume index (from $50 \pm 24-32 \pm 12$ ml/M^2) with no significant change in EF (0.66 ± 0.1 -vs- 0.62 ± 0.1). They suggested that those findings contrast with other studies reported in comparable patients who had MVR with no improvement in volume indices and a decline in EF postoperatively. Bonchek and associates considered that some LV dysfunction observed after MVR may be due simply to excision of the native valve and its tethering apparatus. Mitral repair retained the tethering effect and may thus prevent postoperative LV dilation. Others have suggested that retaining the mitral leaflet chordae papillary muscle complex when replacing the valve also results in less depression of LV performance than does routine mitral valve resection when replacing the valve. Bonchek and associates have provided useful information regarding preservation of LV function in those patients with mitral valve repair; however, the mean EF preoperatively in the 10 patients reported was normal (0.66 ± 0.1). It is not this group in which EF decreases postoperatively. Rather it is in that group with a preoperative EF <0.40 in whom postoperatively further depression of LV function is seen. Thus, additional evaluation of patients having mitral repair with lower preoperative EF is needed to make a convincing argument that saving the mitral tethering apparatus preserves LV function.

Predictors of success of mitral valve replacement

Zile and associates[3] from Boston, Massachusetts, studied 20 patients with chronic MR to determine the effect of MVR on LV volume, mass, function, and clinical symptoms. Pre- and postoperative echo demonstrated that LV dimension at end-diastole was reduced to normal postoperatively in 16 patients and was unchanged in 4. Those patients with a reduction in LV end-diastolic diameter also had a marked reduction in LV mass and decrease in clinical symptoms; however, no change in LV mass was found in the patients who did not change their LV end-diastolic diameter and all 4 remained symptomatic despite medical therapy. The echo data revealed that when LV dimension at end-systole exceeded 2.6 cm/M^2, fractional shortening was $<31\%$, or end-systolic wall stress exceeded 195 mmHg postoperative improvement was not likely to occur.

MITRAL VALVE PROLAPSE

Echo observations

To assess the reliability of M-mode echo patterns of MVP in detection of morphologic evidence of MVP, Waller and associates[4] from Bethesda, Mary-

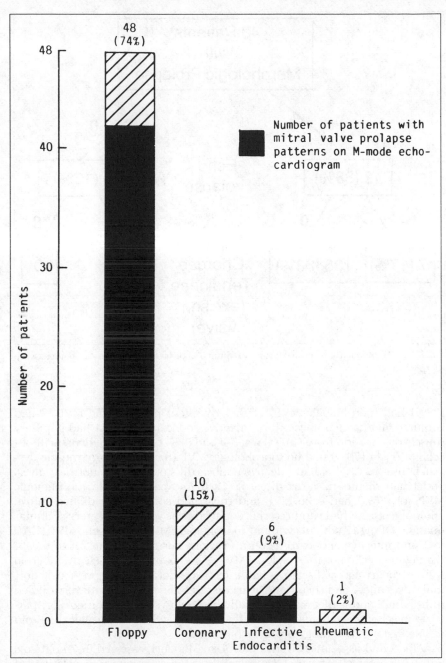

Fig. 5-1. The etiology of isolated pure MR and number of patients and frequency of echo MVP in the 65 patients.

land, studied operatively excised mitral valves and corresponding M-mode echoes from 65 patients with clinically isolated chronic, severe pure MR (Fig. 5-1). Of the 65 patients, 45 (69%) had echo MVP (either holosystolic or mid to late systolic prolapse patterns on preoperative M-mode echoes) and 42

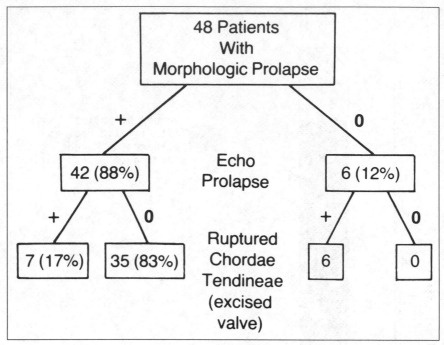

Fig. 5-2. The frequency of echo MVP and ruptured chordae tendineae in the patients with morphologic MVP.

(93%) had morphologic MVP; of the 3 without morphologic MVP, 2 had ruptured chordae tendineae from infective endocarditis and 1 had papillary muscle dysfunction from CAD (Figs. 5-2 and 5-3). Of the 20 patients without echo MVP, 14 (70%) had no morphologic MVP (9 had papillary muscle dysfunction from CAD, 4 had infective endocarditis on previous normal valves, and 1 had rheumatic heart disease). Of the 48 patients with morphologic MVP, 42 (88%) had echo MVP and most had considerably dilated mitral anuli; the other 6 had ruptured chordae tendineae with less degrees of anular dilation. Of the 17 patients without morphologic MVP, 3 had echo MVP (CAD in 1 and infective endocarditis on a previous normal valve in 2); of the 14 with neither echo nor morphologic MVP, 9 had papillary muscle dysfunction from coronary artery disease, 4 had infective endocarditis on previously normal valves and 1 had rheumatic heart disease. The patients with very dilated mitral anuli and leaflet areas generally had holosystolic (hammocking) patterns on echo; the patients with small anuli and leaflet areas usually had mid to late systolic (buckling) prolapse patterns.

Alpert and associates[5] from Columbia, Missouri, assessed in 70 patients with MVP and in 100 normal control subjects the sensitivity and specificity of previously described 2-D echo signs of MVP. Specificity and individual signs were uniformly high, ranging from 88% for excessive motion of the posterior mitral ring to 100% for several signs, including systolic arching in the parasternal long-axis view, excessive posterior coaptation, and diastolic doming of the anterior mitral leaflet. Sensitivity of individual signs was low to moderate, ranging from 1% for whiplike motion of both mitral leaflets to 70% for

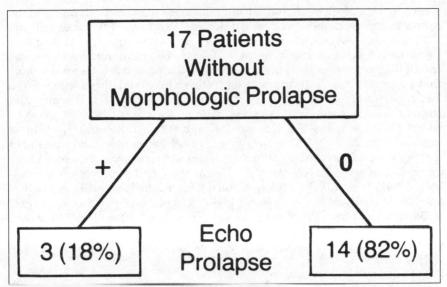

Fig. 5-3. The frequency of echo MVP among the patients without morphologic MVP. Of the 3 patients with echo MVP, 1 had papillary muscle dysfunction from coronary heart disease and 2 had healed infective endocarditis on a previously normal mitral valve. Of the 14 patients without echo MVP, 9 had MR from coronary heart disease, 9 had healed infective endocarditis on previously normal valves, and 1 patient had rheumatic heart disease.

excessive posterior coaptation of the mitral leaflets in the apical 4-chamber view. The highest sensitivity value (87%) was associated with the presence of systolic arching of 1 or both mitral leaflets in the parasternal long-axis view or systolic bowing of 1 or both mitral leaflets in the apical 4-chamber view or excessive posterior coaptation of the mitral leaflets or a combination. This increase in sensitivity was achieved without sacrificing specificity (97%). Thus, the individual 2-D echo signs tested possess uniformly high specificity, but only low to moderate sensitivity; however, sensitivity can be markedly enhanced without sacrificing specificity by using selected combinations of echo signs.

Arvan and Tunick[6] from Pittsburgh, Pennsylvania, examined the relation between the valvular abnormalities and auscultatory findings of patients with MVP. Forty patients with typical auscultatory and 2-D echo findings were studied. Eleven of 14 patients with anterior leaflet MVP (group I) had mid to late systolic clicks without murmurs of MR, whereas 8 of 9 patients with posterior MVP (group II) and 13 of 17 patients with combined anterior and posterior MVP (group III) had murmurs of MR. In each subgroup the mitral anulus size was greater than a control group (group I, 3.8 ± 0.1 cm, p < 0.025; group II, 3.9 ± 0.1 cm, p < 0.005; group III, 4.2 ± 0.2 cm, p < 0.001; and control, 3.4 ± 0.1 cm), but the largest anulus was present in patients with combined MVP. As demonstrated by 2D echo, prolapse of a single mitral leaflet may occur in many instances of MVP. Murmurs of MR occur frequently when the posterior mitral leaflet alone prolapses, whereas isolated clicks are found with anterior MVP.

Two-D echo was performed in 86 consecutive patients with MVP and in 25 normal subjects by Chandraratna and associates[7] from Los Angeles, California. In normal subjects, mitral leaflet thickness was 3.5 ± 0.8 mm and the mitral leaflet thickness/aortic wall thickness ratio was 1.0 ± 2.0. Patients with MVP were separated into 2 groups: those with normal mitral thickness (≤mean + 2 SD observed in normal subjects, i.e., ≤5.1 mm) and normal mitral thickness/aortic wall thickness ratio (≤mean + 2 SD observed in normal subjects, i.e., ≤1.4; group I) and others in whom these values were increased (group II). In group I, mitral thickness was 3.6 ± 0.6 mm and mitral thickness/aortic wall thickness ratio was 1.1 ± 0.1, and in group II, mitral thickness was 8.8 ± 1.2 mm and mitral thickness/aortic wall thickness ratio was 2.2 ± 0.5. The only significant cardiovascular abnormalities in group I were MR in 2 patients and tricuspid valve prolapse in 1 patient. In group II, 7 patients had clinically significant MR, 8 had aortic root abnormalities, 4 had tricuspid valve prolapse, and 6 had the Marfan syndrome. Cardiovascular abnormalities were present in 60% (18 of 30) of patients in group II and in 6% (3 of 56) of patients in group I (p < 0.001). Two-D echo enabled the identification of a subset of patients with MVP who had thickened mitral leaflets. These patients had an increased incidence of cardiovascular abnormalities.

Arrhythmias and/or electrophysiologic studies

Kavey and associates[8] from Syracuse, New York, studied 103 consecutive children with MVP confirmed by echo. Patients ranged in age from 6–18 years and were evaluated with treadmill exercise and ambulatory ECG. Findings were compared with 50 normal children without clinical ECG or echo evidence of heart disease. For MVP patients, 16 of 103 had VPC with exercise and 39 of 103 VPC on ambulatory ECG. High grade ventricular ectopic activity was recorded in 4 patients with MVP during exercise and in 8 with ambulatory ECG. In contrast, no control patient had VPC with exercise and only 4 of 50 had rare uniform VPC on ambulatory ECGs. Neither physical examination, standard ECG results, nor symptoms correlated with VPC in MVP patients. Although MVP is usually a benign condition in children, this study indicates a significant incidence of ventricular ectopic activity that occurred in 19% of the patients studied with exercise and ambulatory ECG. The study points to the need for detailed investigation in any patient with MVP who presents with even suggestive evidence of arrhythmia.

To assess the contribution of bias in subject selection to the prevalence of arrhythmias in patients with MVP, Kramer and associates[9] from New York City and Framingham, Massachusetts, compared ambulatory arrhythmias in 63 patients with MVP and 28 symptom-matched control subjects. All subjects were in sinus rhythm. Mean 24-hour heart rate of the prolapse population was lower than that of the control group (76 -vs- 82 beats/min). Mean atrial premature complex (APC) density per 1,000 beats (0.9 -vs- 0.7 for patients with MVP and control subjects, respectively) and mean VPC density per 1,000 total beats (1.2 -vs- 1.5) did not differ between groups (Table 5-1). Small differences between groups in APC and VPC complexity did not reach statistical significance. Our findings suggest that, compared with similarly symptomatic controls, patients with MVP do not have as high an excess prevalence of arrhythmias as previously believed. This article was followed by an editorial by Alpert[10] from Worcester, Massachusetts.

TABLE 5-1. *Comparative prevalence of arrhythmias in MVP and control groups.* *
Reproduced with permission from Kramer et al.[9]

	APCs (%)	PAT (%)	VPC (%)	COMPLEX VPC (%*)
Present study				
MVP (n, 63)	81	32	63	43
Control (n, 28)	82	18	50	32
Savage et al				
MVP (n, 61)	90	24	89	56
Control (n, 176)	89	15	68	42
DeMaria et al				
MVP (n, 31)	35	3	68	52
Control (n, 40)	10	0	25	8
Winkle et al				
MVP (n, 24)	63	29	75	50
Campbell et al				
MVP (n, 20)		10	80	75

*Definitions of "complex VPC" vary among studies. For the present study, complex VPC are defined as Lown grades 3 or higher (other studies include frequent VPC of Lown grade 2).
PAT = paroxysmal atrial tachycardia.

Morady and associates[11] from San Francisco, California, performed programmed ventricular stimulation with 3 extrastimuli in 36 patients with MVP. Among 11 patients without transient cerebral symptoms, none had inducible VT or VF whether or not sustained VT or VPC were present during ambulatory ECG recordings. These patients remained well without antiarrhythmic drug therapy for 6–57 months (mean, 23) of follow-up. Two patients with recurrent unexplained syncope and no documented ventricular arrhythmia during ECG monitoring also had no inducible VT or VF. Among 20 patients with syncope or presyncope and documented nonsustained VT or VPC during ECG monitoring, polymorphic nonsustained VT was induced in 8, sustained unimorphic VT in 2, and VF in 3. In 1 patient who had inducible polymorphic nonsustained VT, ECG monitoring during syncope showed sinus rhythm. Among 3 patients with a history of sustained VT or VF, unimorphic VT was induced in each. Patients with MVP who have asymptomatic ventricular ectopic activity and no inducible VT may have a benign prognosis without treatment. In patients who have transient cerebral symptoms and documented nonsustained VT or VPC, VT or VF is inducible in 65%, most often polymorphic VT. It is unclear in which patients this finding is clinically significant and in which it is a nonspecific response to programmed stimulation.

Ware and associates[12] from Houston, Texas, and Chicago, Illinois, examined the site of AV block in 60 patients with MVP by electrophysiologic study: 49 had documented arrhythmias and 28 had syncope. Eight patients had spontaneous second- or third-degree AV block and 10 had chronic BBB. Electrophysiologic study revealed abnormal sinus node function in 8 patients, prolonged HV interval in 10, intra-His delay in 9, and functional BBB in 15. Dual AV nodal pathways were demonstrated in 24 patients. Comparison with 101 similarly symptomatic patients without MVP revealed a greater prevalence of dual AV nodal pathways in the MVP patients. Infranodal conduction abnormalities and dual AV nodal pathways are frequently revealed by electrophysiologic testing in symptomatic patients with MVP.

Infective endocarditis prophylaxis

Antimicrobial prophylaxis against infective endocarditis in patients with MVP is controversial. The benefits and risk of prophylactic practice for these patients has been analyzed on the basis of published data and responses to a questionnaire survey of leading authorities on infective endocarditis by Bor and Himmelstein[13] from Cambridge and Boston, Massachusetts. Among 10 million patients with MVP undergoing a dental procedure, an estimated 47 nonfatal cases and 2 fatal cases of infective endocarditis would occur if no prophylaxis were given, 5 cases of infective endocarditis and 175 deaths due to drug reactions would occur if all patients were given prophylaxis with a penicillin, and 12 nonfatal cases and 1 fatal case of infective endocarditis would be expected if a policy of prophylaxis with erythromycin were adopted. Even using assumptions most favorable to the penicillin regimen, this analysis predicts that no prophylaxis and penicillin prophylaxis would result in a similar number of deaths. No prophylaxis or prophylaxis with erythromycin appears preferable to prophylaxis with a penicillin.

MITRAL STENOSIS

Relation of level of total serum cholesterol to amount of calcific deposits in stenotic mitral valves

Mitral stenosis has been observed in persons residing in every continent and in every country on earth. In persons with MS living in Western countries, calcific deposits are usually found in stenotic mitral valves, and often, these deposits are quite heavy. In persons with MS living in undeveloped countries, in contrast, calcific deposits are usually not found in stenotic mitral valves and, when present, they are usually small. A major measurable difference between persons residing in developed Western countries and those residing in undeveloped countries is the serum total cholesterol (TC) level. Day and Roberts[14] from Bethesda, Maryland, theorized that persons with calcific deposits, and particularly those with heavy deposits in stenotic mitral valves, would have higher TC levels than persons with MS and absent or small calcific deposits. To try to substantiate this thesis, they analyzed 155 patients with rheumatic MS in whom the operatively excised mitral valve was x-rayed to determine the presence of and the extent of calcific deposits and the preoperative level of serum TC. The amount of mitral calcium was graded 0 to 4 + , and the average TC for each of the 5 groups was: 0 deposits, 21 patients (14%; TC, 188 mg/dl); 1 +, 50 patients (32%; TC, 196 mg/dl); 2 +, 22 patients 14%; TC, 198 mg/dl); 3 +, 37 patients (24%; TC, 205 mg/dl); 4 +, 25 patients (16%; TC, 184 mg/dl) (Fig. 5-4). These average values of TC and

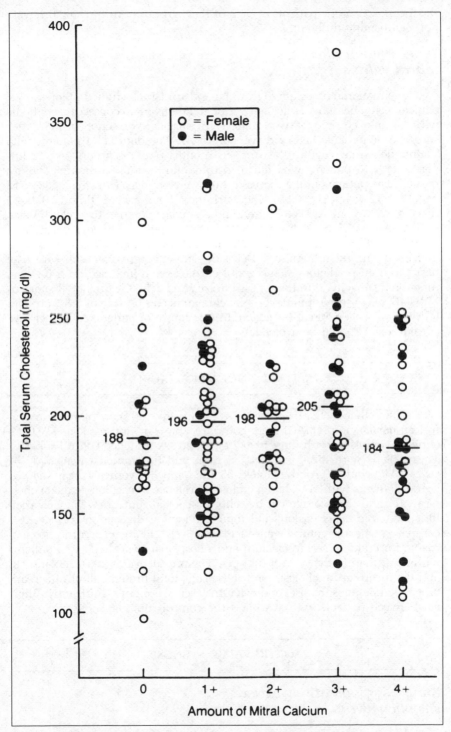

Fig. 5-4. Relation of total serum cholesterol level to the amount of calcific deposits in the stenotic mitral valves of the 155 patients.

the mean ages of the patients in each of the 5 groups of mitral calcium were not significantly different.

Sinus rhythm after mitral valve surgery

Flugelman and associates[15] from Jerusalem, Israel, studied preoperative, clinical, echo, hemodynamic, and surgical data from 40 consecutive patients with MS and chronic AF who underwent surgical correction of MS. After surgery, the patients had cardioversion of AF. The data of 24 patients who maintained sinus rhythm (SR) for >3 months (success group) were compared with 16 patients who failed to maintain SR for >3 months (failure group). The patients in the success group were younger (mean age, 38 ± 12 -vs- 47 ± 13 years, p < 0.05), had symptoms for a shorter time (3.0 ± 4.3 -vs- 6.4 ± 5.0 years, p < 0.02), and had a smaller preoperative echo LA size (4.9 ± 0.9 -vs- 5.5 ± 1.0 cm, p < 0.03). The correlation between duration of SR after cardioversion (range, 0–12 months) and the preoperative data were examined with the use of the "all-possible-subsets-regression" software. The best subset of predictors of successful cardioversion included echo LA size, functional capacity, duration of symptoms, and echo LV fractional shortening. Patients with symptoms for >3 years and echo LA size of >5.2 cm had low rate of successful cardioversion; in this subset of patients, postoperative cardioversion should be avoided.

MITRAL ANULAR CALCIUM

Certain clinical characteristics of 107 patients <60 years of age with mitral anular calcium (MAC) were compared by Nair and associates[16] from Omaha, Nebraska, with those of 107 age- and sex-matched control subjects. The patients with MAC included 55 men and 52 women (mean age, 51 years). The control group included 55 men and 52 women (mean age, 51 years). Patients with MAC had a higher prevalence of cardiomegaly on chest x-ray, LA and LV enlargement by echo, precordial murmurs, diabetes mellitus, systemic hypertension, and total conduction defects on surface ECG compared with the control subjects (Table 5-2). The mean serum phosphorus and product of serum calcium and phosphorus were higher in patients with MAC than in the control subjects. The prevalence of CAD, AS, and HC and the mean serum cholesterol, triglyceride, total protein, albumin, creatinine, alkaline phosphatase, and calcium levels were not significantly different between patients with MAC and the control subjects.

AORTIC VALVE STENOSIS

Analysis of operatively excised stenotic valves

Subramanian and associates[17] from Rochester, Minnesota, reviewed gross morphologic features in 374 operatively excised stenotic aortic valves in pa-

TABLE 5-2. *Clinical data of patients younger than 60 years with mitral anular calcification and the control group*

	PATIENTS WITH MAC		CONTROL PATIENTS	
	N	%	N	%
Total	107		107	
Cardiomegaly on chest x-ray	68	64*	5	5
Echo chamber size				
LA enlargement	76	71*	6	6
LV enlargement	72	67*	2	2
Precordial murmurs	27	25*	2	2
Diabetes mellitus	29	27*	6	6
Systemic hypertension	39	36†	23	22
CAD	22	21	18	17
Aortic stenosis	1	1	0	0
HC	3	3	2	2
Total conduction defects	43	40*	13	12
Sinoatrial disease	12	11†	4	4
AV block	15	14	7	7
BBB, left anterior hemiblock, or intraventricular conduction defect	26	24*	5	5
Serum phosphorus (mg/dl)	3.75§		3.39	
Product of serum calcium and phosphorus	34.7§		31.2	

* p < 0.0001.
† p < 0.025.
‡ p < 0.05.
§ p < 0.0025. Data in 89 patients with MAC and 89 age- and sex-matched controls.

tients who had AVR at the Mayo Clinic during the years 1965, 1970, 1975, and 1980. A congenitally bicuspid aortic valve was found in 46% of the patients. In the remainder, AS was produced by postinflammatory fibrocalcific disease (including rheumatic disease) in 35%, by degenerative calcium of an aging valve in 10%, and by calcium of a congenitally unicommissural valve in 6%. The cause of AS was indeterminate in 4%. Calcium deposits tended to occur more extensively and at a younger age in men than in women. It tended to produce AS and to necessitate AVR earliest in patients with unicommissural valves (mean age, 48 years), later in those with bicuspid or postinflammatory valves (mean age, 59 and 60 years) and latest in those with degenerative AS (mean age, 72 years). The relative incidence of postinflammatory AS remained unchanged from 1965 to 1980, despite the steadily decreasing incidence of acute rheumatic fever reported in western countries during that period. In 36 (28% of the 130 patients with postinflammatory AS), the mitral valve was either stenotic (15 patients) or regurgitant (11 patients) or both stenotic and regurgitant (10 patients). The mitral valve was operatively replaced in 25 of these 36 patients and was considered postinflammatory in each. The mitral valve had also been replaced in 6 patients with noninflammatory AS. Four patients with degenerative AS had MR (2 floppy mitral valves and 2 of indeterminant type). One patient had a stenotic congenitally bicuspid aortic valve and a regurgitant mitral valve of indeterminant type, and 1 patient with a stenotic congenitally unicommissural aortic valve had a regurgitant floppy mitral valve.

Detecting valvular calcium

Dancy and associates[18] from London, England, estimated the density of aortic valve calcific deposits using cinefluoroscopy and M-mode echo in 86 patients with AS, all >30 years of age and AR, if present, was hemodynamically insignificant. None of the 86 patients had either clinical or echo evidence of mitral valve disease. The morphology of the aortic valve was known in 55 of the 86 patients: in 49 the aortic valve was bicuspid and in 5 it was tricuspid. Cinefluoroscopy estimates of aortic valve calcific deposits correlated well with measured peak systolic pressure gradient between left ventricle and aorta. The echo results were less accurate. Echo, however, gave accurate information about the distribution of calcium within the cusps, but this was not of value in predicting the severity of obstruction. Thus, the amount of calcium in stenotic aortic valves can be assessed by simple cinefluoroscopy, and this is a useful guide to the severity of the AS in persons >30 years of age.

Echo (including Doppler) determination of severity

Berger and associates[19] from New York City evaluated 24 patients with suspected AS by continuous wave Doppler ultrasound. Twenty normal subjects served as controls. Maximal velocity measurements in the ascending aorta ranged from 3.0–5.8 m/s (mean, 4.34 ± 0.65) in patients with AS compared with 1.0–1.6 m/s (mean, 1.28 ± 0.16) in normal controls. Peak pressure gradient across the aortic valve was calculated from the maximal velocity using the Bernoulli equation in patients with suspected AS and the results correlated well with peak aortic valve gradients obtained at cardiac catheterization. In 20 of the 24 patients with suspected AS, the peak Doppler gradient was within 25% of the gradient at cardiac catheterization. In 3 patients, the Doppler study underestimated the gradient by slightly >25%, but still identified the presence of significant AS. The Doppler technique failed to identify critical AS in only 1 patient. Overestimation of the gradient by Doppler measurement did not occur in any patient. Thus, these data suggest that continuous wave Doppler ultrasound provides a reliable estimate of the valvular gradient in many patients with AS.

To determine if a combination of noninvasive variables would be useful in the prediction of the severity of isolated AS, 53 patients (mean age, 63 ± 11 years) were evaluated by Nakamura and associates[20] from Palo Alto, California, using the following criteria: aortic valve calcium in the plain chest x-ray film; LV hypertrophy by ECG and M-mode echo; faint or absent aortic closure sound; timing of the peak of the systolic murmur; half-rise time (T time) of the carotid pulse; and ejection time index. A numeric scoring system and a logistic regression model employing these variables were developed. The total maximum score was 16 points. Sensitivity and specificity for each variable were determined. Patients with clinically evident CAD and significant AR were excluded. All patients underwent hemodynamic studies and coronary arteriography. Thirty-two patients had severe AS (aortic valve area, <0.75 cm²) and 21 had mild to moderate AS (aortic valve area >0.75 cm²). Significant CAD (≥50% reduction in luminal diameter) was present in 55% of patients. A total score of ≥5 occurred in 59% (19 of 32) of patients with severe AS compared with 5% (1 of 21) of patients with mild AS. The presence of subclinical CAD moderately reduced the accuracy of the scoring system, principally by its effect on the timing of the systolic murmur and the ejection time. Combining the scoring system with the presence or absence of symptoms improved the identification of severe AS in patients with a low score. It was concluded that a point scoring system and a logistic regression model employing 6 noninvasive variables combined with the clinical evaluation of symptoms provides a useful method of assessing the severity of isolated AS in an older age population.

Warth and colleagues[21] from Boston, Massachusetts, utilized Doppler ultrasound to obtain direct measurements of blood velocity in cardiac chambers and applied this technique to study 16 patients with suspected AS after cardiac catheterization. Aortic valve area (AVA) was calculated with the equation:

$$AVA = CO/(SEP \times \text{mean velocity})$$

where CO is cardiac output measured by thermodilution and SEP is the systolic ejection period derived from the Doppler tracings. The resulting value was compared with valve area calculated from cardiac catheterization and an excellent correlation was noted. This study demonstrated that Doppler ultrasound can be used to measure accurately aortic valve area without the need for left-sided heart catheterization. The investigators pointed out that a limitation is the possible inability to obtain adequate Doppler recordings of the high velocity aortic jet and, as with the Gorlin equation, the new method will overestimate the severity of AS in the presence of AR.

Conduction defects and electrophysiologic studies

Nair and associates[22] from Omaha, Nebraska, investigated the prevalence of conduction defects in 51 patients >60 years old with AS who had AVR. Of the 51 patients, 31 (61%) had associated mitral anular calcium (MAC). The mean age and prevalence of CAD, systemic hypertension, and diabetes mellitus were similar in both groups. The prevalence of conduction defects (AV block, sinoatrial disease, BBB, left anterior hemiblock, or intraventricular conduction defect) was 18 of 31 (58%) in patients with MAC and 5 of 20 (25%) in patients without MAC. Thus, patients >60 years of age with AS have a high prevalence of MAC and the prevalence of conduction defects is higher in patients >60 years with combined AS and MAC than in patients with AS without MAC.

Rasmussen and associates[23] from Aarhus, Denmark, performed intracardiac electrography and 24-hour ambulatory ECG monitoring in 20 patients with isolated AS unassociated with signs of AR and without involvement of other cardiac valves. The peak systolic pressure gradient between left ventricle and systemic artery ranged from 37–128 mmHg (mean, 86). Intracardiac ECG showed impaired sinus node function in 5 patients and a prolonged (≥50 ms) HV interval in 11 patients but there was no difference in the findings of 13 patients with syncope and in 7 without. Ambulatory monitoring showed short pauses in 3 patients and brief episodes of tachycardia in 4, but there was no difference in the findings of patients with and without syncope. The HV interval correlated inversely with the LV EF, whereas no correlation was found between the HV interval and the pressure gradient. Nine patients were reevaluated 15 months after AVR and no change was found in sinus node function, but the HV interval had increased by 7.8 ms. The investigators concluded that in AS in patients aged ≥40 years (mean, 61) neither bradycardia nor tachycardia is shown to be a frequent cause of syncope, a prolonged HV interval is a frequent finding, and further prolongation occurs after AVR. Contractility and conductivity appear to deteriorate in parallel. Coronary angiography was performed in 10 of their 20 patients, all of whom had chest pain, and in 5 narrowing >50% in diameter was found in ≥1 coronary artery.

Frequency of associated coronary arterial narrowing

Exadactylos and associates[24] from London, England, investigated the prevalence of significant (>50% diameter reduction) CAD among 88 consecutive patients with AS requiring AVR. Patients with multiple valve disease, those <35 years of age, those with peak systolic pressure gradients across the aortic valve of <40 mmHg, those with AR more than grade 1/4 from aortic root aortogram and those in whom it was not possible to intubate the coronary arteries were excluded. Twenty-two patients (25%) had significant CAD. Nineteen (45% of 42 patients) with typical angina had CAD; 3 (15% of 20 patients) with atypical chest pain had CAD; and none of 26 patients free of chest pain had significant CAD. Risk factors for CAD were equally distributed among patients with and without significant CAD. The investigators concluded that patients with AS who are free of chest pain did not require routine coronary angiography before AVR. (I [WCR] disagree with that recommendation.)

AORTIC REGURGITATION

Analysis of operatively excised, purely regurgitant valves

Olson and associates[25] from Rochester, Minnesota, reviewed operatively excised aortic valves in 225 patients who had undergone AVR during 4 years (1965, 1970, 1975, and 1980) for pure AR. The 4 most common causes of AR were postinflammatory disease (46%), aortic root dilation (21%), incomplete closure of a congenitally bicuspid aortic valve (20%), and infective endocarditis (9%). Other causes included AR associated with VSD (2%), quadricuspid aortic valve (1%), and undetermined etiology (1%). The mean age of patients at AVR was about 50 years for all etiologies except VSD. The incidence of postinflammatory cause before 1980 was 51% and during 1980, 29%; aortic root dilation was the cause in 17% of patients before 1980 and 37% in 1980. The investigators found aortic root dilation to be the most common cause of pure AR in their patients undergoing AVR. Of interest to me (WCR) was that 54 of the operatively excised aortic valves were bicuspid and the AR resulted entirely from the bicuspid state of the valve in 45 patients; it was secondary to involvement by infective endocarditis in the other 9. The incompetence of the bicuspid valve unassociated with infection was associated with aortic root dilation in 14 patients (31%) of the 45 without infection and with dissection of the ascending aorta in 3 (7%). In the remaining 28 patients (62%), AR apparently occurred primarily because of cuspal prolapse. Of the 21 patients with AR secondary to infective endocarditis, 9 (43%) involved congenitally bicuspid aortic valves. Of the 225 patients, 80 (36%) also underwent MVR at the same time that they underwent AVR. Postinflammatory changes were observed in both the aortic and mitral valves in 69 (86%) of these 80 cases. The mitral valve was stenotic in 11 (16%), regurgitant in 19 (28%), and both in 39 (57%). In each of the remaining 11 patients, the mitral valve was regurgitant. Floppy mitral leaflets were observed in 4 patients with aortic root dilation and in 5 patients with congenitally bicuspid aortic valves. Among the 30 patients in whom the aortic and mitral valves were both excised for pure regurgitation, 19 (63%) were postinflammatory and 9 (30%) were floppy with either bicuspid aortic valves or aortic root dilation.

Prevalence of purely regurgitant bicuspid valves

Although aortic valve prolapse (AVP) has been suggested as a cause of AR in patients with bicuspid aortic valve, neither the frequency of AVP nor its relation to AR in this setting has been defined. To assess these relations, Stewart and associates[26] from Boston, Massachusetts, studied 64 patients with bicuspid aortic valves diagnosed by 2-D echo and in 20 normal subjects, similarly distributed according to age and sex. The presence and degree of AVP were defined using 3 quantitative terms: aortic valve prolapse distance (AVPD), area (AVPA), and volume (AVPV). Each was corrected (c) for patient size with reference to the diameter of the aorta at the level of insertion of the valve cusps. In normal subjects, the $AVPD_c$ averaged 0.09 ± 0.06 cm (range, 0–0.16) and the $AVPA_c$ averaged 0.08 ± 0.06 cm (range, 0–0.15). In patients with bicuspid aortic valves, the $AVPD_c$ averaged 0.26 ± 0.10 (range, 0.11–0.59; p = 0.00005 -vs- normal subjects), whereas the $AVPA_c$ averaged 0.35 ± 0.17 cm (range, 0.05–0.90; p = 0.00005 -vs- normal subjects). When the $AVPD_c$ criteria were used, 81% of the bicuspid valves were abnormal; when the $AVPA_c$ criteria were used, 87% were abnormal. The degree of prolapse defined by the $AVPV_c$, which considers both cusp area and degree of apical displacement, was significantly greater for patients with bicuspid aortic valve with clinical AR than for those without. However, because of the overlap between groups, there was no point at which this measure uniquely separated patients with and without AR. There was no relation between the degree of prolapse and either age or degree of cusp asymmetry. The degree of AVP was greater in bicuspid valves with vertical -vs- those with horizontal commissures. Therefore AVP occurs often in patients with bicuspid aortic valves; however, neither the presence nor the degree of AVP can be used to predict clinical AR.

Associated with HLA-B27 disease

Bergfeldt and associates[27] from Huddinge, Sweden, performed electrophysiologic studies in 12 patients with spontaneous complete heart block and HLA-B27 associated disease, of whom 8 had ankylosing spondylitis, 10 had supra-His second- or third-degree AV block, and 1 had infra-His block. One patient with narrow QRS complexes during complete heart block 3 months earlier had normal findings. Three patients also had sinus node malfunction and 6 had fascicular or BBB. In HLA-B27 associated disease, the AV block seems to be preferentially located in the AV node, although the conduction system may be widely affected. The findings in this study indicate a further cause of high degree AV block with a predominately supra-His location in addition to inferior AMI, digitalis intoxication, and heart block.

Determining severity by Doppler echo

Veyrat and colleagues[28] from Paris, France, measured the spatial extent of the regurgitant jet in the LV outflow tract with a 3 MHz 2-D echo-pulsed Doppler device to assess the severity of AR. The procedure included detection of diastolic disturbances in the LV outflow tract and mapping these disturbances. Length (L) and height (H) were measured with calculation of the product (L × H) in the long-axis view and width (W) in the short-axis view with calculation of the LV outflow tract regurgitant index (LVOTRI) as (L × H) × W. Twelve normal subjects and a group of 83 patients, including 40 patients with AR proved by aortography, were investigated. Diagnostic reliability ranged between 90% for specificity and 95% for sensitivity. Correlations between the grading provided by the LVOTRI and those provided by aortography on a 3-grade scale showed a correlation coefficient between 0.67 (linear model, p < 0.01) and 0.80 (exponential model) because of the high values of the index in cases of severe AR. Reliability of the LV outflow tract investigation in AR requires the use of information from 2 combined scan planes and quantitative rather than qualitative data. Main limitations of the procedure are due to the presence of associated mitral lesions.

LV function

In patients with AR, the LV EF may not adequately reflect depressions of myocardial contractility due to aortic impedance. The sensitivity of end-systolic pressure-volume relations and stress-volume relations in detecting myocardial depression in patients with AR was studied by Mehmel and associates[29] from Heidelberg, West Germany. In 12 patients with normal valvular function but with varying LV dysfunction (due to CAD in 9 patients and dilated cardiomyopathy in 3 patients) (group I), and in 8 patients with AR (group 2), LV angiography was performed before and after sublingual application of isosorbide dinitrate. Heart rate was kept constant by RA pacing. In group 1, the slope k of the end-systolic pressure-volume relation was to EF at rest: $k = 0.091.e^{0.051 \; EF}$; r = 0.88. In AR, this relation was shifted significantly to the right: $k = 0.018.e^{0.066 \; EF}$; r = 0.92. This shift persisted when the end-systolic stress-volume relation instead of the end-systolic pressure-vol-

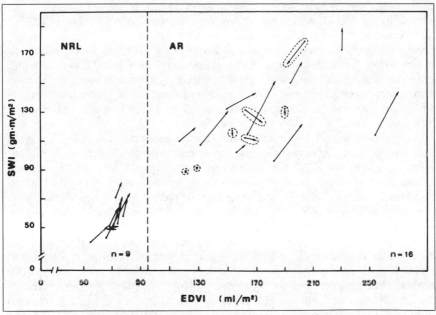

Fig. 5-5. Response of relation of stroke work index (SWI) and end-diastolic volume index (EDVI) to angiotensin in the patients with AR and in the normal subjects (NRL). The dotted outlines identify the patients who showed an abnormal function curve. Reproduced with permission from Branzi et al.[30]

ume relation was calculated. Thus, in patients with AR the end-systolic pressure-volume relation is flatter than that in patients with intact valvular function at a given EF. The same is true for the end-systolic stress-volume relation. The data indicate that EF overestimates myocardial contractility in AR compared with end-systolic pressure-volume or stress-volume relations. This overestimation is probably a result of decreased aortic impedance in AR.

Branzi and colleagues[30] from Bologna, Italy, evaluated the response to afterload stress determined by angiotensin challenge and the end-systolic pressure-volume relation that was determined by echo in 16 asymptomatic or mildly symptomatic patients with severe AR. The ages ranged from 15–56 years and 9 normal subjects of similar ages served as controls. In the group with AR, end-systolic dimensions were >55 mm in 5 of 16 patients and fractional shortening was ≤25% in 2 of 16. In the control group, angiotensin caused a decrease of stroke volume index in 6 of 9 patients and a mild increase in 3. In the patients with AR, stroke volume index decreased ≥15% of the basal value in 9 of 16 patients and increased or decreased by <15% in 7 of 16 (Fig. 5-5). The EF decreased in both groups. Ventricular function curves were derived by relating end-diastolic volume index to stroke work index. Seven of 16 patients had abnormal responses, reflecting an afterload mismatch. Considering all the tested indexes of ventricular performance, the rank order of incidence of abnormal findings in the group with AR was as follows: basal fractional shortening (13%), basal end-systolic dimension

(31%), angiotensin-induced decrease of stroke work index (41%) and stroke volume index (56%), and the end-systolic pressure-volume relation (75%). These investigators concluded that in young asymptomatic or mildly symptomatic patients with chronic severe AR that: (1) the end-systolic pressure-volume relation derived from noninvasive measurement of systolic pressure and echo parameters is the most sensitive index of myocardial dysfunction among those considered and (2) depression of contractility is frequently present before end-systolic dimension reaches 55 mm and fractional shortening decreases <25%.

Vandebossche and coworkers[31] from San Francisco, California, evaluated the usefulness of 2-D echo in asymptomatic or minimally symptomatic patients with significant AR and LV enlargement. The LV size and functional measurements were obtained with a nongeometric technique and gated blood pool radionuclide ventriculography and were compared with measurements made by several 2-D echo methods in 20 patients. The LV size was best assessed by an apical biplane modified Simpson's rule algorithm obtained by computer-assisted planimetry; for end-diastolic volume, r = 0.95 and standard error of the estimate was 25 ml; for end-systolic volume, r = 0.94 and standard error of the estimate was 16 ml. A newly introduced simplified 2-D method obviating the need for planimetry using multiple axis measurements yielded satisfactory results, but volumes >300 ml were markedly underestimated. A single minor axis measured directly from 2-D images and M-mode tracings obtained under 2-D echo control were inadequate for the estimation of volumes. The EF was assessed accurately by the modified Simpson's rule method and by a simplified 2-D method. The M-mode approach using a corrected cube formula also provided an accurate estimation of EF. Thus, these data indicate that 2-D echo provides an accurate means for the assessment of LV size and function in patients with chronic AR.

Goldman and coworkers[32] from New York City examined the role of systolic wall stress at rest in determining LV functional performance during exercise in patients with AR. Thirty patients, 19 men and 11 women (mean age, 47 years) with chronic AR referred for noninvasive studies were evaluated. Each patient had isolated AR without evidence of associated AS or CAD. Fourteen patients had symptoms of CHF (11 in New York Heart functional class II, 2 in class III, and 1 in class IV). Sixteen patients were asymptomatic. Systolic wall stress was measured by M-mode echo and was related to changes in LV function during maximal exercise as detected by radionuclide ventriculography. In these 30 patients, 7 had a normal EF response to exercise, as was evident from an absolute increase in EF $\geq 5\%$ (group I) and 23 had abnormal exercise responses (group II). These data demonstrate that patients in group I had a significantly lower radius/wall thickness ratio (2.5 ± 0.2 -vs- 3.1 ± 0.1, $p < 0.01$) and lower peak systolic wall stress (123 ± 11 -vs- $211 \pm 12 \times 10^3$ dynes/cm^2, $p < 0.01$) than patients in group II. Six of 9 patients with normal systolic wall stress at rest ($<150 \times 10^3$ dynes/cm^2) increased their EF during exercise, but this occurred in only 1 of 21 patients with elevated systolic wall stress ($p < 0.001$). Peak systolic wall stress at rest varied linearly and inversely with changes in LV EF during exercise ($r = 0.60$, $p < 0.001$). There was no difference in EF at rest between patients in groups I and II nor was there any difference in clinical symptoms or maximal workload achieved.

Frequency of associated coronary arterial narrowing

A number of articles have focused on the frequency and extent of coronary arterial narrowing and of angina pectoris in patients with AS. Surprisingly, relatively little angiographic and no necropsy information is available on the frequency and extent of coronary narrowing in patients with pure AR. To fill this void, Day and associates[33] from Bethesda, Maryland, determined at necropsy in 37 patients (30 men and 7 women) aged 34–77 years (mean, 54) with severe isolated, chronic, pure AR the degree of cross-sectional area (XSA) narrowing by atherosclerotic plaque in each of the 4 major epicardial coronary arteries (right, LM, LAD, and LC). In 7 patients (19%), ≥1 major coronary artery was narrowed 76–100% in XSA at some point (Fig. 5-6). Of the 148 major coronary arteries examined in the 37 patients, 12 arteries (8%) were narrowed at some point 76–100% in XSA. Each of the 148 major coronary arteries were divided into 5 mm segments (average, 53 per patient) and a histologic section from each segment was examined. Of the 1,977 segments, 1,087 were narrowed 0–25%; 669 (34%), 26–50%; 170 (9%), 51–75%; 48 (2%), 76–95%; and 3 (0.001%), 96–100% (Fig. 5-7). The average amount of XSA narrowing by atherosclerotic plaque per segment was about 28%. Of the 37 patients, 9 had had angina pectoris, 2 of whom had signifi

Fig. 5-6. Number of necropsy patients by age decade and sex with severe pure AR in whom ≥1 major epicardial coronary artery (right, LM, LAD, and LC) was narrowed 76–100% in cross-sectional area at some point by atherosclerotic plaques.

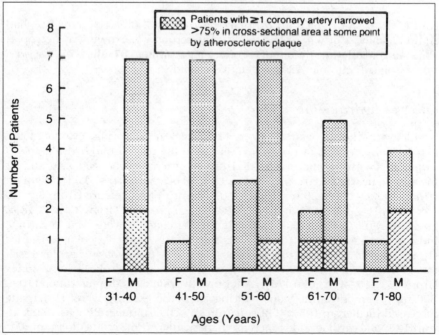

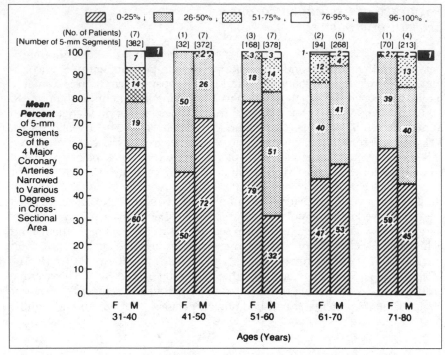

Fig. 5-7. Number and percent of 1,977 5 mm segments of the 4 major epicardial coronary arteries narrowed to various degrees by atherosclerotic plaques in 37 patients (30 men, 7 women) aged 34–77 years with severe pure AR.

cant (>75% XSA reduction) coronary narrowing; 2 other patients had had AMI clinically, 1 of whom had significant coronary narrowing at necropsy. Thus, in general, the amount of coronary narrowing in 37 adults with severe, pure, isolated, chronic AR was relatively mild.

Effect of hydralazine

Elkayam and associates[34] from Los Angeles, California, evaluated the hemodynamic effects of isometric exercise in the response to hydralazine in 11 patients with chronic, severe AR. Isometric exercise produced a significant increase in heart rate (from 78 ± 11–93 ± 19 beats/min, $p < 0.05$), mean BP (from 83 ± 8–104 ± 20 mmHg, $p < 0.05$), mean RA pressure (from 3 ± 2–7 ± 5 mmHg, $p < 0.05$) and mean PA wedge pressure (from 12 ± 7–18 ± 10 mmHg, $p < 0.05$). Small and insignificant changes were seen in cardiac index (from 3.4 ± 0.8–3.9 ± 1.0 liters/min/M^2), systemic vascular resistance (from $1,097 \pm 257$–$1,171 \pm 284$ dynes s cm^{-5}), pulmonary vascular resistance (from 120 ± 76–130 ± 89 dynes s cm^{-5}) and stroke volume index (from 44 ± 10–43 ± 12 ml/M^2). After oral hydralazine administration (100–300 mg), hemodynamic values during isometric exercise were: Heart rate increased further, to 105 ± 14 beats/min ($p < 0.05$), mean BP was 102 ± 16 mmHg (NS), cardiac index increased markedly, to 5.2 ± 1.4 liters/min/M^2

(p < 0.05), stroke volume index increased to 49 ± 12 ml/M² (p < 0.05), RA pressure decreased slightly, to 5 ± 5 mmHg (NS), PA wedge pressure decreased to 14 ± 7 mmHg (p < 0.05), systemic vascular resistance decreased to 903 ± 288 dynes s cm⁻⁵ (p < 0.05), and pulmonary vascular resistance changed to 100 ± 66 dynes s cm⁻⁵ (NS). Thus, isometric exercise in patients with chronic severe AR is associated with only a slight and insignificant increase in systemic vascular resistance, but a marked increase in PA wedge pressure. Direct arteriolar vasodilation with hydralazine results in a significant attenuation of PA wedge pressure increase during isometric exercise and leads concomitantly to a significant augmentation of stroke volume and cardiac output. These findings substantiate the value of hydralazine therapy in patients with chronic severe AR.

Effect of nifedipine

To examine the effects of nifedipine on LV functional response to isometric exercise in patients with AR, Shen and associates[35] from Sydney, Australia, performed 3 minutes of handgrip exercise at 33% of their maximal voluntary contraction, before and after administration of 20 mg of sublingual nifedipine in 20 patients with isolated, moderate to severe AR. Although handgrip exercise produced similar increases in heart rate and systolic BP before and after nifedipine treatment, heart rate was higher and systolic BP lower with handgrip exercise during nifedipine treatment. The LV end-diastolic volume index was not different during the control period and nifedipine handgrip exercise, but the increase in end-systolic volume index was smaller and the EF was higher during nifedipine handgrip exercise. Nifedi-

Fig. 5-8. Right ventricular forward stroke volume (FSV), total LV stroke volume (LVSV), and systemic vascular resistance (SVR) at rest and during exercise before (C) and after nifedipine (N) administration. D.S.CM-5 = dynes·s·cm⁻⁵. Reproduced with permission from Shen et al.[36]

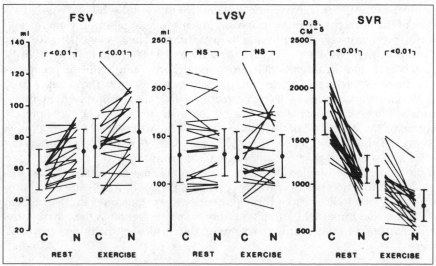

pine reduces afterload and ameliorates handgrip exercise-induced LV dysfunction in patients with AR.

Shen and coworkers[36] from Sydney, Australia, evaluated the influence of nifedipine (20 mg sublingually) on hemodynamics and cardiac function at rest and during supine bicycle exercise in 20 patients with AR. Administration of nifedipine increased heart rate at rest by 13%, systemic vascular resistance decreased by 34%, and regurgitant index decreased by 17%. Changes in systemic vascular resistance were related to initial rest values ($r = 0.82$) and to changes in forward cardiac output ($r = 0.58$) and regurgitant index ($r = 0.60$). The LV end-diastolic and end-systolic volumes, stroke volume, and EF were unchanged, but RV EF increased after nifedipine at rest. During exercise, nifedipine further increased heart rate by 8% and decreased systemic vascular resistance by 19%. Forward stroke volume and cardiac output increased, but total LV stroke volume was unchanged, resulting in a significant decrease in regurgitant index. The LV end-diastolic volumes slightly decreased, end-systolic volume did not change, and EF was higher after nifedipine than during control exercise ($p < 0.01$) (Fig. 5-8). Thus, these data indicate that the acute administration of nifedipine improves cardiac performance and reduces AR at rest and during exercise by reducing afterload and increasing heart rate. The data do not indicate whether similar beneficial effects occur long-term following nifedipine.

Determining prognosis after AVR

Stone and coworkers[37] from San Francisco, California, evaluated 113 consecutive patients with AR who underwent surgical correction between 1962 and 1977 to establish determinants of prognosis. Survivors were followed for a mean interval of 4.6 ± 3.3 years. Clinical and hemodynamic examinations were made in all patients before the operation; echoes were performed in 44 patients preoperatively and in 36 patients postoperatively. Perioperative or postoperative death due to CHF occurred in 8 patients (19%). No statistically significant predictors of total mortality or death due to CHF were found in analysis of the preoperative clinical, hemodynamic, and echo findings. Survivors of the operation demonstrated significant functional improvement (Fig. 5-9). Preoperatively, 77% of patients were in functional class III or IV and postoperatively, 84% were in class I or II ($p < 0.0001$). Statistically significant correlations of functional improvement were found with the preoperative presence of increased cardiac diameter on the chest radiograph ($p < 0.05$) and the severity of LV hypertrophy ($p < 0.05$). Improvement in LV function appeared most closely related to the degree of preoperative preservation of LV function. Specifically, patients with M-mode echo preoperative fractional shortening of the minor diameter >26%, end-systolic dimension <55 mm, and end-diastolic dimension <80 mm were most likely to have more normal LV function after the operation. These data suggest that improved LV function postoperatively correlates best with mildly impaired preoperative echo indices. Even those patients with serious preoperative clinical disability and impaired LV function may have a reduction in their symptoms and an improved quality of life following the surgical correction of their AR.

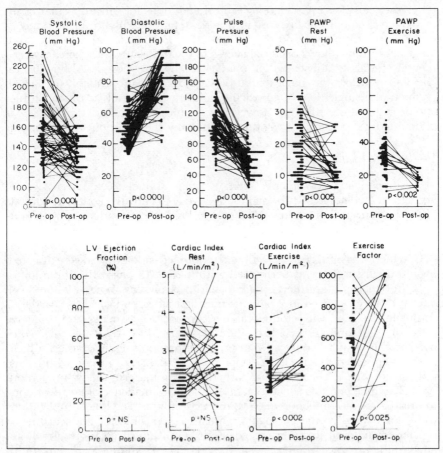

Fig. 5-9.   Preoperative (Pre-op) and postoperative (Post-op) hemodynamic profile of patients with AR. PAWP = PA wedge pressure. Reproduced with permission from Stone et al.[37]

INFECTIVE ENDOCARDITIS

Relation to dental procedures

Guntheroth[38] from Seattle, Washington, reviewed findings in 18 pediatric patients with infective endocarditis (IE) for "failure" of chemoprophylaxis; none had had a previous dental procedure. Guntheroth also reviewed previously published reports and found a surprisingly similarly low prevalence of dental extractions preceding IE, only 3.6% for 1,322 cases. Although bacteremia was associated with 40% of 2,403 reported extractions, it also was found in 38% of patients after mastication, and in 11% of patients with oral sepsis and no intervention. In a hypothetical month, ending with a single dental extraction, the cumulative exposure to these "physiologic" sources of bacteremia is nearly 1,000 times greater than it is from extraction. The current American Heart Association recommendations for intramuscular or intravenous chemoprophylaxis are impractical, and the discomfort and inconvenience may impede good dental care. The Committee also implies that gingival bleeding allows bacterial access to the bloodstream, whereas experimental studies establish the lymphatics as the only access. Although oral chemoprophylaxis for major dental procedures appears prudent, the British regimen of a single dose of amoxicillin administered orally is much simpler and probably more effective. However, scrupulous oral and dental hygiene is undoubtedly superior in preventing IE than any chemoprophylaxis regimen.

In drug addicts

Silverman and coworkers[39] from Chicago, Illinois, evaluated 72 drug abusers treated surgically for acute infective endocarditis. Fourteen patients (19%) had surgical procedures on 2 valves. Predominant infective organisms were *Staphylococcus aureus* and *Pseudomonas aeruginosa* (29%). The most common operative indication in patients with multivalve involvement was CHF, which was uniformly present when both left-sided valves were affected. Even though surgery was performed within 20 ± 13 days after initiation of antibiotic therapy, 7 of the 14 patients had perivalvular abscesses. Both MVR and AVR were required in 9 patients with left-sided endocarditis. Partial or complete tricuspid valvectomy was performed in 5 patients with bilateral infection in combination with 1 AVR and 4 with MVR. Tricuspid valve competence was established by valve insertion or anuloplasty in 2 patients; these patients appeared to have less perioperative CHF than did those with tricuspid excision alone. There were no early deaths. Long-term follow-up demonstrated an incidence of reoperation of 21% and an incidence of late death due to prosthetic valve infection at 3–18 months of 36%. The late complications were not related to the etiologic organism responsible for endocarditis or prosthetic material in the tricuspid anulus, but appeared more closely related to the presence of intracardiac abscess. These data indicate that multiple valve infection does not preclude successful early surgical therapy, reinfection in the addict population increases late mortality, and reinfection may be at least in part related to the presence of myocardial abscesses.

As consequence of flow-directed PA catheterization

Rowley and associates[40] from New Haven, Connecticut, described 55 patients who had flow directed PA catheterization and at necropsy 29 (53%) of them had ≥1 right-sided endocardial lesions: 12 (22%) had subendocardial hemorrhages; 11 (20%), sterile thrombi; 2 (4%), hemorrhage and thrombus; and 4 (7%), infective endocarditis. Of 41 lesions seen in the 29 patients, 23 (56%) were located on the pulmonic valve; 6 (15%), on the tricuspid valve; 6 (15%), in the right atrium; 4 (10%), in the right ventricle; and 2 (5%), in the pulmonary trunk. All 4 patients with infective endocarditis had had positive antemortem blood cultures while the catheter was in place, but in only 1 had the diagnosis of endocarditis been suspected clinically. The unusual locations of the infected vegetations (on the pulmonic valve in 3 and in the right atrium in 1) and the similar location of the uninfected lesions suggest that the infective endocarditis was a consequence of catheter-induced endocardial damage with concurrent or subsequent bacteremia. Among the 87 noncatheterized patients, there were 2 subendocardial hemorrhages and 1 resolving RA thrombus. The investigators concluded that endocardial damage from flow-directed PA catheterization is common and that right-sided infective endocarditis should be suspected in bacteremic catheterized patients.

From enterococcus

Enterococcal endocarditis accounts for an increasing proportion of cases of active infective endocarditis in recent years. The combination of penicillin and an aminoglycoside has become an accepted standard of treatment for enterococcal endocarditis. The optimal choice of antibiotics, duration of therapy, and timing of surgical intervention, however, remain controversial. Herzstein and associates[11] from New Haven, Connecticut, reviewed the presentation, clinical course, treatment, and outcome in 37 patients with 42 separate episodes of enterococcal endocarditis at 4 Yale University hospitals. Patients treated with aminoglycosides and penicillins or vancomycin had significantly better outcomes than those who did not receive aminoglycosides. The duration of aminoglycoside therapy (>4 -vs- <4 weeks) did not appear to affect outcome significantly. These results suggest that excellent cure rates may be achieved after treatment for <4 weeks with an aminoglycoside in combination with penicillin or vancomycin, thus potentially avoiding significant renal and vestibular toxicity.

TRICUSPID VALVE DISEASE

Assessment of tricuspid regurgitation by Doppler

Pennestri and associates[42] from Rome, Italy, tested pulsed Doppler echo to assess the degree of TR classified by right ventriculography in 47 patients. Forty-eight subjects without TR served as controls (39 with sinus rhythm and 9 with atrial fibrillation). Two Doppler methods were used: the distance of systolic turbulence within the right atrium from the tricuspid plane and the quantitative analysis of the flow velocity traces from the hepatic veins (HVs). The RA systolic turbulence was found in 41 of 47 patients with TR and in none of the control subjects and moderately correlated with the angiographic grading (Fig. 5-10). In control subjects, TR flow-velocity traces from the HVs showed 2 antegrade flow waves, systolic and diastolic. The ratio of antegrade systolic/antegrade diastolic velocity was more than 0.6 in 38 subjects with sinus rhythm and in 8 with AF. Twenty-two control subjects had a positive wave (designated as "v") coincident with the end of the T wave. In 30 patients with TR, a retrograde holosystolic wave was present. Of the remaining patients, 12 had a ratio of antegrade systolic/antegrade diastolic velocity <0.6. Fifteen had an end-systolic "v-like" wave that occurred earlier than the v wave in control subjects. In patients with TR, maximal velocities of the antegrade diastolic and retrograde systolic flow correlated with angiographic

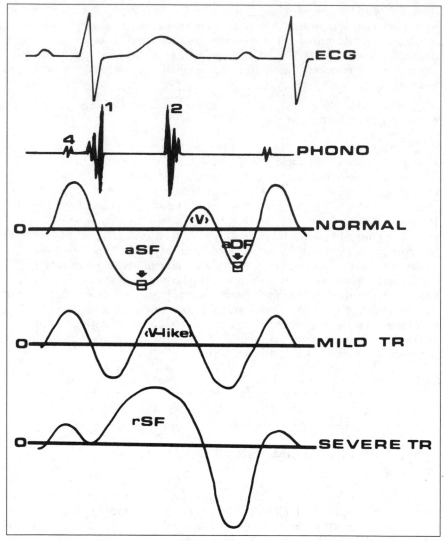

Fig. 5-10. The flow velocity curve pattern in the hepatic veins in normal subjects and in patients with mild and severe TR. The reference line for flow velocity curves is the 0 Doppler deviation line. Points above this line indicate flow toward the transducer and away from the heart. Points below the line indicate flow away from the transducer and toward the heart. A phonocardiographic signal (PHONO) is presented to illustrate timing of Doppler curve events. Fourth, first, and second sounds are labeled 4, 1, and 2, respectively. Arrows indicate points of measurements of maximal Doppler frequency shift. "a" = "a-like" flow wave; aSF = antegrade systolic flow wave; aDF = antegrade diastolic flow wave; "v" = "v-like" (in patients with TR) or "v" (in normal subjects) flow wave.

grading. An antegrade diastolic flow velocity >26 cm/s and a retrograde systolic flow velocity >16 cm/s excluded mild TR. Analysis of Doppler recordings of the HVs is valuable to assess TR semiquantitatively, complementing the RA Doppler findings.

Sakai and associates[43] from Tokyo, Japan, evaluated TR by observing the blood flow pattern in the HV, inferior vena cava (IVC) dimension, and HV dimension with the use of a combined system of pulsed Doppler technique and 2-D echo in 60 patients with valvular heart disease. For comparison, all patients underwent right ventriculography, by which TR was classified as mild, moderate, or severe. The IVC and HV dimensions of the group with severe TR were significantly larger than those of the other groups (p < 0.005). Several types of abnormal blood flow patterns in the HVs were demonstrated in patients with AF. By these flow patterns, the severe or moderate TR groups could be differentiated from the mild TR group, because 21 of the 26 patients (81%) in the former group showed reverse HV flow during systole. Also, the Doppler shifts from baseline in the sound spectrogram correlated well with RA pressure and RV end-diastolic pressure. This method is useful for rapidly evaluating considerable TR and for estimating RA pressure and RV end-diastolic pressure noninvasively.

Comparison of echo and hemodynamic diagnosis of tricuspid stenosis

Guyer and coworkers[44] from Boston, Massachusetts, used 2-D echo to evaluate 147 patients with rheumatic heart disease to identify the utility of echo in recognizing rheumatic tricuspid stenosis (TS). Thirty-eight of these patients also underwent hemodynamic evaluation. The TS was defined by echo as diastolic anterior leaflet doming, thickening and restricted excursion of the other 2 tricuspid leaflets, and decreased separation of the leaflet tips. Using these criteria, the sensitivity and specificity of echo in detecting TS were 69 and 96%, respectively, in the 38 patients who had both echo and hemodynamic evaluations. In the 17 patients who had simultaneous RA and RV pressure recordings, there was excellent agreement between echo and hemodynamic data. These data suggest that 2-D echo provides a sensitive and relatively specific means for recognizing TS, which was found in 14 (9.5%) of the 147 patients who had 2-D echo and in 10 (26.3%) of the 38 patients who had both echo and hemodynamic evaluations.

Predictors of survival after tricuspid valve surgery

Baughman and associates[45] from Boston, Massachusetts, analyzed the long-term survival rate of 74 consecutive patients who underwent multiple cardiac valve surgery, including tricuspid valve surgery, to identify predictive preoperative clinical variables. Univariate analysis revealed that male sex (p < 0.04), symptoms of New York Heart Association functional class IV CHF (p < 0.004), ascites or pulmonary edema (p < 0.01), high preoperative bilirubin level (p < 0.012), mean PA pressure <40 mmHG (p < 0.038), and pulmonary vascular resistance <6 Wood units (p < 0.02) were each associated with an increased risk of death after surgery (Fig. 5-11). Stepwise multivariate analysis indicated that severity of preoperative edema and mean PA pressure were the most predictive combination of independent variables. These 2 variables were used to calculate an estimated probability of 1-year survival after surgery for patients with multivalvular cardiac decompensation.

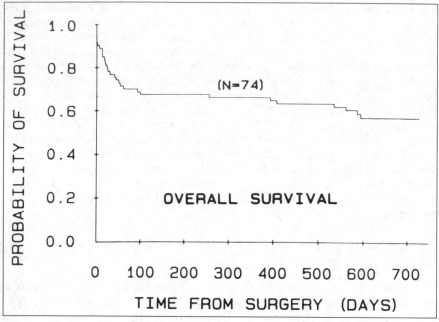

Fig. 5-11. Postoperative life-table analysis of survival after tricuspid and multivalvular surgery in 74 consecutive patients.

MISCELLANEOUS TOPICS

Myocardial performance in chronic AR -vs- chronic MR

Wisenbaugh and coworkers[46] from Philadelphia, Pennsylvania, evaluated patients with chronic MR and AR to determine whether load alterations helped to explain differences in ventricular function between these patients. Ventricular mechanics were compared in 9 patients with severe AR, 8 patients with severe MR, and 7 normal subjects. The amount of volume overload was similar in both groups of patients. In both AR and MR, ejection performance was reduced compared with findings in normal subjects. Preload estimated as end-diastolic stress was comparably elevated above normal in both groups with regurgitation. In patients with MR, end-diastolic stress was 69 ± 24 dynes $\times 10^3/cm^2$ compared with 81 ± 34 dynes $\times 10^3/cm^2$ in AR and 36 ± 11 dynes $\times 10^3/cm^2$ in normal subjects. However, afterload estimated as mean systolic stress was normal in MR (186 ± 34 dynes $10^3/cm^2$), but markedly elevated in patients with AR (260 ± 41 dynes $\times 10^3/cm^2$) ($p < 0.01$). Contractile depression tended to be more severe in patients with MR despite similar ejection performance in patients with MR and AR. These data suggest that patients with chronic MR have more favorable loading conditions and patients with AR with excessive afterload increase have reduced ventricular function. These differences in loading conditions may account for previously observed differences in ventricular function after valve replacement.

Cardiac, skeletal and ocular abnormalities with the Marfan syndrome and in their relatives and comparison with cardiac abnormalities in kyphoscoliosis

Bruno and associates[47] from Milan, Italy, performed apex cardiograms and carotid pulse tracings and M-mode echo in 34 symptomatic patients with the Marfan syndrome, in 32 of their relatives, and in 34 young patients with kyphoscoliosis. The polygraphic test showed significant changes in all patients with the Marfan syndrome: 74 had an apical systolic click and a systolic murmur typical of MVP; 48% had a diastolic murmur of AR; 52% had isolated MVP, and 26% had isolated AR, and 22% had both. Echo changes also were present in all patients: 79% had aortic root dilations; 48% had fluttering of the anterior mitral leaflet; 79% had MVP, mostly pansystolic; 34% had both MVP and aortic root dilation, and 34% had LV dilation. The high prevalence of MVP did not vary with age or sex in patients with the Marfan syndrome or in their relatives: MVP was present in 38% and aortic root dilation, with or without AR, in 14%. Four relatives had the Marfan syndrome and at least 4 others had the forme fruste variety. The metacarpal index was abnormal in 41% of the relatives but ocular abnormalities were rare. In the patients with kyphoscoliosis, only an increase in the prevalence of MVP was found: 18% of the women and in none of the men.

Ventricular arrhythmias in aortic valve disease

Klein[48] from Davis, California, and Albuquerque, New Mexico, determined by 24-hour ambulatory ECG monitoring the frequency and grade of ventricular arrhythmias in patients with AS or pure AR. The occurrence of ventricular arrhythmias in the patients with aortic valve disease was compared with that in matched control subjects without aortic valve disease. Complex arrhythmias were significantly more frequent in patients with valve disease than in control subjects (40 of 102 -vs- 19 of 102); the significant difference occurred in patients without concomitant CAD. In patients with valve disease without CAD, complex arrhythmias were significantly more common than in normal control subjects (22 of 65 -vs- 4 of 64); in the presence of CAD, complex arrhythmias were as prevalent in those with aortic valve disease as in those without it (18 of 37 -vs- 15 of 37, respectively). Among patients with AS or AR, arrhythmia occurrence and grade of ventricular ectopic activity were not related to the degree of AS or AR, ventricular hemodynamics, or the presence or absence of concomitant CAD.

CARDIAC VALVE REPLACEMENT

Aortic root size before AVR

Mukharji and associates[49] from Dallas, Texas, determined the internal diameter of the aortic root by biplane ventriculography in 12 patients who

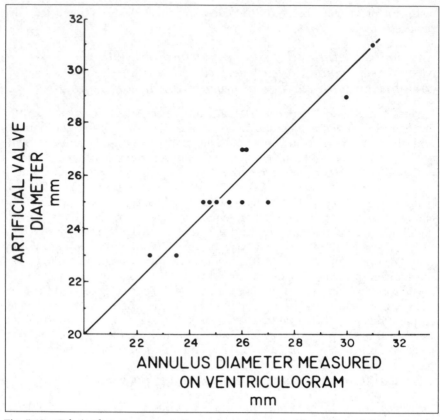

Fig. 5-12.   Relation between preoperative root measurement and artificial valve diameter.

subsequently had AVR with Carpentier-Edwards biprostheses. The artificial valve diameter was predicted with a correlation coefficient of 0.93, a standard error of estimate of 0.89 mm, and an average absolute difference between preoperative measurement and valve diameter of 0.69 mm (Fig. 5-12). Therefore the aortic root diameter can be accurately measured from the ventriculogram, thus detecting the patient preoperatively who will have a small aortic root.

Ventricular performance after AVR

Improved prosthetic aortic valves have reduced the incidence of complications to a point where it can be hypothesized that functional class I subjects after AVR should adapt to a vigorous training program without a significant increase of hemolytic activity or clinical signs of prosthetic malfunction. To test this hypothesis, Landry and associates[50] from Quebec City, Canada, studied 10 men (mean age, 52 years) who had undergone AVR (tilting disk prosthesis) and submitted them to an 8-week training program on ergometer, 3 times a week, from 60–80% of individual maximal heart rate. Ten other men who had undergone AVR but did not participate in the training program were control subjects. The exercise program produced significant improvements in post-training maximum tolerated ergometer work load, in maximum total body oxygen consumption, and in total product at submaximal work load. After training, hemoglobin increased by about 1 g/dl and hematocrit, reticulocyte counts, and haptoglobin did not change significantly. Serum LDH and serum AST levels did not increase. Pre- and post-training echoes did not show detectable alterations. Thus, patients with AVR who are in functional class I can adapt to a physical exercise program without significant adverse effects.

In patients with AR, preoperative LV systolic function is an important predictor of postoperative prognosis. Although LV dysfunction is reversible after AVR to a great extent in patients with good preoperative exercise capacity compared with patients with impaired exercise capacity, not all patients with preserved exercise capacity improve LV function after AVR. To determine the influence of duration of preoperative LV dysfunction on postoperative reversal of LV dysfunction, Bonow and colleagues[51] from Bethesda, Maryland, studied 37 patients with AR who preoperatively had LV dysfunction, defined as subnormal echo fractional shortening ($<29\%$) and good preoperative exercise capacity defined as completion of stage I of the NIH treadmill protocol without limiting symptoms. Eight patients were asymptomatic, 11 had LV dysfunction documented 18–57 months preoperatively, 10 patients developed LV dysfunction in an interval of 14 months or less preoperatively, and in 16 patients the duration of LV dysfunction was unknown. Patients with brief -vs- those with prolonged LV dysfunction did not differ with respect to severity of preoperative symptoms or exercise tolerance, echo determined LV dimensions or fractional shortening, or RNA EF. After AVR, patients with brief LV dysfunction developed a smaller LV diastolic dimension and higher EF than patients with prolonged LV dysfunction (Fig. 5-13). Postoperative EF was intermediate in patients with unknown duration of preoperative LV dysfunction. All deaths occurred in patients with either prolonged or unknown duration of LV dysfunction. Thus, these results suggest the duration of preoperative LV dysfunction in patients with AR is an important determinant of the reversibility of LV dysfunction after AVR.

A persistent question after mechanical unloading of the left ventricle consequent to valve replacement has been whether changes in the structure of hypertrophied myocardium occur and if these changes influence the passive diastolic properties of the postoperative LV myocardium. Hess and colleagues[52] from Zurich, Switzerland, determined passive diastolic properties in 10 control patients and 21 patients with aortic valve disease before and 18 months after successful AVR. Ten patients had severe AS, 5 had combined AS and AR, and 6 had severe AR. A LV endomyocardial biopsy was obtained before and after AVR. Simultaneous echo and high fidelity pressure measurements were made in all patients, and LV chamber stiffness was calculated from a viscoelastic pressure-circumference relation and LV myocardial stiffness from a viscoelastic stress-strain relation. The constant of chamber stiffness was slightly, although not significantly, increased in patients with AS, but was normal in those with AS and AR and slightly decreased in those with AR compared with control subjects. The constant of myocardial stiffness was normal in subjects with AS, AS and AR, and AR before AVR compared with those in the control group. Myocardial morphologic changes showed a significant decrease in muscle fiber diameter in patients with AS, AS and AR, and AR and a significant increase in interstitial fibrosis from 15–26% in those

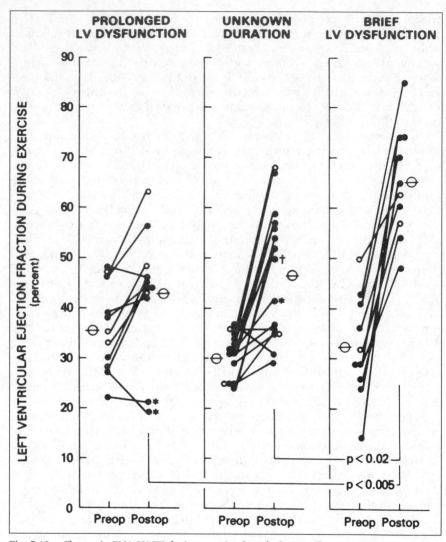

Fig. 5-13.   Change in RNA LV EF during exercise from before to after operation. 0 = patients with no preoperative symptoms; *=3 patients who subsequently died with symptoms of CHF; †=1 patient who subsequently died from prosthetic valve dysfunction; ⊝=mean values. Reproduced with permission from Bonow et al.[51]

with AS and from 15–22% in those with AS and AR, and from 19–24% in those with AR. The LV fibrous content (LV muscle mass index multiplied by interstitial fibrosis) remained unchanged in all 3 groups after AVR. In conclusion, LV chamber stiffness is increased in AS but decreased in AR, whereas LV myocardial stiffness is normal in patients with aortic valve disease before AVR. After AVR, LV myocardial stiffness increased significantly in AS patients but remained unchanged in those with AR. Postoperative changes in myocardial structure were characterized by a decrease in muscle fiber diameter and a relative increase in interstitial fibrosis, whereas fibrous content remained unchanged. Thus, regression of myocardial hypertrophy in aortic valve disease is accompanied by an increase of myocardial stiffness in concentric hypertrophy that is not seen in eccentric hypertrophy. These investigators showed from these sophisticated studies that relief of the LV overload that results in hypertrophy of the myocardium cannot morphologically return to normal since there is an added component of fibrosis of the various pressure and volume overload conditions. Time of optimal AVR should consider not only the potential for regression of myocardial hypertrophy but prevention of significant myocardial fibrosis.

Ventricular arrhythmias before and after AVR

Olshausen and associates[53] from Heidelburg, West Germany, studied the influence of AVR on the incidence of ventricular arrhythmias determined by 24-hour Holter ECG monitoring in 45 patients immediately before and 14 ± 7 months after operation. Ventricular arrhythmias were graded according to the Lown criteria. Preoperative LV EF was determined by angiography and postoperative LV EF by gated blood pool scintigraphy. Repetitive ventricular arrhythmias (Lown grade 4A/B) were associated with a reduced LV EF (<55%) before and after operation. In 24 patients with preoperative normal LV EF (>55%) (group A), mean LV EF remained unchanged after operation 72 -vs- 71%). Pre- and postoperative VPC frequency (45 ± 99 -vs- 39 ± 94 VPC/24 hours) and grade (1.3 -vs- 1.4) were not significantly different. However, in 17 patients with preoperative impaired LV EF (<55%) (group B, LV EF preoperatively 40 ± 8%) and marked postoperative improvement (>10%) (LV EF postoperatively 64 ± 7%), mean VPC frequently decreased from 536–69 VPC/24 hours and mean VPC grade was reduced from 3.8–1.5. Complex VPC were found preoperatively in all 17 patients of group B, but in only 5 patients after operation. Four patients had a reduced LV EF preoperatively, and it did not improve postoperatively (group C). Postoperative Holter monitoring detected VT in all 4 patients. This study indicates that repetitive VPC are infrequent in patients with normal LV EF before and late after AVR. In patients with impaired LV EF and complex VPC preoperatively, the postoperative improvement of LV function is usually accompanied by a reduction of frequent and complex VPC.

Results for regurgitation

McGoon and coworkers[54] from Rochester, Minnesota, evaluated the long-term course of 336 patients with valvular regurgitation who had received Starr-Edwards prostheses between 1962 and 1971. These patients were followed for a mean of 15 years. Eighteen patients (10%) after AVR and 24 (16%) after MVR died early. Mortality remained high (31%) in the first 3 years after AVR and was highest in the first year after MVR, and then it approached the normal rate. The most common mode of death was sudden after AVR and CHF after MVR (Fig. 5-14). At long-term follow-up, 76% of the survivors were improved symptomatically. Three instances of primary valve malfunction occurred. Freedom from thromboembolism at 15 years postoperatively was 56% after AVR and 52% after MVR. These data suggest that the Starr-Edwards ball valve prosthesis is durable but that thromboembolism remains a continuing problem.

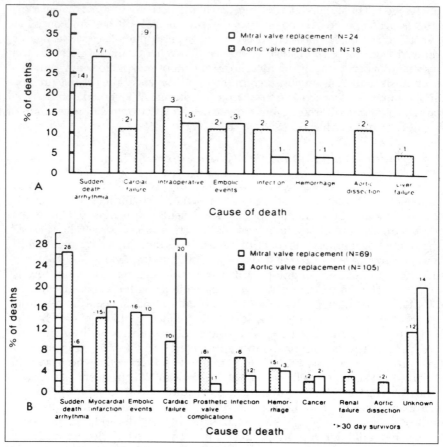

Fig. 5-14. Causes of (A) early postoperative mortality (death within 30 days after Starr-Edwards valve implantation) and (B) late mortality. Reproduced with permission from McGoon et al.[54]

St. Jude medical prosthesis

Chaux and associates[55] from Los Angeles, California, reported a 5-year experience with the St. Jude medical valve: 198 patients received 233 such valves. Total follow-up was 4,896 patient-months: survivors were followed 1–5 years (mean, 35 months). Operative mortality was 11% for MVR, 3% for AVR, and 3% for MVR and AVR. The actuarial survival rate at 4 years was 67% after MVR, 79% after AVR, and 79% after double valve replacement. Ischemic mitral valve disease was associated with an early mortality of 27% and a 4-year survival rate of 34%. Without this high risk subset, early mortality was 3% and the 4-year survival rate was 77% after MVR. Increased postoperative mortality was associated with 3 preoperative patient characteristics: ischemic mitral valve disease, a depressed LV EF and advanced New York Heart Association class. Valve-related complications occurred in 14 patients (3%/patient-year). There were no instances of primary structural failure or hemolysis. Thromboembolism occurred in 9 patients, 2%/patient-year. Thromboembolism occurred more frequently in 12 patients receiving aspirin and dipyridamole than in 173 patients receiving warfarin (2%/patient-year). Of survivors, 90% improved by ≥1 New York Heart Association functional class. The St. Jude medical valve has excellent hemodynamic performance. In addition there were no instances of primary structural failure or hemolysis in this group. The data support warfarin anticoagulation for all such patients.

Bioprostheses

Gonzalez-Lavin and colleagues[56] report a novel and interesting study on the risk of thromboembolism after MVR using 2 types of bioprosthesis. This was a multicenter and retrospective study over an 8-year period (Fig. 5-15). Group I included 206 patients undergoing MVR with a porcine xenograft (169 Hancock and 37 Carpentier-Edwards valves); they were placed on a regimen of long-term oral anticoagulation (mean, 6 months). Group II included 322 patients having MVR with a bovine pericardial valve (Ionescu-Shiley); they were placed on a program of short-term anticoagulation (6 weeks). The decision regarding the type of bioprosthesis inserted in a given patient was based primarily on the preference of the operating surgeon. Either bioprosthesis was inserted with interrupted or running sutures or with a combination of both. In group I there were 24 thromboembolic events (4.6%/patient-year, 4 of which were fatal). Actuarially, 87% ± 4% are free of thromboembolism at 8 years. There were 12 instances of major bleeding episodes for linearized incidence of 2.5%/patient-year. In group II there were 4 thromboembolic episodes, an incidence of 0.36%/patient-year. There were 7 bleeding episodes, an incidence of 0.63%/patient-year. The difference between groups I and II was significant (p < 0.001); there was no significant difference in thromboembolic risk factors between groups I and II. The patients receiving either a porcine or bovine pericardial valve had a similar profile regarding disease severity, functional derangement, associated

Fig. 5-15. Actuarial curves depicting freedom from thromboembolism in groups I and II patients at risk (p < 0.001). BPV = bovine pericardial valve; PXV = porcine xenograft valve. Reproduced with permission from Gonzalez-Lavin et al.[56]

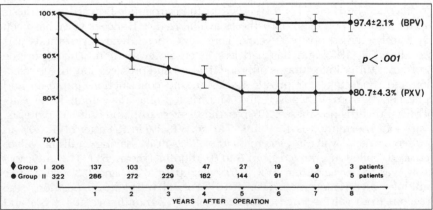

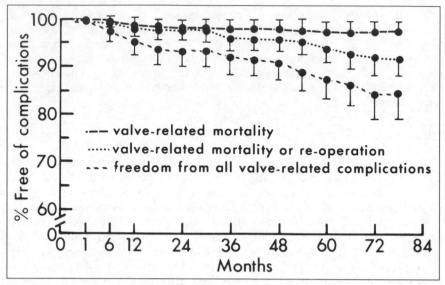

Fig. 5-16.   Freedom from valve-related death and complications. Reproduced with permission from Jamieson et al.[57]

thromboembolic risk factors and concomitant procedures. The operations were performed during the same time interval by the same surgeons. The most crucial difference between the 2 groups lay in the nature of the valve substitute. The study suggests that there is a difference in thrombogenicity, perhaps related to the construction of the bioprosthesis, lack of impairment of blood flow through the bovine bioprosthesis, or bioprosthetic performance. The investigators contend that the superiority of the bovine pericardial bioprosthesis is related to its hydraulic and hemodynamic characteristics. Higher residual gradients were found in patients with porcine bioprostheses. In vitro, flow through the pericardial bioprosthesis is smooth and nonturbulent as opposed to the marked fluttering seen in the orifice of the porcine bioprosthesis.

The glutaraldehyde-preserved porcine bioprosthesis was introduced in 1969 to reduce the risk of thromboembolism associated with mechanical prostheses. The Hancock prosthesis and the Carpentier-Edwards prosthesis are the 2 major porcine bioprostheses available. The Hancock valve has been extensively studied up to 10 years. The Carpentier-Edwards prosthesis was introduced in 1975 and has had less extensive evaluation. The 2 porcine prostheses differ in technique of tissue fixation and preservation, tissue selection and mounting, and prosthesis design and construction. Jamieson and colleagues[57] from Vancouver and Montreal, Canada, evaluated the Carpentier-Edwards prostheses: 397 prostheses were implanted in 355 patients. Thirty-day mortality was 4.5% in 155 after AVR, 9% in 154 after MVR, 20% in 5 after tricuspid valve replacement and 22% in 41 having multiple valves replaced. Follow-up ranged from 6 to 81 months (mean, 51). The late mortality was 3.4%/year after AVR, 3.6%/year after MVR, and 6.3%/year after multiple valve replacement (Fig. 5-16). For all valves in all positions, the freedom from valve-related complications at 72 months was 84 ± 5% and

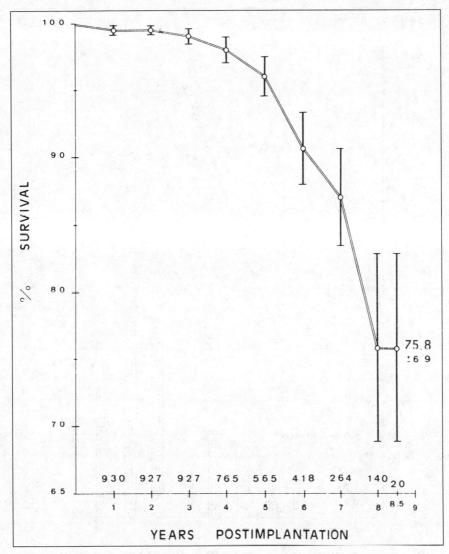

Fig. 5-17. Actuarial rates of freedom from primary tissue failure in patients with Hancock and Carpentier valves, implanted in mitral, aortic, tricuspid, and pulmonary positions. The number of valves at risk per postoperative year is shown.

the freedom from reoperation was 94 ± 4%. There were 21 postoperative thromboembolic events in the total patient population, 7 in AVR patients, 10 in MVR patients, and 4 in multiple valve patients. The embolic rate in the overall group of patients was 1.5%/patient-year. Most patients with aortic bioprosthesis were not anticoagulated. Most patients with a mitral valve bioprosthesis were anticoagulated (in the presence of chronic AF, intracardiac thrombus, or dilated left atrium). Primary tissue failure occurred in 9 patients (0.66%/patient-year); once in AVR, 6 times in MVR, and 2 in multiple valve replacement. Eight patients had reoperation for tissue failure with no deaths. The Carpentier-Edwards bioprosthesis compares favorably with

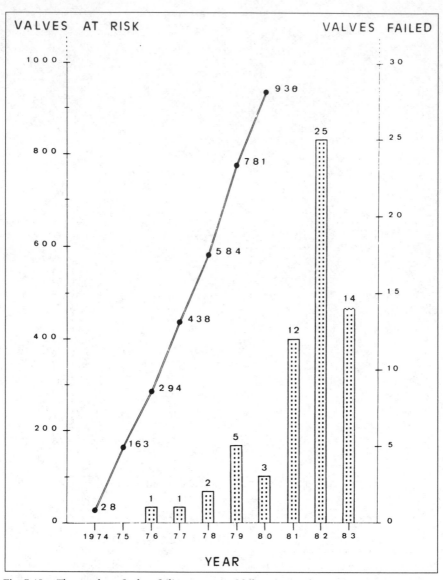

Fig. 5-18.   The number of valves failing per year of follow-up -vs- the number of valves at risk.

the Hancock bioprosthesis and with other mechanical prostheses. Freedom from valve-related complication was approximately 84% at the 6-year interval. This report provides valuable intermediate-term follow-up on this bioprosthesis.

From June 1974 through December 1980, Gallo and associates[58] from Santander, Spain, implanted 938 porcine bioprostheses in 794 patients who survived the operation and were therefore at risk for primary tissue valve failure (Fig. 5-17). Sixty-three instances of primary tissue valve degeneration occurred in 59 of the 794 patients. In patients operated on 9 years ago, 29% of the valves implanted in the mitral position (5 of 17) and 27% in the aortic

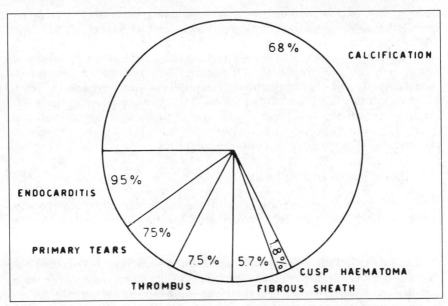

Fig. 5-19. Causes of intrinsic dysfunction in 53 porcine bioprostheses. Calcification accounts for 68% of cases of failure.

position (3 of 11) failed (Fig. 5-18). These percentages decreased to 18% (14 of 80) and 20% (11 of 54) for those implanted in 1975, 8% (6 of 73) and 14% (7 of 51) for those implanted in 1976, 9% (6 of 68) and 5% (4 of 76) for 1977, and 4% (3 of 79) and 3% (2 of 63) for 1978. The average interval between valve placement and explantation or death was 56 months (range, 10–98) for valves in the mitral position and 68 months (range, 12–92) for valves in the aortic position. The rate of valve survival without degeneration was 98 ± 1% at 4 years, 96 ± 2% at 5 years, 90 ± 3% at 6 years, 87 ± 4% at 7 years, and 76 ± 7% at 8 and 9 years. Until 1978, 4 valves failed, 8 failed in 1979–1980, 12 in 1981, 25 in 1982, and 14 have already failed from January–May 1983. The results show a progressive increase in valve degeneration with the passing of time, and no leveling of this failure rate has so far been observed.

Milano and associates[59] from Padova, Italy, examined 67 glutaraldehyde-processed porcine bioprostheses recovered at autopsy or reoperation from 65 patients. Each excised bioprosthesis was x-rayed. Seven of the 65 patients with 8 bioprostheses were <20 years of age. The time interval of function was 2–138 months (average, 62). Pathologically, 53 explants had signs of intrinsic dysfunction, which was ascribed to calcification in 36 (68%) (Fig. 5-19). By x-ray examination, calcific deposits were found in 55 of 67 bioprostheses (82%). The mean duration of function was 70 ± 32 months in calcified -vs- 27 ± 18 months in noncalcified porcine bioprostheses; all 26 that had been in place for >6 years were calcified. In 45 the calcific deposits were considered severe (mean time of function, 76 ± 32 months) and mild in 10 (mean time of function, 44 ± 22 months). The calcific deposits were located at the commissures in 54 bioprostheses (98%), in the body of cusps in 41 (75%), at the free margin in 37 (67%), and at the aortic wall in 37 (67%). When mild, calcific deposits involved the commissures in 90% of cases, the body of cusps in 30%, and the free margin only in 10%. Forty-seven calcified bioprostheses were mounted on flexible stents, and 8 had a rigid stent, with an average time of function of 63 ± 28 and 113 ± 18 months, respectively. Calcific dysfunction occurred earlier in the aortic than in the mitral position (59 ± 19 -vs- 86 ± 35 months). All the porcine bioprostheses explanted from young patients and 47 of 59 removed from adult patients were calcified, with an average time of function of 50 ± 21 -vs- 73 ± 33 months, respectively. The duration in patients >35 years of age and in those aged 20–35 years was identical. Chronic anticoagulant therapy with warfarin did not influence the occurrence and severity of calcium degeneration.

Prosthetic valve endocarditis

Prosthetic valve endocarditis (PVE) remains a potential risk for patients undergoing cardiac valve replacement and has been reported to occur in 1–9% of patients. Ivert and coworkers[60] from Birmingham, Alabama, studied 53 of 1,465 consecutive in-hospital survivors of valve replacement from 1975 to July 1979 (aortic, mitral, or aortic and mitral, only 1 untraced) who developed PVE. Risk factors for developing PVE included native valve endocarditis, black race, mechanical prosthesis (-vs- bioprosthesis), male sex, and long cardiopulmonary bypass time. The hazard function for developing PVE was greatest at 3 weeks after valve replacement. Patients with native valve endocarditis had a tendency to develop PVE early after valve replacement, as did patients in whom mechanical protheses were used. A PVE associated with *Staphylococcus epidermidis* tended to appear within 6 months of valve replacement, whereas streptococcal PVE tended to appear later. Although PVE took an atypical form in some patients, patients with possible PVE had the same findings as those with certain PVE. Bacteriologic confirmation of PVE was not obtained in 11 patients. The typical prosthetic and periprosthetic characteristics of PVE were present in 30 of the 40 cases in whom observations were possible. Of the 53 patients, 43 (64%) died. Most deaths occurred within 3 months of the first evidence of PVE. Recovery of some patients remains possible with appropriate medical and surgical treatment, but the investigators strongly recommended more intense preventive measures. This large study demonstrates the importance of aggressive treatment of this complication.

Occasionally PVE at the aortic area results in the formation of root abscesses, fistulous communications, septal ulceration, or perforations of the anterior mitral leaflet. Replacement of the prosthesis may not control the problem and recurrent PVE occurs. In this situation a persistent finding is ventricular-aortic discontinuity. Attempts to further place prostheses in the orthotopic position result in persistent infection and persistent perivalvular leak. Lau and colleagues[61] from London, England, reported the successful surgical treatment of 6 patients with PVE and uncontrolled bacteremia using a method whereby the aortic root is replaced with a preserved homograft aortic valve. Ventricular aortic continuity is established with a centrally flowing valve together with its attached aorta (Fig. 5-20). The weakened aortic and associated root abscesses are thereby excluded from the systemic circulation. The infected tissues, including the aortic root, are "disarticulated" from the LV base. The aortic homograft is sewn in place onto the ventricular septum, anterior mitral leaflet, and LV base proximally and to the

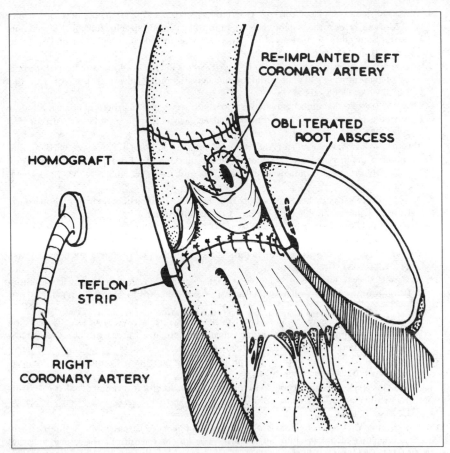

RE-IMPLANTED LEFT
CORONARY ARTERY

OBLITERATED
ROOT ABSCESS

HOMOGRAFT

TEFLON
STRIP

RIGHT
CORONARY ARTERY

Fig, 5-20. Aortic root replacement with a homograft showing the reimplanted left coronary artery. Reproduced with permission from Lau et al.[61]

nondiseased distal ascending aorta distally. The coronary arteries are mobilized and reimplanted into the aortic homograft. There were no deaths, 2 patients had conduction disturbances, and all patients are well with no further evidence of infection.

References

1. GROSE R, STRAIN J, COHEN MV: Pulmonary arterial V waves in mitral regurgitation: clinical and experimental observations. Circulation 69:214–222, Feb 1984.
2. BONCHEK LI, OLINGER GN, SIEGEL R, TRESCH DD, KEELAN MH JR: Left ventricular performance after mitral reconstruction for mitral regurgitation. Thorac Cardiovasc Surg 88:122–127, July 1984.
3. ZILE MR, GAASCH WH, CARROLL JD, LEVINE HJ: Chronic mitral regurgitation: predictive value of preoperative echocardiographic indexes of left ventricular function and wall stress. J Am Coll Cardiol 3:235–242, Feb 1984.

4. WALLER BF, MARON BJ, DEL NEGRO AA, GOTTDIENER JS, ROBERTS WC: Frequency and significance of M-mode echocardiographic evidence of mitral valve prolapse in clinically isolated pure mitral regurgitation: analysis of 65 patients having mitral valve replacement. Am J Cardiol 53:139–147, Jan 1, 1984.

5. ALPERT MA, CARNEY RJ, FLAKER GC, SANFELIPPO JF, WEBEL RR, KELLY DL: Sensitivity and specificity of two-dimensional echocardiographic signs of mitral valve prolapse. Am J Cardiol 54:792–796, Oct 1, 1984.

6. ARVAN S, TUNICK S: Relationship between auscultatory events and structural abnormalities in mitral valve prolapse: a two-dimensional echocardiographic evaluation. Am Heart J 108:1298–1306, Nov 1984.

7. CHANDRARATNA PA, NIMALASURIYA A, KAWANISHI D, DUNCAN P, ROSIN B, RAHIMTOOLA SH: Identification of the increased frequency of cardiovascular abnormalities associated with mitral valve prolapse by two-dimensional echocardiography. Am J Cardiol 54:1283–1285, Dec 1, 1984.

8. KAVEY R-EW, BLACKMAN MS, SONDHEIMER HM, BYRUM CJ: Ventricular arrhythmias in mitral valve prolapse in childhood. J Pediatr 105:885–890, 1984.

9. KRAMER HM, KLIGFIELD P, DEVEREUX RB, SAVAGE DD, KRAMER-FOX R: Arrhythmias in mitral valve prolapse: Effect of selection bias. Arch Intern Med 144:2360–2364, Dec 1984.

10. ALPERT JS: Association between arrhythmias and mitral valve prolapse. Arch Intern Med 144:2333–2334, Dec 1984.

11. MORADY F, SHEN E, BHANDARI A, SCHWARTZ A, SCHEINMAN MM: Programmed ventricular stimulation in mitral valve prolapse: analysis of 36 patients. Am J Cardiol 53:135–138, Jan 1, 1984.

12. WARE JA, MAGRO SA, LUCK JC, MANN DE, NIELSEN AP, ROSEN KM, WYNDHAM CRC: Conduction system abnormalities in symptomatic mitral valve prolapse: an electrophysiologic analysis of 60 patients. Am J Cardiol 53:1075–1078, Apr 1, 1984.

13. BOR DH, HIMMELSTEIN DU: Endocarditis prophylaxis for patients with mitral valve prolapse. Am J Med 76:711–717, Apr 1984.

14. DAY PJ, ROBERTS WC: Relation of level of total serum cholesterol to amount of calcific deposits in operatively excised stenotic mitral valves: analysis of 155 cases. Am J Cardiol 53:157–159, Jan 1, 1984.

15. FLUGELMAN MY, HASIN Y, KATZNELSON N, KRIWISKY M, SHEFER A, GOTSMAN MS: Restoration and maintenance of sinus rhythm after mitral valve surgery for mitral stenosis. Am J Cardiol 54:617–619, Sept 1, 1984.

16. NAIR CK, SUDHAKARAN C, ARONOW WS, THOMSON W, WOODRUFF MP, SKETCH MH: Clinical characteristics of patients younger than 60 years with mitral anular calcium: comparison with age- and sex-matched control subjects. Am J Cardiol 54:1286–1287, Dec 1, 1984.

17. SUBRAMANIAN R, OLSON LJ, EDWARDS WD: Surgical pathology of pure aortic stenosis: a study of 374 cases. Mayo Clin Proc 59:683–690, Oct 1984.

18. DANCY M, LEECH G, LEATHAM A: Comparison of cinefluoroscopy and M mode echocardiography for detecting aortic valve calcification: correlation with severity of stenosis of non-rheumatic aetiology. Br Heart J 51:416–420, Apr 1984.

19. BERGER M, BERDOFF RL, GALLERSTEIN PE, GOLDBERG E: Evaluation of aortic stenosis by continuous wave Doppler ultrasound. J Am Coll Cardiol 3:150–156, Jan 1984.

20. NAKAMURA T, HULTGREN HN, SHETTIGAR UR, FOWLES RE: Noninvasive evaluation of the severity of aortic stenosis in adult patients. Am Heart J 107:959–966, May 1984.

21. WARTH DC, STEWART WJ, BLOCK PC, WEYMAN AE: A new method to calculate aortic valve area without left heart catheterization. Circulation 70:978–983, Dec 1984.

22. NAIR CK, ARONOW WS, STOKKE K, MOHIUDDIN SM, THOMSON W, SKETCH MH: Cardiac conduction defects in patients older than 60 years with aortic stenosis with and without mitral anular calcium. Am J Cardiol 53:169–172, Jan 1, 1984.

23. RASMUSSEN K, THOMSEN PEB, BAGGER JP: HV interval in calcific aortic stenosis: relation to left ventricular function and effect of valve replacement. Br Heart J 52:82–86, July 1984.

24. EXADACTYLOS N, SUGRUE DD, OAKLEY CM: Prevalence of coronary artery disease in patients with isolated aortic valve stenosis. Br Heart J 51:121–124, Feb 1984.

25. OLSON LJ, SUBRAMANIAN R, EDWARDS WD: Surgical pathology of pure aortic insufficiency: a study of 225 cases. Mayo Clin Proc 59:835–841, Dec 1984.

26. STEWART WJ, KING ME, GILLAM LD, GUYER DE, WEYMAN AE: Prevalence of aortic valve prolapse with bicuspid aortic valve and its relation to aortic regurgitation: a cross-sectional echocardiographic study. Am J Cardiol 54:1277–1282, Dec 1, 1984.

27. BERGFELDT L, VALLIN H, EDHAG O: Complete heart block in HLA B27 associated disease: electrophysiological and clinical characteristics. Br Heart J 51:184–188, Feb 1984.

28. VEYRAT C, AMEUR A, GOURTCHIGLOUIAN C, LESSANA A, ABITBOL G, KALMANSON D: Calculation of pulsed Doppler left ventricular outflow tract regurgitant index for grading the severity of aortic regurgitation. Am Heart J 108:507–515, Sept 1984.

29. MEHMEL HC, OLSHAUSEN KV, SCHULER G, SCHWARZ F, KUBLER W: Estimation of left ventricular myocardial function by the ejection fraction in isolated, chronic, pure aortic regurgitation. Am J Cardiol 54:610–616, Sept 1, 1984.

30. BRANZI A, CINZIA L, PIOVACCARI G, RAPEZZI C, BINETTI G, SPECCHIA S, ZANNOLI R, MAGNANI B: Echocardiographic evaluation of the response to afterload stress test in young asymptomatic patients with chronic severe aortic regurgitation: sensitivity of the left ventricular end-systolic pressure-volume relationship. Circulation 70:561–569, Oct 1984.

31. VANDENBOSSCHE J-L, KRAMER BL, MASSIE BM, MORRIS DL, KARLINER JS, ANDERSON C, LOGE D: Two-dimensional echocardiographic evaluation of the size, function and shape of the left ventricle in chronic aortic regurgitation: comparison with radionuclide angiography. J Am Coll Cardiol 4:1195–1206, Dec 1984.

32. GOLDMAN ME, PACKER M, HOROWITZ SF, MELLER J, PATTERSON RE, KUKIN M, TEICHHOLZ LE, GORLIN R: Relation between exercise-induced changes in ejection fraction and systolic loading conditions at rest in aortic regurgitation. J Am Coll Cardiol 3:924–929, Apr 1984.

33. DAY PJ, McMANUS BM, ROBERTS WC: Amounts of coronary arterial narrowing by atherosclerotic plaques in clinically isolated, chronic, pure aortic regurgitation: analysis of 37 necropsy patients older than 30 years. Am J Cardiol 53:173–177, Jan 1, 1984.

34. ELKAYAM U, McKAY CR, WEBER L, EISENBERG D, RAHIMTOOLA SH: Favorable effects of hydralazine on the hemodynamic response to isometric exercise in chronic severe aortic regurgitation. Am J Cardiol 53:1603–1607, June 1, 1984.

35. SHEN WF, ROUBIN GS, HIRASAWA K, UREN RF, HUTTON BF, HARRIS PJ, FLETCHER PJ, KELLY DT: Abnormal left ventricular response to isometric exercise in pure, isolated aortic regurgitation: beneficial effects of nifedipine. Am J Cardiol 54:605–609, Sept 1, 1984.

36. SHEN WF, ROUBIN GS, HIRASAWA K, UREN RF, HUTTON BF, HARRIS PJ, FLETCHER PJ, KELLY DT: Noninvasive assessment of acute effects of nifedipine on rest and exercise hemodynamics and cardiac function in patients with aortic regurgitation. J Am Coll Cardiol 4:902–907, Nov 1984.

37. STONE PH, CLARK RD, GOLDSCHLAGER N, SELZER A, COHN K: Determination of prognosis of patients with aortic regurgitation who undergo aortic valve replacement. J Am Coll Cardiol 3:1118–1126, May 1984.

38. GUNTHEROTH WG: How important are dental procedures as a cause of infective endocarditis? Am J Cardiol 54:797–801, Oct 1, 1984.

39. SILVERMAN NA, LEVITSKY S, MAMMANA R: Acute endocarditis in drug addicts: surgical treatment for multiple valve infection. J Am Coll Cardiol 4:680–684, Oct 1984.

40. ROWLEY KM, CLUBB KS, SMITH GJ, CABIN HS: Right-sided infective endocarditis as a consequence of flow-directed pulmonary-artery catheterization: a clinicopathological study of 55 autopsied patients. N Engl J Med 311:1152–1156, Nov 1, 1984.

41. HERZSTEIN J, RYAN JL, MANGI RJ, GRECO TP, ANDRIOLE VT: Optimal therapy for enterococcal endocarditis. Am J Med 76:186–191, Feb 1984.

42. PENNESTRI F, LOPERFIDO F, SALVATORI MP, MONGIARDO R, FERRAZZA A, GUCCIONE P, MANZOLI U: Assessment of tricuspid regurgitation by pulsed Doppler ultrasonography of the hepatic veins. Am J Cardiol 54:363–368, Aug 1, 1984.

43. SAKAI K, NAKAMURA K, SATOMI G, KONDO M, HIROSAWA K: Evaluation of tricuspid regurgitation by blood flow pattern in the hepatic vein using pulsed Doppler technique. Am Heart J 108:516–523, Sept 1984.

44. GUYER DE, GILLAM LD, FOALE RA, CLARK MC, DINSMORE R, PALACIOS I, BLOCK P, KING ME, WEYMAN AE: Comparison of the echocardiographic and hemodynamic diagnosis of rheumatic tricuspid stenosis. J Am Coll Cardiol 3:1135–1144, May 1984.

45. BAUGHMAN KL, KALLMAN CH, YURCHAK PM, DAGGETT WM, BUCKLEY MJ: Predictors of survival after tricuspid valve surgery. Am J Cardiol 54:137–141, July 1, 1984.

46. WISENBAUGH T, SPANN JF, CARABELLO BL: Differences in myocardial performance and load between patients with similar amounts of chronic aortic versus chronic mitral regurgitation. J Am Coll Cardiol 3:916–923, Apr 1984.

47. BRUNO L, TREDICI S, MANGIAVACCHI M, COLOMBO V, MAZZOTTA GF, SIRTORI CR: Cardiac, skeletal, and ocular abnormalities in patients with Marfan's syndrome and in their relatives: comparison with the cardiac abnormalities in patients with kyphoscoliosis. Br Heart J 51:220–230, Feb 1984.

48. KLEIN RC: Ventricular arrhythmias in aortic valve disease: Analysis of 102 patients. Am J Cardiol 53:1079–1083, Apr 1, 1984.

49. MUKHARJI J, SLOAN TJ, ESTRERA AS, LIPSCOMB KM: Measurement of aortic root size by biplane angiography before cardiac valve replacement. Am J Cardiol 53:1084–1086, Apr 1, 1984.

50. LANDRY F, HABEL C, DESAULNIERS D, DAGENAIS GR, MOISAN A, COTE L: Vigorous physical training after aortic valve replacement: analysis of 10 patients. Am J Cardiol 53:562–566, Feb 1, 1984.

51. BONOW RO, ROSING DR, MARON BJ, McINTOSH CL, JONES M, BACHARACH SL, GREEN MV, CLARK RE, EPSTEIN SE: Reversal of left ventricular dysfunction after aortic valve replacement for chronic aortic regurgitation: influence of duration of preoperative left ventricular dysfunction. Circulation 70:570–579, Oct 1984.

52. HESS OM, RITTER M, SCHNEIDER J, GRIMM J, TURINA M, KRAYENBUEHL HP: Diastolic stiffness and myocardial structure in aortic valve disease before and after valve replacement. Circulation 69:855–865, May 1984.

53. OLSHAUSEN KV, AMANN E, HOFMANN M, SCHWARZ F, MEHMEL HC, KUBLER W: Ventricular arrhythmias before and late after aortic valve replacement. Am J Cardiol 53:142–146, July 1, 1984.

54. McGOON MD, FUSTER V, McGOON DC, PUMPHREY CW, PLUTH JR, ELVEBACK LR: Aortic and mitral valve incompetence: Long-term follow-up (10 to 19 years) of patients treated with the Starr-Edwards prosthesis. J Am Coll Cardiol 3:930–938, Apr 1984.

55. CHAUX A, CZER LSC, MATLOFF JM, DEROBERTIS MA, STEWART ME, BATEMAN TM, MASS RM, LEE ME, GRAY RJ: The St. Jude medical bileaflet valve prosthesis: a five year experience. J Thorac Cardiovasc Surg 88:706–717, Nov 1984.

56. GONZALEZ-LAVIN L, TANDON AP, CHI S, BLAIR RC, McFADDEN PM, LEWIS B, DAUGHTERS G, IONESCU M: The risk of thromboembolism and hemorrhage following mitral valve replacement. J Thorac Cardiovasc Surg 87:340–351, March 1984.

57. JAMIESON WRE, PELLETIER LC, JANUSZ MT, CHAITMAN BR, TYERS GF, MIYAGISHIMA RT: Five-year evaluation of the Carpentier-Edwards porcine bioprosthesis. J Thorac Cardiovasc Surg 88:324–333, Sept 1984.

58. GALLO I, RUIZ B, NISTAL F, DURAN CMG: Degeneration in porcine bioprosthetic cardiac valves: incidence of primary tissue failures among 938 bioprostheses at risk. Am J Cardiol 53:1061–1065, Apr 1, 1984.

59. MILANO A, BORTOLOTTI U, TALENTI E, VALFRE C, ARBUSTINI E, VALENTE M, MAZZUCCO A, GALLUCCI V, THIENE G: Calcific degeneration as the main cause of porcine bioprosthetic valve failure. Am J Cardiol 53:1066–1070, Apr 1, 1984.

60. IVERT TSA, DISMUKES WE, COBBS CG, BLACKSTONE EH, KIRKLIN JW, BERGDAHL LAL: Prosthetic valve endocarditis. Circulation 69:223–232, Feb 1984.

61. LAU JKH, ROBLES A, CHERIAN A, ROSS DN: Surgical treatment of prosthetic endocarditis: aortic root replacement using a homograft. J Thorac Cardiovasc Surg 87:712–716, May 1984.

6

Myocardial Heart Disease

IDIOPATHIC DILATED CARDIOMYOPATHY

Frequency in Denmark

Bagger and associates[1] from Aarhus, Odense, and Saalborg Sygehus, Denmark, performed a retrospective study to assess the incidence of cardiomyopathy in western Denmark (population, 2.8 million) during a 2-year period (1980–1981). The WHO/ISCF classification was followed, and rigid criteria for exclusion and inclusion of patients were adopted. Thus, cases in which specific heart muscle disorders (such as myocarditis, alcoholic heart disease, hypertension) were merely suspected were excluded. Forty-one patients had idiopathic dilated cardiomyopathy (IDC) (overall incidence, $7.3/10^6$ population/year) and 20 HC (overall incidence, $3.6/10^6$ population/year). In men aged 49–59 years, the occurrence of IDC was $23.4/10^6$ population/year. Only 1 case of Löffler's endomyocardial disease was diagnosed during the study period. Since the investigation was retrospective and was a study of diseased persons and not a population, and since a specific set of criteria for exclusion and inclusion was rigidly applied, the results represent the minimum frequency of these diseases.

Endomyocardial biopsy

Zee-Cheng and associates[2] from St. Louis, Missouri, evaluated 35 patients with unexplained CHF to determine the frequency of abnormalities in endomyocardial biopsies. Microscopic, ultrastructural, and immunofluorescent studies allowed a classification of myocyte changes ranging from no inflammation to active lymphocytic myocarditis. Twenty-two (63%) patients had inflammatory changes on endomyocardial biopsy. Eighteen of these had low grade inflammation and some were treated with immunosuppressive agents with improvement in 5 and stabilization in 1. One patient died of progressive CHF. Three of 4 patients with high grade inflammatory change died after a progressively deteriorating clinical course. Thus, these data suggest that inflammatory myocarditis is more common than previously suspected and indicate that there may be ongoing myocardial inflammation in some patients with idiopathic dilated cardiomyopathy.

With endomyocardial biopsy a subset of patients with idiopathic dilated cardiomyopathy (IDC) have unsuspected myocarditis histologically. Endomyocardial biopsy, however, lacks sensitivity due to sampling error if the inflammation is patchy or focal. In such a situation, inflammation-sensitive radioisotopic imaging may be a useful adjunct in the diagnosis of myocarditis. O'Connell and coworkers[3] from Hines, Illinois, evaluated the applicability of gallium-67 myocardial imaging as an adjunct to endomyocardial biopsy for diagnosis of myocarditis. Sixty-eight consecutive patients referred for evaluation of IDC underwent 71 parallel studies with gallium-67 imaging and biopsies. Histologic myocarditis was identified in 8% of biopsy specimens. Clinical and hemodynamic parameters could not be used to predict the presence of myocarditis. Five of 6 biopsy samples with myocarditis had dense gallium-67 uptake, whereas 9 of 65 negative biopsy samples (14%) were paired with equivocally positive gallium-67 scans. The 1 patient with myocarditis and no myocardial gallium-67 uptake had dense mediastinal lymph node uptake that may have obscured cardiac uptake. The frequency of myocarditis on biopsy with a positive gallium-67 scan was 36% (5 of 14); however, the frequency of myocarditis with a negative gallium-67 scan was only 2% (1 of 57). Follow-up scans in 3 patients showed close correlation of gallium-67 uptake with myocarditis on biopsy. These investigators concluded that gallium-67 may be a useful screening test for identifying patients with a high yield of myocarditis on biopsy, and serial scans may eliminate the need for frequent biopsies in patients with proved myocarditis.

HLA and DR typing

Several autoimmune diseases have been associated with increased frequencies of various histocompatibility antigen (HLA) types that may be linked to immune response genes. Idiopathic dilated cardiomyopathy (IDC) has been proposed as a disease with autoimmune features, but HLA associations have not been evaluated. Anderson and associates[4] from Salt Lake City, Utah, performed HLA typing in 37 consecutive patients with IDC. Patients with habitual alcoholism were excluded. Results showed that no single HLA type could account for most cases; IDC is a genetically heterogeneous disease. However, uneven distributions were noted for certain types. Haplotype frequency of B27 was 0.145 in patients -vs- 0.033 in 5,726 local control subjects. Other A and B frequencies (except A2) were evenly distributed. HLA-DR typing also revealed differences. The DR4 locus was present in 54% (19 of 35) of patients -vs- 32% (26 of 82) of blood bank control subjects. The associated relative risk of DR4 was 2.2 and the etiologic fraction, 0.29. Sex, disease chronicity, functional class, EF, and biopsy evidence of myocarditis did not distinguish DR4 positive from DR4 negative patients, but they were older (54 ± 12 -vs- 42 ± 14 years). Of note, 68% were positive for DR4, B27, or both. HLA-DR6Y was underrepresented; it was present in 9% (3 of 35) of patients -vs- 26% (21 of 82) of control subjects. The relative risk of DR6Y was 0.27 and the preventive fraction, 0.19. These associations will require independent confirmation. However, they suggest that genetically determined immune response factors associated with HLA loci may play a role in pathogenesis in certain patients with IDC.

Mechanism of decompensation

Hirota and associates[5] from Takatsuki, Japan, evaluated LV function in 32 patients with idiopathic dilated cardiomyopathy (IDC) who underwent cardiac catheterization during the past 6 years (group 4), and the results were compared with the data of 30 normal subjects (group 1). The patients were divided into mildly (group 2, 12 patients) and severely symptomatic subgroups (group 3, 20 patients). IDC was characterized by dilated and poorly contracting LV with increased muscle mass, reduced cardiac output, and elevated systemic vascular resistance. The LV volume was larger, EF was lower, and end-diastolic and end-systolic stresses were higher in group 3 than in groups 1 and 2. No significant differences were seen in LV muscle mass and wall thickness between groups 2 and 3. A significant inverse correlation was seen between EF and end-systolic stress in patients with IDC. The slope of the correlation line between end-systolic stress and volume in DC was less steep than that of normal subjects. These observations indicate that the primary problem of IDC is depressed contractility. Although afterload elevation and LV dilatation without further increase in wall thickness may be the sequelae of further deterioration of contractility, reduction of fiber shortening, and longer end-systolic fiber length in association with elevated afterload (so-called afterload mismatch) secondary to the absence of adequate hypertrophy, seen in group 3, appears to have an important role in the development of CHF in patients with IDC.

Ventricular arrhythmias

Olshausen and associates[6] from Heidelberg, West Germany, recorded a 24-hour ambulatory ECG in 60 patients with idiopathic dilated cardiomyopathy (IDC). All patients had an LV EF <55%; in 39 it was <40%. The VPC were evident in all patients. Multiform VPC were recorded in 57 patients (95%), paired VPC in 47 (78%), and nonsustained VT consisting of 3–19 beats in 25 (42%). Eight patients had >5 episodes of VT a day. Patients with AF had the same frequency and grade of ventricular arrhythmias as did those with sinus rhythm. Patients with infrequent and frequent VPC could not be differentiated on the basis of clinical or hemodynamic findings. The mean values of New York Heart Association functional class, cardiac index, LV end-diastolic pressure, and EF were significantly different in patients with and without VT. During follow-up of 12 ± 5 months, 7 patients died; all 7 had EF <40%. The investigators concluded that high grade ventricular arrhythmias are often seen in patients with IDC, that patients with VT have more impairment of LV function than do patients without VT, and that ambulatory monitoring appears to be of little help in identifying patients at increased risk of sudden death.

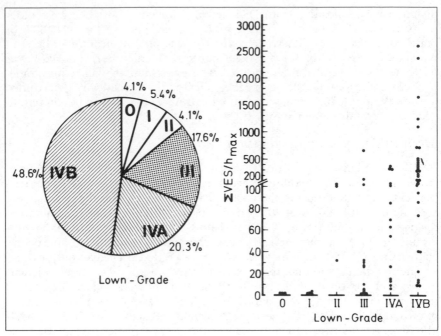

Fig. 6-1. Prevalence of ventricular arrhythmias by the Lown classification during 24-hour monitoring in 74 patients with idiopathic dilated cardiomyopathy (left), and relation between frequency and grade of VPC (right).

Meinertz and associates[7] from Mainz, West Germany, prospectively assessed in 74 patients with IDC the incidence and prognostic significance of ventricular arrhythmias identified by 24-hour ambulatory ECG (Holter). Holter monitoring was performed at the time of entry into the study. Patients were followed for 2–21 months (mean, 11 ± 3). Frequent VPC (>1,000/24 hours) were seen in 35%, and complex VPC (Lown grades III and IV) in 87% of the patients; 49% had nonsustained VT consisting of 3–32 beats with rates from 110–230 beats/min, and 20% had ventricular pairs (Fig. 6-1). No correlation was found between clinical symptoms or the degree of LV impairment and the number of ventricular pairs or episodes of VT. During follow-up, 19 patients died, 7 from CHF and 12 suddenly. Patients who died suddenly had significantly more episodes of VT, ventricular pairs, or total VPC (p < 0.01 each) compared with survivors and those who died from CHF. No significant differences were found between patients who died from CHF or suddenly with respect to LV end-diastolic pressure, LV end-diastolic volume index, LV EF and cardiac index. A linear stepwise discriminant function analysis using hemodynamic (LV EF and cardiac index) and arrhythmic (number of VT episodes and ventricular pairs) variables resulted in a meaningful separation between survivors and patients who died from CHF or suddenly (Table 6-1). Thus, patients with IDC and a reduced LV EF (<40%) in whom frequent episodes of VT or ventricular pairs were detected by 24-hour Holter monitoring are at high risk of dying suddenly.

Although programmed electrical stimulation in the response to serial antiarrhythmic drug testing has been helpful in the management of ventric-

TABLE 6-1.   *Relation between LV EF and ventricular arrhythmias**

LV EF	<35%	35–50%	>50%	*H* TEST
VPC/24 h	848 (225/	346 (17/	21 (1/	p < 0.01
	4,084)	2,193)	712)	
Ventricular				
pairs/24 h	3 (0/66)	0 (0/15)	0 (0/7)	NS
VT/24 h	1 (0/7)	0 (0/1)	0 (0/7)	NS

* The values of the arrhythmic variables are given as median values with the Q_{25} and Q_{75} quantil in parentheses. The Kruskal-Wallis test (*H* test) was used to compare the 3 subgroups.

ular arrhythmias associated with CAD, experience in patients with IDC is limited. Poll and coworkers[8] from Philadelphia, Pennsylvania, studied 11 consecutive patients with IDC and spontaneous, sustained VT of uniform morphology with programmed ventricular stimulation and serial antiarrhythmic drug testing. Mean EF was 30% and sustained VT was induced by programmed electrical stimulation in all 11 patients. A mean of 3.7 antiarrhythmic drugs was evaluated by programmed stimulation, including at least 1 experimental agent in 8 patients. In 9 of 11 patients VT remained inducible on all drug therapy. During a follow-up period of 21 months, there were 4 sudden deaths and 2 patients had recurrences of VT. In all 6 patients with sudden death or recurrence of VT, the arrhythmia remained inducible on drug therapy. Three patients who died suddenly had a hemodynamically stable, induced tachycardia on antiarrhythmic therapy. Of 8 patients treated with amiodarone, only 2 were successful. These investigators concluded that in patients with sustained VT and IDC, VT can be induced by programmed electrical stimulation. The VT will usually remain inducible on antiarrhythmic therapy, and sudden death can occur despite slowing and improved tolerance of the induced arrhythmia. In IDC, amiodarone may have limited efficacy, and more aggressive therapy, such as surgery or implantation of an automatic internal defibrillator, should be considered in these patients.

Factors influencing prognosis

Unverferth and associates[9] from Columbus, Ohio, determined prognostic risk factors of idiopathic dilated cardiomyopathy (IDC) in 69 patients. Each patient had a physical examination (including a history), ECG, echo, cardiac catheterization, 24-hour monitoring, and endomyocardial biopsy. The mortality rate at 1 year was 35% (24 deaths). Univariate analysis revealed that the most powerful predictor of prognosis was the left intraventricular conduction delay (p = 0.003). The PA wedge pressure was also predictive of mortality (p = 0.005). Other significant factors, in order of importance, were ventricular arrhythmias (p = 0.007), mean RA pressure (p = 0.008), angiographic EF (p = 0.03), AF or flutter (p = 0.01), and the presence of an S_3 gallop (p = 0.05). Factors such as duration of symptoms, presence of MR, end-diastolic diameter, myocardial cell size, percent fibrosis in the biopsy, and treatment with vasodilators, antiarrhythmic and anticoagulant drugs were not significant predictors. Multivariate analysis was used to determine which combination of factors could most accurately predict survival and death. The most important factors were left conduction delay, ventricular

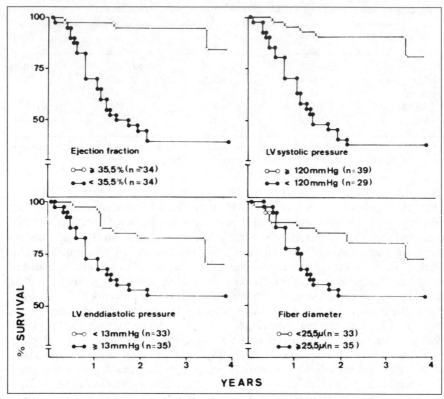

Fig. 6-2. Actuarial survival curves (Kaplan-Meier) of patients with idiopathic dilated cardiomyopathy dichotomized according to LV EF (upper left), LV systolic pressure (upper right), LV end-diastolic pressure (lower left), and fiber diameter of myocardial cells (lower right). Univariate analysis disclosed significant differences for all 4 variables, but the Cox analysis identified LV EF ($p < 0.0001$) and left ventricular systolic pressure ($p < 0.01$) as the only independent predictors of death. Reproduced with permission from Schwarz et al.[10]

arrhythmias and mean RA pressure. An equation was derived that can be applied to the prognosis of patients with IDC. Thus, the clinical assessment of patients with IDC can accurately predict the probability of surviving or dying in 1 year.

Although several morphologic features of the myocardium in patients with IDC have been described, the significance of quantitative morphometric data as independent predictors of survival has not been analyzed. Schwarz and coinvestigators[10] from Heidelberg, West Germany, analyzed data from 68 consecutive patients with IDC to evaluate the prognostic significance of quantitative morphologic findings in LV myocardium compared with the prognostic significance of LV hemodynamics. The LV endomyocardial biopsy specimens were obtained from all patients during cardiac catheterization. Myocardial fiber diameter, volume fraction of interstitial fibrosis, and intracellular volume fraction of myofibrils were determined by light-microscopic morphometry. All patients had normal coronary arteriograms, but reduced LV EF. There were 23 deaths during a mean follow-up of 1,124 days. Multivariate regression analysis by the Cox model revealed that LV EF and LV systolic pressure, but not morphometric findings in biopsy specimens were independent predictors of cardiac death (Fig. 6-2). Thus, these investigators found that morphologic findings in LV myocardium do not contribute significantly to the prognostic evaluation in patients with IDC studied by hemodynamic and angiographic methods.

Wallis and coworkers[11] from Maywood, Illinois, evaluated 50 patients with IDC to determine the frequency and the importance of segmental wall motion abnormalities detected by radionuclide ventriculography: 64% of the patients had segmental and 36% had diffuse wall motion abnormalities. Those patients with segmental abnormalities were older (p < 0.001), had less severe CHF by New York Heart Association classification (p < 0.01), had lower PA wedge pressures (p < 0.001), and had smaller left ventricles (p < 0.001) and better preserved cardiac index and EF (p < 0.001). Those patients with diffuse wall motion abnormalities had more extensive histologic findings based on myocardial biopsy and a higher short-term mortality at 1 year (p < 0.05). Thus, the presence of segmental wall motion abnormalities is a more favorable prognostic finding in patients with IDC. Segmental wall motion abnormalities occur commonly in such patients.

Predominant RV involvement

Fitchett and associates[12] from London, England, described findings in 14 patients aged 9–62 years (mean, 28) with predominately right-sided idiopathic dilated cardiomyopathy (IDC). Five of the 14 died suddenly. Nine were males. Initial symptoms reflected arrhythmia in 10 patients and 4 patients had CHF from the onset, 3 later. The VT caused syncope in 6 patients and SVT resulted in palpitations in 4. Eight patients had no signs of right-sided CHF. The surface ECG was typical of a left BBB pattern. Three patients were examined at necropsy, and 2 of the 3 were brothers. (I [WCR] have never seen a case of IDC involving almost exclusively the right ventricle, and I have seen nearly 200 cases of IDC at necropsy.)

Hydralazine therapy

Magorien and associates[13] from Columbus, Ohio, evaluated central and regional hemodynamic variables at baseline and after 3 months of placebo or hydralazine therapy (100 mg orally every 8 hours) and 20 patients with idiopathic dialated cardiomyopathy (IDC). Both control (placebo) and hydralazine groups were comparable with respect to functional classification (New York Heart Association classes III and IV) and baseline hemodynamic variables. In the hydralazine group, cardiac index increased 25% (2.4 ± 0.4–3.0 ± 0.5 liters/min/M^2), renal blood flow increased 26% (648 ± 199–815 ± 229 ml/min), and limb blood flow was augmented by 35% (6.8 ± 3.0–9.2 ± 4.6 ml/dl/min) with long-term therapy. These changes were significant when compared with both baseline values and values in the control group. Both central and regional hemodynamic parameters remained unaltered in the control group. Long-term hydralazine therapy (3 months) elicited a favorable circulatory response in this group of patients with chronic CHF. Central or regional hemodynamic tolerance to oral hydralazine failed to develop in most patients.

Patterns of inheritance

To determine the mode of inheritance of HC, Maron and associates[14] from Bethesda, Maryland, studied by M-mode and cross-sectional echo 367 relatives from 70 families with HC. Inspection of individual family pedigrees suggested that HC was genetically transmitted in 39 pedigrees (56%) and probably sporadic in 31 (44%) (Fig. 6-3). Of the 39 pedigrees with familial occurrence, 30 had patterns of inheritance that were most consistent with autosomal dominant transmission. A complex mathematical pedigree analysis determined that patterns of genetic transmission observed in the overall study group were not consistent with known models of autosomal dominant, autosomal recessive, or X-linked inheritance and did not support a unified concept of single-gene mendelian transmission for all families (Fig. 6-4). The

Fig. 6-3. Prevalence of different modes of inheritance in 70 families with HC, based on inspection of individual pedigrees.

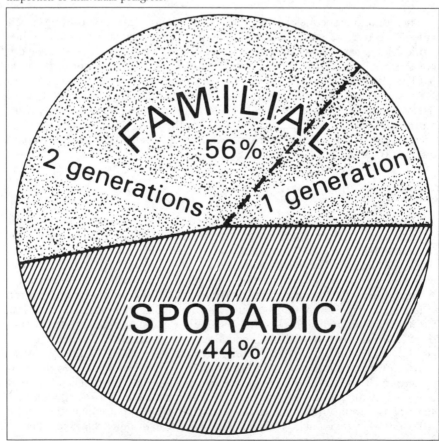

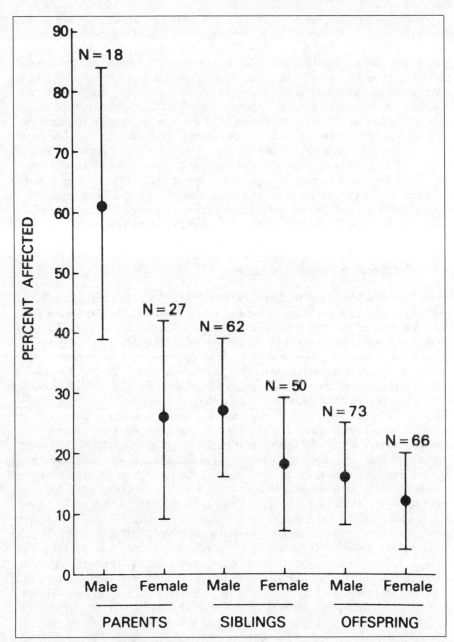

Fig. 6-4.   Proportion of relatives affected by HC (segregation ratio), plotted as mean values with 95% confidence intervals. Shown separately by sex for parents, siblings, and offspring of the proband.

proportion of first-degree relatives affected by HC was 22%, with HC most common in fathers of the proband and least common in offspring. About 20% of the affected relatives (10 of 53) appeared to have inherited a "subclinical" form of HC, in which the sole evidence of HC was the morphologic expression detectable only with echo. Probands and affected relatives differed distinctly with regard to the expression of HC. Probands most often showed functional limitation (81%), subaortic obstruction at rest (53%), particularly diffuse distribution of LV hypertrophy (59%), and marked septal thickening (mean, 23 mm). In contrast, affected relatives were characterized by absence of functional limitation (72%) and subaortic obstruction (94%), localized and unusual sites of hypertrophy (60%), and only modest septal thickening (mean, 17 mm). Probands with the familial or sporadic forms of HC did not differ with regard to the phenotypic expression (clinical or morphologic) of their disease. In conclusion, no single mode of inheritance was typical of HC, although autosomal dominant transmission was most common; a variety of phenotypic expressions occur that appear to have both genetic and nongenetic causes, suggesting that HC may not be a single etiologically distinct disease, and genetic counseling recommendations should be influenced by the particular pattern of inheritance demonstrated in each family.

Miscellaneous echo observations

It has been suggested that the adynamic or hypodynamic appearance of the ventricular septum is a unique echo feature of HC. To determine how characteristic of HC the adynamic septum is, Ciro and associates[15] from Bethesda, Maryland, studied by echo 70 patients with HC and 31 patients with other cardiac diseases that produce LV hypertrophy and pressure overload (AS or systemic hypertension). On M-mode echo, 53 of 70 patients (75%) with HC had an abnormally low value for percent systolic thickening of the septum associated with either reduced or normal septal excursion; however, 17 patients (25%) showed normal septal dynamics. Twenty of 31 patients (64%) with other cardiac diseases that produce pressure overload showed normal septal thickening and excursion, and 11 (36%) had reduced systolic thickening associated with either diminished or normal excursion. Greatly reduced values for percent systolic thickening of the septum were present both in patients with HC ($13 \pm 1\%$) and in patients with other cardiac diseases ($21 \pm 2\%$) (Fig. 6-5). However, differences in systolic septal thickening between the 2 groups were largely a manifestation of the greater absolute diastolic septal thickness in patients with HC (Fig. 6-6). When values for percent systolic thickening were normalized for diastolic septal thickness, or when systolic thickening was compared in only patients with similar diastolic septal thicknesses, differences in septal thickening between patients with HC and those with other cardiac diseases were not significant. Hence, the adynamic or hypocontractile ventricular septum is a frequent, but not invariable morphologic feature of HC, and it occurs commonly in patients with other cardiac diseases that produce LV hypertrophy and pressure overload. Therefore, it is not a specific diagnostic marker for HC.

Suzuki and associates[16] from Kyoto, Japan, evaluated the configuration of the hypertrophied myocardium by thallium-201 emission-computed tomography and 2-D sector scan in 10 patients with obstructive HC, 10 with nonobstructive HC with giant negative T waves, and 10 with concentric LV hypertrophy. Thallium-201 myocardial imaging was reconstructed into multiple 12 mm thick slices in 3 planes. The thickness ratio of the ventricular septum and the LV posterior wall in the short-axis plane and the ratio of the ventricu-

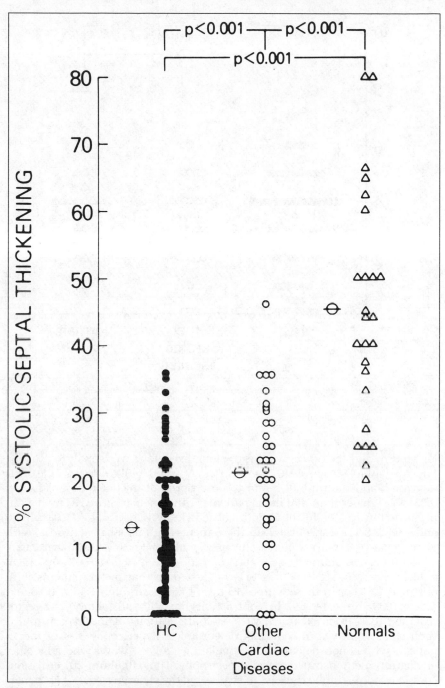

Fig. 6-5. Percent systolic thickening of the ventricular septum in 70 patients with HC, 31 patients with other cardiac diseases that produce LV pressure overload (aortic stenosis and systemic hypertension), and 25 subjects with normal hearts. The mean values are indicated by the slashed circles.

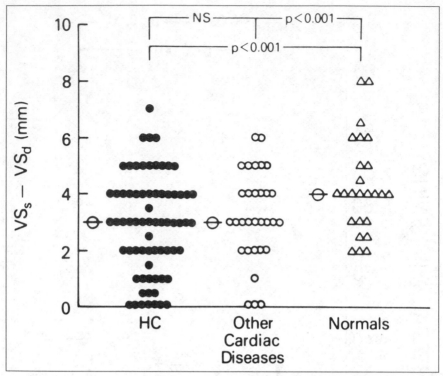

Fig. 6-6.   Absolute change in ventricular septal thickness between systole and diastole ($VS_s - VS_d$) in 70 patients with HC, 31 patients with other cardiac diseases that produce LV pressure overload, and 25 normal subjects.

lar septum and the apical wall in the long-axis plane were analyzed. In the patients with obstructive HC, the ventricular septal wall thickness index was increased, and the ratio of septal to posterior wall thickness index (1.45 ± 0.23) was greater than that in the patients with nonobstructive HC with giant negative T waves or in those with concentric LV hypertrophy (1.03 ± 0.20 and 0.98 ± 0.11, respectively). In the patients with nonobstructive HC with giant negative T waves, increased apical wall thickness with apical cavity obliteration was characteristic, and the ratio of ventricular septal to apical wall thickness index (0.66 ± 0.14) was less than that in the patients with obstructive HC or in those with concentric LV hypertrophy (1.46 ± 0.38 and 1.04 ± 0.09, respectively). In contrast, technically satisfactory 2-D sector scanning (83%) demonstrated various configurations of the hypertrophied ventricular septum, but could not detect apical hypertrophy in 4 of the 10 patients with nonobstructive HC with giant negative T waves whose LV cine-angiograms demonstrated apical hypertrophy. Thus, thallium-201 emission-computed tomography is useful in evaluating the characteristics of LV hypertrophy and assists 2-D sector scan, especially in patients with apical hypertrophy in HC.

Spirito and Maron[17] from Bethesda, Maryland, identified a variety of patterns of systolic anterior motion (SAM) of the mitral valve by real-time 2-D echo in 62 patients with HC (Table 6-2; Fig. 6-7). In 36 patients (58%) both

TABLE 6-2. *Relation of M-mode echo findings to patterns of mitral systolic anterior motion identified by 2-D echo*

			M-MODE ECHO			
					SAM	
PATTERNS OF		VS THICKNESS		MV POSITION		
SAM (2-D ECHO)	# PTS.	(MM)	VS/FW	INDEX*	MODERATE	SEVERE
AML + PML	36	20 ± 6	1.8 ± 0.6	0.9 ± 0.6	13 (36%)	23 (64%)
AML	6	20 ± 1	1.8 ± 0.5	0.9 ± 0.2	3 (50%)	3 (50%)
PML	19	23 ± 4	2.0 ± 0.4	0.9 ± 0.4	15 (79%)	4 (21%)
Chordal	1	24	1.3	0.6	1	0

* Position of the mitral valve in the LV cavity was assessed at the point of closure of the valve leaflets at the onset of systole. Mitral valve position index was calculated by dividing the distance between mitral valve and posterior LV free wall by the distance between mitral valve and ventricular septum.
AML = anterior mitral leaflet; MV = mitral valve; PML = posterior mitral leaflet; SAM = systolic anterior motion of mitral valve; VS = ventricular septum; VS/FW = ventricular septal to left ventricular free wall thickness ratio.

the anterior and posterior mitral leaflets appeared to participate importantly in SAM, although the anterior leaflet actually contacted or most closely approached the ventricular septum during systole because of its anterior anatomic position. In 19 patients (31%), SAM was produced selectively by the posterior mitral leaflet. In only 6 patients (10%) was the anterior leaflet alone responsible for SAM. In just 1 patient did the chordae tendineae appear to be primarily responsible for the SAM. In 51 patients (82%), only the distal portion of the anterior or posterior mitral leaflet (and possibly the attached proximal chordae tendineae) approached or contacted the septum in systole; in 10 patients both the body and tip regions of the anterior leaflet produced mitral-septal apposition. Hence, in obstructive HC the morphologic structures responsible for moderate to severe SAM are not identical in all patients, and a variety of patterns of SAM occurs; the posterior mitral leaflet plays an important role in SAM in almost 90% of patients, either by producing SAM alone (31%) or by moving anteriorly in concert with the anterior leaflet

Fig. 6-7. The variety of patterns of mitral systolic anterior motion (SAM) identified in patients with HC. Most often, both the anterior and posterior mitral leaflets (AML and PML) are responsible for SAM, with or without the contribution of the attached proximal portion of chordae tendineae (AML + PML); in other patients SAM is due to the PML alone, or the AML alone, or rarely to only the chordae tendineae.

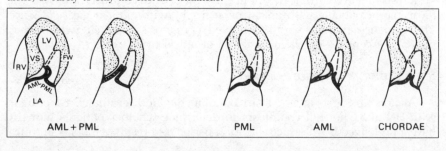

(58%); SAM produced selectively by the anterior mitral leaflet is relatively uncommon; and SAM is usually produced primarily by the distal portions of the mitral leaflets (with or without the attached chordae tendineae).

Changes in outflow gradient

Ciro and associates[18] from Bethesda, Maryland, analyzed, by >1 preoperative hemodynamic study, changes in LV outflow pressure gradient in 409 patients with HC. Basal LV outflow tract obstruction either spontaneously appeared (or increased) or disappeared (or decreased) in 19 nonoperated patients (about 5%). Changes in the hemodynamic state were shown by serial cardiac catheterization in 17 patients and by catheterization and M-mode echo in 2 patients. In most patients (12 of 19), subaortic obstruction under basal conditions appeared or increased; 8 became more symptomatic and in 4 the condition remained stable. Reduction or loss of LV outflow gradient occurred in 7 patients; in 5 their condition deteriorated and in 2 it did not change. Hence, in 13 of the 19 patients (70%), spontaneous changes in the magnitude of the basal LV outflow gradient were associated with symptomatic progression. The mechanism of the decrease or disappearance of subaortic obstruction in those patients who deteriorated appeared to be related in 4 patients to impaired global and/or segmental LV function. Chronic AF probably contributed to the worsening clinical condition in 2 of these patients and in 2 others. In conclusion, substantial changes in the magnitude of basal subaortic obstruction may occur in a small proportion of patients with HC as part of the natural history of their disease, and such hemodynamic alterations are usually associated with clinical deterioration. It is exceedingly rare for the hemodynamic state of a patient with HC to change from totally nonobstructive to obstructive or vice versa, because such patients usually retain the capacity to generate gradients with provocative maneuvers.

Prognostic factors

Koga and associates[19] from Kurume, Japan, followed 136 patients with HC for 1–17 years; 21 had died: 14 suddenly, 2 from CHF, 2 from cerebral embolism, and 3 from noncardiac causes. Life-table analysis revealed that sudden death was significantly associated with age <20 years (relative risk [rr] = 8.63, when compared with those >40 years) and with positive Master's single 2-step test (rr = 3.55). In patients with positive Master's single test (rr = 4.27) and with LV end-diastolic pressure >20 mmHg (rr = 2.58) CHF was more frequent. Observed in 15 patients, AF was a poor prognostic sign, resulting in 5 cardiac deaths and 7 with CHF. In contrast, prognosis was favorable in patients with apical hypertrophy with giant negative T wave. Thus, Japanese patients with HC showed a prognosis consistent with Western patients, except for excellent outcome of apical hypertrophy.

Isovolumic relaxation period

Alvares and associates[20] from London, England, evaluated 84 patients with HC in 31 normal volunteers to determine whether patients with HC have a prolonged isovolumic relaxation period as a result of a delay in mitral valve opening. Isovolumic relaxation was measured as the period from the aortic closure sound to the opening of the mitral valve on echo. In these patients, the isovolumic relaxation period ranged from 0–160 ms (mean, 71 ± 32 ms), and this was not significantly different from that found in the normal controls (63 ± 11 ms). Fifteen patients had an extremely short isovolumic relaxation period caused by marked delay in aortic valve closure. Thus, some patients with HC have an altered timing and sequence of ventricular relaxation.

Ventricular arrhythmias

Frank and associates[21] from Augusta, Georgia, assessed the prevalence of essentially lethal arrhythmias in 50 patients with HC, and also the rate at which the arrhythmias developed during a 2–14-year (mean, 6) follow-up (Fig. 6-8). Sixteen potentially lethal arrhythmias detected at the beginning of observation were excluded from actuarial analysis for new potentially lethal arrhythmias. Twenty-one patients had 24 new potentially lethal arrhythmias (7 with conduction system disease, 1 with sustained SVT, 6 with VPC couplets, and 10 with VT); only 43% of these potentially lethal arrhythmias were heralded by new symptoms. In 6 patients the arrhythmia caused symptoms and was identified by a routine ECG. The 3 patients with His-ventricular disease presented with syncope and required electrophysiologic confirmation of this diagnosis. In only 1 patient was a potentially lethal arrhythmia (VPC couplets) detected only by exercise testing. All other ventricular arrhythmias

Fig. 6-8. Adjusted event-free rate of potentially lethal arrhythmias (PLA) in HC cohort (n, 50). S.E.E. = standard error of the estimate.

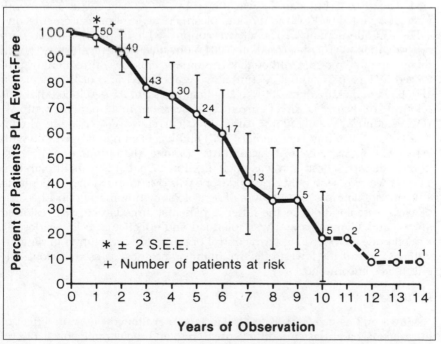

were detected by Holter monitoring. The incidence of conduction system disease in 47 patients free of this condition at entry was 26% at 5 years and 75% at 10 years, and the incidence of VT only was 18% at 5 years and 40% at 10 years. The incidence of all categories of new potentially lethal arrhythmias in the 50 patients was 32% at 5 years and 81% at 10 years. Because new potentially lethal arrhythmias are frequent during long-term follow-up, and most cannot be detected adequately without surveillance, periodic Holter monitoring, at least on an annual basis, is recommended.

Kowey and associates[22] from Philadelphia, Pennsylvania, prospectively evaluated whether induced sustained arrhythmia could explain episodes of cerebral dysfunction in patients with HC. Seven consecutive symptomatic patients (6 of whom had a LV outflow track gradient of 40–130 mmHG) were subjected to atrial and ventricular stimulation. An electrophysiologic abnormality that would explain the symptoms was identified in every patient; SVT was present in 2, sustained VT in 3, VF in 1, and a prolonged QT interval and dispersion of ventricular refractoriness in 1. Antiarrhythmic drugs were selected on the basis of the response to electrophysiologic testing. There has been no recurrence of symptoms in 120 patient-months of follow-up. This experience suggests that arrhythmias are the principal cause of syncope or sudden death in obstructive HC and that electrophysiologic study may be useful in selecting prophylactic therapy.

Amiodarone

McKenna and associates[23] from London, England reviewed findings in 53 patients with HC who had serious arrhythmias (45 patients), refractory chest pain (5 patients), or a high risk of sudden death (3 patients) for 6–96 months (median, 18) after completion of a loading and an initial maintenance period. The dose of amiodarone was altered by 50–200 mg/day at 3–6-month intervals, guided by ECG monitoring, plasma drug level measurements, and side-effect questionnaires. The VT was suppressed in 24 patients (92%) with doses of 100–400 mg/day (median, 300); none died suddenly during a mean follow-up of 27 months. Although symptomatic episodes of frequent or prolonged SVT or paroxysmal AF/flutter were abolished in 8 of 9 patients on 100–600 mg/day (median, 300), in 1 patient incessant AF developed that was relatively refractory to direct current cardioversion. In 11 patients with AF, sinus rhythm was restored in 7 (after direct current cardioversion in 3) with doses of 100–600 mg/day (median, 300) and has been maintained in 5 with associated improvement in symptoms. Despite discontinuation of beta blocker therapy, chest pain was unchanged in 17 patients, was impaired in 11, and was worse in only 2. Amiodarone was discontinued in 3 patients; in 1 because of hair loss, in 1 because of neurologic symptoms, and in 1 because of facial discoloration; in the latter 2 patients, amiodarone was restarted after 1 and 14 months and was tolerated and effective at a lower dosage. Amiodarone provides long-term control of refractory arrhythmia in patients with HC, and if the lowest effective maintenance dose is used, serious side effects are uncommon.

Diltiazem

Suwa and associates[24] from Osaka, Japan, evaluated the acute effect of intravenously administered diltiazem, 10 mg, and the chronic effects of oral diltiazem, 180 mg/day, and propranolol, 60–120 mg/day, administered for 2 weeks in 13 patients with HC. The systolic and diastolic LV function was evaluated. Intravenous injection of diltiazem reduced isovolumic relaxation time from 114 ± 26–99 ± 21 ms and the time to peak rate of LV dimensional lengthening from 166 ± 17–133 ± 10 ms, without significant changes of LV dimensions or fractional shortening. No significant changes were observed in LV dimensions or fractional shortening, but a significant increase in peak rate of LV dimensional lengthening (from 4.1 ± 1.5–4.8 ± 1.6/s), and a reduction in isovolumic relaxation time (from 105 ± 26–77 ± 23 ms) and the time to peak rate of LV dimensional lengthening (from 156 ± 23–124 ± 1220 ms) occurred during the oral administration of diltiazem. In contrast, propranolol caused no significant changes in these values. Thus, diltiazem improves LV relaxation and diastolic filling without altering LV systolic function in patients with HC.

Verapamil

Spicer and associates[25] from Ann Arbor, Michigan, administered verapamil (5.2 ± 1.1 mg/kg/age; range, 2.8–7) to 13 pediatric patients with HC for 13 ± 6 months (range, 2–20). The patients had significant symptomatic improvement on verapamil therapy. Murmur intensity diminished in 6 patients during therapy and LV electromotive forces on the ECG diminished in 4, increased in 5, and did not change in 4. Exercise endurance increased from 8.4 ± 3.9–10.9 ± 2.8 minutes (p < 0.01). Seven patients had ST-segment depression (0.38 ± 0.28 mV) before verapamil therapy, which improved after verapamil therapy in 5 (0.24 ± 0.17 mV, p < 0.02). Of 4 patients with exercise-induced ventricular ectopic activity, 3 had diminution or abolishment of ectopy after verapamil. By echo, the patients had an increase in LV end-diastolic dimension from 3.4 ± 0.7–3.9 ± 0.8 cm (p < 0.01), with no significant change in shortening fraction (46.1 ± 8.0% -vs- 44.6 ± 8.0%). When adjusted for body size and age, there was a significant decrease in LV septal thickness (from 106 ± 70–45 ± 52% of predicted normal values, p < 0.05) and LV posterior wall thickness (from 40 ± 45–5 ± 26% of predicted normal values, p = 0.05) after verapamil. Isovolumic relaxation time decreased from 69 ± 26–42 ± 19 ms after verapamil (p < 0.01). Systolic anterior motion of the anterior mitral leaflet disappeared in 5 of 8 patients and midsystolic closure of the aortic valve was no longer present in 4 of 8. Chronic oral verapamil appears to be an effective therapy for pediatric patients with HC.

Anderson and associates[26] from San Francisco, California, evaluated changes in LV systolic and diastolic function in outflow gradient in 15 patients with obstructive HC after intravenous acute treatment with verapamil and in 11 patients after 6 months of oral chronic treatment. All patients had severe symptoms despite beta blockade and the condition of all but 2 improved after chronic treatment with verapamil. Resting LV outflow tract gradient decreased in 6 of 15 patients after intravenous verapamil, and in 5 of 11 patients after long-term treatment, but there was no change in provocable gradients nor any correlation between changes in gradient and improvement in symptoms. The LV ejection rate did not change after intravenous or oral treatment. End-systolic pressure and end-systolic volume index remained unchanged after oral verapamil treatment. Whereas LV total stroke volume index and end-diastolic volume index increased without any significant change in LV end-diastolic pressure, indicating improved LV diastolic function. In some patients the LV diastolic pressure-volume curve shifted downward or to the right or both. These findings suggest that improvement in symptoms with verapamil in patients with obstructive HC is unlikely to be related to changes in LV outflow gradient or in systolic function and may be related to improved diastolic function.

Observations after operation

To define LV morphologic features after ventricular septal myotomy-myectomy and to elucidate the structural changes associated with a postoperative reduction in the pressure gradient, Spirito and coworkers[27] from Bethesda, Maryland, studied 28 patients with obstructive HC with M-mode and qualitative and quantitative 2-D echo. Nine patients with a marked reduction in the pressure gradient had a marked reduction in septal thickness after surgery (23–13 mm), a concomitant increase in septal to mitral valve distance (20–30 mm), and a loss or substantial decrease in the magnitude of systolic anterior motion of the mitral valve. Two-D echo results demonstrated an increase of >100% in the cross-sectional area of the LV tract at onset of systole (2.2–5.5 cm^2). In 6 patients, postoperative paradoxical septal motion appeared to contribute importantly to the increased size of the outflow tract during ventricular systole. In contrast, 9 patients with little or no change in the pressure gradient demonstrated a less marked decrease in septal thickness and no significant change in septal to mitral valve distance or magnitude of mitral systolic anterior motion. Ten patients with only provocable subaortic gradients after operation showed postoperative LV outflow tract dimensions intermediate between those in patients with either residual basal gradient or no residual gradient. On the basis of this echo assessment of septal myotomy-myectomy, the investigators concluded that abolition or reduction of the subaortic gradient after operation in patients with obstructive HC is largely the consequence of surgical enlargement of the LV outflow tract area.

Fighali and coworkers[28] from Houston, Texas, evaluated 36 patients with HC to determine the long-term results of septal myotomy-myomectomy, MVR, or both. Patients were followed for 5–67 months (mean, 48) postoperatively. Mean LV outflow tract gradient at rest decreased postoperatively in all 3 patient groups (Fig. 6-9). Specifically, mean LV outflow gradient decreased from 60 mmHg (range, 17–160) preoperatively to 3 mmHg (range, 0–20) postoperatively (p < 0.001) in the 13 patients who underwent MVR alone; the outflow tract gradient decreased from 69 mmHg (range, 18–140) to 35 mmHg (range, 20–50) (p < 0.05) in the 12 patients who underwent myotomy-myomectomy alone, and from 89 mmHg (range, 60–165) to 4 mmHg (range, 0–27) (p < 0.001) in 11 patients who underwent myomectomy plus MVR. There was also a marked reduction in symptoms related to outflow tract obstruction after all 3 surgical procedures. There were no operative deaths. The postoperative annual mortality rate was 1.6%. Patients with severe CHF, significantly elevated LV end-diastolic pressure, or AF had a less favorable long-term postoperative course. These data suggest that septal myotomy-myomectomy is the procedure of choice for most patients with HC, because it improves hemodynamics and alleviates symptoms and it avoids

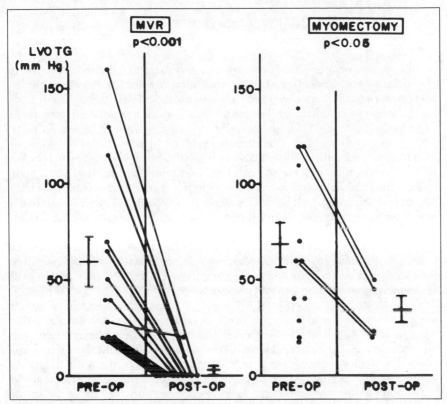

Fig. 6-9.   Mean LV outflow tract gradient (LVOTG) at rest before (PRE-OP) and after (POST-OP) MVR or myotomy and myomectomy. Reproduced with permission from Fighali et al.[28]

the complications of a valve prosthesis. However, the data obtained in this study also suggest that MVR should be considered for patients with associated severe MR and in those patients in whom a previous myotomy-myomectomy has failed to lessen symptoms and/or relieve the LV outflow obstruction.

Laser myoplasty

Isner and associates[29] from Boston, Massachusetts, performed laser myoplasty intraoperatively in 1 patient with HC using a 200 μ fiber interfaced with an argon laser. Measured laser power was 1.5 W; cumulative exposure was <4 minutes; the myoplasty was 4 × 1 × 0.5 cm. These investigations established the feasibility of using laser therapy to create a myoplasty trough that is similar in appearance to that typically achieved by the conventional blade technique. Illumination of the intraventricular operative field and precise modeling of the myoplasty trough constitute the principal advantages of laser myoplasty for HC. Follow-up data on their patient is essential to learn if this new procedure was indeed beneficial.

CARDIAC AMYLOIDOSIS

Falk and associates[30] from Boston, Massachusetts, evaluated 27 patients with primary amyloidosis and 6 with familial amyloid polyneuropathy to determine the prevalence of cardiac arrhythmias. Twenty-four hour ECG monitoring was obtained and echo studies (M-mode and 2-D) also were performed. In these patients, clinically significant bradyarrhythmias were rare. Complex ventricular arrhythmias occurred in 14 patients (47%) with primary amyloid and in 3 patients with familial amyloid polyneuropathy. Cardiac arrhythmias correlated with CHF and with an abnormal ECG. Four patients died suddenly and each had an abnormal echo and complex ventricular arrhythmias. Thus, these data suggest that complex ventricular arrhythmias are common in patients with cardiac amyloidosis and may be a predictor of subsequent sudden cardiac death.

The presence of amyloid infiltration has been described in 5–10% of patients with cardiomyopathies. Nicolosi and coworkers[31] from Pordenone, Italy, designed a study to determine whether changes in myocardial wall echogenicity that suggest amyloid disease could be prospectively identified by a qualitative analysis of 2-D echo images: 2,078 consecutive echoes obtained over a 14-month period were prospectively analyzed. The myocardial walls of 30 patients had multiple, discrete, small, and highly refractive echoes; amyloid disease was not known or suspected in any of them. It was recommended that all 30 patients undergo gingival biopsy to confirm the diagnosis and biopsy was performed in 15 patients. The recommendation for biopsy was made only on the basis of 2-D echo changes and was independent of findings regarding thickness of the walls or the dimensions of the cardiac chambers. Results of biopsy were positive in 11 patients and negative in 4. The investigators concluded that qualitative evaluation of 2-D echo images can identify changes in myocardial wall echogenicity that correlate with the result of gingival biopsy positive for amyloidosis. In patients who have a typical myocardial texture by 2-D echo and a positive gingival biopsy result, cardiac amyloidosis should be strongly suspected. Thus, echo is a useful noninvasive tool for detection of cardiac amyloid, which could then be definitively diagnosed by biopsy.

Serial echo studies are lacking in patients with primary amyloidosis. To see whether serial echo studies could detect early changes of amyloid infiltration of the heart and substantiate progression of cardiac amyloid infiltration, Cueto-Garcia and associates[32] from Rochester, Minnesota, performed serial echoes in 27 patients with primary systemic amyloidosis. Thirteen patients had no clinical cardiac deterioration between the 2 echo studies (group 1), whereas in 14 patients (group 2) CHF or arrhythmia or both appeared or worsened during a mean observation period of 19 months (Table 6-3). The only echo changes in group 1 were a mild increase in LV mass and a mild decrease in LV wall systolic thickening. Patients in group 2 had significant changes in LV wall thickness (mean increase, 34%), in LV mass (mean increase, 42%), in RV wall thickness (mean increase, 78%), in LA size (mean increase, 19%), in LV mass/voltage ratio (mean increase, 68%), in LV radius/thickness ratio (mean decrease, 29%), and in LV fractional shortening (mean decrease, 13%). Significant correlations were found in group 2 between

TABLE 6-3. *Serial echo findings in patients without (group 1) and with (group 2) clinical cardiac deterioration.* Reproduced with permission from Cueto-Garcia et al.*[32]

	GROUP I (n, 13)			GROUP 2 (n, 14)		
	FIRST STUDY	SECOND STUDY	P	FIRST STUDY	SECOND STUDY	P
Interval (mo)	20.1 ± 6.7			18.6 ± 8.3		NS
LVWTd (mm)	11.5 ± 1.6	12.02 ± 2.10	NS	12.36 ± 2.60	16.60 ± 2.27	<0.001
LVWTs (mm)	17.0 ± 2.0	17.0 ± 1.9	NS	17.7 ± 3.2	20.5 ± 2.7	<0.001
LVWTST (%)	53.2 ± 7.3	43.9 ± 16	<0.02	46.6 ± 21.0	24.1 ± 20.0	<0.001
VSTd (mm)	10.5 ± 1.9	11.6 ± 2.5	NS	12.6 ± 2.7	17.0 ± 2.9	<0.001
VSTs (mm)	14.6 ± 2.0	15.5 ± 1.9	NS	16.5 ± 3.0	20.4 ± 2.9	<0.001
VSTST (%)	40 ± 16	37 ± 20	NS	31.9 ± 12.9	20.3 ± 11.0	<0.001
LVDd (mm)	42.1 ± 3.5	43.0 ± 3.3	NS	41.5 ± 2.2†	38.9 ± 5.6†	NS
LVDs (mm)	26.1 ± 2.9	28.1 ± 2.9	NS	26.8 ± 4.4†	27.0 ± 6.2†	NS
LVM (g)	180 ± 42	213 ± 56	<0.02	233 ± 69†	331 ± 87†	<0.001
RVWT (mm)	3.1 ± 2.1	3.1 ± 2.0	NS	4.6 ± 2.8§	8.2 ± 2.7§	<0.01
LAS (mm)‖	33 ± 6	34 ± 5.4	NS	36.1 ± 7.0	43.0 ± 6.0	<0.001
LAS/Ao	1.2 ± 0.27	1.3 ± 0.25	NS	1.4 ± 0.24†	1.6 ± 0.24†	<0.05
FS (%)	37.6 ± 6.1	35.0 ± 6.4	NS	34.9 ± 9.9†	30.3 ± 12.0†	<0.01
Mass/voltage	1.55 ± 0.46	1.70 ± 0.56	NS	2.20 ± 0.80‡	3.69 ± 1.20‡	<0.001
Radius/thickness	2.0 ± 0.4	1.9 ± 0.4	NS	1.7 ± 0.4†	1.2 ± 0.4†	<0.001

* FS = fractional shortening; LAS = left atrial size; LAS/Ao = left atrial size/aortic root dimension; LVDd = LV end-diastolic dimension; LVDs = LV end-systolic dimension; LVM = LV mass; LVWTd = LV wall thickness at end diastole; LVWTs = LV wall thickness at end-systole; LVWTST = systolic thickening of LV posterior wall; RVWT = RV wall thickness; VSTd = ventricular septal thickness at end-diastole; VSTs = ventricular septal thickness at end-systole; VSTST = systolic thickening of ventricular septum.

changes in systolic and diastolic BP and changes in ventricular wall thickness and mass. Changes in LV systolic function did not correlate significantly with changes in other clinical, ECG, or echo measurements. In 6 cases (2 in group 1), in which amyloid infiltration of the heart was proved by myocardial biopsy or autopsy, the only echo abnormality when the patients were asymptomatic was a moderate increase in LV or RV wall thickness. Thus, M-mode and 2-D echo examinations can substantiate progressive amyloid infiltration of the heart and are useful tools for the noninvasive serial assessment of patients with primary systemic amyloidosis.

IDIOPATHIC RESTRICTIVE CARDIOMYOPATHY

Siegel and associates[33] from Los Angeles, California, described clinical, hemodynamic, and morphologic data from 4 patients with a primary restrictive cardiomyopathy. Symptoms of CHF, jugular venous distention, and murmurs of MR and TR were present in all patients. The 4 patients also had pacemakers, 3 for the brady-tachy syndrome and 1 for complete heart block. Echo examination documented LA enlargement in all patients along with normal LV internal dimensions. Global LV systolic function was preserved in all patients and LV, and RV filling pressures were elevated in 3 individuals. A dip in plateau pattern was present in the pressure tracings of 2 of the 3 patients. No specific morphologic cause for the condition was found at necropsy. Thus, a restrictive hemodynamic profile can be observed in the absence of specific infiltrative disorders and affected individuals may have a prolonged clinical course from about 4–14 years. The congestive heart failure that is common in this disorder responded poorly to medical therapy.

MYOCARDITIS

Chiale and associates[34] from Buenos Aires, Argentina, administered oral amiodarone to 24 patients with chronic chagasic myocarditis (CCM) and malignant arrhythmias. Control 24-hour Holter recordings revealed frequent VPC (157–2,572/h; mean, 714 ± 125), multiform VPC, and countless numbers of ventricular couplets in all patients, R-on-T phenomenon in 17 patients, and VT in 21 patients. Amiodarone caused total and persistent suppression of ventricular couplets and VT and >93% reduction of VPC number in 22 patients, during a follow-up of 27 months (range, 2–55). In 1 patient, ventricular couplets and VT persisted despite a 98% reduction of VPC number, and this was the only patient in the whole group who died suddenly. The maximal antiarrhythmic effect was attained gradually after 3–26 weeks (mean, 7). In 4 patients in whom treatment was discontinued after 3–12 months, the antiarrhythmic protection lasted 4–9 weeks. In 9 patients the dose of amiodarone was 600–800 mg/day. In 15 patients the dose had to be increased to 800–1,000 mg/day. Despite the presence of CHF in 7 patients and intraventricular block in 17 patients, no limiting side effects were observed. Amiodarone proved to be effective and safe against the most malignant ventricular arrhythmias.

Vignola and coworkers[35] from Miami Beach, Florida, evaluated 65 patients with either aborted out of hospital sudden death, VT resistant to standard clinically directed antiarrhythmic medication, or high grade ventricular arrhythmia with or without syncope. Among these patients, 17 were identified in whom no obvious cardiac disease was found. Twelve of the 17 underwent RV endomyocardial biopsy. Six of the 12 biopsies demonstrated lymphocytic myocarditis (group A). In 3 of the remaining 6 biopsies, there was evidence of an early cardiomyopathy and the last 3 biopsies were completely normal (group B). No clinical, laboratory, electrophysiologic, hemodynamic, or angiographic criteria identified patients in groups A and B selectively. All group A patients were treated with prednisone and azathioprine. After 6 months of immunosuppression, all patients with myocarditis were reevaluated. Neither VT or VF could be provoked in the laboratory during repeat electrophysiologic testing in 5 of the 6 patients. Repeat myocardial biopsy after immunosuppressive therapy had been discontinued failed to demonstrate evidence of inflammation, but did demonstrate varying degrees of residual interstitial fibrosis. These data indicate that lymphocytic myocarditis can result in a patient presenting with life-threatening ventricular arrhythmias. Diagnosis is made by endomyocardial biopsy and it appears that some of these patients may respond to immunosuppressive therapy.

Although transvenous endomyocardial biopsy is an accepted method to evaluate cardiac transplant rejection, the clinical diagnostic value of the technique for other forms of heart disease has not been established. Parrillo and coworkers[36] from Bethesda, Maryland, performed biopsies in 100 consecutive patients without significant complications. Pathologic diagnostic information obtained was judged to be useful to the clinician in 54 and not useful in 46. In 74 patients with CHF of unknown etiology and a dilated heart, useful diagnoses included myocarditis, vasculitis, doxorubicin cardiomyopathy, and idiopathic dilated cardiomyopathy. In most patients with biopsy findings of myocarditis there were no other clinical or laboratory findings indicating its presence, and the diagnosis of myocarditis would have been overlooked without biopsy. In 26 patients in whom there was clinical evidence of constrictive or restrictive cardiovascular physiologic characteristics, useful biopsy diagnoses included radiation-induced cardiomyopathy, endomyocardial fibrosis, amyloidosis, or no myocardial disease. In the patients without myocardial disease, thoracotomy was performed for constrictive pericarditis. Thus, transvenous endomyocardial biopsy can provide clinically useful information in the evaluation of diseases of the myocardium.

ASSOCIATION WITH A CONDITION AFFECTING PRIMARILY A NONCARDIAC STRUCTURE

Duchenne's muscular dystrophy

In the cardiomyopathy of Duchenne's muscular dystrophy, an ECG in early childhood suggests involvement of the posterobasal LV segment, and necropsy studies have confirmed these regions as sites of myocardial fibrosis in the absence of small vessel coronary disease. Perloff and coworkers[37] from Los Angeles, California, used positron emission computed tomography to study regional LV myocardium with ^{18}F 2-fluorodeoxyglucose and metabolism and/or perfusion with ^{13}NH$_3$. All subjects had thallium-201 scans, technetium-99m multiple-gated equilibrium blood pool imaging, ECG, vectorcardiograms, and M-mode and 2-D echo. ^{18}F 2-fluorodeoxyglucose activity was selectively increased in the posterobasal and posterolateral LV wall in 11 of 12 patients with technically adequate images, indicating accelerated regional exogenous glucose utilization. ^{13}NH$_3$ activity was selectively decreased in the same areas in 13 of 15 patients, indicating either a regional metabolic alteration in uptake and trapping, a reduction in regional blood flow, or both. These data identify a myocardial metabolic abnormality concentrated in specific areas of the LV free wall in living patients with Duchenne's dystrophy.

Perloff and associates[38] from Los Angeles, California, performed ECG, 24-hour ambulatory ECG, vectorcardiography, chest radiographs, echo, electrophysiologic studies, and technetium-99m angiography in 25 patients with myotonic muscular dystrophy to determine the presence, degree, and frequency of disorders of cardiac conduction and rhythm and of regional or global myocardial dystrophy or myotonia. Involvement is relatively specific, primarily assigned to the His-Purkinje system. The cardiac muscle disorder takes the form of dystrophy rather than myotonia and is not selective, appearing with approximately equal distribution in all 4 chambers. Myocardial dystrophy seldom results in clinically overt ventricular failure, but may be responsible for atrial and ventricular arrhythmias. Since myotonic dystrophy is genetically transmitted, a primary biochemical defect has been proposed with complete expression of the gene toward striated muscle tissue, whether skeletal or cardiac. Specialized cardiac tissue and myocardium have close, if not identical, embryologic origins, so it is not surprising that the genetic marker affects both. Cardiac involvement is therefore an integral part of myotonic dystrophy, targeting particularly the infranodal conduction system, to a lesser extent the sinus node, and still less specifically, the myocardium.

Hemosiderosis

Dabestani and associates[39] from Los Angeles, California, performed M-mode and 2-D echo in gated equilibrium blood pool imaging in 10 patients with primary hemochromatosis to characterize the spectrum of pathophysiologic abnormalities of the cardiac ventricles and to determine the response to chronic therapeutic phlebotomy. Dilated and restrictive cardiomyopathic patterns were identified in 1 patient each, but the data did not permit conclusions on when in the natural history a given pattern becomes overt. On entry into the study, 3 patients had normal ventricles and 7 had ventricular abnormalities on echo and blood pool angiography. In 2 of the latter patients, biventricular dysfunction and increased LV mass normalized after phlebotomy; 1 patient achieved a normal LV response to exercise. Of the 4 patients with isolated abnormal LV EF responses to exercise, the EF normalized in 2 after phlebotomy. In 1 patient, isolated RV enlargement and dysfunction (echo and radionuclide imaging) normalized after phlebotomy. Thus, primary hemochromatosis can affect LV and RV size and function; clinically occult cardiac involvement can be identified by echo and equilibrium blood pool imaging; therapeutic phlebotomy can ameliorate or reverse the deleterious effects of excess cardiac iron deposition that appears to exert its harm, at least in part, by a mechanism other than irreversible connective tissue replacement.

Systemic lupus erythematosus

Accelerated CAD and AMI in young patients with systemic lupus erythematosus (SLE) is well documented. The prevalence, however, of CAD is unknown. Accordingly, Hosenpud and associates[40] from Portland, Oregon, selected 26 patients with SLE irrespective of previous cardiac history and performed exercise thallium-201 cardiac scintigraphy. Segmental perfusion abnormalities were present in 10 of the 26 patients (39%). Five patients had reversible defects suggesting ischemia, 4 patients had persistent defects consistent with scar, and 1 patient had both reversible and persistent defects in 2 areas. There was no correlation between positive thallium results and duration of disease, amount of corticosteroid treatment, major organ system involvement, or age. Only a history of pericarditis appeared to be associated with positive thallium-201 results. It was concluded that segmental myocardial perfusion abnormalities are common in patients with SLE. Whether this reflects large-vessel or small-vessel CAD abnormalities remains to be determined.

Scleroderma and CREST

To investigate cardiopulmonary function in progressive systemic sclerosis (scleroderma), Follansbee and associates[41] from Pittsburgh, Pennsylvania, studied 26 patients with maximal exercise and redistribution thallium scans, rest and exercise radionuclide ventriculography, pulmonary function testing, and chest roentgenograms. Although only 6 patients had clinical evidence of cardiac involvement, 20 had abnormal thallium scans, including 10 with reversible exercise-induced defects and 18 with fixed defects (8 had both). Seven of the 10 patients who had exercise-induced defects and underwent cardiac catheterization had normal coronary angiograms. Mean resting LV EF and mean resting RV EF were lower in patients with postexercise LV thallium defect scores above the median (59 ± 13% -vs- 69 ± 6% [p < 0.025], and 36 ± 12 -vs- 47 ± 7% [p < 0.025], respectively). The investigators concluded that abnormalities of myocardial perfusion are common in patients with scleroderma and appear to be due to a disturbance of myocardial microcirculation. Both RV and LV dysfunction appear to be related to this circulatory disturbance, suggesting ischemically mediated injury.

Siegel and associates[42] from Torrance, California, evaluated LV function in 10 scleroderma patients with signs and symptoms suggestive of CHF. M-mode and 2-D echo demonstrated normal to increased systolic function in all patients. The presence of pulmonary venous congestion on the chest radiograph was not useful in assessing LV systolic function. Five of 9 patients with normal to increased LV EF had increased cardiothoracic ratios and increased pulmonary vascular markings. The LV hypertrophy was associated with a worse New York Heart Association functional class, more pulmonary vascular congestion, and greater LA size. In the presence of normal systolic function and LV hypertrophy, diminished LV diastolic compliance may account for the cardiac dysfunction in these patients. Cold pressor testing induced peripheral Raynaud's phenomenon in 9 of 9 patients; however, no ST segment changes or chest pain was provoked. In 7 of 9 patients there was no abnormal decrease in LV EF. Little was found to suggest that a myocardial Raynaud's phenomenon affects LV perfusion or systolic function. Clinical signs and symptoms of CHF and chest radiographs were poor indicators of impaired systolic function. Based on these findings, it appears that evaluation of LV systolic function should include echo or angiographic study before such patients are treated for CHF with inotropic agents.

Follansbee and associates[43] from Pittsburgh, Pennsylvania, evaluated myocardial function and perfusion in 22 patients with progressive systemic sclerosis with the CREST syndrome using exercise and radionuclide techniques, pulmonary function tests, and chest roentgenograms. The results were compared with a similar study of 26 patients with progressive systemic sclerosis with diffuse scleroderma. The prevalence of thallium perfusion abnormalities was similar in the groups with CREST syndrome and diffuse scleroderma, (64 -vs- 77%), but the defects were significantly smaller in the CREST syndrome. Reperfusion thallium defects in the absence of extramural CAD were seen in 38% of patients with diffuse scleroderma. This finding was not seen in any of the patients with the CREST syndrome. In diffuse sclero-derma, abnormalities of both RV and LV function were related to larger thallium perfusion defects. In the CREST syndrome, abnormalities of LV function were minor, were seen only during exercise, and were unrelated to thallium perfusion defects. Abnormal resting RV function was seen in 36% of the patients with the CREST syndrome and was associated with an isolated decrease in diffusing capacity of carbon monoxide. It is concluded that the cardiac manifestations of the CREST syndrome are distinct from those found in diffuse scleroderma. Unlike diffuse scleroderma, abnormalities of LV function in the CREST syndrome are minor and are unrelated to abnormalities of coronary perfusion. The RV dysfunction in the CREST syndrome appears to be primarily related to pulmonary vascular disease.

Diabetes mellitus

Until recently, cardiac dysfunction in patients with diabetes mellitus has been believed to be due solely to CAD. Several recent studies have suggested a unique type of cardiomyopathy in patients with diabetes unrelated to ob-structive CAD. Friedman and associates[44] from New York City determined whether type I diabetics without clinically apparent heart disease had abnor-malities of the cardiovascular response to stress and whether blood glucose control, reflected by hemoglobin A_{1c}, was associated with these abnormali-ties. Although diabetics had a normal LV EF (66% ± 6%), they showed a trend toward smaller LV cavities. Their cardiovascular response to a cold pressor test was abnormal and cardiac function after the cold pressor test correlated with hemoglobin A_{1c} levels. Average hemoglobin A_{1c} was inversely related to EF and early filling volume and directly related to the ratio of preejection period/ejection time (PEP/LV ET) after a cold pressor test. Hemo-globin A_{1c} at the time of study correlated more closely with PEP/LV ET after a cold pressor test than did the 6-month average hemoglobin A_{1c} level, sug-gesting that cardiac function fluctuates with recent changes in blood glucose control. Thus, even when diabetics have a normal LV EF, an abnormal cardi-ovascular response to stress may still be present, and such abnormalities correlate with blood glucose control.

Mildenberger and coworkers[45] from Toronto, Canada, evaluated ventric-ular function at rest and during supine bicycle exercise using gated radionu-clide ventriculography in 20 diabetic patients and 18 normal subjects without clinical evidence of heart disease. Ages of the diabetic patients were 21–44 years and all except 1 received insulin therapy. During exercise, no subject developed chest pain or ECG changes suggestive of ischemia. Individuals in both groups had a similar rest and exercise heart rate and BP and achieved similar workloads. Control subjects had an EF at rest of 65 ± 6% (mean ± SD) and only 1 of 18 demonstrated a decrease in EF with exercise. Diabetic patients had a mean EF at rest of 64 ± 7% but 7 of 20 showed a decrease during exercise and the mean EF response was significantly lower than that of the control group (p < 0.01). The EF response to exercise in the diabetic patients varied widely and the magnitude and direction of the response did not correlate with age, sex, duration of diabetes, cigarette smoking, retinopa-thy, exercise heart rate, BP, or rate-pressure product. Neither did it correlate with the workload achieved or the EF at rest. These data indicate that approximately one third of patients with diabetes have subclinical LV dysfunction. The etiology of this LV dysfunction remains uncertain.

Alcoholic hepatic cirrhosis

Kelbaek and associates[46] from Frederiksberg, Denmark, investigated by noninvasive means cardiac performance in 15 patients (mean age, 47 years) with biopsy proved alcoholic hepatic cirrhosis and no cardiac symptoms and who had abstained from alcohol drinking for ≥2 months. They also studied 12 healthy persons of the same age as controls. Heart rate at rest was significantly elevated in the patient group, median 90 beats/minute (range, 62–128) -vs- 73 beats/minute (range, 61–89; p < 0.02). No significant differences were found in physical work capacity and systolic time intervals, and echo parameters did not differ with the exception of LA dimension (median, 36 mm [range, 22–47] in the patient group and 31 mm [range, 17–38] in the control subjects, p < 0.05). No significant difference was found in LV EF at rest. During exercise, however, the median LV EF increased only 6% in the patients -vs- 14% in the control subjects (p < 0.05). These results suggest that patients with alcoholic cirrhosis, although free of cardiac symptoms, may have a latent or preclinical cardiomyopathy that is manifested during physical stress.

Ahmed and coworkers[47] from Newark, New Jersey, determined whether cardiac and hepatic abnormalities occur together in alcoholics hospitalized with liver or cardiovascular disease, and elucidated factors that determine the cardiac response to therapeutic modalities for patients with cirrhosis that may alter cardiac function. Thirteen normal subjects (group I) were matched for age, sex, and cardiac size with 37 patients with hepatic cirrhosis (group II). An additional group of 32 alcoholics without cirrhosis (group III) who had cardiac symptoms but no cardiomegaly or CHF also were evaluated. Patients with cirrhosis did not differ from the normal subjects in regard to LV filling pressure or cardiac index. However, 21 patients with cirrhosis had a stroke index significantly less than normal, whereas the remaining 16 patients had a significantly increased stroke index with a diminished systemic arterial resistance. In alcoholics without obvious cirrhosis (group III), LV end-diastolic and mean aortic pressures were significantly elevated compared with values in normal subjects and cardiac index was abnormal. Further analysis revealed that patients with cirrhosis and a reduced stroke index had abnormal filling pressures in response to volume or pressure increments. These data suggest that although obvious cardiomyopathy is infrequent in patients with cirrhosis, relatively asymptomatic myocardial disease may assume clinical importance during periods of stress.

References

1. BAGGER JP, BAANDRUP U, RASMUSSEN K, MOLLER M, VESTERLUNDS T: Cardiomyopathy in western Denmark. Br Heart J 52:327–331, Sept 1984.
2. ZEE-CHENG C, TSAI CC, PALMER DC, CODD JE, PENNINGTON DG, WILLIAMS GA: High incidence of myocarditis by endomyocardial biopsy in patients with idiopathic congestive cardiomyopathy. J Am Coll Cardiol 3:63–70, Jan 1984.

myocarditis by endomyocardial biopsy in patients with idiopathic congestive cardiomyopathy. J Am Coll Cardiol 3:63–70, Jan 1984.

3. O'CONNELL JB, HENKIN RE, ROBINSON JA, SUBRAMANIAN R, SCANLON PJ, GUNNAR RM: Gallium-67 imaging in patients with dilated cardiomyopathy and biopsy-proven myocarditis. Circulation 70:58–62, July 1984.

4. ANDERSON JL, CARLQUIST JF, LUTZ JR, DEWITT CW, HAMMOND EH: HLA A, B and DR typing in idiopathic dilated cardiomyopathy: a search for immune response factors. Am J Cardiol 53:1326–1330, May 1, 1984.

5. HIROTA Y, SHIMIZU G, KAKU K, SAITO T, KINO M, KAWAMURA K: Mechanisms of compensation and decompensation in dilated cardiomyopathy. Am J Cardiol 54:1033–1038, Nov 1, 1984.

6. OLSHAUSEN K, SCHAFER A, MEHMEL HC, SCHWARZ F, SENGES J, JUBLER W: Ventricular arrhythmias in idiopathic dilated cardiomyopathy. Br Heart J 51:195–201, Feb 1984.

7. MEINERTZ T, HOFMANN T, KASPER W, TREESE N, BECHTOLD H, STIENEN U, POP T, LEITNER E, ANDRESEN D, MEYER J: Significance of ventricular arrhythmias in idiopathic dilated cardiomyopathy. Am J Cardiol 53:902–907, March 15, 1984.

8. POLL DS, MARCHLINSKI FE, BUXTON AE, DOHERTY JU, WAXMAN HL, JOSEPHSON ME: Sustained ventricular tachycardia in patients with idiopathic dilated cardiomyopathy: electrophysiologic testing and lack of response to antiarrhythmic drug therapy. Circulation 70:451–456, Sept 1984.

9. UNVERFERTH DV, MAGORIEN RD, MOESCHBERGER ML, BAKER PB, FETTERS JK, LEIER CV: Factors influencing the one-year mortality of dilated cardiomyopathy. Am J Cardiol 54:147–152, July 1, 1984.

10. SCHWARZ F, MALL G, ZEBE H, SCHMITZER E, MANTHEY J, SCHEURLEN H, KUBLER W: Determinants of survival in patients with congestive cardiomyopathy: quantitative morphologic findings and left ventricular hemodynamics. Circulation 70:923–928, Dec 1984.

11. WALLIS DE, O'CONNELL JB, HENKIN RE, COSTANZO-NORDIN MR, SCANLON PJ: Segmental wall motion abnormalities in dilated cardiomyopathy: a common finding and good prognostic sign. J Am Coll Cardiol 4:674–679, Oct 1984.

12. FITCHETT DH, SUGRUE DD, MACARTHUR CG, OAKLEY CM: Right ventricular dilated cardiomyopathy. Br Heart J 51:25–29, Jan 1984.

13. MAGORIEN RD, UNVERFERTH DV, LEIER CV: Hydralazine therapy in chronic congestive heart failure: sustained central and regional hemodynamic responses. Am J Med 77:267–274, Aug 1984.

14. MARON BJ, NICHOLS PF, PICKLE LW, WELSEY YE, MULVHILL JJ: Patterns of inheritance in hypertrophic cardiomyopathy: assessment by M-mode and two-dimensional echocardiography. Am J Cardiol 53:1087–1094, Apr 1, 1984.

15. CIRO E, MAIONE S, GIUNTA A, MARON BJ: Echocardiographic Analysis of ventricular septal dynamics in hypertrophic cardiomyopathy and other diseases. Am J Cardiol 53:187–193, Jan 1, 1984.

16. SUZUKI Y, KADOTA K, NOHARA R, TAMAKI S, KAMBARA H, YOSHIDA A, MURAKAMI T, OSAKADA G, KAWAI C, TAMAKI N, MUKAI T, TORIZUKA K: Recognition of regional hypertrophy in hypertrophic cardiomyopathy using thallium-201 emission computed tomography: comparison with two-dimensional echocardiography. Am J Cardiol 53:1095–1102, Apr 1, 1984.

17. SPIRITO P, MARON BJ: Patterns of systolic anterior motion of the mitral valve in hypertrophic cardiomyopathy: assessment by two-dimensional echocardiography. Am J Cardiol 54:1039–1046, Nov 1, 1984.

18. CIRO E, MARON BJ, BONOW RO, CANNON RO, EPSTEIN SE: Relation between marked changes in left ventricular outflow tract gradient and disease progression in hypertrophic cardiomyopathy. Am J Cardiol 53:1103–1109, Apr 1, 1984.

19. KOGA Y, ITAYA K, TOSHIMA H: Prognosis in hypertrophic cardiomyopathy. Am Heart J 108:351–359, Aug 1984.

20. ALVARES RF, SHAVER JA, GAMBLE WH, GOODWIN JF: Isovolumic relaxation period in hypertrophic cardiomyopathy. J Am Coll Cardiol 3:71–81, Jan 1984.

21. FRANK MJ, WATKINS LO, PRISANT M, STEFADOUROS MA, ABDULLA AM: Potentially lethal arrhythmias and their management in hypertrophic cardiomyopathy. Am J Cardiol 53:1608–1613, June 1, 1984.

22. Kowey PR, Eisenberg R, Engel TR: Sustained arrhythmias in hypertrophic obstructive cardio-myopathy. N Engl J Med 310:1566–1569, June 14, 1984.

23. McKenna WJ, Harris L, Rowland E, Kleinebenne A, Krikler DM, Oakley CM, Goodwin JF: Amiodarone for long-term management of patients with hypertrophic cardiomyopathy. Am J Cardiol 54:802–810, Oct 1, 1984.

24. Suwa M, Hirota Y, Kawamura K: Improvement in LV diastolic function during intravenous and oral diltiazem therapy in patients with hypertrophic cardiomyopathy: an echocardio-graphic study. Am J Cardiol 54:1047–1053, Nov 1, 1984.

25. Spicer RL, Rocchini AP, Crowley DC, Rosenthal A: Chronic verapamil therapy in pediatric and young adult patients with hypertrophic cardiomyopathy. Am J Cardiol 53:1614–1619, June 1984.

26. Anderson DM, Raff GL, Ports TA, Brundage BH, Parmley WW, Chatterjee K: Hypertrophic obstructive cardiomyopathy: effects of acute and chronic verapamil treatment on left ventricular systolic and diastolic function. Br Heart J 51:523–529, May 1984.

27. Spirito P, Maron BJ, Rosing DR: Morphologic determinants of hemodynamic state after ven-tricular septal myotomy-myectomy in patients with obstructive hypertrophic cardiomy-opathy: M mode and two-dimensional echocardiographic assessment. Circulation 70:984–995, Dec 1984.

28. Fighali S, Krajcer Z, Leachman RD: Septal myomectomy and mitral valve replacement for idiopathic hypertrophic subaortic stenosis: short- and long-term follow-up. J Am Coll Cardiol 3:1127–1134, May 1984.

29. Isner JM, Clarke RH, Pandian NG, Donaldson RF, Salem DN, Konstam MA, Payne DD, Cleve-land RJ, Bonin JD, Lolfski FW, Ahron A: Laser myoplasty for hypertrophic cardiomyopa-thy. Am J Cardiol 53:1620–1625, June 1, 1984.

30. Falk RH, Rubinow A, Cohen AS: Cardiac arrhythmias in systemic amyloidosis: correlation with echocardiographic abnormalities. J Am Coll Cardiol 3:107–113, Jan 1984.

31. Nicolosi GL, Pavan D, Lestuzzi C, Burelli C, Zardo F, Zanuttini D: Prospective identification of patients with amyloid heart disease by two-dimensional echocardiography. Circulation 70:432–437, Sept 1984.

32. Cueto-Garcia L, Tajik AJ, Kyle RA, Edwards WD, Greipp PR, Callahan JA, Shub C, Seward JB: Serial echocardiographic observations in patients with primary systemic amyloidosis: an introduction to the concept of early (asymptomatic) amyloid infiltration of the heart. Mayo Clin Proc 59:589–597, Sept 1984.

33. Siegel RJ, Shah PK, Fishbein MC: Idiopathic restrictive cardiomyopathy. Circulation 70:165–169, Aug 1984.

34. Chiale PA, Halpern MS, Nau GJ, Tambussi AM, Przybylski J, Lazzari JO, Elizari MV, Rosenbaum MB: Efficacy of amiodarone during long-term treatment of malignant ventricular ar-rhythmias in patients with chronic chagasic myocarditis. Am Heart J 107:656–665, Apr 1984.

35. Vignola PA, Aonuma K, Swaye PS, Rozanski JJ, Blankstein RL, Benson J, Gosselin AJ, Lister JW: Lymphocytic myocarditis presenting as unexplained ventricular arrhythmias: diagnosis with endomyocardial biopsy and response to immunosuppression. J Am Coll Cardiol 4:812–819, Oct 1984.

36. Parrillo JE, Aretz HT, Placios I, Fallon JT, Block PC: The results of transvenous endomyo-cardial biopsy can frequently be used to diagnose myocardial diseases in patients with idiopathic heart failure. Endomyocardial biopsies in 100 consecutive patients revealed a substantial incidence of myocarditis. Circulation 69:93–101, Jan 1984.

37. Perloff JK, Henze E, Schelbert HR: Alterations in regional myocardial metabolism, perfu-sion, and wall motion in Duchenne muscular dystrophy studied by radionuclide imaging. Circulation 69:33–42, Jan 1984.

38. Perloff JK, Stevenson WG, Roberts NK, Cabeen W, Weiss J: Cardiac involvement in myotonic muscular dystrophy (Steinert's disease): a prospective study of 25 patients. Am J Cardiol 54:1074–1081, Nov 1, 1984.

39. Dabestani A, Child JS, Henze E, Perloff JK, Schon H, Figueroa WG, Schelbert HR, Thes-somboon S: Primary hemochromatosis: anatomic and physiologic characteristics of the cardiac ventricles and their response to phlebotomy. Am J Cardiol 54:153–159, July 1, 1984.

40. HOSENPUD JD, MONTANARO A, HART MV, HAINES JE, SPECHT HD, BENNETT RM, KLOSTER FE: Myocardial perfusion abnormalities in asymptomatic patients with systemic lupus erythematosus. Am J Med 77:286–292, Aug 1984.

41. FOLLANSBEE WP, CURTISS EI, MEDSGER TA, STEEN VD, URETSKY BF, OWENS GR, RODNAN GP: Physiologic abnormalities of cardiac function in progressive systemic sclerosis with diffuse scleroderma. N Engl J Med 319:142–148, Jan 19, 1984.

42. SIEGEL RJ, O'CONNOR B, MENA I, CRILEY JM: Left ventricular function at rest and during Raynaud's phenomenon in patients with scleroderma. Am Heart J 108:1469–1476, Dec 1984.

43. FOLLANSBEE WP, CURTISS EI, MEDSGER TA, OWENS GR, STEEN VD, RODNAN GP: Myocardial function and perfusion in the CREST syndrome variant of progressive systemic sclerosis. Am J Med 77:489–496, Sept 1984.

44. FRIEDMAN HS, SACERDOTE A, BANDU I, JUBAY F, HERRERA AG, VASAVADA BC, BLEICHER SJ: Abnormalities of the cardiovascular response to cold pressor test in Type I diabetes: correlation with blood glucose control. Arch Intern Med 144:43–47, Jan 1984.

45. MILDENBERGER RR, BAR-SHLOMO B, DRUCK MN, JABLONSKY G, MORCH JE, HILTON JD, KENSHOLE AB, FORBATH N, McLAUGHLIN PR: Clinically unrecognized ventricular dysfunction in young diabetic patients. J Am Coll Cardiol 4:234–238, Aug 1984.

46. KELBAEK H, ERIKSEN J, BRYNJOLF I, RABOEL A, LUND JO, MUNCK O, BONNEVIE O, GODTFREDSEN J: Cardiac performance in patients with asymptomatic alcoholic cirrhosis of the liver. Am J Cardiol 54:852–855, Oct 1, 1984.

47. AHMED SS, HOWARD M, TEN HOVE W, LEEVY CM, REGAN TJ: Cardiac function in alcoholics with cirrhosis: absence of overt cardiomyopathy—myth or fact? J Am Coll Cardiol 3:696–702, March 1984.

7

Congenital Heart Disease

Frequency and size of
patent foramen ovale with aging

Hagen and associates[1] from Rochester, Minnesota, studied the incidence and size of the patent foramen ovale in 965 necropsy human hearts and reviewed previous reports (Table 7-1). Neither incidence nor size of the defect was significantly different between male and female subjects. The overall incidence was 27%, but it progressively declined with increasing age from 34% during the first 3 decades of life to 25% during the decades 4–8 and to 20% during the ninth and tenth decades. Among the 263 specimens with patency, the foramen ovale ranged from 1–19 mm (mean, 5) in maximal potential diameter. The size tended to increase with increasing age from a mean of 3.4 mm in the first decade to 5.8 mm in the tenth decade of life.

RA and LA pressures

Parikh and associates[2] from New York City, studied the pattern of RA and LA pressure waves in 40 adults and 55 children in sinus rhythm with an isolated secundum ASD. In adults, 20% of patients had prominent RA "v" waves (v > a) compared with 63% of children. In adults this pattern occurred in the younger patients with higher RA and RV end-diastolic pressure.

TABLE 7-1. *Incidence of patent foramen ovale (PFO) in various studies. Reproduced with permission from Hagen et al.[1]*

YEAR	AUTHORS	# HEARTS	INCIDENCE OF PFO (%)	AGE (YR) OF PATIENTS
1897	Parsons and Keith	399	26	All ages
1900	Fawcett and Blachford	306	31.7	>10
1918	Scammon and Norris	1,809*	29	>1
1931	Patten	4,083*	24.6	Mostly adults
1934	Seib	500	17	>20
1948	Wright et al	492	22.9	Mostly adults
1972	Schroeckenstein et al	144	35.4	>20
1979	Sweeney and Rosenquist	64	31	>10
1984	Hagen et al	965	27.3	>1

* Combined review of literature.

In children no age-related or hemodynamic determinations for the "v" > "a" pattern were found. These investigators clearly show that the "left atrialization" of the RA pressure wave is not a common hemodynamic sign of ASD in adults. The relative paucity of prominent right atrial "v" waves in adults suggests that phasic flow across the ASD during systole may diminish with age, possibly associated with progressive alteration and compliance of a chronically dilated right atrium or ventricle.

Estimating shunt by Doppler

Kitabatake and associates[3] from Osaka, Japan, utilized duplex Doppler to estimate RV and LV stroke volumes in 10 normal subjects and in 22 patients with ASD. Patients ages ranged from 3–66 years and comparisons were made with catheterization data obtained within 1 week in 15 of 22 patients. Doppler estimates of flow velocities were obtained in the RV outflow tract and at the aortic orifice of the LV outflow tract. There was an excellent correlation between Qp/Qs by oximetry at cardiac catheterization with that obtained by Doppler measurements (r = 0.92). Qp/Qs for normal patients averaged 0.99 ± 0.05 and for patients with ASD, 2.20 ± 0.80. These studies indicate that with careful attention to details of the measurement and adequate imaging of outflow orifices, noninvasive estimates of pulmonary/systemic flow ratio are possible. There remains some scatter in terms of values in patients with left-to-right shunts and further work needs to be done to detect clearly the sensitivity, specificity, and diagnostic accuracy of this approach.

Necessity of preoperative catheterization

Freed and associates[4] from Boston, Massachusetts, reviewed data on 161 patients aged 4 months to 33 years (median, 5 years) who were considered clinically to have an ASD: 109 (69%) underwent surgery without catheterization with the diagnosis made by clinical examination alone in 5, RNA in 5,

M-mode echo in 13, and 2-D echo in 43. Both M-mode echo and RNA were used in 24 and 2-D echo plus RNA in 19. Of the 52 patients who underwent catheterization, 47 (90%) had the diagnosis confirmed at surgery. Two patients thought to have a secundum defect had a sinus venosus defect, one had a sinus venosus defect with partial anomalous venous connection, 1 had a coronary sinus septal defect instead of a secundum defect, and 1 had unrecognized partial anomalous pulmonary venous connection without an ASD. The diagnostic accuracy in the group without catheterization was 84% (92 of 109). Nine patients thought to have a secundum defect had a sinus venosus defect and 2 had partial anomalous pulmonary venous connection without an ASD. In 5 of 10 patients suspected of having a sinus venosus defect, 3 had additional unrecognized anomalous pulmonary veins and 2 had anomalous pulmonary venous connection without an ASD. Finally, 1 patient thought to have a primum defect had a secundum defect at surgery. The clinical course and complications at surgery were similar in both groups and in no patient did the surgeon feel that the diagnostic error caused any intraoperative problems.

VENTRICULAR SEPTAL DEFECT

Yeager and associates[5] from Boston, Massachusetts, presented surgical results and follow-up data on 128 patients <1 year of age who underwent primary repair of VSD for failure to thrive, CHF, or PA hypertension. The hospital mortality rate was 8% and the late mortality rate was 2%. Mortality was highest among younger infants with preexisting respiratory problems or hemodynamically significant residual lesions postoperatively. Complications included large residual shunt in 6%, transient neurologic problems in 4%, and persistent complete heart block in 2%. Complete right BBB developed in 64% and bifascicular, in 9%. Recatheterization in 55% showed normal PA pressures in all but 2 patients and these patients had large residual shunts. Complete closure of the VSD had been achieved in 70% of those catheterized and an hemodynamically insignificant shunt was present in 27%. Patients without significant hemodynamic residua were asymptomatic and tended to accelerate growth after surgery. Risk factors for poor results included preoperative error in diagnosis, multiple VSD, and possibly age at surgery or complicating features, such as respiratory failure or systemic infection. Although the mortality figures are a little higher than in older patients, surgery in infancy may be required to avoid death or severe complications. The PA hypertension regressed completely in all patients even in the presence of abnormal histologic morphometric findings of pulmonary vascular disease. Postoperative heart block occurred in 3 patients and in 1 this occurred several years after the operation. Right BBB occurred in 62% of the patients, despite predominantly transatrial closure.

Momma and associates[6] from Tokyo, Japan, studied development of aortic valvular deformities retrospectively in 395 inpatients with subarterial infundibular VSD. Aortic valvular deformities included prolapse into the VSD without AR (77 patients), prolapse and AR (95 patients), and aneurysm of the sinus of Valsalva (36 patients). No aortic valvular deformity was found and 111 of these 187 patients had associated PA hypertension. Prolapse and regurgitation of the aortic valve developed most frequently at ages 5–8 years. Sinus of Valsalva aneurysm was not found before age 10 years, but began to develop during the teens and was diagnosed most frequently in the 20s. Only 1 patient with PA hypertension developed an aortic valvular deformity. All inpatients with VSD and without PA hypertension over age 30 years had developed some aortic valvular deformities.

PULMONIC VALVE STENOSIS

Isolated "critical" PS is rare and its surgical management currently remains controversial. Coles and coworkers[7] from Toronto, Canada, reported their experience with 36 neonates <1 month of age. Each underwent pulmonary valvotomy, which was isolated in 22 (12 deaths, 54%), plus a systemic-PA shunt in 8 (2 deaths), and in 5 patients associated with perioperative infusion of prostaglandin E_1 (PGE_1; 0 deaths). There was significant improvement in hospital mortality in those receiving a systemic-PA shunt or perioperative PGE_1 when compared with those undergoing isolated valvotomy ($p < 0.05$). Late postoperative angiography demonstrated RV growth in most patients, but important residual abnormalities of the RV outflow tract necessitated secondary surgical procedures in many. The actuarial rate of freedom from reoperation was 73% at 5 years and 42% at 10 years. The investigators current protocol for management of critical PS involves the perioperative administration of PGE_1 combined with urgent transarterial valvotomy performed with inflow occlusion. If there is evidence of postoperative deterioration in the clinical status of a patient during weaning from PGE_1 (continued for 24–48 hours postoperatively), a systemic-PA shunt is constructed.

Johnson and coworkers[8] from Lexington, Kentucky, studied 15 consecutive patients aged 3 months to 35 years with PS or RV outflow obstruction from an aneurysm of the membraneous septum. A Doppler system capable of both pulsed and continuous wave recording was used. Gradients estimated from Doppler correlated well with those measured at cardiac catheterization with a correlation coefficient of 0.95 and an SEE of 8 mmHg. There was a trend to underestimation of gradient in more severe obstruction. These authors and others indicate the usefulness for Doppler in estimating the severity of PS. Clearly, experience in close contention to examination technique with minimalization of angle of incidence and precise localization of the area of maximum flow velocity are required to prevent errors with this technique.

Kan and associates[9] from Baltimore, Maryland, reported on transluminal balloon valvuloplasty for treatment of 20 patients with PS aged 3 months to 56 years. Follow-up catheterization was performed in 11 patients 2–12 months after the procedure. Peak systolic gradient decreased from 68 ± 27 to 27 ± 5 mmHg ($p < 0.001$, after valvuloplasty), and was 22 ± 5 mmHg in 9 patients studied 6–12 months after valvuloplasty. All patients with typical PS had an excellent result. One patient with a very thick dysplastic valve and a second patient who was dilated 11 months after a closed valvulotomy for pulmonary atresia had initial decreases in gradient that subsequently reverted to near prevalvuloplasty values. These investigators, who have been instrumental in developing this technique, demonstrated excellent results for valvuloplasty for typical PS. The results have been duplicated in a number of centers, and this method will probably become the treatment of choice for the typical patient with PS. The very thick nodular dysplastic valve in most cases has not been treated successfully by this method. It is still unclear as to which patients with moderately dysplastic valves can be treated adequately with balloon valvuloplasty.

Rocchini and coworkers[10] from Ann Arbor, Michigan, performed percutaneous balloon pulmonary valvuloplasty in 7 children with moderate to severe PS with RV to PA gradients >15 mmHg. All patients had a decrease in RV peak systolic pressure from 108 ± 30–60 ± 6 mmHg. All patients tolerated the procedure well with no serious complications. Two patients underwent exercise testing before and after valvuloplasty. Maximal exercise RV pressure was 212 and 175 mmHg before and 140 and 125 mmHg after valvuloplasty. These investigators presented further evidence for the efficacy of this procedure. The RV pressure generally increases to supra-systemic pressure during this procedure with RV end-diastolic pressure increasing usually only to a mild degree. These investigators showed no changes in angiographic RV end-diastolic volume or EF before or after valvuloplasty.

TETRALOGY OF FALLOT

Ventricular arrhythmias

Deanfield and associates[11] from London, England, studied 48-hour ECG in 145 TF patients: 60 were aged 30 months to 46 years and were studied before repair and 85 were studied from 4–22 years after repair: 20% of the uncorrected group had ventricular arrhythmia and the incidence increased significantly from 0% in patients <8 years to 50% in those 8–16 years of age. In the corrected group, 44% had ventricular arrhythmia. The incidence of arrhythmia was associated with an older age at repair but not with postoperative hemodynamic status, duration of follow-up, or era of surgery. Deanfield and associates have made an excellent contribution to the continuing problem of ventricular arrhythmia and TF. In contrast to other investigators, they have not shown an association between arrhythmia and residual hemodynamic problems or abnormalities in function assessed by RNA. As with other investigators, they found an association with older age at repair. They have not treated their patients and as yet have not reported morbidity or mortality. Further follow-up will be useful.

Kavey and associates[12] from Syracuse, New York, studied 38 postoperative TF patients by RNA, echo, exercise testing, and ambulatory ECG monitoring. Patients were divided into groups 1 (n, 18; VPC) and 2 (n, 20; no VPC). Age at surgery was 7.1 years in group 1 and 6.2 years in group 2, with age at study being 18 and 16 years, respectively. There were no significant differences in types of surgical repair, presence of pulmonary regurgitation murmur, or postoperative RV systolic or diastolic pressure. The RV EF was decreased in both groups and not significantly different. The LV EF was significantly lower for group 1, 45 -vs- 55%, with considerable overlap between the 2 groups. In addition, echo RV/LV diastolic dimension ratio was increased in both groups, in group 1 > 2. These investigators demonstrated decreased resting LV and RV EF in a large number of their postoperative TF patients. These patients all underwent repair at a mean age of 6.4 years and at a time when myocardial preservation techniques were not routinely used. As the investigators indicated, both the older age at repair with prolonged hypoxia and polycythemia or intraoperative global ischemia may have contributed to the resting ventricular dysfunction. The data do indicate that a larger right ventricle and a more depressed LV EF are more commonly associated with ventricular arrhythmia, although there was considerable overlap in these measurements between the 2 groups. Fortunately, ventricular arrhythmia in TF appears to be less of a problem in patients repaired in recent years. Continued follow-up of these patients is indicated in an attempt to identify those who may be at risk for serious ventricular arrhythmia to initiate appropriate medical or surgical therapy.

Dunnigan and associates[13] from Minneapolis, Minnesota, performed electrophysiologic evaluation in 3 patients (average age, 25 years) who had repair of TF in childhood. All 3 had had a cardiac arrest or transit neurologic disturbance associated with ventricular arrhythmia. All 3 patients had an excellent hemodynamic result from surgery as judged by cardiac catheterization. Ambulatory ECG and stress testing were normal in 2 patients and showed complex VPC in 1. During invasive electrophysiologic studies, all patients had inducible VT with adverse hemodynamic effects. These data indicate that rapid VT inducible in the catheterization laboratory may occur despite an apparent excellent surgical result in TF.

Late results of operation

Klinner and coworkers[14] from Munich, Germany, reported a 25-year postoperative follow-up of 642 patients who survived repair of TF between 1958 and 1980. A valveless transanular patch was employed in 140. The average age at operation was 10 years. In the transanular patch group, there were 25 (18%) late deaths compared with 33 (7%) in the nonpatch group. Two-thirds of the deaths in each group were cardiac in origin. Actuarial survival at 20 years was 80% for those receiving a patch and 93% in the nonpatch group. The New York Heart Association functional class of each group was similar, most being class I or II. The investigators concluded that patients with a valveless RV outflow patch should be observed carefully in the follow-up period and the presence of increasing cardiomegaly postoperatively should indicate thorough evaluation and consideration for implantation of an orthotopic pulmonary valve. Although there are many differences in the intraoperative methods employed during the early years of this study when compared with operations performed in the modern era, the evidence presented in this study is against the indiscriminate use of transanular patching during TF repair. In addition, it clouds some of the current enthusiasm for the use of nonvalved extracardiac conduits in the repair of other congenital defects.

Lorgeril and associates[15] from Geneva, Switzerland, studied LV function after repair of TF in 84 patients aged 1.5–16 years at a mean of 4.6 months after operation. The postoperative LV EF was decreased in 46%. The variable most significantly associated with altered LV function was a history of hypoxic spells. Although no correlation was found between the duration of cardiopulmonary bypass and LV EF, bypass times >120 minutes were associated with a decreased EF. These investigators demonstrated a relatively large number of patients with altered LV EF after TF repair. These data suggest that factors other than duration of preoperative hypoxia and cardiopulmonary bypass time are associated with LV dysfunction. Relatively severe hypoxia that can occur intermittently with hypoxic spells may have accounted for a significant part of the LV dysfunction. Factors relating to myocardial protection rather than bypass time also may have played a role as yet undefined.

COMPLETE TRANSPOSITION
OF THE GREAT ARTERIES

LV outflow tract by echo

Subpulmonic stenosis in complete TGA is a frequently associated malformation, the precise diagnosis of which is essential for optimal medical and surgical treatment. Sixteen patients with TGA and RV outflow obstruction were studied by M-mode and 2-D echo and cardiac catheterization in an investigation carried out by Vitarelli and associates[16] from Rome, Italy. Dynamic obstruction was found in 6 patients and fixed stenosis in 10. Systolic anterior motion of the mitral valve without fixed obstruction of the LV outflow tract was present in patients with dynamic stenosis. Measurements of LV end-diastolic posterior wall thickness/minor semiaxis ratio correlated well (p < 0.001) with the pressure gradient across the LV outflow tract. In addition, it was possible to delineate various types of anatomic fixed obstruction. M-mode echo provided assessment of dynamic obstruction but did not allow quantitative evaluation of the length of the narrowed segment. The latter can be achieved by 2D echo, which offers improved definition of different anatomic types.

Balloon septostomy

Powell and associates[17] from Liverpool, England, assessed palliation afforded by balloon septostomy in 124 infants with TGA. Successful palliation was defined as survival after initial septostomy to 6 months of age without any further palliative or definitive procedures other than surgery for associated anomalies. By this definition, failure was significantly affected by the presence of VSD, LV outflow obstruction, or PDA. In addition, the maximum volume of the balloon used to perform the septostomy also was related significantly to successful palliation and the size of the ASD found in subsequent surgery or necropsy. The use of larger balloon volumes (up to 6 ml) for balloon atrial septostomy has been an available technique for several years. These investigators are the first to show definite improvement in the size of the defect produced associated with balloon volumes between 3.5 and 6 mm. In addition, they do not indicate an excessive incidence of complications compared with smaller balloons. They recommend beginning septostomy with volumes of 2–2.5 mm and subsequently increasing to a maximum of

4–4.5 mm. Echo can frequently provide evidence of how large the foramen ovale is and what balloon size may be useful. It is obvious that only the "flap" of the atrial defect can be torn and the muscular edges underneath cannot be ruptured successfully with a balloon.

Venous switch operation

Venous switching can be accomplished by either the Senning or Mustard operations. Living autologous atrial tissue is used in the former, whereas a baffle of either parietal pericardium or synthetic material is used in the latter. Cobanoglu and colleagues[18] from Portland, Oregon, reviewed their results with 75 patients with TGA and essentially intact ventricular septum who underwent Mustard's operation with a pericardial baffle between 1965 and 1983. The operations were standardized in that a rectangular patch of pericardium was used for the baffle and the pulmonary venous chamber was enlarged with a triangular patch of pericardium. There were 16 deaths within 30 days and 12 late deaths. Late follow-up included 45 survivors (97%) and at 9 years actuarial survival for those operated between 0 and 6 months of age (group I) was 48%, 7–12 months (group II), 55%, and >12 months (group III), 68%. Thirteen patients underwent reoperation for baffle dysfunction, superior vena cava obstruction in 11, baffle leak in 2. The reoperation-free rates at 4 years for group I was 59%, group II, 78%, and group III, 95%. At 9 years, this was 59, 60, and 95%, respectively. Before 1973, 1 of 3 patients reoperated on died early and 1 at 4 months postoperatively. Since then, there have been no operative deaths and 1 late death in the 10 patients reoperated on. The investigators concluded that the incidence of reoperation remains higher in patients <1 year of age and even though reoperation carries a low risk, they now favor the Senning procedure in this younger age group. The use of the arterial switch operation in some medical centers during the first few weeks of life for patients with TGA, and intact ventricular septum introduces new controversy to the surgical management of these patients. Careful analysis of early and late results, such as presented by these investigators, is mandatory to provide an objective basis for determining the most appropriate surgical management program for these patients.

Ramsey and associates[19] from Melbourne, Australia, evaluated RV and LV function in 25 children after a Mustard repair of TGA. Mean age at operation was 2.6 years and mean age at study was 12.2 years. First-pass and gated equilibrium RNA was performed on all patients at rest and during supine bicycle exercise. First-pass studies showed a slightly higher RV EF but with neither technique did the mean RV EF increase with exercise. With the equilibrium technique, 71% had an abnormal exercise response and with the first-pass technique 61% had abnormal results. Although the mean LV EF increased significantly with exercise, 35% of patients had an abnormal LV exercise response with equilibrium technique and 41% with the first-pass technique. These investigators present similar data on rest and exercise function in postoperative TGA patients to that previously reported by three other groups. (Benson et al., *Circulation* 65: 1052–1059, 1982; Parrish et al., *Circulation* 67: 178–183, 1983; and Murphy et al., *Am J Cardiol* 51: 1520–1526, 1983). They have demonstrated that similar conclusions can be made on RV EV using either equilibrium or first-pass studies in these patients. In addition, they have found a significant incidence of abnormal LV function with exercise as previously reported. These data have been seen commonly in patients with little or no clinical symptoms. Close follow-up of a large number of these patients will be important to determine long-term effects of these abnormalities in patients with an atrial repair of TGA.

Arterial switch operation

Venous switching has become the classic management of patients with TGA and intact ventricular septum. Concern remains regarding the occurrence of late RV failure or TR and the development of atrial arrhythmias after this procedure. Arterial switching is successful when the left ventricle is used to systemic afterload and in TGA intact ventricular septum, this is present in the neonatal period or may be later induced by preliminary banding of the pulmonary trunk. Castaneda and coworkers[20] from Boston, Massachusetts, reported their experience with 14 neonates, 18 hours to 32 days of age, who underwent arterial switching. The mean preoperative LV/RV systolic pressure ratio was 0.92, and echo showed a ventricular septum that was centrally positioned in 10 and displaced rightward in 4. There was 1 (7%) hospital death and 2 patients required later reoperation for supravalvular PS. This experience demonstrates the capacity of the neonatal left ventricle effectively to assume the systemic circulation. The investigators indicate that a longer follow-up is needed to assess late ventricular function, coronary ostial and anastomotic growth, and delayed function of the "new" aortic valve. This is a superb surgical experience that has raised major questions regarding the best management program for this subset of patients with TGA.

A variety of arterial switch operations has been developed for patients with TGA and certain types of double-outlet right ventricle (DORV). The most common of these is the extracardiac arterial switch procedure first performed successfully by Jatene. Another developed by Damus, Stansel, and Kaye consists of dividing the pulmonary trunk, connecting its proximal end to the ascending aorta, and reestablishing continuity of the distal PA, with the right ventricle usually incorporating a valved extracardiac conduit. Ceithaml and coworkers[21] from Rochester, Minnesota, reviewed their experience with this procedure in 20 patients operated on between 1975 and 1982. They ranged in age from 6 days to 20 years (median, 13 months); 20 with TGA and associated VSD in 10, and 4 with DORV and subpulmonary VSD. There were 14 (58%) hospital deaths, 13 occurring among 17 patients with ≥1 of the following risk factors: age <18 months, weight <10 kg, LV peak systolic pressure <75% of systemic. Follow-up of the 10 operative survivors ranged from 12–87 months (mean, 57). There was 1 late death from RV failure 2 years after repair and the remaining 9 patients are asymptomatic. Two reoperations to replace stenotic conduits were performed and an additional patient awaits this. The investigators believe this procedure is of value in this subset of patients when coronary artery translocation necessary in the Jatene procedure is restricted by anatomic factors. Results are best in patients with TGA or DORV and subpulmonary VSD who are >18 months of age and have a "prepared" left ventricle.

Borow and associates[22] from Middlesex, England, and Boston, Massachusetts, studied 12 children who had undergone anatomic repair for TGA. The ages at anatomic correction ranged from 0.2–2.9 years and 8 had prior pulmonary trunk banding. The interval from repair to study averaged 2.3 ± 1.4

years and ranged from 0.4–4.8 years. Patients were studied noninvasively after sedation with the use of echo to estimate LV wall stress and percent shortening of the LV minor axis before and during afterload stress with methoxamine. Data were compared with 9 control subjects whose ages ranged from 6–16 years and who had normal findings on cardiac physical examination and echo. Ten of 12 patients had normal end-systolic pressure-dimension relations and normal values for percent LV shortening as normalized for end-systolic wall stress. There was an inverse relation between the age at anatomic correction and the end-systolic pressure dimension slope value for these patients. These intriguing data indicate that most patients studied after early anatomic correction of TGA have normal values for contractile state as estimated from end-systolic pressure dimension and percent LV shortening as normalized for wall stress. There appears to be a relation between age at repair and contractile state as estimated with these methods. The methods for estimation of contractile state, however, remain, since this same group (Colan et al, *J Am Coll Cardiol* Sept, 1984) showed that percent LV shortening may be influenced by preload changes during afterload stress. Nevertheless, such data as these remain important in attempting to evaluate short- and long-term results after repair of complex congenital heart defects. With increasing surgical proficiency with anatomic repair of TGA, this alternative will become available for more patients. Early results indicate a higher surgical mortality, but perhaps less short-term morbidity. Whether or not long-term abnormalities will be found remains to be determined.

LEFT VENTRICULAR
OUTFLOW OBSTRUCTION

Aortic stenosis in infancy

Huhta and associates[23] from Houston, Texas, used echo to diagnose infants with critical AS. There were no false positive or negative results. Criteria for diagnosis included immobile aortic valve cusps and LV hypertrophy with increased echo density of the LV papillary muscles and mitral valve support apparatus. Patients without other aortic obstruction had poststenotic dilation of the ascending aorta with a ratio of the ascending aorta/aortic anulus >1.7. Disturbed Doppler signal in the aorta supported the presence of AS. These investigators and others have demonstrated the ability to make an accurate diagnosis of critical AS in infancy and avoid catheterization. They demonstrated their method for measurement of the poststenotic dilation, which can be a helpful adjunct. The only other information that can be helpful in deciding whether or not valvulotomy is feasible is data regarding LV size. Previous data from Houston (*Am J Cardiol* 48:887–891, 1981) suggest that an LV cross-sectional area of ⩾1.8 cm^2 is probably a reasonable index of sufficient LV size to be able to pump systemic blood flow after operation. The LV end-diastolic volume by biplane angiogram should be ⩾60% of predicted normal to survive this operation and to be able to pump systemic blood flow.

Waller and associates[24] from Indianapolis, Indiana, present data on a 2-day-old infant who died after undergoing balloon angioplasty for critical

AS. At necropsy, a circumferential transverse aortic tear was found. Six additional infants aged 1–7 days underwent postmortem angioplasty within 1 hour of death. Transverse wall tears occurred in aortas with similar aortic and balloon diameters; no aortic wall damage occurred with rupture of undersize balloons, but aortic rupture resulted with the use of oversize balloons. These investigators suggest that angioplasty balloon diameters ≥1 mm smaller than the diameters of the aortic anulus should be used if this technique is to be applied clinically. Most infants with critical AS have such small orifices that it seems unlikely that many angiographers will be able to get such a catheter across the valve in a reasonable period of time. Thus, application of this technique in the young infant with AS may be limited.

Surgical treatment is manditory for survival of infants with AS who present with severe LV failure. In the past, diagnosis has been made by cardiac catheterization and direct aortic valvotomy performed using cardiopulmonary bypass methods, or inflow occlusion or indirectly by a closed method employing transventricular dilation. Sink and colleagues[25] from London, England, presented their current protocol for these ill infants. When the clinical diagnosis and absence of major associated cardiac anomalies is confirmed by 2-D echo, aortic valvotomy under inflow occlusion is performed without cardiac catheterization studies. Eight infants (6 < 2 weeks of age) were operated on by this method and 5 were diagnosed by 2-D echo alone. There were 2 hospital deaths each in patients with severe endocardial fibroelastosis. The authors concluded that the diagnosis of critical AS in the infant can be accurately made by 2-D echo, obviating the need for invasive studies. They believe the technique of inflow occlusion is best for these seriously ill infants. This technique of inflow occlusion has been used by many groups for aortic valvotomy. I (ADP) believe that a more precise valvotomy can be accomplished using cardiopulmonary bypass methods that are probably as safe except in profoundly ill infants. A selective approach to the surgical management of these infants seems appropriate.

Hospital mortality for neonates undergoing aortic valvotomy has ranged from 29–71%. A variety of surgical methods are available to perform this procedure, including the use of blind transventricular dilation, direct valvotomy by inflow stasis or cardiopulmonary bypass (CPB), or profound hypothermia and total circulatory arrest. In an effort to determine current hospital mortality and the early prognosis of these patients, Messina and coworkers[26] from San Francisco, California, reviewed their experience with 11 neonates <30 days of age who underwent aortic valvotomy between 1976 and 1983. Valvotomy was performed during CPB using a cold blood prime and moderate hypothermia with a mean CPB time of 21 minutes and a mean aortic cross-clamp time of 6.4 minutes. There was 1 hospital death, which occurred in a patient with a small LV cavity and associated aortic coarctation and mitral stenosis. There were no late deaths over a mean follow-up period of 2.2 years and each patient was free of heart failure. Mild or moderate residual stenosis was present in 3 of 4 patients who were restudied late postoperatively. The other had severe residual stenosis and underwent successful repeat valvotomy. The remaining 6 patients were judged by clinical criteria to have mild residual stenosis in 4 and moderate in 2. A new murmur of mild AR was present in 4 of the 10 patients late postoperatively. The investigators concluded that neonates with severe AS can undergo valvotomy using CPB with low hospital risk and a favorable early prognosis.

Subaortic stenosis

There is little information regarding the late prognosis after localized resection of discrete or tunnel type LV outflow obstruction. Thus, Moses and colleagues[27] from Bethesda, Maryland, studied the late follow-up status of 41 of 56 patients who underwent transaortic resection of LV outflow obstruction. There was 1 hospital death (2%) among 42 with discrete and 2 (14.3%) among 14 with tunnel LV outflow obstruction. In the discrete group, 21 patients were in New York Heart Association class I and 5 in class II, compared with 1 and 4, respectively, in the tunnel group (p < 0.05). Postoperative cardiac catheterization was performed in 32 patients within 4 years of operation and the peak systolic gradient was 22 mmHg in the discrete group (25 patients) and 98 mmHg in the tunnel group (7 patients), p < 0.02. Postoperative actuarial survival at 20 years was 82 ± 9% in the discrete group and 40 ± 19% in the tunnel group, p < 0.10. Late survival without an adverse event (death, reoperation, residual gradient >50 mmHg, significant AR, infective endocarditis, or complete heart block) for the discrete group was 43% at 4 years, 36% at 10 years, and 15% at 20 years compared with 0% at 4 years for the tunnel group, p < 0.02. These data indicate that patients with tunnel LV outflow obstruction will have an unsatisfactory result from local resection, whereas those with discrete obstruction will survive and be relieved of symptoms but will have clinically significant adverse events early and late postoperatively. Careful and continued long-term follow-up evaluations are therefore necessary. This careful study provides useful information regarding the late prognosis. The late results in the discrete group are less good than anticipated and this may in part be related to the relatively older age at operation (mean age, 18 ± 2 years) or to the possibility that this is a more complicated lesion than previously believed, an idea supported by other studies. The tunnel type of obstruction should be managed by methods other than transaortic resection.

Vouhe and colleagues[28] from Paris and Amiens, France, described a new surgical approach to permit adequate resection of diffuse subvalvar aortic stenosis with preservation of the aortic valve. The aorta, right ventricle, and septum are incised in the same way as during the aortoventriculoplasty described by Konno and also by Rastan (procedures that include AVR) with the exception that the aortic anulus is carefully divided through the commissure between the left and right aortic valve cusps. The septostomy is extended beyond the limits of the obstruction, and fibrous or muscular tissue is removed from each edge of the septal incision. The various incisions are then closed and the aortic valve reconstructed. This procedure was accomplished in 2 patients, 1 aged 13 years with a tunnel-type subaortic stenosis. Preoperatively, he had a 100 mm gradient between the LV and aorta and trivial AR. Postoperatively, there was no change in the degree of AR and the gradient was reduced to 30 mmHg. The second patient was treated for HC at age 14 years. Preoperatively, there was a gradient of 100 mmHg and a postoperative catheterization study at 1 month showed no gradient and no AR. The investigators caution that this procedure is useful for diffuse subaortic stenosis when the aortic valve and anulus are normal and a dominant septal coronary artery has been excluded by coronary angiography. They believe this may be the procedure of choice in the treatment of diffuse subaortic stenosis, whereas the aortoventriculoplasty and apicoaortic valved conduit operations should be employed when the valvar or supravalvar aortic levels are involved. This procedure will probably become an established one for selected patients with diffuse subaortic stenosis. It provides optimal surgical exposure for resection, is designed to preserve the aortic valve, but, nevertheless, it risks injury to the aortic valve leaflets and the ventricular septum.

Severe anular with or without subvalvar aortic stenosis may be treated by placing a valved extracardiac conduit from the left ventricle to the aorta. DiDonato and coworkers[29] from Rochester, Minnesota, reviewed their experience with 13 patients receiving this procedure between 1974 and 1982. The distal anastomosis was placed to the ascending aorta in 7 and to the abdominal aorta in 6. The conduit was sutured directly to the left ventricle in 6 and in 7 a stented right-angle connector was employed. The mean preoperative LV-aortic gradient was 127 mmHg preoperatively and was reduced to 4 mmHg postoperatively. There were 4 hospital deaths, including each of the 3 < 2 years of age who had associated endocardial fibroelastosis and only 1 among 10 who were between 2 and 18 years of age. Reoperation was required in 7 of 9 survivors between 2.7 and 5.2 years postoperatively for conduit valve failure in 5, progression of native AR in 1, and both of these in 1 patient. An additional patient required a second reoperation for rereplacement of the conduit valve. There was 1 death among these 7. The investigators concluded that although LV-aortic conduits provide excellent relief of LV outflow tract obstruction, the high incidence of late complications argues against this procedure and in favor of management by aortoventriculoplasty.

AORTIC ISTHMIC COARCTATION

Mitral valve abnormalities

Celano and coworkers[30] from Buffalo, New York, performed 2-D echo in 56 consecutive patients with coarctation of the aorta (C of A) ranging in age from 1 day to 33 years. Patients with hypoplastic left heart syndrome or mitral atresia were excluded. Data were compared with 20 normal subjects aged 23 days to 32 years. Associated lesions other than mitral valve abnormalities were present in 28. In 23 patients the mitral valve was normal, 21 had minor anomalies, and 12 had major anomalies, including supravalve MS, valvular MS, MVP, and parachute mitral valve. Minor anomalies included abnormalities of the papillary muscles, chordae tendineae, or both. These data are similar to a report by Rosenquist (*Circulation* 49: 985, 1970) who demonstrated a 58% frequency of mitral malformations in patients with C of A detected at autopsy. The minor anomalies included normally formed small valves with restrictive free margin of the anterior leaflet, underdeveloped space between the papillary muscles and ventricular wall, and abnormal leaflet attachment to papillary muscles or anomalous LV chords. Minor abnormalities of the mitral valve during auscultation are often heard before and after repair of simple C of A. Such abnormalities could be detected by meticulous echo investigation. Although most of these minor lesions cause no symptoms, long-term follow-up is advisable in an attempt to determine which if any of the lesions will become significant at a later age.

Subclavian or synthetic arterioplasty

Coarctation of the aorta (C of A) may be surgically repaired by resection with end-to-end anastomosis, the use of prosthetic patch angioplasty and by subclavian flap repair. The latter repair has been advocated for neonates in the hope that this autogenous tissue will grow appropriately and minimize the chance of recoarctation. Moulton and coworkers[31] from Baltimore, Maryland, reviewed their experience with 29 patients who underwent subclavian flap repair. Each of the 4 early deaths occurred in patients with major associated cardiac anomalies who were operated on during the first 5 days of life. One late death occurred 6 months postoperatively in a patient with a hypoplastic left ventricle. Postoperative follow-up ranged from 3–45 months (mean, 26) and each patient had normal leg pulses and was normotensive. Simultaneous arm and leg BP measured by Doppler showed a gradient >10 mmHg in 1 patient. Postoperative cardiac catheterization studies were performed in 7, and a gradient across the area of repair (5 mm) was found in 1 patient. The investigators concluded that the subclavian flap repair can be performed safely with a mortality determined by the presence of major associated cardiac defects. Intermediate results suggested appropriate growth of the repaired area, but longer follow-up and postoperative exercise testing is planned. This article has a good discussion of the surgical problems and results of C of A repair by various methods.

Some infants with C of A present during the neonatal period with severe CHF. Many have major associated cardiac defects and for these reasons operative mortality has been higher than that for elective repair at an older age. When repair is performed by resection and end-to-end anastomosis in infancy, recurrence or persistence of C of A has been estimated at between 16 and 60%. Penkoske and colleagues[32] from Toronto, Canada, reported their experience with 106 infants <1 year of age who underwent C of A repair by subclavian flap angioplasty between 1977 and 1982. There was 1 (3%) death among 34 group I patients with isolated C of A, 3 (11%) among 27 group II patients with associated VSD, and 21 (47%) among 45 group III patients with various intracardiac defects other than simple VSD. Ninety-six of the infants were operated on during the first 3 months of life, 60 in the first month. Nineteen of the 25 deaths occurred during the first month of life and there were no deaths after age 6 months. Among group II infants, there were 3 deaths among 14 having pulmonary trunk banding compared with no deaths in 13 infants without this (p = 0.12), but the VSD tended to be larger in the banded group. Additional operative procedures were performed in 18 group III patients with 8 deaths (44%), compared with 13 (48%) deaths among 27 patients undergoing isolated C of A repair. The actuarial survival rate of 81 patients dismissed from the hospital was 97% at 2 years, 1 late death occurring in group II and 1 in group III. Nineteen infants had significant arm-leg pressure gradients during the first 18 months after repair, but 11 of these subsequently lost the pressure gradient and became normotensive. Recurrent C of A was present in 5 of 81 infants and 2 reoperations were required. One patient in group I was reoperated on 4 years after repair and a large recurrent posterior shelf was found despite previous resection. This patient and a second patient in group II who was reoperated on at 6 months had a short subclavian patch with stenosis at the distal suture line. The investigators believe that although further information is necessary to provide a definitive recommendation, these clinical results suggest consideration be given to repair of asymptomatic C of A by subclavian flap angioplasty when the infant is 6–12 months of age. For those with an associated VSD, they recommend C of A repair alone and early VSD repair perioperatively should this become necessary.

The timing of elective C of A repair remains controversial. Earlier repair seems to reduce the late development of systemic hypertension, but when performed in small symptomatic infants, it has a higher mortality and a greater incidence of restenosis. Campbell and coworkers[33] from Hershey, Pennsylvania, reviewed their experience with 53 patients <1 year of age who underwent the subclavian flap repair between 1974 and 1984. Thirty-five (66%) were <1 month of age. There were 2 (4%) hospital deaths and no deaths among patients >4 days of age. Invasive follow-up studies were performed in 11 patients and demonstrated residual systolic gradients <20 mmHg in 3 of the 4 in whom a continuous nonabsorbable suture technique was used. No gradient was present in the fourth patient, or in the 7 who had repair using an interrupted nonabsorbable suture technique. Noninvasive evaluation of 9 patients in whom an absorbable continuous suture technique was used suggest no residual gradients. The authors currently favor prompt subclavian flap repair of C of A in all infants with or without symptoms and the use of an interrupted suture technique when absorbable vascular suture is unavailable.

Some infants present with CHF in the neonatal period from C of A and require early operation. Some surgeons are recommending elective repair of C of A in the first year of life in an effort to reduce the frequency of late arterial systemic hypertension. In an effort to answer questions regarding possible long-term growth of the hypoplastic aortic arch and of the intact posterior wall after prosthestic patch aortoplasty for C of A, Sade and colleagues[34] from Charleston, South Carolina, evaluated 21 patients between 1 day to 2 years (mean, 8 months) at operation. Seventeen received a Gore Tex patch and 4 a Dacron patch aortoplasty. Nine patients underwent recatheterization between 2 months and 5 years (mean, 27 months) after repair. There were 2 hospital and 4 late deaths. Systolic BP in the remainder declined from 140 mmHg preoperatively to 101 mmHg postoperatively; right arm-left leg systolic pressure gradients declined from 66–5 mmHg, respectively. The diameter of the transverse aortic arch increased in 6 of 9 patients who underwent postoperative cardiac catheterization. Two patients have evidence of narrowing of the aorta at the patch and 1 patient evaluated 8 years after operation by angiography, has an aortic diameter at the C of A greater than that of either the transverse arch or the descending aorta. The investigators concluded that there is evidence that both the hypoplastic and intact posterior wall of the aorta can grow after patch repair of C of A in infancy. I (ADP) remain concerned regarding the late development of aneurysm formation at the site of prosthetic patch aortoplasty, which has been reported by others in 5 patients >10 years after repair. Although the true late incidence of this important complication is not well defined, I believe caution should be exercised in the use of this method of C of A repair.

Smith and associates[35] from Charleston, South Carolina, studied 50 patients with end-to-end (26 patients) versus synthetic patch aortoplasty (24 patients) repair of C of A. Age at operation was 6.6 ± 3.3 years in the end-to-end group and 7.2 ± 3 years in the patch group. Age at exercise was 14 ± 4 years and 10 ± 3 years, respectively. Systolic BP was significantly higher before and at peak exercise in the end-to-end -vs- the patch repaired group. In addition, arm-leg gradient measured immediately after exercise averaged 32 ± 27 mmHg in the end-to-end group and 10 ± 20 in the patch aortoplasty group. These investigators showed significant differences between 2 types of C of A repair in patients whose repair was outside of the infancy age group. The longer time of follow-up for the end-to-end anastomosis group and the older age at study probably does not account for all of the differences seen. These data indicate that significant postoperative gradients may be brought on by the stress of exercise testing and that such testing can be useful to detect significant residual obstruction in these patients. The control data in this report from 20 subjects is also useful in terms of assessing normal findings.

Spinal cord injury during repair

The incidence of spinal cord complications after coarctation of the aorta (C of A) surgery varies between 0.4 and 1.5%. The youngest previously reported patient in whom this occurred was 3 years of age. Crawford and Sade[36] from Charleston, South Carolina, reported the occurrence of paraplegia after C of A repair in 2 patients aged 2 years and 1 aged 6 months. Each had a large VSD and a PDA supplying the distal aortic flow. Patient temperature during repair varied between 38 and 40°C. The authors speculated that the presence of a large PDA supplying the distal aortic flow may retard the development of arterial collaterals and increase the risk of spinal cord ischemia during aortic cross-clamping. The presence of the VSD may have led to increased left-to-right shunting during aortic cross-clamping, thereby reducing systemic blood flow and contributing to spinal cord ischemia. Hyperthermia may have increased the metabolic demand of the spinal cord tissue at a time of decreased oxygen supply during aortic cross-clamping. The investigators believe that C of A operations should not be performed in individuals who are febrile preoperatively and that body temperature should be measured and kept at normal or less than normal during the period of repair.

ECHOCARDIOGRAPHY

Intrauterine

St.-John Sutton and associates[37] from Philadelphia, Pennsylvania, studied 16 normal fetuses at 4-week intervals from 20-weeks gestation to term using echo. They found that cardiac chamber dimensions, wall thickness, and ventricular muscle mass increased linearly and not exponentially with gestational age. In addition, the ratios of RV/LV diameters and relative wall thickness maintained a fixed relation with gestational age, LV fractional shortening remained constant throughout gestation, and LV mass assessed by echo corresponded closely with postmortem anatomic LV weights. The RV and LV dimensions and wall thicknesses and free wall weights were similar throughout gestation. These studies, in contrast to animal investigations, did not show an RV dominance during fetal life. Because of the relatively higher brain blood flow in the human fetus in contrast to the lamb, it is not only possible but likely that RV and LV stroke volumes during fetal life are more nearly equal than are those reported for the lamb fetus. These studies are valuable in understanding fetal cardiac physiology and alterations that can occur as a result of congenital or acquired cardiovascular disease in the fetus and in the neonate.

Allan and associates[38] from London, England, diagnosed 34 cases of congenital heart disease in 1,600 pregnancies studied with fetal echo. In each case echo diagnosis was confirmed by anatomic study. There were 8 errors in echo diagnosis, including both false-positive prediction of ASD or VSD and false-negative prediction of absence of ASD, VSD, TF, and TGA. Factors contributing to the errors were believed to be small defect size, maternal obesity, only 1 examination, and oligohydramnios. The investigators have an excellent record for correct fetal echo diagnosis of congenital heart disease. Subsequent to their failure to diagnose TGA, no subsequent study was accepted as ruling out this abnormality unless the aortic arch had been identified and a "crossing over" of the 2 great arteries seen. In addition, they subsequently required that septal defects be seen in 2 planes before making the diagnosis and thereafter have not made a false prediction of VSD. With experience in the technique, they feel that it is possible to obtain adequate images in about 95% of pregnancies between 16-weeks gestation and term, although the examination is difficult in the last 8 weeks of pregnancy. These data provide an excellent example of the accuracy of this technique in a large number of patients. When the images are clear, information can be of definite use in obstetric management and decisions regarding pregnancy termination.

For quantifying shunts

Barron and associates[30] from Tucson, Arizona, used Doppler echo for quantifying Qp/Qs ratios in 21 patients. Diagnoses included PDA, ASD, and VSD. Flow estimations were obtained for pulmonary trunk, RV outflow tract, ascending aorta, and mitral valve area. Control data were obtained in 25 normal subjects, 2 months to 12 years, without evidence of cardiac disease. Patients' ages ranged from 2 months to 13 years. Comparison of shunts were made in 18 patients with catheterization data and 3 with radionuclide scintigraphy. For patients with PDA, Qp was calculated at the mitral area and Qs at the RV outflow tract. For ASD patients, Qp was measured in the pulmonary trunk, and Qs at the mitral and ascending aorta areas. For patients with VSD, Qp was determined from the mitral area and Qs in the aorta. Comparison of the Doppler and catheterization data revealed an r value of 0.85 with a SEE of 0.48 for the Qp/Qs ratio. These investigators found a reasonably good correlation of oximetry data with these noninvasive estimates of Qp/Qs ratio. Meticulous attention to detail in obtaining these measurements is important. There was some scatter of the data with the Doppler estimation tending to be lower than the catheterization measurements. This technique, however, continues to show promise in estimating Qp/Qs. A prospective study to determine sensitivity, specificity, and diagnostic accuracy is indicated.

For estimating pulmonary arterial pressure

Stevenson and coworkers[40] used routine M-mode echo in 95 infants and children with congenital heart disease to estimate peak PA pressure measured at catheterization. The interval from pulmonary valve closure to tricuspid valve opening, the period of isovolumic diastole, was measured and plotted on a modified table relating the interval heart rate and predicted peak PA pressure. The correlation for all patients was good (r = 0.86, SEE = 15) but was considerably better in 33 patients whose echo was performed with sedation (r = 0.97, SEE = 6). In patients whose heart rate was >155 beats/minute there was a poor correlation between predicted and measured peak PA pressure. These authors have provided another noninvasive measurement for estimating PA pressure. Other indices that have initially showed promise have included RV preejection/ejection time and more recently the time from onset to maximal PA velocity of flow. The present method has the advantage over systolic time intervals in not requiring a clear definition of the onset of the ECG, only measurement of the same point of the ECG for each patient. In addition, the present method can be used in patients with right BBB. Further testing of this methodology would be helpful to determine if it is going to be clinically useful.

Pulmonic regurgitation

To determine whether pulmonic regurgitation (PR) can be reliably diagnosed using contrast echo, Meltzer and associates[41] from New York City and Tel Hashomer, Israel, studied 24 individuals using echo during intravenous injections of 5% dextrose solution. Twelve were without PR and 12 had PR (10 after intracardiac repair of TF, 1 after a Brock procedure for PS, and 1 after insertion of a RV-PA conduit for pseudotruncus arteriosus). M-mode echoes spatially oriented to the RV outflow tract were obtained. Two blinded independent observers correctly diagnosed PR in all patients when it was present, and correctly excluded it in 11 of 12 of the patients without PR. They disagreed in 1 patient who had an unusual contrast pattern during diastole. Four postoperative patients had PR by contrast echo despite the absence of a cardiac murmur at the time of study. It was concluded that contrast echo is a practical, sensitive, and specific noninvasive method for diagnosing PR.

Congenital mitral stenosis

To define the use of 2-D echo and Doppler methods for diagnosis of forms of congenital MS, Grenadier and associates[42] from Tucson, Arizona, and Haifa, Israel, studied 16 children (age range, 2 months to 13 years) with congenital deformities of the mitral valve documented at cardiac catheterization. Thirteen had additional congenital heart defects, most commonly AS or aortic coarctation. In 8 patients features of mitral valve anatomy were observed and described during cardiac surgery and in 1 child the anatomy was verified by necropsy. Two-D echo studies allowed anatomic subclassification of 10 valves that had asymmetric or single dominant papillary muscles (parachute) and 6 that had arcade mitral valve attached by short chords to multiple diminutive papillary muscle heads. In each patient echoes demonstrated shortened and thickened mitral chordae and doming of the mitral leaflets during diastole, and 7 children had restricted mitral orifices imaged on the short-axis imaging plane. All 7 patients studied by Doppler echo had increased maximal transmitral inflow velocity (range, 111–260 cm/s) greater than the 95% confidence limits for mitral flow velocities in 34 normal children who served as the control group. This investigation suggests that 2-D echo, especially when combined with Doppler interrogation, are sensitive for defining forms of congenital MS.

Overriding and straddling atrioventricular valves

Vargas Barron and associates[43] from Tucson, Arizona, and Mexico City, Mexico, studied 21 patients with positional abnormalities of the AV valves associated with complex congenital heart disease by 2-D echo. Eighteen patients had an inlet VSD with tricuspid valve overriding identified angiographically. On 2D echo, the inlet VSD was visualized, and 10 of the 18 had tricuspid valve overriding with chordal attachments of the tricuspid valve crossing the septum into the contralateral ventricle, that is, overriding with straddling. Three of these were verified intraoperatively or at necropsy. Eight patients had 2-D echo diagnosis of tricuspid valve overriding without straddling, 4 verified at surgery and 1 at necropsy. In 1 patient, an echo diagnosis of valve overriding was missed because chords were not imaged crossing the defect and straddling was verified at surgery. Three patients had mitral valve overriding angiographically; 2 had an echo suggestion of mitral valve overriding with straddling, the other had criss-cross heart with mitral and tricuspid valve overriding by echo and angiography. One patient with mitral valve overriding and straddling had the anatomy confirmed at necropsy. This study suggests that 2-D echo is effective for evaluating and clarifying surgically important abnormalities of the AV valve associated with congenital heart disease.

Aortic stenosis, pulmonic stenosis, or aortic coarctation

Stevenson and Kawabori[44] from Seattle, Washington, used pulsed Doppler echo to estimate aortic and pulmonary gradients in 39 infants and children aged 1 day to 10 years with AS, PS, or pulmonary trunk band. A multiple sample volume method with increased pulse repetition frequency was employed and angle correction not used. There was excellent agreement between Doppler prediction and actual gradients for differences up to 100 mmHg (r = 0.9). These investigators indicate that pulsed Doppler echo can be used to obtain reasonable noninvasive estimates of gradients with the multiple sample volume method and increased pulsed repetition frequency. This method is somewhat difficult to employ in practice for large gradients but certainly gives reasonable estimates for mild and moderate gradients, providing a good echo window can be found with minimal intercept angle and meticulous searching for the highest velocity is performed.

Robinson and associates[45] from London, England, used cross-sectional echo and continuous wave Doppler measurements in the ascending and descending aorta in 6 neonates presenting with reduced or absent pulses to determine the site of obstruction. Abnormal high velocity jets in the ascending aorta in 3 patients with normal descending velocities suggested AS. In the other 3 patients, velocity in the ascending aorta was normal but high in the descending aorta, suggesting coarctation. The Doppler diagnosis was confirmed in 5 patients who required surgery. Two patients had residual high velocity just after valvulotomy and had good agreement between gradients predicted by Doppler and subsequent catheterization-confirmed gradients. Infants with coarctation frequently have an abnormal aortic valve. Determination of the important site of obstruction is certainly extremely useful since the operative approach is vastly different.

Pulmonary arterial and aortic anomalies

Huhta and associates[46] from Houston, Texas, compared 2-D echo with angiogram results in 261 consecutive infants and children with congenital heart disease (aged 1 day to 20 years; mean, 3.3 years). Complete visualization of ascending and descending aorta and arch branches was possible by echo in 255 patients (98%). One or more arch anomalies were present on angiogram in 116 patients (46%) and were detected by echo in 110 of 116 (sensitivity, 95%; specificity, 99%). Anomalies detected by echo included ascending aortic hypoplasia (4 of 4), truncus (3 of 3), right arch (31 of 31), anomalous subclavian artery (11 of 16), coarctation (27 of 29), and PDA (53 of 57). These investigators present excellent results using 2-D echo to determine aortic anatomy. With meticulous attention to detail, as discussed, most aortic anomalies can be detected noninvasively in younger patients.

Gutgesell and associates[47] from Houston, Texas, performed a prospective 2-D echo evaluation in 20 consecutive cyanotic infants to evaluate PA and aortic arch anatomy. Qualitative assessment was compared with angiograms and was as follows: detection of left arch (13 of 13), detection of right arch (7 of 7), PDA identification (13 of 13; 1 false positive echo), identification of right PA (20 of 20), identification of left PA (19 of 20), identification of confluence of pulmonary arteries (19 of 20), and identification of pulmonary trunk (14 of 16; 2 false positive echo diagnoses). Echo estimates of arterial diameters were slightly smaller than those obtained by angiogram. Echo angiogram diameters were: aortic arch, 8.6/10.6 mm; pulmonary trunk, 5.7/6.3; right PA 4.1/4.2; and left PA, 4.2/3.9. These investigators demonstrated superb detail in assessing the aortic arch and innominate artery, the PDA and PA. This article and the figures should be studied in detail by clinicians who deal with cyanotic infants. They concluded that selected infants could undergo systemic-PA shunts without catheterization when the echo data are clear. Further testing of the hypothesis that these infants can be handled effectively without angiogram would be of value.

Anomalous pulmonary venous connection

Cooper and associates[48] from San Francisco, California, studied 6 neonates with the infradiaphragmatic form of total anomalus pulmonary venous connection (TAPVC) with echo Doppler techniques. Three large vascular channels could be observed passing through the diaphragm from the subcostal parasagittal plane. The vessels were identified as the descending aorta closest to the spine, inferior vena cava farthest from the spine, and the anomalous pulmonary venous channel between these 2 vessels. Pulsed Doppler revealed characteristically normal signals in the aorta and inferior vena cava and a continuous venous signal from the anomalous pulmonary vein. These investigators prospectively made the diagnosis of TAPVC below the diaphragm in all 6 patients. This diagnosis is usually possible with 2-D echo without the use of Doppler. Occasionally, however, the findings can be somewhat confusing and this is a good demonstration of the use of Doppler to verify the anomalous vascular channel.

Anomalous coronary artery

Robinson and associates[49] from London, England, studied 3 infants with anomalous origin of the left coronary from the pulmonary trunk. In all 3 cases, an echo-free linear structure apparently arising from the aorta and resembling a normal left coronary was imaged. This false positive simulation of a normal left coronary was believed to be due to the tranverse sinus of the pericardium. Identification of the anomalous origin of the left coronary from the pulmonary trunk appears to be the only reliable echo finding in this condition and is not readily found in many patients with this condition. Contrast angiography remains the procedure of choice for this diagnosis, and echo has not proved to be a feasible alternative at this time.

After the Fontan procedure

Nakazawa and associates[50] from Tokyo, Japan, studied 7 patients after the Fontan procedure with the use of a catheter tip velocity transducer, Doppler echo, and angiocardiography. Patients ranged in age from 2 19 years at the time of surgery and were studied from 1 month to 4 years after repair. Five studies were within 1 month after operation. No patient had valves inserted at repair. The RA contraction caused forward flow in the PA and backward flow in the inferior vena cava. Backward flow to the superior vena cava was minimal. During RA relaxation, a rapid forward flow occurred at inferior and superior vena cava and a small amount of pulmonary regurgitation was seen. Subsequently, forward flow was observed at the cava and PA during RA diastole. Angiographically determined RA stroke volume was <40% of LV stroke volume in 3 patients in whom the postoperative increase in atrial "A" wave (Δa) was $\geq$8 mmHg while it was >LV stroke volume in 4 patients in whom Δa was <6 mmHg. The LV end-diastolic volume was normal or mildly elevated in all patients, but EF was low, averaging 0.53 $\pm$ 0.7 with a reduced cardiac index (2.8 $\pm$ 0.7). There was no correlation between RA stroke volume or RA EF and cardiac index. These data indicate that RA contraction causes forward flow to the PA, and pulmonary regurgitation is insignificant even when valves are not inserted. The postoperative increase in RA afterload may depress RA function and the contribution of atrial contraction to output of the right side of the heart may not be a major determinant of cardiac output. These investigators present interesting data on dynamics of right-sided heart flow in patients after the Fontan procedure. Various studies have indicated that the insertion of valves are probably not necessary in most patients and may actually impede right-sided heart forward flow both early and certainly with time as valve function becomes abnormal. These investigators also demonstrated very high RA pressure, depressed cardiac output, and low LV EF after surgery. The data indicate the need for further studies after the Fontan procedure in an attempt to determine what patients benefit most from the procedure and at what age and with what modifications the operation should be performed.

DiSessa and associates[51] from San Francisco, California, studied flow patterns in the vena cava, and PA using pulsed Doppler techniques. Seven patients had tricuspid atresia and 8 had single ventricle with ages ranging from 5–38 years. Studies were performed between 1 and 6 months after surgery. Ten patients had nonvalved RA-PA connections, 4 had nonvalved RA-RV communication, and an RA-RV valved conduit was used in one patient. In 14 of 15, forward flow in the PA was biphasic, with flow beginning at the end of the T wave (early ventricular diastole), peaking at or before the T wave (atrial systole), and returned to baseline by the peak of the R wave. The second phase of forward flow commenced at the peak of the R wave (ventricular systole) and returned to baseline at the end of the T wave. Caval flow during atrial systole was reversed in 8, absent in 3, and forward in 1 patient. Forward caval flow occurred between the peak of the R wave and the end of the T wave and was either continuous or biphasic. The PA and caval flow patterns were not different for tricuspid atresia -vs- single ventricle patients nor were they dependent on the type of communication used at surgery. These investigators have presented interesting data on Doppler flow profiles in patients with Fontan's operation. There has been considerable speculation that use of the small RV chamber in patients with tricuspid atresia could result in augmentation of pulmonary blood flow and might result in a better functional and clinical result. It has been difficult to demonstrate augmentation of pulmonary flow due to this RV chamber in a number of subjects. Further data, such as this using noninvasive techniques correlated with catheterization demonstration of nonobstructed RA to RV connection and nonobstructed RV to PA outflow in patients with reasonable-sized right ventricles would be useful to demonstrate whether or not use of this small chamber can ever be convincingly demonstrated to augment pulmonary blood flow. It certainly seems logical that such would be the case in those patients in whom a wide anastomosis can be made between right atrium and right ventricle, such as with the Björk modification.

Extracardiac conduits

Reeder and associates[52] from Rochester, Minnesota, studied 23 patients with prior extra cardiac RV-PA conduit. Patients ages ranged from 5–39 years (mean, 18). A valved conduit had been placed in 22 patients. The mean interval from prior surgery was 66 months (range, 21–140). Portions of the conduit were seen in all 23 patients, but the entire conduit could be visualized in none. In 11 patients, ≥1 cusps of the prosthetic valve were visualized and were normal in only 1. Continuous wave Doppler examination was possible in 20 patients and was used to estimate gradient. In addition, 9 patients had TR, and RV pressure was estimated using the peak regurgitant velocity. There was an excellent correlation between estimated RV pressure and conduit gradient measured at catheterization or by Doppler (r = 0.90). These investigators have had considerable experience with conduits in complex congenital heart disease. As has been the experience in other centers, visualization of the entire conduit and obtaining anatomic detail about the conduit is difficult. The correlation, however, of estimated gradients and estimated RV pressure in patients with TR provides a reasonable tool for following these patients. There still remains the problem of identifying at what point intervention in the young child with an obstructed conduit and no symptoms should be done.

Intracardiac masses

Marx and associates[53] from Boston, Massachusetts, reviewed echoes on 741 infants <2 years of age and identified intracardiac masses prospectively in 6 patients. All patients presented with unexplained murmurs that were associated with either hemodynamic instability, arrhythmia, or systemic emboli. Masses identified included: a vegetation from infective endocarditis, mural thrombus, rhabdomyomas, and 1 fibro-fatty nodule adjacent to the tricuspid valve anulus. Although intracardiac masses have been readily identified in older patients and adults, this is one of the first series to review a large number of echoes and present data regarding confirmed diagnosis in infants. This technique can be important in diagnosis to provide guidance in both medical and surgical treatment of patients with intracardiac masses.

Meningococcemia

Boucek and associates[54] from Nashville, Tennessee, assessed myocardial function clinically and with echo in 12 children with meningococcemia. Echo evidence of cardiac dysfunction was found in 7 (58%) as defined by depressed LV shortening fraction (SF). The mean LV SF in these 7 children was 0.25 ± 0.03 compared with 0.39 ± 0.07 in the remaining 5 children. The LV SF estimate of myocardial function correlated strongly with cardiac output by thermodilution ($r = 0.98$, $p < 0.01$). Meningococcemia was not fatal in those children with no evidence of myocardial dysfunction. In contrast, 3 of 7 with myocardial dysfunction died. In children with an initially low LV SF, recovery was associated with normalization of this variable. These studies clearly show evidence of myocardial dysfunction in almost 60% of children admitted with meningococcemia. The echo evidence of the low SF was not due to a low preload or increased afterload, since patients with or without echo evidence of a low SF had similar values for end-diastolic dimension and systemic resistance and similar values for central venous pressure. The implications of the study are that efforts toward performing myocardial performance early in the course of the disease should accompany efforts to be certain that adequate intravascular volume is maintained.

MISCELLANEOUS TOPICS IN PEDIATRIC CARDIOLOGY

Fetal growth

St. John Sutton and associates[55] from Philadelphia, Pennsylvania, quantified the growth patterns of the normal fetal right and left ventricles from postmortem hearts obtained from 55 spontaneously aborted human fetuses from the completion of cardiogenesis to term. Fetal age was assessed by menstrual history and fetal measurements. Each heart was perfused and fixed at constant pressure and dissected to obtain RV and LV free wall, LV, and total heart weights. Total heart and RV and LV wall weights increased linearly with body weight but exponentially with head circumference, crown-rump length, and menstrual history. The RV and LV free-wall weights were similar throughout gestation and the percent that each contributed to total heart weight was constant at 29 ± 2% and 30 ± 2%, respectively. The RV and LV wall thicknesses also did not differ significantly. Finally, the surface areas of RV and LV free walls were indistinguishable throughout the period of gestation. The similarities in RV and LV weights and size indicate a similar growth rate of both ventricles from completion of cardiogenesis to term and do not support the presence of RV dominance in the developing human fetal heart. These studies represent a follow-up of echo measurements by these investigators and others. Prior fetal studies in the lamb have indicated definite RV dominance with the right ventricle pumping from 1.5–2 times as much blood during gestation as the left ventricle. There has been speculation as to whether or not this differential size and blood flow is present in the human fetus. Because there is considerably greater cerebral blood flow in the human fetus than the lamb, the possibility has been entertained that right and left ventricles are similar in size and similar in the amount of blood pumped before gestation. These studies would appear to indicate that such is the case.

Pulmonic valve atresia

Baker and associates[56] from London, England, used radionuclide labeled microspheres to demonstrate the distribution of pulmonary perfusion in 5 patients with pulmonary atresia associated with VSD. Selective injection into pulmonary arteries or systemic pulmonary collateral arteries was performed and subtracted images used to detect those portions of each lung that were supplied by both the PA and collateral vessels. These studies can be helpful in assessing the possibility for ligating or embolizing collateral arteries in patients with multifocal pulmonary perfusion. When collateral vessels are ligated in which there is no other source of perfusion, pulmonary infarction results—usually with disastrous results.

"Absent" pulmonary artery

Presbitero and associates[57] from London, England, reported 12 patients with an angiographic diagnosis of "absent" PA. At subsequent surgery, 10 of 11 had a PA. In 5 of 10 there was a intrapericardial artery and in 5 of 10 the artery was patent only at the hilum. In those without a intrapericardial vessel, the occult artery was on the side opposite the aortic arch and there was evidence of a ductus coming from the innominant artery. The occult artery when identified at operation was usually joined to the systemic circulation in order that continuity between right ventricle and pulmonary trunk might be established surgically at a later date. These investigators presented excellent data on the so-called absent or occult PA. The truly absent PA is rare and as is pointed out surgical exploration is indicated in most patients as early as possible to provide flow through the PA and achieve sufficient growth so that subsequent reconstructive surgery might be performed.

Exercise testing in functional single ventricle

Driscoll and coworkers[58] from Rochester, Minnesota, studied 27 patients, aged 6.5–17 years, with tricuspid atresia univentricular heart and complete AV canal with common atrium with upright bicycle exercise. Of the 27 patients, 12 had 1 previous shunt procedure, 6 had 2 previous shunt procedures, and 1 had a prior pulmonary trunk band. Operations were performed ≥ 1 year before exercise testing. The mean maximal voluntary ventilation was $90 \pm 18\%$ of predicted, and forced vital capacity was 77%. Total work performed, maximal power obtained, and duration of exercise were reduced by an average of 2.3 and 2.8 SD from predicted values, respectively. Maximum oxygen consumption rate as a ratio of predicted values ranged from 24 to 58% of normal. With increasing age, there was significant decrease in work performed. Maximum heart rate during exercise was 3 SD below the predicted normal. The average systemic oxygen saturation was 83% at rest and decreased to 57% during exercise. ST-segment depression of ≥ 1 mm during exercise was found in 11 of 25 and was more common in patients >10 years of age. Arrhythmia was found during or after exercise in 12 of 27 and consisted of single or multiple VPC. Only 1 of 6 patients >10 years had arrhythmia, whereas 11 of 21 >10 years had ventricular arrhythmia. Finally, patients had excessive ventilation at rest and during exercise. These investigators provided excellent quantitative data regarding the reduced exercise response in patients with functional single ventricle. Multiple factors undoubtedly contribute to the abnormal exercise response, including inability adequately to increase pulmonary blood flow, rapid occurrence of metabolic acidosis, inability to increase heart rate normally, abnormal ventilatory response, and ventricular arrhythmia. It will be important to provide comparative data on patients who have had Fontan type operations to determine if there has been a significant improvement in these parameters with this type of palliative repair.

Magnetic resonance imaging

Higgins and associates[59] from San Francisco, California, studied 22 patients with a variety of congenital and cardiovascular anomalies with magnetic resonance imaging (MRI), which detected 11 of 11 abnormalities of great vessels, 6 of 6 atrial septal abnormalities, and 10 of 11 VSD. Complex anomalies such as double-outlet right ventricle, uncorrected transposition, single AV valve, single ventricle, and common ventricle were clearly shown by MRI. These investigators have been pioneers in the use of MRI in various heart defects. These studies demonstrate excellent anatomic detail in patients with known cardiovascular anomalies, including TF and Ebstein's anomaly. Further comparison with other noninvasive modalities such as echo will be useful in defining specific indications for these studies.

Jacobstein and associates[60] from Cleveland, Ohio, studied 17 palliative systemic-PA shunts in 11 patients using ECG gated MRI, which successfully imaged 5 of 9 Blalock-Taussig shunts, 4 of 6 Glenn shunts, and 2 of 2 aortico-

PA shunts. This technique permits assessment of the relative size, course, patency, and distribution of shunts and the size and morphology of proximal pulmonary arteries. These techniques can be useful in older patients with congenital heart disease in whom echo images of aorta and PA are more difficult than in the infant and young child. These images now can be obtained in approximately 20 minutes in most patients. Further data are needed to determine the usefulness, limitations, and cost/benefit ratio for these studies.

Prostaglandin E_1

Teixeira and associates[61] from Toronto, Canada, used prostaglandin E_1 (PGE_1) intravenously for an average of 39 days (range, 8–104 days) in 17 neonates with congenital heart defects. Seven patients had TGA with intact ventricular septum or small VSD, 8 had ductus-dependent pulmonary flow due to right-sided heart obstructive lesions, and 2 had aortic coarctation. Beginning dose was 0.05 μg/kg/minute and the dose was decreased in all patients when this was feasible to as low as 0.00625 μg/kg/minute for continued infusion. Patients with TGA or right-sided heart obstructed lesions had an increase in arterial oxygen tension and the 2 patients with coarctation had an improvement in lower limb BP and restoration of renal function. Adverse effects included CHF in some patients due to increased ductal flow; this provided a difficult management problem in only 1 patient. Mild pyrexia, diarrhea, and apnea or seizures were usually handled easily by reduction in dose. Three patients died and had morphologic examination of the PDA. The changes found were believed to be changes similar to the normally closed ductus and not attributable to PGE_1 therapy. Cortical hyperostosis of long bones of the limbs was seen in 5 patients and was manifested by swelling and tenderness in 3 and detected radiologically in 2. These changes were seen after 3 weeks of therapy and appeared to be dose related. This complication reversed spontaneously when treatment was discontinued. The initial worry about abnormal histologic changes in the ductus with long-term therapy no longer appears to be a major problem. The bone changes are worrisome but do appear to regress completely after therapy is discontinued. Fortunately, in most situations therapy only needs to be given on a short-term basis before surgical intervention is possible.

Venous angioplasty

Lock and associates[62] from Minneapolis, Minnesota, and Philadelphia, Pennsylvania, reported results of balloon angioplasty in 10 infants and children with severe congenital or operative "venous" obstructions. In 5 patients the obstructions were "vena caval" and followed repair for TGA or liver transplant. In 4 patients, balloon angioplasty relieved the obstruction, decreasing the average gradient from 16–5 mmHg and increasing the average diameter from 3–9 mm. Five infants had obstructed pulmonary veins: 3 with congenitally narrowed vessels, 1 with acquired stenosis, and 1 with postoperative obstruction after repair of anomalous venous connections. One patient had a tear in a common pulmonary vein with a modest mediastinal hemorrhage and 1 patient had acute hemoptysis. The balloon dilatation was not believed to be the cause of significant morbidity or death in any of the patients. Whether or not these results will be long-term benefits is still undetermined. Three of the TGA patients had follow-up from 4–6 months with resolution of edema or hepatomegaly. The inability to treat pulmonary venous stenosis successfully is similar to results by other investigators using both operative and balloon dilation techniques.

Occluding vascular anomalies

Fuhrman and coworkers[63] from Minneapolis, Minnesota, reported successful embolization of 15 of 17 vessels in 5 patients aged 5 months to 12 years. Steel coils coated with thrombogenic Dacron strands were inserted through no. 5 or 6 F end-hole catheters. Anomalies successfully occluded were pulmonary AV malformations, systemic-pulmonary collateral arteries, left superior vena cava, and PDA. There were no complications or errors in placement of coils. These investigators present excellent results with coil embolization. Other methods of transcatheter embolization include the use of bucrylate adhesive and attachable silicone balloons. The methodology reported herein has been used sporadically previously and is a technique that should be available at all pediatric cardiac centers that care for a significant number of patients with complex cardiovascular disease.

Amiodarone for arrhythmias

Garson coworkers[64] from Houston, Texas, used amiodarone in 39 patients whose ages ranged from 6 weeks to 30 years (mean, 12 years) with arrhythmias unresponsive to conventional treatment. The most common diagnosis was congenital heart disease and dilated cardiomyopathy was the second most common. Only 3 patients had an otherwise normal heart. Elimination of arrhythmia on 24-hour ECG occurred in 15 of 16 patients with atrial flutter, 11 of 14 with VT, and 5 of 9 with SVT. Symptomatic side effects were rash, headache, nausea, and peripheral neuropathy. Seven patients had asymptomatic corneal deposits that became normal after the drug was discontinued. No side effects occurred in patients <10 years of age. Heart rate decreased in all patients with an average change from 86 ± 12–70 ± 11. The QTc interval increased markedly from 0.38 ± 0.01–0.48 ± 0.02. There were no significant changes in indices of hematologic, renal, or hepatic function. During follow-up from 6 months to 3 years, 21 of 39 continued to take amiodarone with complete control of arrhythmias, 9 were no longer taking the drug, and 9 died. There were 2 sudden deaths, 1 possibly related to the drug and the other definitely related to the drug. These investigators have shown excellent results in treatment of resistant arrhythmias in patients who for the most part had very abnormal hearts. The lack of severe side effects is encouraging, although toxicity still remains a real or potential problem and further follow-up studies are certainly indicated. The drug usually does not worsen CHF and is therefore excellent for treatment of patients with reduced myocardial function. Bradycardia can be a severe problem in patients with known or suspected sinus node or AV node disease and may need pacemaker therapy.

Pulmonary vascular changes after operations

Rabinovitch and associates[65] from Boston, Massachusetts, correlated pulmonary vascular changes assessed morphometrically and also according to the Heath-Edwards classification in patients undergoing repair of congenital cardiac defect. Diagnoses included VSD, TGA, endocardial cushion defect, ASD, aortico-PA shunts, and left-sided valvular disease. Correlations were performed in 74 patients with PA pressure measured 1 day after repair and with pressure and/or pulmonary resistance measured 1 year after repair in 74 and 67 patients, respectively. One year after repair, mean PA pressure or resistance was normal in all patients whose conditions were repaired before 9 months of age regardless of the severity of pulmonary vascular changes. Values also were normal in patients whose conditions were repaired at 9 months or later who had grade A (mild) morphometric findings associated with any Heath-Edwards grade. The PA pressure or resistance, however, was increased in 50% of patients with grade B (severe) morphometric findings and Heath-Edwards grade II or with either mild or severe morphometric changes and Heath-Edwards grades I or II alterations. The PA pressure and resistance were increased in all patients whose conditions were repaired after 2 years of age with grade C morphometric findings and to a severe degree if associated with Heath-Edwards grade III. These data indicate that early reparative surgery is the best safeguard against the persistence or progression of pulmonary vascular disease. Future investigations should be aimed at determining how to induce regression of structural changes, such as extension of muscle into peripheral arteries, medial hypertrophy, and mild intimal hyperplasia, as well as how to stimulate growth of new vessels.

MISCELLANEOUS TOPICS IN PEDIATRIC CARDIAC SURGERY

Cardioplegic protection

Intraoperative myocardial protection with various cardioplegic methods has been extensively studied in adult cardiac surgery, but a paucity of information is available in children. Bull and coworkers[66] from London, England, compared their experience with the St. Thomas Hospital cardioplegic solution used in 200 patients operated on between 1977 and 1981 and 200 patients who received intermittent coronary perfusion between May 1974 and 1977. A large variety of congenital cardiac defects were corrected and were similar in the 2 groups. There was a tendency to accept longer ischemic times in the cardioplegic group ($p < 0.01$). Mortality increased sharply in the perfusion group after 60 minutes and in the cardioplegic group after 85 minutes. Cytochemical and biophysical assessment of 129 pairs of RV biopsy specimens taken before and after ischemia in the cardioplegic group demonstrated deterioration of myocardium despite its use. Poor scores were predictive of hospital death. Overall, about 50% of hospital deaths in the cardioplegic group were attributable to inadequate myocardial protection.

The authors concluded that the use of cardioplegia did not confer substantially greater myocardial protection over the alternative technique of intermittent cross-clamping in the pediatric age group.

Patent ductus arteriosus

Two hundred sixty-eight premature infants with birth weights <1,750 g underwent surgical closure of a PDA as part of a national collaborative study on the management of PDA in premature infants. Wagner[67] from Philadelphia, Pennsylvania, and others reported on this subset of patients, which was part of 752 infants diagnosed as having a hemodynamically significant PDA in 13 participating neonatal intensive care units. Four hundred twenty-one patients were eligible to enter a randomized double blind trial comparing indomethacin and placebo. One hundred forty-six of these infants underwent closure of the PDA because of unsuccessful medical treatment, as did 122 infants who did not enter the randomized trial because of a contraindication to indomethacin in 98, lack of parental consent in 16, and the urgent advisability of operation in 8. No patient died during the operation, which was done at a median age of 10 days, 8 (3%) died within 36 hours of operation, and death in 1 of these was directly related to the surgical procedure (ductal tear with hemorrhage). Overall hospital mortality was 23% but was largely related to the usual problems of prematurity, including bronchopulmonary dysplasia, pneumothorax, and sepsis. The findings indicate that operation is an effective and safe treatment for hemodynamically significant PDA in premature infants. The surgical results are not influenced by birth weight, age at operation, degree of preexisting pulmonary disease, or the prior use of indomethacin.

Ebstein's anomaly

Silver and associates[68] from Bethesda, Maryland, described late clinical and hemodynamic observations in 6 patients who had either tricuspid valve anuloplasty (TVA; 2 patients) or tricuspid valve replacement (TVR; 4 patients) 5–132 months earlier for Ebstein's anomaly of the tricuspid valve unassociated with RV outflow obstruction. Of the 6 patients, 4 had improved postoperatively by 1 New York Heart Association functional class and 2 had improved by 2 functional classes. The cardiothoracic ratio decreased 5–12 months after either TVR or TVA in all 6 patients (from a mean of 0.72–0.62). Repeat cardiac catheterization 5–12 months after TVA or TVR disclosed that the RA mean pressure had increased from a median of 4–11 mmHg (p = 0.05); the RV peak systolic pressure had increased from 19–32 mmHg (p = 0.02); the RV end-diastolic pressure had increased from 5–9 mmHg (p = 0.05); the systemic arterial peak systolic pressure had increased from 115–123 mmHg (p = 0.03); and the cardiac index had increased (in all 4 patients in whom both pre- and postoperative values were available) from 1.7–2.9 liters/min/M^2 (p = 0.06). Thus, the tricuspid valve operations in the 6 patients with Ebstein's anomaly were associated with a decrease in symptoms of cardiac dysfunction, a decrease in cardiac size, an increase in cardiac index, and an increase in RV and RA pressures. The elevation of the RA pressures postoperatively may have resulted from increased RV filling pressures, persistent TR, or bioprosthetic stenosis.

Aortic arch interruption

Most patients with aortic arch interruption have associated intracardiac abnormalities and untreated die in the first few months of life from severe CHF. Whether their surgical management should be by primary complete repair or initial palliative procedures and secondary repair remains controversial. Fowler and colleagues[69] from Oklahoma City, Oklahoma, reported their experience with 17 children 2 days to 4 years of age (13, <3 months). There were 3 patients with isolated aortic arch interruption who survived repair by end-to-end reconstruction. The remaining 14 had associated intracardiac defects and received initial palliation by anastomosis of the left subclavian artery to the aorta in 2, interposition of a Dacron tube graft in 1, and placement of a polytetrafluoroethylene (PTFE) graft with division of PDA and pulmonary trunk banding in 11. Ten (71%) survived initial palliation and among 5 with associated VSD, 3 subsequently underwent successful VSD closure. Six of the group of 14 who had palliation and each of the 3 who had correction are long-term survivors. The investigators concluded that patients with isolated aortic arch interruption should undergo repair with end-to-end reconstruction, whereas those with associated intracardiac anomalies should be palliated by PTFE interposition, division of PDA, and pulmonary trunk banding.

Univentricular heart

Patients with double-inlet ventricle or a "common ventricle" who do not have PS often require surgical treatment early in life. Septation of this heart is an attractive option but there has been little experience with it during the first year of life. Ebert[70] described a staged partitioning procedure accomplished in 5 patients with "common ventricle." The first stage operation was done between ages 2 and 10 months, at which time 2 patches of Teflon felt were placed to separately partition the apical and basal portions of the heart, leaving an opening between them. If the pulmonary trunk was not already banded, a band was placed to reduce pulmonary blood flow. Each survived the first stage procedure and returned 3–8 months later for final closure of the remaining interventricular communication and removal of the band. Each survived this procedure and maintained normal sinus rhythm. Fibrous ingrowth into this synthetic material was present, which stiffened it and prevented paradoxical motion which normally exists after primary septation. Fewer sutures than usual were employed at the first stage and, despite this, at the second stage procedure the patches appeared to be firmly attached to the intervening myocardium. The author believed that further experience is necessary to determine if the septation procedure in infants will prove better than waiting until the children are older and employing either primary septation or the more traditional Fontan-type procedure. This important work clearly places staged septation within the surgical options available to treat patients with double-inlet ventricles. Classically, the septation procedure has been employed in older patients with double-inlet left ventricle and a rudimentary outlet chamber. It has been associated with a high incidence of surgically induced complete heart block. Although this innovative work by Ebert was employed in a different type of heart, it may well be applicable to other morphologic types of double-inlet and holds the promise of markedly reducing the risk of complete heart block in the most common subset of these malformations.

Subaortic stenosis can occur naturally in patients with a univentricular AV connection or may be acquired often after pulmonary trunk banding. Untreated, these patients will die of marked ventricular hypertrophy, cavity obliteration, and subendomyocardial ischemia. Penkoske and coworkers[71] from Toronto, Canada, reviewed their experience with 17 patients, 4 with tricuspid atresia and 11 with double-inlet left ventricle. The diagnosis of subaortic stenosis was made between 11 days and 15 years (median, 2.3 years) after banding in 15. It was present in 1 patient with naturally occurring PS and 1 with pulmonary atresia. The following surgical procedures were performed: extracardiac conduit from LV to aorta in 1 patient (died), creation of an aorto-PA window proximal to the band and tightening of the band in 3 patients (2 deaths), enlargement of the VSD in 3 patients (2 deaths), Fontan procedure in 5 patients (3 deaths), and Fontan procedure plus arterial switch in 2 survivors. The investigators currently recommend initial pulmonary trunk banding followed by early enlargement of the VSD at any sign of narrowing as assessed clinically and by echo. The best long-term results have been achieved in only 2 patients by an atrio-PA operation in addition to arterial repair of the transposed great arteries.

Systemic-pulmonary arterial anastomoses

Various types of systemic-PA shunts are available to palliate cyanotic infants. Woolf and coworkers[72] from Philadelphia, Pennsylvania, Baltimore, Maryland, and Groningen, The Netherlands, compared the results in 3 institutions with the classic Blalock-Taussig, Waterston, and polytetrafluoroethylene (PTFE) interposition shunts among 67 cyanotic infants <2 weeks of age. Early shunt failure (14%), mortality after revision for this (0%), and overall hospital mortality (5%) were lowest for 21 patients who received the PTFE shunt. Postoperative CHF from excessive flow was similar for the Blalock-Taussig and PTFE shunts, both of which were lower than the Waterston shunt. Cummulative probabilities of late shunt adequacy at 1 year were similar for each method (<80%), but probability of late shunt failure was highest for the PTFE shunt at 3.5 years (p = 0.04). These results suggest that the PTFE shunt may be safest in neonates but that secondary shunting or total repair should be considered between 1 and 2 years of age.

Despite general agreement that primary corrective operations are preferable for most patients with correctable congenital cardiac defects, a definite place for systemic-PA shunts persists. The interposition of a PTFE conduit between the subclavian and PA may be a suitable alternative to the classic Blalock-Taussig shunt. Bove and coworkers[73] from Syracuse, New York, evaluated 20 patients, 1 day to 15 years of age, who underwent PTFE interposition shunts. Eleven were <14 days of age and 9 were prostaglandin dependent. A 5 mm graft was used in 18 patients <27 months of age and 6 mm grafts in the 2 older patients. Intraoperative heparinization was employed. One shunt was revised early postoperatively because of twisting of the subclavian artery. There were no hospital deaths, 2 late deaths unrelated to the shunt, no late reoperations, and good palliation in each of the 18 survivors followed between 7 and 29 months (mean, 19). Recatheterization studies in 11 patients demonstrated normal PA pressures, good PA growth, and absence of vessel distortion. The investigators concluded that PTFE shunts should be used selectively and that in neonates with small subclavian or pulmonary arteries better palliation may be achieved than with the classic Blalock-Taussig shunts. The intermediate-term results of PTFE shunts are good, but the long-term results remain undefined. I (ADP) believe this is the shunt of choice for neonates and for older subjects in whom the need for a functioning shunt will not persist >2–4 years. I continue to prefer the classic Blalock-Taussig shunt in older patients when long-term shunt patency is desired.

Ilbawi and coworkers[74] from Chicago, Illinois, reviewed their experience with PTFE interposition shunts in 30 neonates with a variety of congenital defects associated with PS or pulmonary atresia who were <30 days of age (mean, 9 days). The shunt was made through a right thoracotomy in 18, through a left thoracotomy in 9, and through a median sternotomy in 3. A 5 mm graft was employed in 21 and a 6 mm graft in 9. Early shunt occlusion occurred in 3% and hospital mortality was also 3%. There were no deaths or reoperations related to shunt failure in patients followed between 2 and 37 months postoperatively. Actuarial functional life of the shunt at 3 years was 91%. Nine patients underwent postoperative cardiac catheterization studies that showed no distortion of the PA and an increase in the ratio of the diameter of the pulmonary trunk and pulmonary valve anulus to that of the descending aorta by 50% (p < 0.001) and 52% (p < 0.05), respectively. The investigators believe the PTFE interposition shunt may be the shunt of choice in patients <1 month of age.

Cavo-pulmonary anastomosis

A total cavo-PA shunt operation was performed by Kawashima and colleagues[75] from Osaka, Japan, in 4 patients with complex congenital heart disease, including azygos or hemiazygos continuation of the inferior vena cava. Each had a double-inlet ventricle with PS and a common AV valve that was incompetent in 3. Repair consisted of closure of the pulmonary trunk, anastomosis of the superior vena cava receiving azygos or hemiazygos continuation, and the contralateral superior vena cava (present in 2) to the left or right PA. The incompetent common AV valve was replaced in 3. One patient died early from low cardiac output and another 2 months postoperatively from hepatitis and septicemia. The remaining 2 patients are in New York Heart Association classes I and II, 30 and 56 months postoperatively with arterial oxygen saturation (SaO$_2$) of 90 and 91%. This type of partial ventricular exclusion operation diverts all of the systemic venous return to the lungs except for that draining via the hepatic veins and coronary sinus. The investigators concluded that this procedure is a promising means of palliation for severely ill patients with uncorrectable cardiac malformations associated with azygos or hemiazygos continuation of the inferior vena cava. This procedure has limited application but results in high SaO$_2$ without increasing cardiac work. The PA size and pulmonary vascular resistance should be normal for its application. It is a useful addition to the surgeon's armamentarium.

RA-PA anastomosis (Fontan)

Positive end-expiratory pressure (PEEP) is commonly used after various cardiac operations in children and adults to improve arterial oxygenation. Cardiac output after Fontan's operation is in part dependent on pulmonary vascular resistance. The hemodynamic effects of PEEP in patients early after Fontan's operation have not been defined. Williams and colleagues[76] from Rochester, Minnesota, studied the effect of increased levels of PEEP in 13 patients 1–2 days after connecting the right atrium directly to the PA or to a rudimentary right ventricle. The patients ranged in age from 5–43 years (mean, 14 years). Preoperatively, each had normal-sized pulmonary arteries and a normal pulmonary vascular resistance. With increasing levels of PEEP from 0–12 cm H_2O, significant positive trends were demonstrated for arterial oxygen tension and pulmonary vascular resistance index and a significant negative trend for cardiac index. No trend was demonstrated for heart rate, mean arterial pressure, RA and LA pressure, systemic vascular resistance index and arterial carbon dioxide tension. These data indicate that PEEP is an effective means of raising arterial oxygen tension after Fontan's operation, but is associated with a progressive decrease in cardiac index that is significant at PEEP >6 cm H_2O. The reduction in cardiac index appears to be mediated by a significant increase in pulmonary vascular resistance index.

The ventricular exclusion operation described by Fontan is being applied to a variety of congenital cardiac defects. Although a number of studies have described the functional status of patients at rest, information is sparse concerning the exercise performance of this group. Thus, Peterson and coworkers[77] from Durham, North Carolina, and Atlanta, Georgia, performed radionuclide angiography at rest and during upright bicycle exercise in 16 patients between 4.5 and 23 years (mean, 13 years). Nine had tricuspid atresia, 2 a hypoplastic tricuspid valve, and a double-inlet ventricle was present in 5. A direct RA-PA anastomosis had been made in 6, an RA-RV connection in 7 (valved in 1), and a porcine valved RA-PA connection in 1. At the time of study, 14 of 16 patients were New York Heart Association class I and 15 were in sinus rhythm. Mean cardiac index was 5.2 liters/min/M^2 at rest and 9.4 liters/min/M^2 during exercise (p < 0.0001) and was similar to that observed in a normal control group. The study group had a lower systemic ventricular EF, and higher resting ventricular end-diastolic volume and stroke volume indices from normal. The data document similar exercise capacity in the Fontan group when compared with the control group and that a large exercise cardiac output can be achieved by these patients without a functioning right ventricle.

The atrio-PA connection operation described by Kreutzer in 1973 included anastomosis of the pulmonary trunk with its intact pulmonary valve to the right atrium. Ishikawa and associates[78] from Auckland, New Zealand, reported the hemodynamics of this procedure 4–7 years postoperatively in 3 patients who underwent repair of tricuspid atresia between 3 and 18 months of age. Each had sinus rhythm, mild hepatomegaly, and was in New York Heart Association class I or II. Resting cardiac index ranged between 2.0 and 2.5 liters/min/M^2 and RA pressure had a mean value between 11 and 14 mmHg in each. A mean pressure gradient between RA and PA of 0–2 mmHg was identified in each. Pulmonary arteriograms demonstrated growth of the pulmonary valve ring in each patient, ranging from 66–118% of preoperative values. Rapid contrast injection into the PA showed competent pulmonary valves with good valve motion. Slow injection of contrast media showed that the pulmonary valve cusps remained in the open position throughout the cardiac cycle. The RA angiograms showed good atrial contractility and considerable reflux of contrast into the hepatic veins and inferior vena cava. Echo showed no valve closure under normal conditions. The investigators believe that this structurally perfect valve remains more or less permanently open and serves no function. Considerable debate remains regarding the specific type of RV exclusion operation that should be employed. Some believe a valve should always be incorporated in any conduit connecting the right atrium to the PA, whereas others believe a direct atrio-PA nonvalved connection should be employed. Although much remains to be learned about this type of surgical procedure, this important article casts significant doubt on the usefulness of a valve interposed between the right atrium and pulmonary trunk. This conclusion may be different when other variations of this surgical procedure are employed.

Extracardiac conduits

Extracardiac conduits can become obstructed from neointimal peel formation, valvular degeneration, anastomotic problems, or mismatch due to increased patient growth. To determine the risks and outcome of conduit replacement, Schaff and coworkers[79] from Rochester, Minnesota, reviewed the records of their first 100 consecutive patients having a mean age of 13 years. The interval between initial repair and reoperation ranged from 3 months to 10 years (mean, 5.4 years). Mean pressure gradients decreased from 81 ± 26 mm preoperatively to 7 ± 8 mm postoperatively. Mortality <30 days was 7% and there were no deaths among 47 patients without associated procedures. The probability of survival at 5 years was $86 \pm 6\%$. The investigators review the surgical methods employed to perform these procedures safely and discuss the various replacement devices available. Their experience demonstrates a low risk of reoperation for conduit obstruction that minimizes the effect of late conduit failure on overall late survival.

Valve prostheses

It has been shown that tissue prostheses to replace diseased cardiac valves in children are not appropriate because of the high incidence of degeneration. Thus, a mechanical prosthesis must be used. Anticoagulants in children with a cardiac prostheses may pose special dangers because of the activity and exposure to trauma in childhood. Pass and colleagues[80] from Charleston, South Carolina, used the St. Jude medical (SJM) cardiac valve prosthesis without postoperative anticoagulation in 34 children undergoing valve replacement. These ranged in age from 9 months to 21 years. There were 3 operative deaths all in infants with complex disease. One patient died suddenly at home 5 weeks after valve replacement, probably due to a ventricular arrhythmia. During the subsequent follow-up of 1–50 months comprising 646 patient months, no thromboembolic complications were observed. The investigators suggest that the SJM prosthesis is hemodynamically satisfactory for children and is associated with a low incidence of thrombosis and thrombo-embolism even in the unanticoagulated state. The mean follow-up period was about 24 months in this group and thus the absence of thrombosis and thromboembolism must be regarded as preliminary data. Recently, several other groups have reported good results in terms of freedom from thrombo-embolism using either no anticoagulation or a variation of aspirin or dipyrid-amole in children. There is also data now on the other side of the question in which there has been relatively low incidence of thromboembolism and low danger of hemorrhagic side effects in children with prosthetic devices having full or moderate anticoagulation using warfarin. Indeed, there may be some inherent protection from thromboembolism in children due either to the presence of sinus rhythm in most patients or rapid heart rates and high flow across the prosthesis. These data have not proved the SJM prosthesis to be superior nor have they proved that absence of anticoagulation is totally ap-propriate with the SJM prosthesis in children.

Premature degeneration and calcification of glutaraldehyde-preserved porcine valve heterografts has made most surgical groups return to pros-thetic devices for valve replacement in children. Iyer and coworkers[81] from New Delhi, India, reviewed their experience with 136 patients between 6 and 20 years of age who underwent valve replacement with the Björk-Shiley pros-thesis: mitral in 61, aortic in 50, and both in 25. Hospital mortality was 10% and late actuarial survival at 8 years was 89%, 82%, and 81% for each group, respectively. Anticoagulation with acenocoumarol was employed in each patient and there were no instances of valve thromboses or fatal thromboem-bolism. Nonfatal embolism, anticoagulated-related hemorrhage, and periprosthetic leak occurred with similar frequency in this group compared with a group of 413 similar patients >20 years of age at operation. At 8 years, actuarial embolism-free survival was 99% and actuarial reoperation-free sur-vival was 99%. Each surviving patient was in New York Heart Association functional class I or II at follow up. The data indicate that Björk-Shiley pros-thetic valve provides good and durable long-term palliation in young pa-tients.

Schaff and coworkers[82] from Rochester, Minnesota, reviewed their experi-ence with 50 children between 6 months and 18 years (mean, 10 years) who received a Starr-Edwards prosthesis between 1963 and 1978. The aortic valve was replaced in 19, mitral in 24, and both in 1. The systemic AV valve was replaced in 6 with congenital defects. Actuarial survival at 10 years was 81% for the entire group, 90% after AVR, and 76% after systemic AV valve replace-ment. Anticoagulation with warfarin was recommended for each patient and major thromboembolism occurred in 7, minor emboli in 5, multiple in 4 of these. Actuarial embolus-free survival after AVR was 91% at 5 years, 66% at 10 years, compared with 95% and 91%, respectively, after systemic AV valve replacement. Hemorrhagic complications of anticoagulation occurred in 7 and were major in 3 patients. Four reoperations were performed because of patient-prosthesis mismatch that resulted from patient growth. Each was successful and permitted insertion of an adult-sized prosthesis. The investi-gators concluded that this experience supports the use of mechanical valves, such as the Starr-Edwards prosthesis, in the pediatric age group. Their over-all results are superior to a previous experience with biologic valves in chil-dren in which 41% required reoperation within 5 years.

Aortic valve homograft

The use of an extracardiac conduit is necessary for the correction of a variety of congenital cardiac defects. Although widespread use of porcine heterograft valved conduits has occurred during the past decade, the incidence of premature valvular degeneration and conduit obstruction has been discouraging and has resulted in the use of nonvalved tubes by some groups. Fontan and coworkers[83] from Bordeaux, France, reported their experience with 103 aortic valved homografts implanted in various positions in patients ranging in age from 7 months to 36 years (mean, 12 years). Early in the experience, 5 were sterilized by betapropiolactone and stored in Hanks' solution at 4°C and since 1971, 98 were obtained sterilely, placed in antibiotic solution, and stored by various methods, most recently in tissue culture medium with dimethyl sulfoxide at −196°C. There were 25 early and 9 late deaths, none related to the aortic valve homograft. Fifty-nine survivors were followed 1 month to 15 years (mean, 4 years), without evidence of homograft valve dysfunction, thromboembolism, or hemolysis; 93% of these patients were in New York Heart Association class I or II. Postoperative cardiac catheterization studies were performed in 53 patients 1 month to 10 years (mean, 2.2 years) later. Of 31 patients with a right atrium-dependent conduit, gradients of 4, 6, 9, and 9 mmHg were measured in 4 patients, absent in 27. Among 21 with a ventricle-PA conduit, a pressure gradient >10 mmHg was found in 14. This was prevalvar in 3, postvalvar in 6, and transvalvar or undetermined in 5. Serial catheterization studies were performed in 19 at a mean of 7 months and 4.6 years postoperatively. No significant difference was found between the mean pressure gradients measured at the valvular level. In 7, the final control catheterization was performed ≥5 years after operation (range, 5–10 years; mean, 8 years) and only 1 had a significant increase in transvalvar gradient and his RV pressure remained <65 mmHg. Most patients had a variable degree of calcium in the wall of the aortic valve homograft but not in the cusps. There were no reoperations for homograft valve failure, but 1 reoperation was performed because of an outgrown and stretched conduit with a RV-PA gradient of 70 mmHg, 10 years after initial placement. The investigators are encouraged that the homograft valved conduit functioned well over the 15-year follow-up period of this study.

References

1. HAGEN PT, SCHOLZ DG, EDWARDS WD: Incidence and size of patent foramen ovale during the first 10 decades of life: an autopsy study of 965 normal hearts. Mayo Clinic Proc 59:17–20, Jan 1984.
2. PARIKH DN, FISHER J, MOSES JW, GOLDBERG HL, LEVIN AR, ENGEL MA, BORER JS: Determinations and importance of atrial pressure morphology in atrial septal defect. Br Heart J 51:473–479, May 1984.
3. KITABATAKE A, INOVE M, ASAO M, ITO H, MASUYAMA T, TANOUCHI J, MORITA T, HORI M, YOSHIMA H, OHMISHI K, ABE H: Noninvasive evaluation of the ratio of pulmonary to systemic flow in atrial septal defect by duplex Doppler echocardiography. Circulation 69:73–79, Jan 1984.
4. FREED MD, NADAS AS, NORWOOD WI, CASTANEDA AR: Is routine preoperative cardiac catheteri-

zation necessary before repair of secundum and sinus venosus atrial septal defects? J Am Coll Cardiol 4:333–336, Aug 1984.

5. YEAGER SB, FREED MD, KEANE JF, NORWOOD WI, CASTANEDA AR: Primary surgical closure of ventricular septal defect in the first year of life: results of 128 infants. J Am Coll Cardiol 3:1269–1276, May 1984.

6. MOMMA K, TOYAMA K, TAKAO A, ANDO M, NAKAZAWA M, HIROSAWA K, IMAI Y: Natural history of subarterial infundibular ventricular septal defect. Am Heart J 108:1312–1318, Nov 1984.

7. COLES JG, FREEDOM RM, OLLEY PM, COCEANI F, WILLIAMS WG, TRUSLER GA: Surgical management of critical pulmonary stenosis in the neonate. Ann Thorac Surg 38:458–465, Nov 1984.

8. JOHNSON GI, KWIAN OL, HANDSHO ES, NOONAN JA, DeMARIA AN: Accuracy of combined two-dimensional echocardiography in continuous wave Doppler recordings and estimation of pressure gradient in right ventricular outlet obstruction. J Am Coll Cardiol 3:1013–1018, Apr 1984.

9. KAN JS, WHITE RI JR, MITCHELL SE, ANDERSON JH, GARDNER TJ: Percutaneous transluminal balloon valvuloplasty for pulmonary valve stenosis. Circulation 69:554–561, March 1984.

10. ROCCHINI AP, KVESLIS DA, CROWLEY D, DICK M, ROSENTHAL A: Percutaneous balloon valvuloplasty for treatment of congenital pulmonary valvular stenosis in children. J Am Coll Cardiol 3:1005–1012, Apr 1984.

11. DEANFIELD JE, McKENNA WJ, PRESBITERO P, ENGLAND D, GRAHAM GR, HALLADIE-SMITH K: Ventricular arrhythmia in unrepaired and repaired tetralogy of the lobe. Br Heart J, 52:77–81, July 1984.

12. KAVEY R-EW, THOMAS FD, BYRUM CJ, BLACKMAN MS, SONDHEIMER HM, BOVE EL: Ventricular arrhythmias and bi-ventricular dysfunction after repair of tetralogy of Fallot. J Am Coll Cardiol 4:126–131, July 1984.

13. DUNNIGAN A, PRITZECKER MR, BENNITT G, BENSON DW: Life threatening ventricular tachycardias in late survivors of surgically corrected tetralogy of Fallot. Br Heart J 52:198–206, Aug 1984.

14. KLINNER W, REICHART B, PFALLER M, HATZ R: Late results after correction of tetralogy of Fallot necessitating outflow tract reconstruction. Comparison with results after correction without outflow tract patch. Thorac Cardiovasc Surg 32:244–247, Oct 1984.

15. LORGERIL MD, FRIEDLIO B, ASSIMACOPOULOS A: Factors affecting left ventricular function after correction of tetralogy of Fallot. Br Heart J 52:536–541, Nov 1984.

16. VITARELLI A, D'ADDIO AP, GENTILE R, BURATTINI M: Echocardiographic evaluation of left ventricular outflow tract obstruction in complete transposition of the great arteries. Am Heart J 108:531–538, Sept 1984.

17. POWELL TG, DEWEY M, WEST ER, ARNOLD R: Fate of infants with transposition of the great arteries in relation to balloon atrial septostomy. Br Heart J 51:371–376, Apr 1984.

18. COBANOGLU A, ABBRUZZESE PA, FREIMANIS I, GARCIA CE, GRUNKEMEIER G, STARR A: Pericardial baffle complications following the Mustard operation. Age-related incidence and ease of management. J Thorac Cardiovasc Surg 87:371–378, March 1984.

19. RAMSEY JM, VENEBALES AW, KELLEY MJ, KALFF V: Right and left ventricular functions at rest and with exercise after the Mustard operation for transposition of the great arteries. Br Heart Journal 51:364–370, Apr 1984.

20. CASTANEDA AR, NORWOOD WI, JONAS RA, COLON SD, SANDERS SP, LANG P: Transposition of the great arteries and intact ventricular septum: anatomical repair in the neonate. Ann Thoracic Surg 38:438–443, Nov 1984.

21. CEITHAML EL, PUGA FJ, DANIELSON GK, McGOON DC, RITTER DG: Results of the Damus-Stansel-Kaye procedure for transposition of the great arteries and for double-outlet right ventricle with subpulmonary ventricular septal defect. Ann Thorac Surg 38:433–437, Nov 1984.

22. BOROW KM, ARENSMAN FW, WEBB C, RADLEY-SMITH R, YACOUB AR: Assessment of left ventricular contractile state after anatomic correction of transposition of the great arteries. Circulation 69:106–112, Jan 1984.

23. HUHTA JC, LATSON LA, GUTGESELL HP, COOLEY DA, KEARNEY DL: Echo-cardiography in the diagnosis and management of symptomatic aortic valve stenosis in infants. Circulation 70:438–444, Sept 1984.

24. WALLER BF, GIROD DA, DILLON JC: Transverse aortic wall tears in infants after balloon angio-

plasty for aortic valve stenosis. J Am Coll Cardiol 4:1235–1241, Dec 1984.

25. Sink JD, Smallhorn JF, Macartney FJ, Taylor JFN, Stark J, de Leval MR: Management of critical aortic stenosis in infancy. J Thorac Cardiovasc Surg 87:82–86, Jan 1984.

26. Messina LM, Turley K, Stanger P, Hoffman JIE, Ebert P: Successful aortic valvotomy for severe congenital valvular aortic stenosis in the newborn infant. J Thorac Cardiovasc Surg 88:92–96, July 1984.

27. Moses RD, Barnhart GR, Jones M: The late prognosis after localized resection for fixed (discrete and tunnel) left ventricular outflow tract obstruction. J Thorac Cardiovasc Surg 87:410–420, March 1984.

28. Vouhe PR, Poulain H, Bloch G, Loisance DY, Gamain J, Lombaert M, Quiret JC, Lesbre JP, Bernasconi P, Pietri J, Cachera JP: Aortoseptal approach for optimal resection of diffuse subvalvular aortic stenosis. J Thorac Cardiovasc Surg 87:887–893, June 1984.

29. DiDonato RM, Danielson GK, McGoon DC, Driscoll DJ, Julsrud PR, Edwards WD: Left ventricle-aortic conduits in pediatric patients. J Thorac Cardiovasc Surg 88:82–91, July 1984.

30. Celano V, Pieroni DR, Morera JA, Roland J-MA, Gingell RL: Two-dimensional echocardiographic examination of mitral valve abnormalities associated with coarctation of the aorta. Circulation 69:924–932, May 1984.

31. Moulton AL, Brenner JI, Roberts G, Tavares S, Ali S, Nordenberg A, Burns JE, Ringel R, Berman MA: Subclavian flap repair of coarctation of the aorta in neonates. Realization of growth potential? J Thorac Cardiovasc Surg 87:220–235, Feb 1984.

32. Penkoske PA, Williams WG, Olley PM, LeBlanc J, Trusler GA, Moes CAF, Judakin R, Rowe RD: Subclavian arterioplasty. Repair of coarctation of the aorta in the first year of life. J Thorac Cardiovasc Surg 87:894–900, June 1984.

33. Campbell DB, Waldhausen JA, Pierce WS, Fripp R, Whitman V: Should elective repair of coarctation of the aorta be done in infancy? J Thorac Cardiovasc Surg 88:929–938, Dec 1984.

34. Sade RM, Crawford FA, Hohn AR, Riopel DA, Taylor AB: Growth of the aorta after prosthetic patch aortoplasty for coarctation in infants. Ann Thorac Surg 38:21–25, July 1984.

35. Smith RT Jr, Sade RM, Riopel DA, Taylor AD, Crawford FA Jr, Hohn AR: Stress testing for comparison of synthetic patch aortoplasty with resection and end-to-end anastomosis for repair of coarctation in childhood. J Am Coll Cardiol 4:765–770, Oct 1984.

36. Crawford FA, Sade RM: Spinal cord injury associated with hyperthermia during aortic coarctation repair. J Thorac Cardiovasc Surg 87:616–618, Apr 1984.

37. St.-John Sutton MG, Gewitz MH, Shahab A, Reicher N, Gabbe S, Huff DS: Quantitative assessment of growth and function of the cardiac chambers of the normal human fetus: a prospective longitudinal echocardiographic study. Circulation 69:645–654, Apr 1984.

38. Allan LD, Crawford DC, Anderson RH, Tynan MJ: Echocardiographic and anatomical correlations in fetal congenital heart disease. Br Heart J 52:542–548, Nov 1984.

39. Barron JV, Sahn DJ, Valdes-Cruz LM, Lima CO, Goldberg SJ, Grenadier E, Allen HD: Clinical utility of two-dimensional echocardiographic techniques for estimating pulmonary to systemic blood flow ratios in children with left-to-right shunting atrial septal defect, ventricular septal defect or patent ductus arteriosus. J Am Coll Cardiol 3:169–178, Jan 1984.

40. Stevenson JG, Kawabori I, Guntheroth WG: Non-invasive estimation of peak pulmonary artery pressure by M-mode echocardiography. J Am Coll Cardiol 4:1021–1027, Nov 1984.

41. Meltzer RS, Vered Z, Hegesh T, Benjamin P, Visser CA, Shem-Tov AA, Neufeld NH: Diagnosis of pulmonic regurgitation by contrast echocardiography. Am Heart J 107:102–107, Jan 1984.

42. Grenadier E, Sahn DJ, Valdes-Cruz LM, Allen HD, Lima CO, Goldberg SJ: Two-dimensional echo Doppler study of congenital disorders of the mitral valve. Am Heart J 107:319–325, Feb 1984.

43. Vargas Barron J, Sahn DJ, Valdes-Cruz LM, Lima CO, Grenadier E, Allen HD, Goldberg SJ: Two-dimensional echocardiographic evaluation of overriding and straddling atrioventricular valves associated with complex congenital heart disease. Am Heart J 107:1006–1014, May 1984.

44. Stevenson JG, Kawaborii: Non-invasive determination of pressure gradients in children: two methods of employing pulsed Doppler echocardiography. J Am Coll Cardiol 3:179–192,

Jan 1984.

45. ROBINSON TJ, WYSE RKH, DEANFIELD JE, FRANKLIN R, MACCARTNEY RJ: Continuous wave Doppler velocimetry as an adjunct to cross-sectional echocardiography in diagnosis of critical left heart obstruction in neonates. Br Heart J 52:552–556, Aug 1984.

46. HUHTA JC, GUTGESELL HP, LATSON LA, HUFFINES FD: Two-dimensional echocardiographic assessment of the aorta in infants and children with congenital heart disease. Circulation 70:417–424, Sept 1984.

47. GUTGESELL HP, HUHTA JC, COHEN MH, LATSON LA: Two-dimensional echocardiography assessment of pulmonary artery and aortic arch anatomy in cyanotic infants. J Am Coll Cardiol 4:1242–1246, Dec 1984.

48. COOPER MM, TIETEL DF, SILVERMAN NH, ENDERLAINE MA: Study of the infradiphragmatic total anomalies pulmonary venous connection with cross-sectional and pulsed Doppler echocardiography. Circulation 70:412–416, Feb 1984.

49. ROBINSON PJ, SULLIVAN ID, KUMPANG V, ANDERSON RH, MACARTNEY FJ: Anomalous origin of the left coronary from the pulmonary trunk: potential for false negative diagnosis with cross-sectional echocardiography. Br Heart J 52:272–277, Sept 1984.

50. NAKAZAWA M, NAKANISHI T, OQUD H, SATOMI G, NAKIA S, MININAI Y, TAKAO A: Dynamics of right heart flow in patients after Fontan procedure. Circulation 69:306–312, Feb 1984.

51. DISESSA TG, CHILD JS, PERLOFF JK, WOO L, WILLIAMS RJ, LAKS H, FRIEDMAN WF: Systemic venous and pulmonary arterial flow patterns after Fontan's procedure for tricuspid atresia or single ventricle. Circulation 70:898–902, Nov 1984.

52. REEDER GS, CURRIE PJ, FYFE DA, HAGLER DJ, SEWARD JB, TAJIK AJ: Extra cardiac conduit obstruction: initial experiences in the use of Doppler echocardiography for non invasive estimation of pressure gradient. J Am Coll Cardiol 4:1006–1011, Nov 1984.

53. MARX GR, BIERMAN FC, MATTHEWS E, WILLIAMS R: Two-dimensional echocardiographic diagnosis of intracardiac masses in infancy. J Am Coll Cardiol 3:827–832, March 1984.

54. BOUCEK MM, BOERTH RC, ARTMAN M, GRAHAM TP JR, BOUCEK RJ JR: Myocardial dysfunction in children with acute meningococcemia. J Pediatr 105:538–542, Oct 1984.

55. ST. JOHN SUTTON MG, RAICHLEN AS, REICHEK N, HUFF DS: Quantitative assessment of right and left ventricular growth in the human fetal heart: a pathoanatomic study. Circulation 70:935–941, Dec 1984.

56. BAKER EJ, MALAMIPSI J, JONES OBH, MAISYMER TYNAN MJ: Use of radionuclide labeled microspheres to show the distribution of the pulmonary perfusion with multifocal pulmonary blood supply. Br Heart J 52:72–76, July 1984.

57. PRESBITERO P, BOLD C, HAYWORTH SG, LAVAL MR: Absent or occult pulmonary artery. Br Heart J 52:178–185, Aug 1984.

58. DRISCOLL DG, STATTS BA, HEISE CT, RICE MJ, PUGA FG, DANIELSON GK, RITTER DG: Functional single ventricle: cardiorespiratory response to exercise. J Am Coll Cardiol 4:337–372, Aug 1984.

59. HIGGINS CB, BYRD BF, FARMER DW, OSAKI L, SILVERMAN NH, CHEITLIN MD: Magnetic resonance imaging in patients with congenital heart disease. Circulation 70:851–860, Nov 1984.

60. JACOBSTEIN MD, FLETCHER BD, NELSON D, CLAMPITT M, ALFIEDE RJ, RIEMENSCHNEIDER TA: Magnetic resonance imaging: evaluation of palliative systemic-pulmonary artery shunts. Circulation 70:650–656, Oct 1984.

61. TEIXEIRA OHP, CARPENTER B, MACMURRAY SB, VLAD P: Long term prostoglandin E, therapy on congenital heart defects. J Am Coll Cardiol 3:838–843, March 1984.

62. LOCK JE, BASS JL, CASTANEDA-ZUNIGA W, FUHRMAN BP, RASHKIND WJ, LUCAS RB JR: Dilation angioplasty of congenital or operative narrowings of venous channel. Circulation 70:457–464, Sept 1984.

63. FUHRMAN BP, BASS JL, CASTANEDA-ZUNIGA W, AMPLATZ K, LOCK JE: Coil embolization of congenital thoracic vascular anomalies in infants and children. Circulation 70:285–289, Aug 1984.

64. GARSON A JR, GILLETTE PC, MCVEY P, HESSLEIN PS, PORTER CJ, ANGELL LK, KALDIS LC, HITTNER H: Amiodarone treatment of critical arrhythmias in children and young adults. J Am Coll Cardiol 4:749–755, Oct 1984.

65. RABINOVITCH M, KEANE JF, NORWOOD WI, CASTANEDA A, REID L: Vascular structure in lung tissue

obtained at biopsy correlated with pulmonary hemodynamic findings after repair of congenital heart defects. Circulation 69:655–667, Apr 1984.

66. BULL C, COOPER J, STARK J: Cardioplegic protection of the child's heart. J Thorac Cardiovasc Surg 88:287–293, Aug 1984.

67. WAGNER HR, ELLISON RC, ZIERLER S, LANG P, PUROHIT DM, BEHRENDT D, WALDHAUSEN JA: Surgical closure of patent ductus arteriosus in 268 preterm infants. J Thorac Cardiovasc Surg 87:870–875, June 1984.

68. SILVER MA, COHEN SR, McINTOSH CL, CANNON RO, ROBERTS WC: Late (5 to 132 months) clinical and hemodynamic results after either tricuspid valve replacement or anuloplasty for Ebstein's anomaly of the tricuspid valve. Am J Cardiol 54:627–632, Sept 1, 1984.

69. FOWLER BN, LUCAS SK, RAZOOK JD, THOMPSON WM JR, WILLIAMS GR, ELKINS RC: Interruption of the aortic arch: experience in 17 infants. Ann Thorac Surg 37:25–32, Jan 1984.

70. EBERT PA: Staged partitioning of single ventricle. J Thorac Cardiovasc Surg 88:908–913, Dec 1984.

71. PENKOSKE PA, FREEDOM RM, WILLIAMS WG, TRUSLER GA, ROWE RD: Surgical palliation of subaortic stenosis in the univentricular heart. J Thorac Cardiovasc Surg 87:767–781, May 1984.

72. WOOLF PK, STEPHENSON LW, MEIJBOOM E, BAVINCK JH, GARDNER TJ, DONAHOO JS, EDIE RN, EDMUNDS LH JR: A comparison of Blalock-Taussig, Waterston, and polytetrafluoroethylene shunts in children less than two weeks of age. Ann Thorac Surg 38:26–30, July 1984.

73. BOVE EL, SONDHEIMER HM, KAVEY REW, BYRUM CJ, BLACKMAN MS, PARKER FB JR: Subclavian-pulmonary artery shunts with polytetrafluoroethylene interposition grafts. Ann Thorac Surg 37:88–91, Jan 1984.

74. ILBAWI MN, GRIECO J, DELEON SY, IDRISS FS, MUSTER AJ, BERRY TE, KLICH J: Modified Blalock-Taussig shunt in newborn infants. J Thorac Cardiovasc Surg 88:770–775, Nov 1984.

75. KAWASHIMA Y, KITAMURA S, MATSUDA H, SHIMAZAKI Y, NAKANO S, HIROSE H: Total cavopulmonary shunt operation in complex cardiac anomalies. A new operation. J Thorac Cardiovasc Surg 87:74–81, Jan 1984.

76. WILLIAMS DB, KIERNAN PD, METKE MP, MARSH HM, DANIELSON GK: Hemodynamic response to positive end-expiratory pressure following right atrium-pulmonary artery bypass (Fontan procedure). J Thorac Cardiovasc Surg 87:856–861, June 1984.

77. PETERSON RJ, FRANCH RH, FAJMAN WA, JENNINGS JG, JONES RH: Noninvasive determination of exercise cardiac function following Fontan operation. J Thorac Cardiovasc Surg 88:263–272, Aug 1984.

78. ISHIKAWA T, NEUTZE JM, BRANDT PWT, BARRATT-BOYES BG: Hemodynamics following the Kreutzer procedure for tricuspid atresia in patients under two years of age. J Thorac Cardiovasc Surg 88:373–379, Sept 1984.

79. SCHAFF HV, DIDONATO RM, DANIELSON GK, PUGA FJ, RITTER DG, EDWARDS WD, McGOON DC: Reoperation for obstructed pulmonary ventricle-pulmonary artery conduits. Early and late results. J Thorac Cardiovasc Surg 88:334–343, Sept 1984.

80. PASS HI, SADE RM, CRAWFORD FA, HOHN AR: Cardiac valve prostheses in children without anticoagulation. J Thorac Cardiovasc Surg 87:832–835, June 1984.

81. IYER KS, REDDY KS, RAO IM, VENUGOPAL P, BHATIA ML, GOPINATH N: Valve replacement in children under twenty years of age. Experience with the Björk-Shiley prosthesis. J Thorac Cardiovasc Surg 88:217–224, Aug 1984.

82. SCHAFF HV, DANIELSON GK, DIDONATO RM, PUGA FJ, MAIR DD, McGOON DC: Late results after Starr-Edwards valve replacement in children. J Thorac Cardiovasc Surg 88:583–589, Oct 1984.

83. FONTAN F, CHOUSSAT A, DEVILLE C, DOUTREMEPUICH C, COUPILLAUD J, VOSA C: Aortic valve homografts in the surgical treatment of complex cardiac malformations. J Thorac Cardiovasc Surg 87:649–657, May 1984.

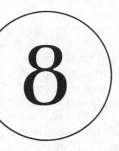

8

Congestive Heart Failure

MISCELLANEOUS TOPICS

Laterality of Pleural Effusion

It has been reported that pleural effusions in patients with pericardial disease were almost always left-sided. It has also been widely believed that pleural effusion in patients with chronic CHF are right-sided. Thus, an accompanying isolated left pleural effusion would place effusive pericardial disease high on the list of possible diagnoses. Given an enlarged cardiac outline, an isolated left, isolated right, or bilateral pleural effusion, what would be the odds that a given patient would have CHF? Weiss and Spodick[1] from Worcester, Massachusetts, attempted to answer this question by studying 70 patients with definite CHF and pleural effusions. Of these, 51 (73%) had pleural effusions: 13 (19%) had only a right and 6 (9%) only a left pleural effusion. Thus, confronted with a patient who has clinical or roentgenographic signs of an enlarged cardiac silhouette, isolated right-sided or bilateral plural effusion would favor a diagnosis of CHF and a left-sided effusion, a diagnosis of pericardial disease.

With normal systolic function

Although there have been isolated reports of CHF with normal systolic function, the prevalence and characteristics of this condition have not previously been described. To fill this void, Dougherty and associates[2] from Houston, Texas, prospectively evaluated 188 patients with CHF undergoing radionuclide ventriculography: 67 (36%) had a normal EF (<0.45) and 121, an abnormal EF (>0.45). Of these, 72 (55 with an abnormal EF [group I] and 17 with a normal EF [group II]) were also reviewed for clinical characteristics. There was no demographic difference between groups, except that systemic hypertension appeared to be a contributing factor in 65% of the patients in group II, compared with 23% of the patients in group I (p < 0.002). Echo LA emptying index, reflecting LV compliance, was determined in 72 patients and 14 normal subjects. The LA emptying index in normal control subjects was 0.93 ± 0.11 compared with 0.41 ± 0.18 in group I and 0.44 ± 0.19 in group II patients (p < 0.001 -vs- control in both groups). Thus, normal systolic function is common among patients with CHF. Diastolic dysfunction, consistent with a noncompliant LV, was found in both CHF groups.

Exercise tolerance

The cause of exercise intolerance in CHF is unclear. Franciosa and associates[3] from Philadelphia, Pennsylvania, measured hemodynamic and ventilatory responses during symptomatic maximal upright bicycle exercise in 28 patients with chronic, severe LV failure who achieved a maximum oxygen uptake of only 12 ± 4 ml/min/kg. All patients reached anaerobic metabolism as the respiratory exchange ratio increased and arterial pH decreased significantly. The PA wedge pressure increased from 20 ± 10 mmHg at rest to 38 ± 9 mmHg at peak exercise and cardiac index increased from 2.51 ± 0.73–4.54 ± 1.65 liters/min/M^2 (both p < 0.001). Systemic vascular resistance decreased, but pulmonary vascular resistance did not change during exercise. Despite the marked pulmonary venous hypertension at peak exercise, blood gases were unchanged (arterial oxygen tension, 96 ± 15 mmHg; arterial carbon dioxide tension, 35 ± 7 mmHg). Systemic arterial oxygen content increased from 16 ± 2–17 ± 2 vol% (p < 0.01). Changes in PA wedge pressure did not correlate with changes in arterial oxygen content. Results were similar whether patients were limited by dyspnea or fatigue. Thus, exercise intolerance in patients with severe LV failure is associated with marked elevation of PA wedge pressure and anaerobic metabolism without hypoxemia or altered carbon dioxide tension. These findings suggest that exercise ability in CHF is more dependent on cardiac output than on ventilatory consequences of pulmonary congestion.

Although the maximal exercise capacity of patients with chronic CHF is frequently reduced, it is yet to be directly demonstrated that perfusion of working skeletal muscle is impaired during upright maximal exercise in such patients. To investigate whether this exercise intolerance is caused by inadequate nutritive flow to skeletal muscle, Wilson and coworkers[4] from Philadelphia, Pennsylvania, compared cardiac outputs, leg blood flow, and leg metabolism during maximal bicycle exercise in 7 patients with normal oxygen uptake and 8 patients with CHF and moderately reduced maximal oxygen uptake. As the severity of exercise increased in the 3 groups, there was a progressive decline in cardiac output and leg blood flow at any given work load accompanied by a progressive decline in maximal cardiac output. All patients terminated exercise because of severe leg fatigue. At termination of exercise all 3 groups had similar marked levels of leg oxygen extraction and high femoral-arterial lactate gradients, suggesting that exercise was limited when a critical level of muscle underperfusion was reached. These data suggest that the reduced maximal exercise capacity of patients with chronic CHF is primarily due to impaired nutritive flow to skeletal muscle and resultant muscular fatigue.

Although the left ventricle is traditionally viewed as the heart's main pumping chamber, no correlation has been shown between LV EF at rest and exercise capacity in patients with chronic LV failure. Because vasodilators with venodilating activity increase exercise capacity more than predominant arterial dilators in patients with LV failure, RV function may relate to exercise capacity in these patients. In 25 patients with chronic LV failure caused by CAD in 12 patients and by idiopathic dilated cardiomyopathy in 13 patients, RV EF and LV EF at rest were measured by radionuclide angiography by Baker and associates[5] from Little Rock, Arkansas. Maximal upright bicycle exercise testing also was performed to determine maximal oxygen consumption, which averaged only 13 ± 14 ml/min/kg. The LV EF at rest was 26 ± 10% and did not correlate with maximal oxygen consumption (r = 0.08). The RV EF was 41 ± 12% and correlated with maximal oxygen consumption in the same patients. The correlation was stronger in patients with CAD than in those with idiopathic dilated cardiomyopathy. Thus, RV EF at rest is more predictive of exercise capacity than LV EF in the same patients with chronic LV failure. These results are consistent with the clinical observation that only venodilating agents increase exercise capacity of patients with chronic LV failure.

The S_3

Although the third heart sound has been regarded as a clinical hallmark of impaired LV function, an early diastolic low frequency sound may be present under different hemodynamic conditions. To explore the pathogenesis of the third heart sound (S_3), Van de Werf and coinvestigators[6] from Brussels, Belgium, studied LV hemodynamics in early diastole during early catheterization in normal adults without an S_3 (group I; n, 12), and in cardiac patients with an S_3 as a result of severe MR (group II; n, 11), idiopathic dilated cardiomyopathy (IDC) (group III; n, 24), or restricted LV filling (group IV; n, 4). The height and steepness of the rise in LV pressure after minimum diastolic pressure (the so-called rapid filling wave), maximum dV/dt, and the time constant of decrease in isovolumetric pressure were measured. Pressure-volume data were fitted to simple elastic and viscoelastic models incorporating inflow rate into the equation. In all patients with S_3 a significantly higher and steeper rapid filling wave was found than in normal adults. Maximum dV/dt was significantly greater in group II than in the other groups. No significant differences in LV chamber elastic properties in the different groups were found. However, intrapatient comparisons of the results of the use of elastic and viscoelastic equations revealed a significantly better curve fit and a much higher viscous constant for group III. Similar results were found in group IV. In patients with S_3 LV relaxation was slower and more complete than in normal adults. In conclusion, the presence of an S_3 was associated with a higher and steeper rapid filling wave on the LV pressure tracing. The increased rapid filling wave could be attributed mainly to an increased filling rate in patients with volume overload (group II) and to impaired relaxation or increased viscous relaxed resistance to filling in patients with myocardial dysfunction (groups III and IV). This increased rapid filling wave may play an important role in the pathogenesis of the S_3, since it causes more rapid deceleration of inflow and since the vibrations of the S_3 occur during this phase of LV filling. Clinicians should appreciate the grouping of these patients, since the investigators indicate the different circumstances for generation of the S_3 sound and severe MR versus IDC and restricted filling. The end-systolic volume also plays an important role in the generation of the S_3 gallop, particularly in the IDC and the restricted LV filling group, whereas in severe MR, the S_3 sound can occur with preservation of LV function.

Regional blood flow

Leithe and coinvestigators[7] from Columbus, Ohio, obtained central and regional hemodynamic data that included hepatic, renal, and limb measurements in a normal population and in patients with CHF. The 64 patients represented a wide spectrum of severity of CHF and various relations between central and regional hemodynamics were analyzed. In patients with CHF blood flow to hepatic, renal, and limb regions is significantly decreased and this decrease is proportional and linearly related to the reduction in cardiac output. Vascular resistances of these regions correlated directly with systemic vascular resistance. Changes in renal vascular resistance and renal blood flow became attenuated as the severity of CHF advanced from moderate to severe and at higher levels of systemic vascular resistance. The investigators found little to no correlation between systemic BP and liver, kidney, and limb blood flow for the range of systemic pressures studied. These findings do not pertain to exercise in CHF patients and a great variation in individual flow values at each level of cardiac output and vascular resistance were observed, reflecting the complex nature of regional blood flow regulation.

Baroreceptor sensitivity

Chronic CHF is associated with neurohumoral excitation, which could result in part from impairment in the inhibitory influence of baroreflexes. Ferguson and coworkers[8] from Iowa City, Iowa, postulated that patients with LV dysfunction have impaired baroreflex modulation of vascular resistance and administration of a digitalis glycoside would immediately restore baroreflex sensitivity. Eleven patients with LV dysfunction and baseline LV EF $18 \pm 2\%$, cardiac index, $2.4 \pm 0.2\%/min/M^2$, and PA wedge pressure, 26.0 ± 3.2 mmHg were compared with 17 normal control subjects. The investigators measured forearm vasoconstrictor responses to simulated orthostatic stress with use of lower body negative pressure to unload cardiopulmonary and arterial baroreceptors. Baseline forearm vascular resistance was higher in patients with LV dysfunction than in normal subjects. During unloading of baroreceptors, normal subjects developed vasoconstriction but patients with LV dysfunction failed to have vasoconstriction and tended to develop vasodilation. Despite high baseline values for forearm vascular resistance (FVR) patients with LV dysfunction developed vasoconstriction during intraarterial infusions of norepinephrine, thereby excluding a nonspecific depression of vascular activity as the mechanism for abnormal responses in patients with LV dysfunction. The short-term effects of a digitalis glycoside, ouabain, or lanatoside C was studied on baroreflex-mediated vasoconstrictor responses to lower body negative pressure in the patients with LV dysfunction. Digitalis glycoside reduced baseline FVR and responses tended to be normalized after administration of the drug. Thus, these patients with LV dysfunction had selective impairment of baroreflex-mediated vasoconstrictor responses to unloading of baroreceptors by simulated orthostatic stress that did not appear to be caused by high baseline vascular resistance or decreased vascular responsiveness. This response is normalized immediately by administration of a digitalis glycoside, possibly because of baroreceptor sensitivity.

Ventricular tachycardia

Maskin and associates[9] from New York City evaluated the prevalence of ventricular arrhythmias in 35 patients with severe CHF in New York Heart Association functional classes III and IV. The etiology of CHF was equally distributed between ischemic and nonischemic cardiomyopathy. The severity of cardiac dysfunction was evident from a LV EF <20%, mean cardiac index 1.75 ± 0.40 liters/min/M^2, PA wedge pressure 28 ± 7 mmHg, and mean exercise capacity 6 ± 4 minutes. During 24-hour ambulatory Holter monitoring, 71% of these patients had repetitive episodes of VT, 92% had multifocal VPC, and 88% had $\geqslant 10$ VPC/1,000 normal heart beats. Within 1–72 weeks of the Holter monitoring, 25 patients died. Death could be attributed to VT in only 1 patient. In all others, death was secondary to worsening CHF. Thus, although asymptomatic malignant ventricular arrhythmia occurred frequently in these CHF patients, sudden death was rarely observed.

Plasma catecholamines

Plasma norepinephrine (NE) levels are increased in patients with chronic CHF, reflecting activation of the sympathetic nervous system. Levels are considerably higher in patients with severe symptoms than in those with mild symptoms. Although the precise mechanism or mechanisms stimulating this sympathetic nervous system in CHF are not fully understood, the magnitude of increase in plasma NE may be a more sensitive indicator of the cardiac functional state than the more traditional measurements of cardiac performance. Cohn and associates[10] from Minneapolis, Minnesota, measured hemodynamics, plasma NE, and plasma renin activity at supine rest in 106 patients (83 men and 23 women) with moderate to severe CHF. During follow-up lasting 1–62 months, 60 patients died (57%); 47% of the deaths were sudden, and 45% were related to progressive CHF. Statistically unrelated to the risk of mortality were cause of disease (60 patients had CAD, and 46 had cardiomyopathy of unspecified type), age (mean, 55 years), cardiac index (mean, 3 liters/min/M^2), PA wedge pressure (mean, 25 mmHg), and mean arterial pressure (mean, 83 mmHg). A multivariate analysis of the 4 significant univariate prognosticators—heart rate (mean, 84 beats/min), plasma renin activity (mean, 15 ng/ml/hour), plasma NE (mean, 700 pg/ml), serum sodium (mean, 136 mM/liter), and stroke-work index (mean, 21 g-m/M^2)— found only plasma NE to be independently related to the subsequent risk of mortality. The NE value also was higher in patients who died from progressive CHF than in those who died suddenly. These data suggest that a single resting venous blood sample showing the plasma NE concentration provides a better guide to prognosis than other commonly measured indexes of cardiac performance.

Prostaglandins

To determine whether prostaglandins are involved in circulatory hemostasis in chronic CHF, Dzau and associates[11] from Boston, Massachusetts, and New York City measured plasma levels of the metabolites of vasodilator prostaglandins I_2 and E_2 in 15 patients with severe chronic CHF. Mean circulating levels of both metabolites were 3–10 times higher than those in normal subjects. Plasma levels of both metabolites correlated directly with plasma renin activity and plasma angiotensin II concentrations. Individual serum sodium concentrations were inversely correlated with levels of prostaglandin E_2 metabolites and plasma renin activity. Of 23 patients with severe CHF challenged with indomethacin (an inhibitor of prostaglandin synthesis), the 9 with hyponatremia had significant decreases in the cardiac index (1.99 ± 0.12–1.72 ± 0.13 liters/min/M^2 of body surface area and significant increases in the PA wedge pressure (17 ± 2–24 ± 2 mmHg) and systemic vascular resistance (1,882 ± 239–2,488 ± 315 dyn · s · cm^{-5}), whereas the 14 patients with a normal serum sodium concentration had no significant hemodynamic changes. The investigators concluded that both vasoconstrictor (renin-angiotensin) and vasodilator (prostaglandin) mechanisms are operative in patients with CHF complicated by hyponatremia and that these mechanisms interact to modulate circulatory homeostasis. This article was followed with an editorial by Braunwald and Colucci[12] from Boston, Massachusetts, and they reviewed the history of vasodilators for patients with chronic CHF.

TREATMENT

Amrinone

Amrinone is an effective inotropic agent, but its electrophysiologic effects in humans have not been determined. Naccarelli and associates[13] from Houston, Texas, performed electrophysiologic studies in 15 patients with CHF after withdrawal of all other cardioactive drugs before and after 10–20 µg/kg/minute of intravenous amrinone (doses that increased cardiac index and decreased PA wedge pressure and systemic vascular resistance). Amrinone caused no change in PR, QRS, QTc, AH, or HV intervals or maximal corrected sinus node recovery time and had no significant effect on the ventricular effective refractory periods. Amrinone decreased the atrial effective refractory period from 256 ± 40–240 ± 38 ms, and the AV nodal functional refractory period from 374 ± 65–356 ± 64 ms, and enhanced maximal 1:1 AV nodal conduction from 371 ± 46–334 ± 47 ms. Nine patients had baseline HV prolongation; this was not affected by amrinone. The frequency of inducible VT was not significantly affected by amrinone. Holter recordings (24–48 hours) were obtained from 10 patients before and after acute oral amrinone dosing 75–150 mg every 8 hours). There was no change in the number of VPC/24 hours (2,197 ± 3,305 -vs- 2,616 ± 2,436) or number of runs of VT/24 hours (10 ± 12 -vs- 12 ± 13); however, the number of ventricular couplets per 24 hours increased from 22 ± 34–52 ± 55. Thus, amrinone is safe to use in patients with intraventricular conduction disturbances. It shortens the atrial effective and AV nodal functional refractory period and enhances AV nodal conduction, and it has minimal effects on ventricular arrhythmogenesis during acute drug administration.

Amrinone increases myocardial contractility, just as does digitalis, in normal and failing hearts and improves cardiac performance in experimental and clinical studies. Although amrinone produces acute hemodynamic improvement in patients with severe chronic CHF, it has not produced clinical benefits in long-term controlled trials. To determine if the administration of subtherapeutic doses of amrinone may account for its lack of efficacy in the studies, Packer and associates[14] from New York City investigated the dose requirements of the drug in 30 patients with severe CHF. Doses of 100 mg of oral amrinone produced moderate increases in cardiac index (0.35 liters/min/M^2) and decreases in PA wedge pressure (7 mmHg) and systemic vascular resistance (16%); these effects, however, were short-lived (<2.5 hours). Doses of 200 mg of oral amrinone produced marked increases in cardiac index (0.56 liters/min/M^2) and substantial decreases in LV filling pressure (10 mmHg) and systemic vascular resistance (30%), and these effects persisted for longer than 4 hours. Only 4 patients showed hemodynamic responses with 100 mg of the drug that were sufficiently marked and long-lasting to merit chronic therapy, whereas 28 patients had such a response with the 200 mg dose. When 200 mg of amrinone was administered orally every 8 hours, sustained hemodynamic benefits were seen for 48 hours. However, 16 of 22 patients who received 600 mg of the drug daily for >1 week had intolerable adverse reactions that required drug withdrawal. In conclusion, hemodynamically effective doses of amrinone (600 mg/day) cannot be tolerated for long periods by most patients with severe chronic CHF. These observations may explain the ineffectiveness of the drug in controlled clinical trials.

Firth and associates[15] from Dallas, Texas, assessed in patients with a range of LV function the hemodynamic effects of graded dose infusions of amrinone (maximal dose 30 μg/kg/min; 10 patients) and isoproterenol (maximum dose, 4 mg/min; 11 patients). The LV EF ranged from 0.13 to 0.77 (mean, 0.47 ± 0.23) among the patients who received amrinone and from 0.24–0.77 (mean, 0.52 ± 0.18) among those who received isoproterenol. Peak dose amrinone produced a reduction in LV filling pressure (from 15 ± 10–10 ± 7 mmHg, but no significant change in heart rate, cardiac output, mean aortic pressure, total systemic vascular resistance (SVR) or LV dP/dt$_{max}$. In contrast, peak dose isoproterenol produced a similar reduction in LV filling pressure (from 17 ± 12–13 ± 13 mmHg), but also caused increases in heart rate, cardiac output, and LV dP/dt$_{max}$ and decreases in mean aortic pressure and SVR. The absolute change in cardiac output and stroke volume correlated closely with the change in SVR in response to amrinone, but not in response to isoproterenol. Although isoproterenol produced a marked increase in cardiac output and LV dP/dt$_{max}$ (not explained by heart rate changes alone) in all patients, amrinone produced an increase in cardiac output only in those with markedly elevated LV filling pressures (who had a reduction in SVR), and an increase in LV dP/dt in a minority.

Packer and associates[16] from New York City treated 31 patients with severe chronic CHF with oral amrinone (600 mg daily) and performed invasive hemodynamic studies during short- and long-term treatment with the drug. Stroke volume and stroke work indexes increased markedly during the first 48 hours of therapy but returned to pretreatment values after 2–10 weeks. On drug withdrawal, both variables deteriorated rapidly to values significantly lower than those observed before treatment with amrinone, despite similar values for LV filling pressure, mean arterial pressure, and systemic vascular resistance. This pattern of response indicated that progression of the underlying heart disease had occurred during treatment with amrinone and contributed importantly to its failure to produce long-term benefits. Progression of LV dysfunction was associated with a progressive increase in heart rate and plasma renin activity and a decline in serum sodium concentration. Clinically, amrinone therapy was complicated by sustained symptomatic VT in 4 patients, worsening myocardial ischemia in 4 patients, and worsening CHF in 8 patients, all of whom had been stable before entry into the study. Only 3 of the 31 patients improved clinically. Ten patients died during the first 2 weeks of treatment, and 16 were dead within 3 months (52%), a mortality rate twice as great as that seen during comparable trials with vasodilating drugs. In conclusion, long-term therapy with amrinone may accelerate progression of LV Dysfunction, exacerbate myocardial ischemia, and provoke life-threatening ventricular tachyarrhythmias, thereby shortening survival in patients with severe chronic CHF. Thus, these investigators warn that prolonged administration of inotropic drugs may achieve short-term gains at the expense of long-term detrimental effects on the myocardium.

DiBianco and associates[17] from Washington, D.C., performed a placebo-controlled study to evaluate the effects of oral amrinone in patients with CHF. After at least 4 weeks of standard treatment of refractory CHF, oral amrinone was added to the treatment regimen of 173 patients: 52% of the patients had ischemic cardiomyopathy and 37% had idiopathic, dilated cardiomyopathy; 40% were in the New York Heart Association functional class II, 59% in class III, and 1% in class IV. The mean LV EF was 25 ± 15%. The addition of amrinone (113 ± 33 mg 3 times daily) resulted in 52 patients (30%) demonstrating a maximal increase in treadmill exercise time >2 minutes; 72 (42%) had a lesser increase in treadmill time, and 24 (14%) developed adverse reactions, including 20 patients who died and 5 who dropped out of the study. Fifty-two responders free of limiting side effects and with a >2-minute increase in exercise time were randomized in a double-blind fashion to continue amrinone or switched to placebo for an additional 12 weeks. In 31 of the 52 responders who continued to receive amrinone compared with 21 patients randomized to placebo, there was no significant difference in LV size or function or maximal exercise time. Follow-up of these patients revealed that episodes of CHF severe enough to mandate termination of the double-blind treatment occurred as frequently in patients taking placebo (18%) as in those taking amrinone (13%). Average symptom score and functional class also remained comparable. Gastrointestinal and central nervous system complaints, reduced platelet counts, and increased liver enzymes were more common in the patients treated with amrinone. Thus, these data indicate that oral amrinone therapy does not importantly improve cardiac function chronically beyond that provided by standard medical therapy.

Thrombocytopenia is an adverse reaction associated with amrinone therapy. Ansell and associates[18] from Worcester, Massachusetts, evaluated the frequency and characteristics of thrombocytopenia resulting from administration of amrinone in 43 patients, 8 of whom developed thrombocytopenia (19%). The thrombocytopenia was due to accelerated peripheral loss of platelets. There appeared to be a dose relation with regard to the rapidity of onset and degree of thrombocytopenia. Although platelet-associated IgG levels were elevated when measured in patients with thrombocytopenia, the clinical features were suggestive of a direct, perhaps nonimmunologic effect of amrinone on platelets. Thrombocytopenia was mild in most cases and bleeding attributable to thrombocytopenia did not occur. Several patients continued amrinone therapy over long periods despite low platelet counts, showing that mild to moderate thrombocytopenia is not necessarily an indication that therapy should be discontinued, but that platelet counts should be observed closely.

Amrinone -vs- nitroprusside

Wilmshurst and associates[19] from London, England, compared the effects of intravenous amrinone and sodium nitroprusside on hemodynamic indices, LV contractility, and myocardial metabolism in 14 patients with chronic CHF secondary to idiopathic dilated cardiomyopathy (IDC) in 8 patients and to CAD in 6 patients. All 14 patients had received 1 dose of each drug and some received serial doses. The responses to the 2 drugs were independent of the etiology of CHF. Both drugs lowered LV end-diastolic pressure and aortocoronary sinus oxygen difference and increased cardiac index and LV efficiency; these effects were dose related. Although the effects of the drugs on peripheral blood substrate concentrations were different, those on myocardial substrate metabolism were identical. Pressure-derived indices of contractility in each group of patients were unaltered by either drug. After amrinone administration, increases in cardiac index were related to plasma amrinone concentration, but alterations in contractility were not. In 4 individual patients increases in contractility were associated with alterations in plasma metabolite concentrations, which suggested that catecholamine release had occurred. For the groups of patients as a whole, however, amrinone had effects that did not differ significantly from those of the pure vasodilator, nitroprusside. There was no evidence that amrinone had a direct positive inotropic effect, since no dose-related changes in indices of contractile function could be established.

Captopril

Although the short-term hemodynamic and clinical responses to angiotensin-converting enzyme inhibition in patients with chronic CHF are well known, little information is available about the long-term results of captopril therapy. Thus, Massie and associates[20] from San Francisco, California, gave captopril to 15 stable outpatients and followed them 6–27 months (mean, 19) with serial clinical assessments and measurements of exercise tolerance, EF, and cardiothoracic ratio. Exercise tolerance on a modified Naughton protocol improved from $10.5 \pm 2.7–12.7 \pm 2.4$ minutes at 3 months, tended to increase progressively up to 12 months, and remained significantly increased even after 24 months (9.7 ± 1.8 -vs- 13.5 ± 4.0 minutes). However, individual responses were variable; 4 patients did not show measurable improvement. The LV EF increased from 0.20 ± 0.06–0.25 ± 0.06 at 3 months and remained higher (0.30 ± 0.12) at latest follow-up. Cardiothoracic ratio decreased from 0.59 ± 0.04–0.56 ± 0.05 at 3 months and remained significantly lower at 12 months and at latest follow-up, although again individual responses were variable. Clinical responses generally correlated with these objective measurements, with clinical classification on a scale modified from the New York Heart Association classification improving from 3.0 ± 0.6–2.3 ± 0.5 at 3 months and remaining improved throughout the follow-up period. Two patients died suddenly after 10 and 14 months and another had a disabling cerebrovascular accident, but survival at 18 months remained 85%. These findings indicate that captopril produces prolonged clinical improvement in many patients with moderately severe CHF.

The short-term hemodynamic benefits have led to the use of vasodilators in the management of patients with chronic CHF. Although a growing body of data supports the clinical value of vasodilator therapy, the role of hemodynamic monitoring during initiation of this form of treatment remains to be defined despite the tremendous potential socioeconomic and clinical ramifications. Massie and colleagues[21] from San Francisco, California, performed resting and exercise hemodynamic studies before and during the initial 48 hours of captopril therapy in 14 stable patients with New York Heart Association class II or III chronic CHF. Their clinical response to therapy was determined by evaluating changes in clinical status and the measured changes in exercise tolerance, heart size, and EF after 3 months. Significant improvement in each of these indexes was found for the group as a whole, but the baseline hemodynamics and the hemodynamic responses to captopril differed little between the patients showing marked improvement and those who had little or no change. Correlations between the hemodynamic measurements and the changes in clinical class, exercise tolerance, heart size, and EF were generally poor. Even when they achieved significance, these correlations were too loose to allow prediction of the clinical efficacy of captopril in individual subjects. These findings indicate that the routine use of invasive hemodynamic monitoring during the initiation of captopril is unnecessary and potentially misleading, although such measurements remain valuable for diagnosis, for the management of patients with complex conditions, and for investigation. The response to captopril may be best evaluated by serial measurements of exercise tolerance and heart size in addition to clinical assessment. These investigators proposed rational considerations for the indications of initial hemodynamic monitoring as prelude for long-term vasodilator therapy.

Mujais and associates[22] from Cleveland, Ohio, assessed the effects of treatment with captopril in 10 patients with resistant normotensive chronic CHF. Administration of this drug in this circumstance is known to cause a pronounced reduction in BP, particularly after the first dose. These investigators assessed the effects of reduction on renal function at the beginning of and during chronic treatment (at 1 and 12 weeks). Renal plasma flow and glomerular filtration rates were measured by isotope clearance during water diuresis. The first dose of captopril (25 mg) led to a pronounced decrease in renal plasma flow and glomerular filtration rates together with a decrease in mean arterial pressure; this decrease correlated with baseline plasma renin activity. These changes were paralleled by decreases in water and sodium excretion. In contrast, by the end of the first week of treatment, a similar decrease in mean arterial pressure occurred together with a pronounced increase in renal plasma flow; the glomerular filtration rate was maintained and there was no decrease in water and sodium excretion. This new response pattern recurred after 3 months of treatment. The difference in response at different stages of treatment may reflect the balance between the different mechanisms influencing kidney dynamics in heart failure and their alteration by converting enzyme inhibition. The sustained increase in renal plasma flow during chronic treatment with captopril may account for the continued control of CHF in these patients.

To determine the efficacy of converting-enzyme inhibition in patients with low renin CHF, Packer and associates[23] from New York City evaluated the long-term hemodynamic and clinical responses to captopril in 26 consecutive patients with severe, chronic CHF whose pretreatment plasma renin activity (PRA) was <2 ng/ml/hour. After 2–8 weeks of continuous treatment with captopril, 14 patients (54%) showed long-term hemodynamic benefits, of whom 13 (50%) improved clinically by at least 1 New York Heart Association functional class. To distinguish responders from nonresponders, patients were grouped based on the presence or absence of sustained reactive hyperreninemia (PRA during chronic therapy >4 ng/ml/hour). After 2–8 weeks of therapy with captopril, 14 patients had sustained reactive hyperreninemia Their cardiac index increased by 0.33 liters/min/M^2 (p < 0.01), LV filling pressure decreased by 12.6 mmHg (p < 0.001), mean RA pressure decreased by 5 mmHg (p < 0.001), and systemic vascular resistance decreased by 529 dyne s cm^{-5} (p < 0.001). Twelve of these 14 patients improved clinically. Twelve other patients had no reactive increase in PRA, and these patients showed no significant improvement in any hemodynamic variable after 2–8 weeks of treatment with captopril; only 1 of the 12 patients improved clinically (p < 0.001 between groups). The 2 groups were otherwise similar with regard to pretreatment demographic, hemodynamic, and hormonal variables. Thus, many patients with severe, chronic CHF associated with a low PRA improve during therapy with captopril, and these patients can be distinguished from nonresponders by the occurrence of reactive hyperreninemia during long-term treatment.

Cleland and associates[24] from Glasgow, Scotland, investigated the effect of captopril on long-term treatment in 20 patients with severe CHF in a double-blind trial. Of the patients, 13 had CAD, 4 had idiopathic dialated cardiomyopathy, and 3 had severe LV dysfunction associated with valvular regurgitation. Of the 20 patients, 14 completed the double-blind trial. Captopril reduced plasma concentrations of angiotensin II and norepinephrine, with a converse increase in active renin concentration. Effective renal plasma flow increased and renal vascular resistance decreased; glomerular filtration rate did not change. Serum urea and creatinine concentrations increased. Both serum and total body potassium contents increased; there were no long-term changes in serum concentration or total body content of sodium. Exercise tolerance was appreciably improved, and dyspnea and fatigue lessened. The LV end-systolic and end-diastolic dimensions were reduced. There was an appreciable reduction in complex VPC. Adverse effects were few: weight gain and fluid retention were evident in 5 patients when captopril was introduced, and 2 patients initially experienced mild postural dizziness; rashes in 2 patients did not recur when the drug was reintroduced at a lower dose;

there was a significant reduction in white cell count overall, but the lowest individual white cell count was $4,000 \times 10^6$/liter. Captopril thus seemed to be of considerable value in the long-term treatment of severe CHF.

Diltiazem

Materne and associates[25] from Liege, Belgium, studied the acute hemodynamic effects of intravenous diltiazem in 8 patients with CAD, LV failure, rest EF < 40%, or a cardiac index < 2.4 liters/min/M^2. Hemodynamic measurements and LV angiograms were performed at rest before and after the administration of diltiazem, 0.5 mg/kg, administered at a speed of 5 mg/minute. Diltiazem treatment induced a decrease in heart rate from 68 ± 12–55 ± 9 beats/minute (p < 0.001). Mean aortic pressure decreased from 94 ± 14–81 ± 15 mmHg (p < 0.05). Thus, the pressure-rate product significantly decreased under the influence of the drug. from 8,791 ± 2,465–6,342 ± 1,808 beats mmHg/min, (p < 0.001). Diltiazem induced no significant change of LV end-diastolic pressure, pulmonary wedge pressure, cardiac index, and LV stroke work index. Systemic vascular resistance decreased (p < 0.01), whereas pulmonary vascular resistance showed no change. End-systolic volume diminished (p < 0.02), which accounts for the increase of stroke volume and EF (p < 0.001). Disorders of regional contractility were not aggravated by diltiazem, and even improved in individual cases. Thus, intravenous diltiazem may be used safely in patients with CHF. However, in view of the marked bradycardiac effects seen in some cases, heart rate should be carefully monitored.

Dobutamine

Liang and coworkers[26] from Boston, Massachusetts, and Rochester, New York, randomly assigned 15 patients with idiopathic dilated cardiomyopathy (IDC) to a protocol in which dobutamine or 5% dextrose in water was infused continuously for 72 hours. The dose of dobutamine was titrated to increase cardiac output to twice the baseline values. The patients were evaluated before infusion, shortly after infusion, and 1, 2, and 4 weeks thereafter. Functional class improved in 6 of 8 dobutamine-treated patients but in only 2 of 7 control patients during the 4-week observation period. Maximal exercise time and LV EF increased significantly above baseline only in the dobutamine group. Neither dobutamine nor placebo infusion produced significant changes shortly after infusion in heart rate, cardiac index, or total peripheral vascular resistance at rest or during exercise at similar workloads. The group receiving dobutamine did demonstrate a reduction in systemic systolic and PA mean and diastolic pressure at rest. Total body oxygen consumption during similar workloads was lower after dobutamine infusion than before. These changes occurred without alteration in plasma catecholamine or arterial blood lactate concentrations. The improvement in resting hemodynamics, exercise tolerance, and symptoms observed for at least several weeks after dobutamine infusion suggests that there is a sustained effect on cardiac function after short-term inotropic stimulation. This may represent an innovative form of long-term therapy for debilitating cardiac failure. Although improvement of myocardial mitochondrial structure and increased adenosine triphosphate/creatinine ratios have been demonstrated in endocardial biopsy specimens in patients reported by others, the mechanism of these mitochondrial changes as well as the time course remains to be elucidated.

The maximal exercise capacity of patients with CHF is frequently reduced, partly because of inadequate skeletal muscle nutritive flow. To investigate whether this altered muscle nutritive flow is a result of inability of the heart to increase output normally during exercise, Wilson and associates[27] from Philadelphia, Pennsylvania, examined the effect of dobutamine on systemic and leg blood flow and metabolism during maximal exercise in 11 patients with CHF. At maximal exercise before dobutamine, all patients were limited by fatigue and had reduced maximal systemic oxygen uptake (11.9 ± 1.1 ml/min/kg) (±SEM), markedly elevated leg oxygen extraction (85 ± 2%) and elevated femoral venous lactate (53 ± 5 mg/dl), consistent with impaired nutritive flow to working muscle. Dobutamine increased the peak cardiac output (from 6.5 ± 0.9–7.4 ± 0.7 liters/min) and peak leg flow (from 1.7 ± 0.3–2.1 ± 0.3 liters/min) during exercise. In contrast, no change occurred in maximal exercise duration (5.5 ± 0.8 -vs- 5.8 ± 0.8 min), peak systemic oxygen consumption (829 ± 97 -vs- 869 ± 77 ml/min), peak arterial lactate (34 ± 2 -vs- 35 ± 4 mg/dl), or peak leg lactate output (248 ± 39 -vs- 275 ± 53 mg/min), whereas peak leg oxygen extraction decreased (85 ± 2–80 ± 2%), suggesting no improvement in muscle nutritive flow. These data suggest that nutritive flow to working skeletal muscle is impaired in patients with CHF and that this impairment is not due simply to an inability of the heart to increase the cardiac output normally during exercise.

Enalapril

Levine and coworkers[28] from Minneapolis, Minnesota, administered enalapril, a new oral angiotensin-converting enzyme inhibitor to 9 patients with severe CHF. Short-term hemodynamic response was noted within 2 hours and persisted for <24 hours. At peak effect mean arterial pressure decreased from 83–72 mmHg, RA pressure from 14–10 mmHg, PA pressure from 39–32 mmHg, PA wedge pressure from 28–22 mmHg, and total pulmonary resistance from 875–697 dynes-s-cm[5]. Cardiac index was not changed, but there was a significant redistribution of regional blood flow with an increase of renal blood flow after enalapril. Plasma renin activity increased significantly, whereas plasma norepinephrine did not change after enalapril. Seven patients were treated with the drug for 4 weeks. Five patients reported symptomatic improvement. Five of six patients tested had an increase in both exercise time and maximum oxygen consumption. Repeat hemodynamic evaluation in 6 patients after long-term enalapril therapy showed a persistent effect with significant reductions in RA pressure from 14–7 mmHg and mean arterial pressure from 83–77 mmHg and a significant increase in cardiac index from 2.1–2.5 liters/min/M^2. Long-term therapy was well tolerated. These investigators concluded that enalapril is a long-acting oral converting-enzyme inhibitor with an acute vasodilatory effect that appears to be well tolerated in long-term administration in patients with CHF. Although the hemodynamic responses are similar to captopril, the results suggest that enalapril has a slower onset and a longer duration of action.

Short-term hemodynamic and symptomatic improvement in patients with CHF have been demonstrated with angiotensin converting-enzyme inhibitors. The long-term efficacy of the oral long-acting converting inhibitor enalapril has not been established in controlled studies. Sharpe and colleagues[29] from Auckland, New Zealand, evaluated enalapril in 36 patients with New York Heart Association functional class II or III CHF who were clinically stable on digoxin and diuretic therapy. After baseline evaluation of symptoms, exercise capacity, results of echo examination, and right-sided heart catheterization, patients were randomly assigned a treatment with 5 mg enalapril twice daily or placebo in a double-blind fashion. The 2 groups had similar clinical, echo, and hemodynamic characteristics before treatment. After 3 months of treatment, the enalapril group showed a significant improvement as judged by subjective patient impression, functional class, and exercise duration. Diuretic dosage was reduced in 6 patients and increased in 1 patient, 1 patient had died, and another had been withdrawn from the study. In the placebo group there was no significant change with respect to patient impression, functional class, or exercise duration; diuretic dosage was increased in 7 patients and 4 patients had died. Echo LV dimensions were significantly reduced and LV shortening fractions significantly increased in the enalapril group, but were unchanged in the placebo group. Hemodynamic assessment showed a significant reduction in LV filling pressure and an increase in stroke volume index in the enalapril group, but no change in the placebo group with LV filling pressure and stroke volume remaining similar. This study provides a basis for the efficacy and safety of enalapril in the treatment of patients with chronic CHF, which provided significant hemodynamic and symptomatic benefit with long-term treatment.

Endralazine

Quyyumi and associates[30] from London, England, made hemodynamic measurements at rest and during submaximal and maximal exercise in 12 patients with chronic CHF before and after oral endralazine. After acute assessment, patients received endralazine, twice daily, for a mean of 2.8 months, when hemodynamic measurements were repeated. The drug was withdrawn for 3–4 days and subsequently reintroduced. Three patients with greatly elevated PA wedge pressures were assessed after 30 mg of isosorbide dinitrate, which was also chronically administered. Resting mean cardiac and stroke volume indexes increased by 44 and 33%, respectively (p < 0.01), with concomitant reduction of the systemic resistance. This improvement was maintained on a long-term basis in 8 of the 11 surviving patients. Withdrawal and subsequent reintroduction of endralazine confirmed that there was worsening of LV dysfunction in the other 3 subjects. Chronic but not acute therapy produced a modest reduction in wedge pressure. At maximal exercise, cardiac and stroke volume indexes increased by 29 and 18%, respectively (p < 0.01), after endralazine; the duration of exercise increased in 7 of the 10 subjects after acute therapy and this was maintained on a long-term basis. Mean creatinine clearance increased by 34% (p < 0.01). The results confirm that endralazine produces acute and long-term hemodynamic and functional improvement without tolerance in CHF.

Hydralazine

In a placebo-controlled trial carried out by Conradson and colleagues[31] from Lund, Sweden, 62 patients with chronic CHF (New York Heart Association class III) had hydralazine (149 ± 11 mg daily) or placebo added to conventional therapy. During 12 months of follow-up, 27 patients dropped out, 15 of 32 in the hydralazine group and 12 of 30 among the control subjects. The 1-year mortality rate was 28% in the hydralazine group compared with 27% in the control group. Symptomatic improvement was noted in both groups; however, it was gradually more pronounced in the actively treated group with a statistically significant difference between the 2 groups at month 12 ($p < 0.05$). The hydralazine patients increased their exercise capacity 25%, from 53 ± 3 W at month 0 to 67 ± 4 W at month 12 ($p < 0.01$). No improvement in exercise capacity took place in the placebo group. A significant improvement in chest x-ray examination was found with hydralazine ($p < 0.01$) in contrast to a significant deterioration among the control subjects ($p < 0.05$). Thus, it was concluded that hydralazine used in chronic CHF has beneficial clinical effects during long-term treatment.

Levodopa

Among the positive inotropic agents available to improve myocardial contractility in CHF, only digitalis glycosides are suitable for oral administration. Rajfer and associates[32] from Chicago, Illinois, administered oral levodopa (1.5–2.0 g), which is decarboxylated to form dopamine, to 10 patients with severe CHF. Peak hemodynamic responses occurred 1 hour after the ingestion of levodopa, with the mean (±SEM) cardiac index increasing from 1.8 ± 0.1–2.4 ± 0.2 liters/min/M^2 of body surface area and systemic vascular resistance declining from 1,905 ± 112–1,513 ± 121 dyn · s · cm^{-5}. These effects persisted for 4–6 hours. The LV filling pressure, heart rate, and mean arterial pressure were unchanged. Plasma concentrations of dopamine rose to a peak level of 34 ± 5 ng/ml 1 hour after drug ingestion and decreased toward baseline over the ensuing 5 hours. A significant correlation was observed between plasma dopamine levels and changes in cardiac index. Five patients enrolled in a trial to evaluate the effectiveness of long-term therapy with levodopa had similar hemodynamic responses to the drug after 6.8 ± 1.7 months of treatment. Thus, oral administration of levodopa to patients with severe CHF produced a sustained improvement in cardiac function. The hemodynamic responses observed can be attributed to the activation of beta$_1$ adrenergic, dopamine$_1$ and dopamine$_2$ receptors by dopamine derived from levodopa. This article was followed by an editorial by LeJemtel and Sonnenblick[33].

MDL 17043

To assess the potential positive inotropic properties of the drug MDL 17043, 10 patients were studied by Crawford and associates[34] from San Antonio, Texas. Each patient had impaired LV performance and each was undergoing diagnostic cardiac catheterization. The LV EF ranged from 16–46%. MDL 17043 was given in repeated intravenous doses of 0.5 mg/kg every 15 minutes until a maximal effect was observed or a total dose of 3 mg/kg was attained. Cardiac output increased from 3.5 ± 1.0–5.3 ± 0.7 liters/minute; PA wedge pressure decreased from 22 ± 4–9 ± 5 mmHg; and total systemic resistance decreased from 2,335 ± 1,147–1,310 ± 365 dyne cm^{-5}. Also, maximal LV dP/dt increased from 1,011 ± 301–1,243 ± 330 mmHg/s. No significant changes in heart rate, systemic BP, routine blood chemistries, complete blood counts, or platelet counts were observed. Thus, MDL 17043 has hemodynamic effects consistent with positive inotropic and vasodilating properties in patients with reduced LV performance. Because this agent is effective orally, further evaluation in patients with overt CHF is warranted.

Martin and coworkers[35] from Philadelphia, Pennsylvania, evaluated the inotropic agent and phosphodiesterase inhibitor MDL 17043 in patients with chronic CHF. Inravenous increments of 0.05 mg/kg (maximal total, 3 mg/kg) were given to determine a peak cardiac output response in 13 patients with New York Heart Association functional class IV CHF secondary to ischemic or myopathic disease. In the patients receiving MDL 17043, there was an increase in cardiac output (3.5–4.6 liters/min), heart rate (86–90 beats/min), and a decrease in PA wedge pressure (25–17 mmHg), mean arterial pressure (85–78 mmHg), and RA pressure (10–7 mmHg). Nine of 12 patients given long-term oral therapy improved ≥1 functional class at 2 weeks, and this improvement was sustained at 20 weeks in 5 patients. Thus, these data suggest that MDL 17043 improves the function of the failing heart acutely. However, larger numbers of patients need to be studied, both acutely and chronically, to determine the ultimate value of this new inotropic agent.

Kereiakes and associates[36] from San Francisco, California, evaluated the mechanisms for improved LV function with MDL 17043 in patients with severe chronic CHF; 24 patients were assessed by simultaneous determination of hemodynamics by right-sided heart catheterization and EF by computerized nuclear probe before and after intravenous administration of MDL 17043 (mean cumulative dose, 3.6 mg/kg). After MDL 17043, there was an increase in cardiac index (+62%), stroke volume index (+42%), and stroke work index (+68%), together with a decrease in PA wedge pressure (−46%), indicating improved LV pump function. There was a marked reduction in systemic vascular resistance (−40%) and a modest reduction in arterial pressure, indicating decreased LV outflow resistance. The ratio of peak systolic BP/calculated LV end-systolic volume tended to increase, but the change was not statistically significant. Despite a marked increment in stroke volume index, LV ejection time corrected for heart rate was shortened, suggesting enhanced contractility. In the group as a whole, the calculated LV end-diastolic volume remained unchanged, but it increased in 14 patients. Since PA wedge pressure decreased in each patient, this suggests improved overall LV distensibility. Thus, decreased LV outflow resistance, and possibly increased contractile function, and improved LV diastolic compliance may all contribute to improved LV pump function with MDL 17043 in patients with severe CHF.

MDL 17043 has been shown to produce salutary hemodynamic effects in severe CHF, but its effects on myocardial metabolism are unknown. Amin and associates[37] from Los Angeles, California, determined whether such hemodynamic effects are associated with adverse effects on the myocardial oxygen demand and supply relation. Intravenous MDL 17043 was given in incremental doses to a mean maximum dose of 2.1 mg/kg to 9 patients with severe chronic CHF. Overall cardiac pump performance was significantly improved by MDL 17043, as reflected by an 88% increase in stroke work index (17 ± 11–32 ± 19 g-m/M^2, $p < 0.001$), a 43% reduction in LV filling pressure (28 ± 4–16 ± 5 mmHg, $p < 0.0001$), a 49% reduction in systemic vascular resistance ($1,832 \pm 490$–937 ± 296 dynes-s-cm^{-5}, $p < 0.0001$) with a slight (11%) decrease in mean arterial pressure (86 ± 17–76 ± 19 mmHg, p = 0.005) and without significant changes in heart rate (88 ± 14–91 ± 12 beats/min,; NS). These hemodynamic effects were associated with an 18% reduction in myocardial oxygen consumption (17 ± 5–14 ± 5 ml/min, p = 0.01), a 17% reduction in myocardial arteriovenous oxygen difference (13 ± 2–11 ± 2 volumes %, p = 0.01), and a 120% improvement in external myocardial efficiency (stroke work index/oxygen consumption) (1.0 ± 0.6– 2.2 ± 0.9; p < 0.0001). There were no overall changes in coronary sinus blood flow (126 ± 31–124 ± 38 ml/min, NS) or percentage of myocardial lactate extraction (38 ± 12–28 ± 19, NS). The decline in myocardial oxygen consumption suggests that concomitant reduction in preload and afterload may have more than offset the increase in myocardial oxygen consumption expected secondary to the known inotropic effect of the drug. It was concluded that short-term intravenous MDL 17043 produces salutary acute hemodynamic effects in severe CHF and that these effects are associated with an improved external myocardial efficiency without adverse effects on global myocardial energetics.

Milrinone

To examine the mechanisms by which a new bipyridine inotropic agent milrinone improves cardiac function, Monrad and coworkers[38] from Boston, Massachusetts, obtained multiple indexes of LV diastolic function before and after administration of milrinone to patients with advanced CHF. In 13 patients LV pressure measurements were made with a micromanometer to permit assessment of peak negative dP/dt and the time constant of LV isovolumic relaxation, T, before and after milrinone. In 9 patients radionuclide ventriculographic studies were performed during left-sided heart catheterization, allowing calculation of LV peak filling rate, volumes, and the diastolic pressure-volume relation before and after milrinone. After intravenous administration of milrinone, peak negative dP/dt increased 18% and T decreased 30%, whereas heart rate increased by only 8%, LV systolic pressure did not change, and mean aortic pressure decreased by 11%. The LV peak filling rate increased despite a decrease in LV filling pressure. There was a decrease in LV end-diastolic pressure from 29–19 mmHg with no significant change in LV end-diastolic volume. This was associated with a downward shift in the LV diastolic pressure-volume relation in most cases. These changes in parameters of LV diastolic relaxation and chamber distensibility after administration of milrinone suggest that improved diastolic function may contribute to the beneficial hemodynamic effect of milrinone in patients with CHF.

Minoxidil

Minoxidil is a potent predominate arterial dilator that improves hemodynamics over the short term in patients with CHF. Franciosa and coworkers[39] from Little Rock, Arkansas, initiated a random double-blind study of 17 patients with chronic CHF; 9 patients were given minoxidil and 8 patients received placebo in addition to digoxin and diuretics for 3 months. Cardiac index and heart rate increased and mean arterial pressure and systemic vascular resistance decreased within 4 hours of minoxidil administration. The

RV and PA pressures were unchanged over the short term, but increased after long-term minoxidil. After 3 months of minoxidil treatment, systemic vascular resistance was still reduced. Hemodynamics were similar at baseline and remained unchanged during placebo treatment. Mean LV EF increased from 30–43% after 3 months of minoxidil treatment but remained unchanged at 25% after 3 months of placebo. Exercise duration and maximal oxygen uptake during exercise were unchanged during minoxidil or placebo treatment. Total clinical events, including increased need for diuretics, angina, ventricular arrhythmias, worsening CHF, and death were all more frequent during minoxidil -vs- placebo administration (21 -vs- 7 total events). Thus, this study revealed that despite improved hemodynamics and LV function, long-term minoxidil administration was associated with a poorer clinical course in patients with chronic LV CHF. These investigators properly emphasized that this experience shows that improvement in LV function alone cannot be reliably interpreted as proof of clinical efficacy of therapeutic interventions in patients with CHF.

Nifedipine

In patients with CHF, depressed cardiac output, diminished coronary perfusion pressure, increased ventricular filling pressures and wall tension, and myocardial hypertrophy are all factors that may interfere with adequate myocardial perfusion. Magorien and coworkers[40] from Columbus, Ohio, assessed resting and exercise systemic hemodynamic parameters, coronary blood flow, and myocardial energetics before and 15 minutes after the sublingual administration of 20 mg of nifedipine in 10 patients with idiopathic dilated cardiomyopathy (IDC). When compared with control, nifedipine increased rest and exercise cardiac index by 37 and 28%, respectively. Peripheral vasodilation was demonstrated by a decrease in systemic arterial pressure, exercise PA wedge pressure, and systemic vascular resistance. The calcium channel blocker did not alter myocardial oxygen consumption. However, coronary blood flow increased by 32% at rest while coronary vascular resistance diminished both at rest and after exercise compared with control. Nifedipine elicited a decrease in the rest and exercise aortocoronary sinus oxygen difference while the coronary sinus oxygen saturation increased. In this group of patients with IDC, nifedipine enhanced myocardial performance while increasing coronary blood flow and favorably altering the myocardial oxygen supply-demand balance. The investigators pointed out that these observations represent short-term responses and may not persist with prolonged drug administration and therefore long-term assessment will be necessary to define the clinical utility of the calcium blocking agent.

In an investigation performed by Leier and associates[41] from Columbus, Ohio, 10 patients with moderate to severe CHF underwent central and regional hemodynamic measurements at rest and central hemodynamic measurements during exercise before and after the oral administration of nifedipine (0.2 mg/kg). Nifedipine significantly decreased systemic BP, systemic vascular resistance, PA pressure, pulmonary vascular resistance, and PA wedge pressure. Stroke volume and cardiac output increased after nifedipine. The measured parameters of LV inotropy did not change significantly for this calcium channel blocker. Although blood flow to renal hepatic, and limb vascular beds increased (p < 0.05 for renal and limb) after nifedipine, only limb blood flow increased in proportion to the increase in cardiac output, suggesting preferential dilation of limb vasculature. Although initial-dose nifedipine did not increase exercise duration, it elicited an improvement in exercise hemodynamics by reducing systemic vascular resistance and PA wedge pressure and increasing stroke volume and cardiac output. The calcium channel blocker, nifedipine, can be administered safely in the setting of ventricular failure and appears to alter resting and exercise hemodynamics favorably. A select number of patients with CHF may benefit from its long-term administration.

Nifedipine -vs- hydralazine

Elkayam and associates[42] from Los Angeles, California, compared the hemodynamic response with a similar reduction of systemic vascular resistance after nifedipine and hydralazine administration in a randomized crossover protocol in patients with severe chronic CHF. All 15 patients had a $\geq 25\%$ reduction in vascular resistance with intravenous hydralazine (5–30 mg) and 11 patients had a similar response with oral nifedipine (20–50 mg). In the latter 11 patients, despite similar reductions in systemic vascular resistance (35 ± 2% with nifedipine and 36 ± 4% with hydralazine, difference not significant), nifedipine resulted in a smaller increase in stroke volume index (from 23 ± 2–30 ± 2 ml/M² and from 24 ± 2–34 ± 2 ml/M² with hydralazine, p < 0.05), cardiac index (from 2.0 ± 0.1 2.6 ± 0.2 liters/min/M² with nifedipine and from 2.0 ± 0.1–2.8 ± 0.2 liters/min/M² with hydralazine, p < 0.05) and stroke work index (from 25 ± 3–27 ± 3 g-m/M² with nifedipine and from 26 ± 2–32 ± 2 g-m/M² with hydralazine, p < 0.05). The decrease in BP after nifedipine was slightly but not significantly larger than that with hydralazine (13 ± 3 -vs- 8 ± 2%). The changes in RA pressure, PA wedge pressure, and pulmonary vascular resistance were similar. The 4 patients who did not reduce their systemic vascular resistance by at least 25% with nifedipine had a worsening of their hemodynamic state, as was evident from 1 or more of the following findings: elevation of vascular resistance, decrease in cardiac index, and increase in PA wedge pressure. These results suggest that nifedipine exerts a clinically important negative inotropic effect in patients with severe chronic CHF that is only partially offset by its strong arteriolar dilatory effect. Hydralazine appears to be better than nifedipine when LV afterload-reducing therapy is indicated in patients with severe CHF.

Nifedipine -vs- nitroprusside

Elkayam and associates[43] from Los Angeles, California, compared the hemodynamic effects of 20–40 mg of oral nifedipine with those of intravenous nitroprusside in 11 patients with severe chronic CHF. In each patient, both drugs were administered to produce similar reduction of systemic vascular resistance (SVR) (29 ± 13% with nifedipine and 29 ± 12% with nitroprusside [NS]). At this comparable decrease in systemic vascular resistance, significant differences in hemodynamic responses to both drugs were noted: Nifedipine caused a smaller increase in cardiac index (20 ± 20 -vs- 40 ± 24%) and a larger decrease in mean BP than nitroprusside (16 ± 9 -vs- 8 ± 10%). In addition, nifedipine produced a smaller decrease in mean PA wedge pressure (13 ± 24 -vs- 36 ± 21%) and pulmonary vascular resistance than nitroprusside (6 ± 42 -vs- 26 ± 46%, NS). Mean RA pressure decreased with nitroprusside, from 10 ± 7–5 ± 3 mmHg, but not with nifedipine (10 ± 7 mmHg before and after nifedipine administration, NS). The LV stroke work index increased with nitroprusside (20 ± 8–27 ± 9 g-m/M²), but did not change with nifedipine (21 ± 9 -vs- 21 ± 10 g-m/M², NS). These data show that nifedipine has an arteriolar dilatatory action in patients with CHF. However, compared with nitroprusside, nifedipine had a significantly larger hypotensive effect and had a lesser effect on right and LV filling pressure, cardiac output, and LV function.

Nitroglycerin

The hemodynamic effects of a new transdermal preparation of nitroglycerin (NTG) were evaluated in 9 patients with chronic CHF by Rajfer and associates[44] from Chicago, Illinois. A graded infusion of NTG was administered initially to establish the dose-response relation for NTG and estimate the dose of topical NTG to be applied. Significant hemodynamic improvement was observed 0.5–1.0 hour after the cutaneous application of the NTG-impregnated polymer. The peak effect occurred at 6 hours with the LV filling pressure decreasing from 24 ± 2–18 ± 1 mmHg (mean ± SE) (p < 0.01) and the cardiac index increasing from 2.0 ± 0.2–2.6 ± 0.2 liters/min/M² (p < 0.01). The systemic vascular resistance decreased from 1,860 ± 198– 1,531 ± 162 dynes s cm⁻⁵ (p < 0.01). Heart rate and mean arterial pressure were unchanged. Significant hemodynamic benefit was observed for 24 hours, and no rebound deterioration occurred upon withdrawal of the drug. The average dose of transdermal NTG applied was 51 ± 6 cm² (1.7 ± 0.2 mg/kg; 6 of the 9 patients received 64 cm²). Thus, topical application of a new NTG-impregnated polymer induces an improvement in cardiac performance that is sustained for 24 hours in patients with chronic CHF. However, substantial doses of the drug may be required to produce a satisfactory hemodynamic response in most patients with CHF.

Nitroprusside

Bencowitz and coworkers[45] from San Diego, California, evaluated the influence of nitroprusside in patients with CHF and respiratory failure. Sodium nitroprusside administration was associated with an increase in cardiac output and decreases in mean arterial pressure, PA pressure, PA wedge pressure, and pulmonary vascular resistance. The partial pressure of oxygen in arterial blood also decreased after nitroprusside in all but 1 patient (mean, 76 ± 15–68 ± 18 mmHg, p = 0.032). Ventilation and perfusion showed increased perfusion of lung units with low ventilation/perfusion ratios in all patients during nitroprusside infusion. The amount of shunt increased in 2 patients, with some shunt present in the baseline measurements. Thus, these data indicate that sodium nitroprusside therapy worsens ventilation/perfusion mismatching while increasing cardiac output and overall oxygen transport in patients with CHF and respiratory failure. The mechanisms responsible for worsening ventilation/perfusion mismatching is probably pulmonary vasodilation, increased cardiac output, or both.

Piroximone (MDL 19205)

Petein and coworkers[46] from Minneapolis, Minnesota, determined the hemodynamic and neurohumoral effects of cumulative intravenous doses of piroximone (MDL 19205), a noncatecholamine, nonglycoside, imidazole derivative with positive inotropic and vasodilating properties. Eight patients with severe CHF were studied; 1.25 mg/kg MDL 19205 was given to 7 patients and 1.75 mg/kg to 1 patient. MDL 19205 increased cardiac index by 75% and decreased systemic vascular resistance by 41%, RA pressure by 66%, and PA wedge pressure by 35% ($p < 0.005$). The administration of MDL 19205 also decreased mean arterial pressure from 78–71 mmHg and forearm blood flow increased by 42%. Plasma norepinephrine decreased from 830–542 pg/ml ($p < 0.05$). Four patients had comparable increases in cardiac index after the administration of dobutamine (15 μg/kg/min) but lesser decreases in PA wedge pressure and an increase in heart rate-BP product. Thus, these data indicate that piroximone is a potent inotropic agent with an hemodynamic responsiveness that may be somewhat more favorable than that of dobutamine. These results should encourage further evaluation of piroximine.

Prenalterol

Although short-term administration of an orally active beta-adrenergic agonist improves hemodynamics in patients with CHF, doubt exists as to the ability of the impaired ventricle to respond to additional long-term adrenergic stimulation. Roubin and colleagues[47] from Sydney, Australia, studied 11 patients with severe LV impairment (mean EF, 24%) and moderate impairment of exercise tolerance with a double-blind, placebo-controlled, crossover trial of the orally administered beta agonist prenalterol. Exercise hemodynamics and tolerance were measured during bicycle and treadmill exercise after 2 weeks of therapy with placebo or prenalterol. Cardiac index, EF, and stroke work index were not improved and exercise duration and peak oxygen consumption were not significantly different during the 2 treatments. During prenalterol treatment, heart rate during exercise was consistently reduced. These results show that prolonged therapy with prenalterol does not improve hemodynamics or exercise tolerance and is associated with a diminished heart rate response to exercise. Although experimental studies have revealed evidence of beta adrenoreceptor down regulation after continuous adrenergic stimulation, such clinical studies may require further assessment of beta-receptors in myocardial biopsies to confirm the observations of the present study.

Wahr and associates[48] from San Francisco, California, determined in patients with chronic CHF the systemic and coronary hemodynamic effects of prenalterol, a beta₁ receptor agonist. These effects were determined in 10 patients initially after intravenous administration and in 8 patients after oral administration. Cardiac index increased by 33 and 30% after intravenous and oral prenalterol, respectively. The increase in stroke volume index and stroke work index and decrease in PA wedge pressure and systemic vascular resistance were not significant. Myocardial oxygen consumption and coronary sinus blood flow increased in most patients, although these changes were not statistically significant. There were no significant changes in transmyocardial norepinephrine or epinephrine balance. The systemic and coronary hemodynamic effects of both intravenous and oral prenalterol were similar. Major side effects included sudden death (2 patients) and hypotension and bradycardia (3 patients) during oral prenalterol treatment. It was concluded that improved LV function after both intravenous and oral prenalterol may be associated with increased myocardial oxygen consumption, and serious adverse effects may occur during prenalterol therapy.

Petch and associates[49] from Edinburgh, Scotland, studied the acute hemodynamic affects of oral prenalterol, a new beta$_1$ adrenoceptor agonist that is active in both the parenteral and oral forms, in 14 patients with severe chronic CHF secondary to CAD. All patients received treatment with digoxin, diuretics, and in most cases vasodilators. Prenalterol was administered at 2 hourly intervals to give cumulative doses of 20, 50, and 100 mg and mean plasma concentrations of 53, 97, and 175 nM/liter. Hemodynamic measurements were made 2 hours after each dose with Swan-Ganz catheterization; cardiac output was measured by thermodilution. There were no significant changes in heart rate, mean arterial pressure, or PA diastolic pressure after the drug. Cardiac index rose significantly after 50 mg and 100 mg prenalterol. Oral prenalterol has a beneficial short-term hemodynamic effect in patients with severe CHF. If this effect is sustained, prenalterol may be of value in the long-term management of patients with this disabling condition.

Saralasin

The renin-angiotensin system has been shown to participate in the pathophysiology of chronic CHF in many patients. However, the immediate assessment of this contribution in individual patients may sometimes be difficult. As a pharmacologic estimate of angiotensin II receptor activity, Cody and associates[50] from New York City infused the angiotensin II analogue, saralasin, in 20 patients with severe chronic CHF. The infusion resulted in BP responses ranging from an agonist pressor response (increased systemic resistance) in patients with low intrinsic renin-angiotensin system activity, to an antagonist depressor response (decreased systemic resistance) in patients with marked activation of the renin-angiotensin system. The ability of the saralasin response pharmacologically to estimate angiotensin II receptor activity in CHF was further revealed by 2 physiologic maneuvers that decrease endogenous circulating angiotensin II and angiotensin II receptor occupancy. Both converting enzyme inhibition with captopril and sodium repletion, factors known to decrease endogenous angiotensin II activity, provoked agonist responses to saralasin infusion. Furthermore, saralasin was able to reverse the orthostatic hypotension precipitated by converting enzyme inhibition of angiotensin-dependent vascular tone. It was concluded that saralasin provides a means to estimate angiotensin receptor activity and may therefore serve as a probe of angiotensin-mediated vasoconstriction in the pathophysiology of chronic CHF.

References

1. WEISS JM, SPODICK DH: Laterality of pleural effusions in chronic congestive heart failure. Am J Cardiol 53:951, March 1984.

2. DOUGHTERTY AH, NACCARELLI GV, GRAY EL, HICKS CH, GOLDSTEIN RA: Congestive heart failure with normal systolic function. Am J Cardiol 54:778–782, Oct 1, 1984.

3. FRANCIOSA JA, LEDDY CL, WILEN M, SCHWARTZ DE: Relation between hemodynamic and ventilatory responses in determining exercise capacity in severe congestive heart failure. Am J Cardiol 53:127–134, Jan 1, 1984.

4. WILSON JR, MARTIN JL, SCHWARTZ D, FERRARO N: Exercise intolerance in patients with chronic heart failure: role in impaired nutritive flow to skeletal muscle. Circulation 69:1079–1087, June 1984.

5. BAKER BJ, WILEN MM, BOYD CM, DINH H, FRANCIOSA JA: Relation of right ventricular ejection fraction to exercise capacity in chronic left ventricular failure. Am J Cardiol 54:596–599, Sept 1, 1984.

6. VANDEWERF F, BOEL A, GEBOERS J, MINTEN J, WILLEMS J, DEGEEST H, KESTELOOT H: Diastolic properties of the left ventricle in normal adults and in patients with third heart sounds. Circulation 69:1070–1078, June 1984.

7. LEITHE ME, MARGORIEN RD, HERMILLER JB, UNVERFERTH DV, LEIER CV: Relationship between central hemodynamics and regional blood flow in normal subjects and in patients with congestive heart failure. Circulation 69:57 64, Jan 1984.

8. FERGUSON DW, ABBOUD FM, MARK AL: Selective impairment of baroreflex-mediated vasoconstrictor responses in patients with ventricular dysfunction. Circulation 69:451–460, March 1984.

9. MASKIN CS, SISKIND SJ, LEJEMTEL TH: High prevalence of nonsustained ventricular tachycardia in severe congestive heart failure. Am Heart J 107:896 901, May 1984.

10. COHN JN, LEVINE TB, OLIVARI MT, GARBERG V, LURA D, FRANCIS GS, SIMON AB, RECTOR T: Plasma norepinephrine as a guide to prognosis in patients with chronic congestive heart failure. N Engl J Med 311:819–823, Sept 27, 1984.

11. DZAU VJ, PACKER M, LILLY LS, SWARTZ SL, HOLLENBERG NK, WILLIAMS GH: Prostaglandins in severe congestive heart failure: Relation to activation of the renin-angiotensin system and hyponatremia. N Engl J Med 310:347–352, Feb 9, 1984.

12. BRAUNWALD E, COLUCCI WS: Vasodilator therapy of heart failure. Has the promissory note been paid? N Engl J Med 310:459–461, Feb 9, 1984.

13. NACCARELLI GV, GRAY EL, DOUGHERTY AH, HANNA JE, GOLDSTEIN RA: Amrinone: acute electrophysiologic and hemodynamic effects in patients with congestive heart failure. Am J Cardiol 54:600–604, Sept 1, 1984.

14. PACKER M, MEDINA N, YUSHAK M: Failure of low doses of amrinone to produce sustained hemodynamic improvement in patients with severe chronic congestive heart failure. Am J Cardiol 54:1025–1029, Nov 1, 1984.

15. FIRTH BG, RATNER AV, GRASSMAN ED, WINNIFORD MD, NICOD P, HILLIS LD: Assessment of the inotropic and vasodilator effects of amrinone versus isoproterenol. Am J Cardiol 54:1331–1336, Dec 1, 1984.

16. PACKER M, MEDINA N, YUSHAK M: Hemodynamic and clinical limitations of long-term inotropic therapy with amrinone in patients with severe chronic heart failure. Circulation 70:1038–1047, Dec 1984.

17. DIBIANCO R, SHABETAI R, SILVERMAN BD, LEIER CV, BENOTTI JR: Oral amrinone for the treatment of chronic congestive heart failure: results of a multicenter randomized double-blind and placebo-controlled withdrawal study. J Am Coll Cardiol 4:855–866, Nov 1984.

18. ANSELL J, TIARKS C, MCCUE J, PARRILLA N, BENOTTI JR: Amrinone-induced thrombocytopenia. Arch Intern Med 144:949–952, May 1984.

19. WILMSHURST PT, THOMPSON DS, JUUL SM, JENKINS BS, COLTART DJ, WEBB-PEPLOE MM: Comparison of the effects of amrinone and sodium nitroprusside on hemodynamics, contractility, and myocardial metabolism in patients with cardiac failure due to coronary artery disease and dilated cardiomyopathy. Br Heart J 52:38–48, July 1984.

20. MASSIE BM, KRAMER BL, TOPIC N: Long-term captopril therapy for chronic congestive heart failure. Am J Cardiol 53:1316–1320, May 1, 1984.

21. MASSIE BM, KRAMER BL, TOPIC N: Lack of relationship between the short-term hemodynamic effects of captopril and subsequent clinical responses. Circulation 69:1135–1141, June 1984.

22. MUJAIS SK, FOUAD FM, TEXTOR SC, TARAZI RC, BRAVO EL, HART N, GIFFORD RW: Transient renal

dysfunction during initial inhibition of converting enzyme in congestive heart failure. Br Heart J 52:63–71, July 1984.

23. PACKER M, MEDINA N, YUSHAK: Efficacy of captopril in low-renin congestive heart failure: importance of sustained reactive hyperreninemia in distinguishing responders from non-responders. Am J Cardiol 54:771–777, Oct 1, 1984.

24. CLELAND JGF, DARGIE HJ, HODSMAN GP, BALL SG, ROBERTSON JIS, MORTON JJ, EAST BW, ROBERTSON I, MURRAY GD, GILLEN G: Captopril in heart failure: a double blind controlled trial. Br Heart J 52:530–535, Nov 1984.

25. MATERNE P, LEGRAND V, VANDORMAEL M, COLLIGNON P, KULBERTUS HE: Hemodynamic effects of intravenous diltiazem with impaired left ventricular function. Am J Cardiol 54:733–737, Oct 1, 1984.

26. LIANG C, SHERMAN LG, DOHERTY JU, WELLINGTON K, LEE VW, HOOD WB: Sustained improvement of cardiac function in patients with congestive heart failure after short term infusion of dobutamine. Circulation 69:113–119, Jan 1984.

27. WILSON JR, MARTIN JL, FERRARO N: Impaired skeletal muscle nutritive flow during exercise in patients with congestive heart failure: role of cardiac pump dysfunction as determined by the effect of dobutamine. Am J Cardiol 53:1308–1315, May 1, 1984.

28. LEVINE TB, OLIVARI MT, GARBERG V, SHARKEY SW, COHN JN: Hemodynamic and clinical response to enalapril, a long-acting converting-enzyme inhibitor, in patients with congestive heart failure. Circulation 69:548–553, March 1984.

29. SHARPE DN, MURPHY J, COXON R, HANNAN SF: Enalapril in patients with chronic heart failure: a placebo-controlled, randomized, double-blind study. Circulation 70:271–278, Aug 1984.

30. QUYYUMI AA, WAGSTAFF D, EVANS TR: Long-term beneficial effects of endralazine, a new arteriolar vasodilator at rest and during exercise capacity in chronic congestive heart failure. Am J Cardiol 54:1020–1024, Nov 1, 1984.

31. CONRADSON T-B, RYDÉN L, AHLMARK G, SAETRE H, PERSSON S, NYQUIST O, WERNERSSON B: Clinical efficacy of hydralazine in chronic heart failure: one-year double-blind placebo-controlled study. Am Heart J 108:1001–1006, Oct 1984.

32. RAJFER SI, ANTON AH, ROSSEN JD, GOLDBERG LI: Beneficial hemodynamic effects of oral levodopa in heart failure: relation to the generation of dopamine. N Engl J Med 310:1357–62, May 24, 1984.

33. LEJEMTEL TH, SONNENBLICK EH: Should the failing heart be stimulated? N Engl J Med 310:1384–1385, May 24, 1984.

34. CRAWFORD MH, RICHARDS KL, SODUMS MT, KENNEDY GT: Positive inotropic and vasodilator effects of MDL 17,043 in patients with reduced left ventricular performance. Am J Cardiol 53:1051–1053, Apr 1, 1984.

35. MARTIN JL, LIKOFF MJ, JANICKI JS, LASKEY WK, HIRSHFELD JW Jr, WEBER KT: Myocardial energetics and clinical response to the cardiotonic agent MDL 17043 in advanced heart failure. J Am Coll Cardiol 4:875–883, Nov 1984.

36. KEREIAKES DJ, VIQUERAT C, LANZER P, BOTVINICK EH, SPANGENBERG R, BUCKINGHAM M, PARMLEY WW, CHATTERJEE K: Mechanisms of improved left ventricular function following intravenous MDL 17,043 in patients with severe chronic heart failure. Am Heart J 108:1278–1284, Nov 1984.

37. AMIN DK, SHAH PK, HULSE S, SHELLOCK FG, SWAN HJC: Myocardial metabolic and hemodynamic effects of intravenous MDL-17,043, a new cardiotonic drug, in patients with chronic severe heart failure. Am Heart J 108:1285–1292, Nov 1984.

38. MONRAD ES, McKAY RG, BAIM DS, COLUCCI WS, FIFER MA, HELLER GV, ROYAL HD, GROSSMAN W: Improvement in indexes of diastolic performance in patients with congestive heart failure treated with milrinone. Circulation 70:1030–1037, Dec 1984.

39. FRANCIOSA JA, JORDAN RA, WILEN MM, LEDDY CL: Minoxidil in patients with chronic left heart failure: contrasting hemodynamic and clinical effects in a controlled trial. Circulation 70:63–68, July 1984.

40. MAGORIEN RD, LEIER CV, KOLIBASH AJ, BARBUSH TJ, UNVERFERTH DV: Beneficial effects of nifedipine on rest and exercise myocardial energetics in patients with congestive heart failure. Circulation 70:884–890, Nov 1984.

41. LEIER CV, PATRICK TJ, HERMILLER J, DALPIAZ PACHT K, HUSS P, MAGORIEN RD, UNVERFERTH DV:

Nifedipine in congestive heart failure: effects on resting and exercise hemodynamics and regional blood flow. Am Heart J 108:1461–1468, Dec 1984.

42. ELKAYAM U, WEBER L, McKAY CR, RAHIMTOOLA SH: Differences in hemodynamic response to vasodilation due to calcium channel antagonism with nifedipine and direct-acting agonism with hydralazine in chronic refractory congestive heart failure. Am J Cardiol 54:126–131, July 1, 1984.

43. ELKAYAM U, WEBER L, TORKAN B, McKAY CR, RAHIMTOOLA SH: Comparison of hemodynamic responses to nifedipine and nitroprusside in severe chronic congestive heart failure. Am J Cardiol 53:1321–1325, May 1, 1984.

44. RAJFER SI, DEMMA FJ, GOLDBERG LI: Sustained beneficial hemodynamic responses to large doses of transdermal nitroglycerin in congestive heart failure and comparison with intravenous nitroglycerin. Am J Cardiol 54:120–125, July 1, 1984.

45. BENCOWITZ HZ, LeWINTER MM, WAGNER PD: Effect of sodium nitroprusside on ventilation-perfusion mismatching in heart failure. J Am Coll Cardiol 4:918–922, Nov 1984.

46. PETEIN M, LEVINE B, COHN JN: Hemodynamic effects of a new inotropic agent, piroximone (MDL 19205), in patients with chronic heart failure. J Am Coll Cardiol 4:364–371, Aug 1984.

47. ROUBIN GS, CHOONG CYP, DEVENISH-MEARES S, SADICK NN, FLETCHER PJ, KELLY DT, HARRIS PJ: β-Adrenergic stimulation of the failing ventricle: a double-blind randomized trial of sustained oral therapy with prenalterol. Circulation 69:955–962, May 1984.

48. WAHR DW, SWEDBERG K, RABBINO M, HOYLE MJ, CURRAN D, PARMLEY WW, CHATTERJEE K: Intravenous and oral prenalterol in congestive heart failure: effects on systemic and coronary hemodynamics and myocardial catecholamine balance. Am J Med 76:999–1005, June 1984.

49. PETCH MC, WISBEY C, ORMEROD O, SCOTT C, GOODFELLOW RM: Acute hemodynamic effects of oral prenalterol in severe heart failure. Br Heart J 52:49–52, July 1984.

50. CODY RJ, COVIT AB, SCHAER GL, LARAGH JH: Estimation of angiotensin II receptor activity in chronic congestive heart failure. Am Heart J 108:81–89, July 1984.

9

Miscellaneous Topics

PERICARDIAL HEART DISEASE

RA and RV collapse in tamponade

Echo is the most sensitive and accurate procedure for detecting pericardial effusion (PE). To determine the hemodynamic derangement associated with RV diastolic collapse and to assess the value of RV and RA collapse in identifying cardiac tamponade, Singh and coinvestigators[1] from Milwaukee, Wisconsin, recored 2-D echo simultaneously with measurement of RA, PA wedge, intrapericardial, and systemic arterial pressures and cardiac output in 16 patients as they underwent pericardiocentesis. Twelve patients (group I) had evidence of RV or RA collapse or both on echo and hemodynamic evidence of cardiac tamponade before pericardiocentesis (Fig. 9-1). All hemodynamic parameters improved after pericardiocentesis. Continuous monitoring during pericardiocentesis in 3 patients showed significant improvement in all parameters except heart rate at the point of disappearance of RV diastolic collapse, with further improvement in cardiac output as pericardiocentesis continued. The RA collapse persisted after RV collapse disappeared, but was no longer present when pericardiocentesis was completed. Three patients (group II) had no RV or RA collapse, no hemodynamic evidence of cardiac tamponade, and no improvement in hemodynamic parameters after pericardiocentesis. A single patient (group III) was found to have elevated right-sided heart pressures and RV hypertrophy before pericardiocentesis. Although there was hemodynamic evidence of cardiac tamponade in this patient, there was no evidence of RV or RA collapse. In this study, the sensi-

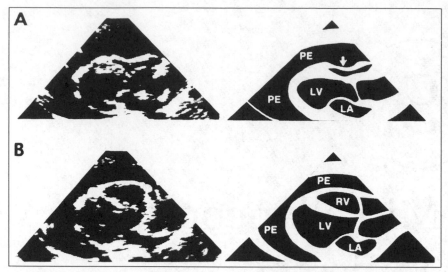

Fig. 9-1. Apical long-axis view from a patient with cardiac tamponade. A: During early diastole, right ventricular collapse is present (arrow). Normal curvature of the right ventricular wall is present during systole (B). LA = left atrium; LV = left ventricle; PE = pericardial effusion; RV = right ventricle. Reproduced with permission from Singh et al.[1]

tivity of RV collapse as a marker for cardiac tamponade was 92%, its specificity, 100%, its accuracy, 94%, and its predictive value, 100%. The sensitivity of RA collapse was 64%, its specificity, 100%, its accuracy, 75%, and its predictive value, 100%. These echo signs should be useful in detecting hemodynamically important PE and assisting in their management.

Pulsatile liver in constriction

In a study of 30 consecutive patients with constrictive pericardial heart disease diagnosed by clinical, radiologic, and echo, 21 (70%) were found by Manga and associates[2] from Durban, South Africa, to have pulsatile hepatomegaly. The pulsations were palpated clinically and confirmed by external hepatic recordings. These pulsations conformed almost identically to the jugular venous pulsations in the neck. The hepatic pulsations disappeared after successful pericardiectomy. Persistence of the hepatic pulsations was associated with poor postoperative relief, suggesting that hepatic pulsations are a useful sign in the assessment of the adequacy of pericardiectomy. Thus, this poorly appreciated clinical finding appears to be present in a higher proportion of patients with constrictive pericardial heart disease.

Chronic drainage in children

To determine the safety and efficacy of chronic percutaneous pericardial drainage in children, Lock and associates[3] from Minneapolis, Minnesota, inserted pigtail catheters over curbed guidewires under fluoroscopic control into the pericardial space in 7 consecutive children with pericardial effusion (PE). Pericardiocentesis was therapeutic (for tamponade) in 1 child, diagnostic in 4, and both therapeutic and diagnostic in 2. The children were 0.5–16 years old and weighed 5—65 kg. Underlying diagnoses included cancer (3 children), congenital heart disease (2 children), and immunodeficiency and hemolytic uremic syndrome (1 each). When unmodified pigtail catheters, designed for angiography, were used (as in the first 3 children), either the catheters clotted within 36 hours, necessitating operative pericardial drainage, or repeated heparin infusions were required to keep the catheter patent. When 8 F catheters were modified by placing 0.050 inch side holes along the distal shaft, the catheters remained patent and effectively drained the pericardial space for 3–7 days. Heparin infusion was not required, no child managed with the modified catheters required subsequent drainage and no complications occurred. In conclusion, percutaneous pericardial drainage is safe, even in small children, and can be effective chronically if catheters with large drainage holes are used.

Dialysis for uremic pericarditis

To identify predictors of success or failure of daily intensive dialysis in uremic patients, De Pace and associates[4] from Philadelphia, Pennsylvania, made a retrospective examination of initial clinical, laboratory, and echo data in 97 patients using univariate and multivariate statistical analysis. In this group, 67 patients had response to intensive dialysis, and 30 patients did not (22 required surgery and 8 died). By univariate analysis, 9 factors correlated with intensive dialysis failure: admission temperature $> 102°F$, rales, admission systolic BP <100 mmHg, jugular venous distension, peritoneal leukocyte count $> 15,000/mm^3$, leukocyte count left shift, large effusion by echo, and both anterior and posterior pericardial effusion (PE) by echo. Echo LV size and function were not useful predictors of success or failure; there was no difference in response to hemodialysis in patients with pericarditis before dialysis (69%) -vs- patients with pericarditis during a maintenance program (67%). By discriminant analysis, a 7-variable function was constructed that divided the patients into 3 groups: those likely to show response to intensive dialysis (48 patients, predictive value of 98%), those with an intermediate (38%) chance of showing response (30 patients), and those unlikely to show response (14 patients, predictive value of 100%). When the function was applied prospectively to 12 patients (8 with success and 4 with failure), all were classified correctly. Thus, discriminant analysis of patients with uremic pericarditis allows improved selection of patients likely to have response to daily intensive dialysis and early consideration of alternative forms of treatment in patients unlikely to show response to intensive dialysis.

After cardiac operation

Pericardial effusion (PE) is common after cardiac surgery and once PE is documented, serial echo studies are frequently performed. Weitzman and coworkers[5] from New York City studied 122 consecutive patients (104 men, 18 women) to determine the incidence and natural history of a PE occurring 2, 5, 10, and 20–50 days. Three patients had a PE before and 103 patients (91 men, 3 women), after surgery. The PE was first recorded on postoperative day 2 in 72 patients, on day 5 in 29 patients, and on day 10 in 2 patients (Table 9-1). In 96 patients, PE reached its maximum size by postoperative

TABLE 9-1. *Size of pericardial effusions in 122 patients.* Reproduced with permission from Weitzman et al.[5]

| | PREOPER-ATIVE | POSTOPERATIVE DAY | | | | |
PE SIZE		2	5	10	20	30–50
No PE	118	40	28	30	13	69
Small	4	57	43	26	10	14
Moderate	0	15	45	40	8	6
Large	0	0	6	12	6	0

* These results are for all echos recorded for the study. Not listed are results from 10 studies on postoperative day 2 and from 1 on postoperative day 10 that were uninterpretable.

day 10. Of the 103 patients with a PE, 66 (64%) were followed to complete resolution. A specific pattern was observed in most resolving effusions. The echo-free space diagnostic of PE became progressively more echo-dense as the PE diminished in size. As the PE became echo-dense, the posterior portion of pericardium, which had been motionless, resumed its normal systolic anterior motion. These investigators concluded that PE occurs frequently after cardiac surgery, but that associated complications are rare.

Echo is frequently performed postoperatively to evaluate patients suspected of having cardiac tamponade or pericarditis. Stevenson and associates[6] from Los Angeles, California, used M-mode and 2-D echo to study 39 stable patients 4–10 days after cardiac surgery: 22 patients (56%) had unequivocal moderate to large PE, which was identified on serial chest radiographs in only 6 patients. The PE was significantly more common after heavy postoperative bleeding and occurred in 16 to 19 patients with >500 ml of total chest tube output and in only 6 of 20 patients with chest tube output <500 ml. There was no correlation of PE by echo with pericardial friction rubs, chest pain, or atrial arrhythmias. Elevated erythrocyte sedimentation rate did not correlate with PE by echo or clinical pericarditis. In 1 of 22 patients with PE, tamponade developed, and the patient required reoperation on day 5; the other 21 were discharged without related therapy. Thus, early postoperative PE is common and related to postoperative bleeding. Because they do not correlate with symptoms of pericarditis and rarely lead to tamponade, their identification is usually of limited clinical significance.

Ribeiro and associates[7] described 3 patients in whom constrictive pericarditis was diagnosed after CABG. The time interval between CABG and the development of features of pericardial or myocardial constriction varied from 2–6 weeks. All 3 patients presented with severe CHF. Hemodynamic findings were characteristic of constrictive pericardial heart disease. One patient had a PE, and surgical pericardial drainage was necessary. One patient underwent pericardiectomy with preservation of the bypass conduits. The investigators suggested that diagnosis of constrictive pericardial heart disease should be considered in patients presenting with unexplained right-sided CHF after cardiac surgery.

Pericardial of mediastinal hemorrhage requiring reoperation occurs in 2–5% of patients, usually early (0–48 hours), after open heart surgery. This hemorrhage may be occult, and resulting cardiac tamponade may easily be misinterpreted as ventricular dysfunction, common early postoperatively. In such cases, appropriate and timely intervention may not occur. Bateman and associates[8] from Los Angeles, California, evaluated 50 patients by technetium-99m red blood cell gated equilibrium RNA because of early postoperative cardiogenic shock of uncertain etiology; 17 had unique scintigraphic images suggestive of intrathoracic hemorrhage. Of these 17, 5 had a generalized "halo" of abnormal radioactivity surrounding small hyperdynamic right and left ventricles, 11 had localized regions of intense blood pool activity outside the cardiac chambers (2 with compression of single chambers), and 1 had marked radionuclide activity in the right hemithorax, (2,000 ml of blood at reoperation). Twelve patients had exploratory reoperation for control of hemorrhage as a direct result of the scintigraphic findings, 3 were successfully treated with fresh frozen plasma and platelet infusions along with medical interventions to optimize cardiac performance, and 2 patients died in cardiogenic shock (presumed tamponade) without reoperation. All 12 reoperated on were confirmed to have active pericardium bleeding. Scintigraphic localization of abnormal blood pools within the pericardium corresponded to the sites at which active bleeding was witnessed at reoperation. The abnormal bleeding was etiologically related to the tamponade state, with marked improvement in hemodynamics after reoperation. Nine additional patients were reoperated on for presumed tamponade after RNA revealed an exaggerated halo of photon deficiency surrounding the cardiac chambers. No patient was observed to have an active bleeding site at reoperation. Thus, abnormal accumulations of radioactivity surrounding the cardiac chambers should be regarded as specific for the presence of active pericardial or mediastinal bleeding. Repeat imaging 30–180 minutes after initial imaging, multiple imaging positions, and acquiring RNA in nonzoomed and zoomed mode were helpful additions to standard imaging protocols for evaluating early postoperative patients for the presence of significant hemorrhage. It was concluded that the utility of technetium-99m red blood cell RNA in evaluating the etiology of early postoperative cardiogenic shock is enhanced by its ability to detect significant but occult pericardial or mediastinal hemorrhage.

PRIMARY PULMONARY HYPERTENSION

Primary pulmonary hypertension (PPH) is considered to be a fatal illness with survival typically <4 years although survival of >10 years has been well confirmed. To assess the characteristics of patients with PPH who survive -vs-those who do not, Rich and Levy[9] followed 12 patients with PPH by serial catheterization (Table 9-2). The survivors, 4 male and 3 female, had their illness for a mean of 5.2 ± 2 years from the time of initial catheterization, with 6 of the 7 alive at the end of the follow-up period. The 5 nonsurvivors, all female, had a mean survival of 0.3 ± 0.2 years. The nonsurviving group had significantly higher RA pressures (17 ± 6 -vs- 6 ± 2 mmHg), lower cardiac indexes (1.2 ± 0.1 -vs- 2.3 ± 0.5 liters/min/M^2), and stroke volume indexes (12 ± 7 -vs- 30 ± 5 ml/beat/M^2), and higher systemic resistances (64 ± 13 -vs- 43 ± 14 U) and pulmonary resistances (57 ± 31 -vs- 20 ± 4 U).

TABLE 9-2. *Hemodynamic findings at initial catheterization in patients with primary pulmonary hypertension.*

PATIENTS	HEART RATE (beats/min)	MEAN SYSTEMIC ARTERIAL PRESSURE (mmHg)	MEAN PULMONARY ARTERY PRESSURE (mmHg)	RIGHT ATRIAL PRESSURE (mmHg)	CARDIAC INDEX (liters/min/M²)	STROKE VOLUME INDEX (ml/beat/M²)	SYSTEMIC VASCULAR RESISTANCE (U)	PULMONARY VASCULAR RESISTANCE (U)
Survivors								
1	50	73	42	3	1.63	33	43	23
2	85	115	60	5	2.53	30	42	20
3	88	95	48	7	2.90	33	30	14
4	70	120	58	8	1.65	24	68	27
5	74	72	58	5	2.91	39	23	17
6	88	105	62	6	2.21	25	45	25
7	74	108	42	6	2.00	27	51	18
Mean ± SD	76 ± 14	98 ± 19	53 ± 9	6 ± 2	2.26 ± 0.53	30 ± 5	43 ± 14	20 ± 4
Nonsurvivors								
1	110	115	63	22	1.18	11	79	44
2	104	115	67	16	1.29	12	77	49
3	85	90	52	8	1.33	16	62	34
4	95	80	120	22	1.04	11	56	110
5	105	80	68	18	1.30	12	48	48
Mean ± SD	100 ± 10	96 ± 18	74 ± 27	17 ± 6	1.23 ± 0.12	12 ± 7	64 ± 13	57 ± 31
p*	< 0.01	NS	NS	< 0.01	< 0.01	< 0.01	< 0.05	< 0.01

* Represents the differences between the survivors and nonsurvivors.

NS = not significant.

The PA pressure did not significantly differ between the groups. Using regression analysis, it was found that stroke volume index and RA pressure were the best independent predictors of survival, with a coefficient of determination (r^2) of 83 and 72, respectively. When the initial and most recent catheterization data were compared among the survivors, no significant differences were found. Determining the stroke volume index and RA pressure of patients with PPH at the time of their initial presentation should help in predicting their clinical course. The hemodynamic changes seen in nonsurviving patients appear to confirm that RV failure is the resultant cause of death. Patients who present with favorable hemodynamic findings seem to maintain a stable clinical course for several years. The marked differences in survival in these 2 groups raise the possibility that PPH hypertension may in fact be more than 1 illness.

The World Health Organization has defined PPH as PA hypertension of unknown cause. Although PPH is not common, it poses a formidable challenge because its cause or causes are obscure, its natural history is ill-defined, and in almost all cases it is rapidly lethal. Fuster and colleagues[10] from Rochester, Minnesota, undertook a long-term retrospective follow-up study of 120 patients (33 male, 87 female) with PPH diagnosed by strict clinical and hemodynamic criteria (Fig. 9-2). The mean age at diagnosis was 34 years (3–64), but only 24 patients (21%) were alive 5 years later. Lung tissue obtained at autopsy from 56 patients revealed 2 major pathologic types: thromboembolic pulmonary hypertension in 32 patients (57%) and plexogenic pulmonary arteriopathy in 18 (32%). Thus, in more than half the patients having autopsy, the major histologic feature was thrombi without any evidence of plexiform lesions. The 2 groups were similar with respect to

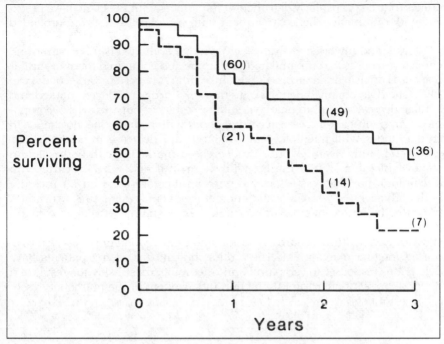

Fig. 9-2.   Observed survival with and without anticoagulant treatment in patients with primary pulmonary hypertension (those who survived diagnostic catheterization). Survival rate was better among 78 patients who received oral anticoagulants (solid line) than among 37 who did not (dashed line) (p = 0.02, log-rank test). Parentheses enclose numbers of patients living and under observation at end of each year. Reproduced with permission from Fuster et al.[10]

their clinical and hemodynamic features and short survival. Of the variables tested for prognostic importance by stepwise multivariate analysis, only 2 were significant: PA oxygen saturation and anticoagulant therapy. Thus, the investigators concluded anticoagulant therapy is recommended for patients with PPH.

Calcium channel blockade provides a logical approach to the treatment of PPH because these drugs exert direct vasodilator effects in the highly constricted pulmonary circulation. To determine the effectiveness of verapamil in treatment of PPH, hemodynamic effects of the drug were evaluated by Packer and associates[11] from New York City in 7 patients with PPH: 10 mg was given intravenously to 6 patents and 120 mg orally to 1 patient. Verapamil produced a 20% decline in pulmonary vascular resistance and a 27% decrease in mean PA pressure without significant changes in systemic vascular resistance. One patient, who received verapamil 480 mg orally daily for 3 months, had sustained hemodynamic and clinical improvement. Concomitant with its beneficial effects on the pulmonary circulation, however, verapamil produced a pronounced decrease in RV stroke work index (42%) and increase in RV filling pressure (50%), indicating a direct depressant effect of the drug on RV function. In 1 patient these cardiodepressant effects were sufficiently pronounced to produce severe hypotension and cardiac arrest. The investigators concluded that although verapamil appears to exert preferential vasodilator effects on the pulmonary circulation, its negative inotropic effects may be particularly detrimental to patients with PPH who have preexisting RV dysfunction; hence, treatment with verapamil is not recommended in such cases.

Packer and coworkers[12] from New York City evaluated hemodynamic and clinical responses to verapamil and nifedipine and compared them to similar responses after hydralazine in 12 patients with PA hypertension secondary to PPH. The data obtained demonstrate that all 3 drugs produced marked and similar decreases in pulmonary vascular resistance, but this was accompanied by a significant increase in cardiac index with hydralazine, no change in cardiac index with nifedipine, and a significant decrease in cardiac index with verapamil. Mean PA pressure decreased markedly with both calcium channel blockers (-16.0 mmHg with verapamil and -14.5 mmHg with nifedipine), but this was associated with an increase in mean RA pressure with both agents. Hydralazine did not change mean RA pressure or mean PA pressure. In some patients, unfavorable hemodynamic effects of calcium channel blockers were accompanied by hypotension and even cardiogenic shock during acute drug administration and exacerbation of right-sided CHF during long-term treatment. These data indicate that some patients have deleterious responses to verapamil and nifedipine, most likely the result of a direct depressant effect on RV function independent of the pulmonary vasodilating influence.

EXERCISING and EXERCISERS

Effect of aging

To evaluate the effect of age on cardiac volumes and function in the absence of overt or occult CAD, Rodeheffer and colleagues[13] from Baltimore, Maryland, performed serial gated blood pool scans at rest and during progressive upright bicycle exercise to exhaustion in 61 participants in the Baltimore Longitudinal Study of Aging. The subjects ranged in age from 25–79 years and were free of cardiac disease according to their histories and results of physical, resting, and stress ECG and stress thallium scintigraphic examinations. Absolute LV volumes were obtained at each work load and there were no age-related changes in cardiac output, end-diastolic or end-systolic volumes, or EF at rest (Fig. 9-3). During vigorous exercise, cardiac output was not related to age. However, there was an age-related increase in end-diastolic volume and stroke volume, and an age-related decrease in heart rate. The dependence of the age-related increase in stroke volume on diastolic filling was emphasized by the fact that at this high work load end-systolic volume was higher and EF lower with increasing age. These findings indicate that although aging does not limit cardiac output in healthy community-dwelling subjects, the hemodynamic profile accompanying exercise is altered by age. These investigators interpret and explain these findings by an age-related diminution in the cardiovascular response to beta adrenergic stimulation. These observations could be further extended as a caution to the use of beta adrenergic agents in an aging population, since effectiveness of

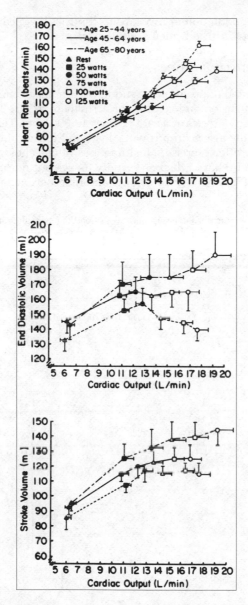

Fig. 9-3. Relationship between heart rate *(A)*, end-diastolic volume (EDV) *(B)*, and stroke volume *(C)*,–vs– cardiac output across range of work loads. The subjects are divided a priori into the three following age groups: 25–44 years old (n, 22), 45–64 years old (n, 23), and 65–79 years old (n, 16). The symbols within each curve correspond to the work load depicted for them in figure 2. In the older age group the same higher cardiac output during exercise is attained with a lower heart rate, higher EDV, and higher stroke volume. The effect of age was significant, by analysis of covariance, for heart rate (p = 0.001), EDV (p = 0.04), and for stroke volume (p = 0.002). The number of subjects able to complete the exercise period decreased with increasing work load; at a work load of 125 W (n, 16 in group 1, n, 15 in group 2, and n, 11 in group 3). When the data were analyzed including only those who were able to achieve 125 W, a similar pattern was observed in all three parameters and the significance of the age effect was unchanged. Reproduced with permission from Rodeheffer et al.[13]

beta adrenergic modulation of myocardial contractility, heart rate, and vascular tone declines with advancing adult age.

Postexercise catecholamines

The phenomenon of postexercise sudden death has been noted for centuries. Serious hypotension and ventricular arrhythemias also have been noted in stress testing laboratories at a rate of 4 per 10,000 tests. The morbid events occur about equally at maximum work load and during the cool-down period immediately after exercise. Most analyses of catecholamines during or shortly after exercise have relied on urinary assays but not plasma samples. The recent availability of radioenzymatic and high-performance liquid chro-

Fig. 9-4. Plasma norepinephrine levels and work load. Means and SDs of plasma norepinephrine levels as affected by exercise work load. Reproduced with permission from Dimsdale et al.[14]

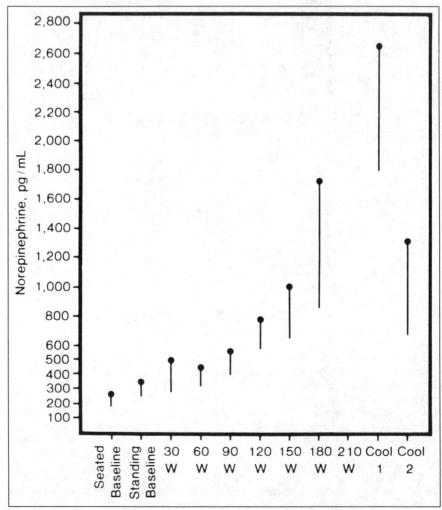

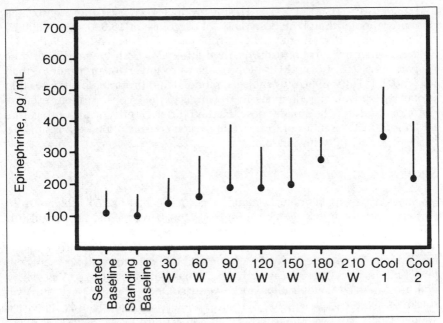

Fig. 9-5. Plasma epinephrine levels and work load. Means and SDs of plasma epinephrine levels as affected by exercise work load. Reproduced with permission from Dimsdale et al.[14]

matographic techniques has now made it possible to measure the plasma catecholamine response in relation to work load, cardiac rhythm, and BP. Dimsdale and associates[14] from Boston, Massachusetts, studied plasma catecholamine levels in 10 healthy men at each work load during exercise testing and during the recovery period after exercise. Both norepinephrine (NE) and epinephrine levels increased in response to exercise, although the response was much more noteworthy for NE (Figs. 9-4 and 9-5). In the recovery period after exercise, both catecholamine levels continued to increase, with the NE level increasing 10-fold over baseline. Such increases may have profound effects, particularly for subjects with preexisting CAD.

Effect of beta blockade

Beta adrenergic receptor blocking drugs with intrinsic sympathomimetic activity may have the advantage of not depressing myocardial function and heart rate (HR) at rest. Little is known about their effects during exercise. Thus, Ades and associates[15] from Denver, Colorado, compared the effects of small and large doses of pindolol, a nonselective beta adrenergic blocking drug with intrinsic sympathomimetic activity, with the effects of small and large doses of propranolol in 13 normal men during treadmill exercise. Compared with placebo, all drug regimens decreased exercise duration. There were no significant differences in duration between pindolol and propranolol, or between the small and large dose of each drug. Maximal oxygen consumption tended to be lower with all preparations compared with placebo. With smaller doses, decrements of maximal HR and HR-BP product were equivalent for pindolol and propranolol (decreases of 46 -vs- 43 beats/min, and 13,000 -vs- 12,000 U). The HR-BP product decreased more with high dose propranolol than high dose pindolol (decrease of 18,000 -vs- 14,800 U) due to a greater decrement in HR with propranolol (decrease of 65 ± 3 -vs- 53 ± 3 beats/min). At both submaximal levels, for both low and high dose preparations, HR, BP, and HR-BP product were lower for propranolol than for pindolol. Thus, in healthy subjects, pindolol and propranolol at doses that produced equivalent reductions in maximal oxygen consumption, exercise duration, and, for the smaller dose, HR had different effects on submaximal HR-BP product, an index of myocardial oxygen consumption, as a result of a higher HR and BP with pindolol.

Studies in athletes

Shapiro[16] from London, England, recorded echos in 154 athletes from various sports (swimming, 33; running, 32; throwing events, 15; weight-lifting, 19; wrestling or judo, 16; canoeing, 14, and ball sports, 28) and 21 ex-athletes and compared findings with those in 40 normal control subjects (nonathletes). Diastolic cavity dimension and LV posterior wall and ventricular septal thickness were measured and LV mass and the ratio of LV posterior wall thickness/LV cavity radius and a ventricular septum/LV posterior wall thickness were calculated. As a group, athletes had significantly increased systolic cavity dimension, posterior wall and septal thickness, and LV mass. The ratio of posterior wall LV thickness/cavity radius was distributed as a single continuous variable with a significantly increased mean, and there was no separate subgroup of shot putters or weight lifters with inappropriate hypertrophy. The mean ratio of septum to posterior wall thickness was normal, but there was a wide range of values up to 2.1:1. Ex-athletes had normal LV dimensions and wall thicknesses. When athletes were categorized by their standard of competition, national standard competitors had a significantly increased posterior wall and septal thickness and LV mass compared with university and noncompetitive sportsmen. The investigators concluded that strenuous activity results in LV hypertrophy that is appropriate to the body size of the athlete and the degree of activity but not to its type.

The ECG of athletes reflects physiologic cardiovascular adaptations that occur in well-conditioned individuals. To clearly define ECG changes seen in predominantly power-trained athletes, the ECG of 289 apparently healthy professional football players were analyzed by Balady and associates[17] from Boston, Massachusetts. The players, aged 21–35 years, one third of whom were black, had a mean body surface area of 2.24 M^2, a mean heart rate at rest of 56 ± 9 beats/minute (with 77% [223] having a rate of <60 beats/ min), and a mean P axis of 30 ± 25°. A wide QRS-T angle (>60°) was present in 14% (41 players) of the group. The mean PR interval was 0.18 ± 0.02 second (>0.21 in 9% [26 players]). Although two thirds of the players had a QRS duration of 0.10 second, only 1 had right BBB and none had left BBB. The sum of S in lead V_1 plus R in lead V_5 averaged 37 ± 9 mm, with 35% (101 players) demonstrating voltage criteria for LV hypertrophy. The S + R value varied inversely with weight. The maximum T height in any lead had a mean of 8.6 ± 3 mm, with 22% (64 players) having a T height ⩾11 mm. U waves were universally present. ST-T changes mimicking ischemia were noted in 39 of 289 players (13%), 22 (58%) of whom were black. The maximal J-point elevation in any lead averaged 1.9 ± 0.9 mm. These findings confirm that the ECG of power-trained athletes has changes similar to those of endurance-trained athletes. These changes most likely reflect the increased vagal tone and ventricular mass observed in conditioned athletes. Large body size masks the voltage changes expected with increased LV mass. Ischemic-like ST-T wave deviations were found predominantly in black athletes.

Northcote and associates[18] from Glasgow, Scotland, described 30 subjects of sudden death (29 men, 1 woman) associated with squash playing. The subjects ranged in age from 22–66 years (mean, 47 ± 10). Necropsy was performed in 27 patients. Significant CAD was found in 23, valvular heart disease in 3, HC in 1, and cardiac arrhythmia (the absence of other morphologic change) in 2. One subject died from intracerebral hemorrhage. Twenty-two of the 30 persons had reported prodromal symptoms, and of those with CAD, 16 had had at least 1 identifiable CAD risk factor. Twelve of the 30 subjects had been known by their family physician to have a medical disorder related to the cardiovascular system.

Osbakken and Locko[19] from Hershey, Pennsylvania, evaluated LV function and coronary perfusion with rest-exercise gated blood pool and stress-redistribution thallium scans in a group of long-distance runners and compared them with a group of catheterization-proved normal subjects. Exercise duration, work load, and oxygen consumption were significantly greater for long-distance runners. Rest end-diastolic volume, end-systolic volume, and stroke volumes were significantly larger in long-distance runners than in control subjects, and EF, cardiac index, and ejection rate were similar in both groups. Exercise end-diastolic volumes increased and end-systolic volumes decreased, producing an increase in stroke volume and EF in long-distance runners. Exercise end-diastolic volume did not change and end-systolic volume decreased less, producing lesser increase in stroke volume and EF in the control group. Qualitative evaluation of thallium scans showed apparent perfusion defects with normal redistribution in 6 myocardial segments in 5 long-distance runners. Quantitative evaluation demonstrated initial defects, which persisted on delay scans, but were associated with normal relative redistribution in 3 ventricular walls in 3 long-distance runners. Thus, LV reserve function was greater in long-distance runners than in control subjects. Endurance exercise can be associated with apparent myocardial perfusion defects, which may be due to uneven ventricular hypertrophy resulting from the pressure and volume loads imposed by exercise.

Fagard and associates[20] from Pellenberg, Belgium, studied by ECG 12 cyclists and 12 long-distance runners matched for age, height, and weight with 2 control groups of 12 nonathletes to evaluate cardiac structure and function. Runners weighed 8 kg less than cyclists, but age and height were similar. Peak oxygen uptake per kilogram body weight was higher in athletes than in the control subjects but was similar in the cyclists and the runners. The athletes' hearts had a larger end-diastolic LV internal diameter, mean wall thickness, and cross-sectional area of the LV wall than those of the respective control subjects. Nevertheless, whereas the LV internal diameter was not different between the cyclists and runners, mean wall thickness and cross-sectional area of the LV wall were greater in the cyclists even after adjustment for weight. The ratio of wall thickness to LV internal radius was significantly larger in cyclists than in their control group, but the ratio was similar in runners and their control group. The echo indices of LV function were similar in the athletes and the control groups. Systolic LV meridional wall stress was lower in the cyclists than in the runners. The data suggest that runners develop an increase in LV wall thickness that is proportionate to the internal diameter but that in cyclists the increase is disproportionate because of the isometric work of the upper part of the body during cycling.

OBESITY

Necropsy study

Although obesity may predispose to cardiovascular disease, few studies have focused on morphologic cardiac findings in massively obese patients. Warnes and Roberts[21] from Bethesda, Maryland, described observations in 12 massively obese patients (5 women, 7 men) aged 25–59 years (mean, 37) who weighed 312–>500 pounds (mean, 381) (Table 9-3). Seven patients had had systemic hypertension, 4 hypersomnia or sleep apnea, 2 diabetes mellitus, and 1 patient symptomatic CAD. Five patients died suddenly from undetermined causes, 2 from right-sided CHF, 1 patient from AMI; 1 from aortic dissection; 1 from intracerebral hemorrhage; 1 from a drug overdose; and 1 soon after an ileal bypass. The heart weight was increased in all 12 patients. The heart weight/body weight ratio expressed as a percent ranged from 0.22–0.61 (mean, 0.37; normal for men, 0.42–0.46, [mean, 0.43]; normal for women, 0.38–0.46 [mean, 0.40]). The LV cavity was dilated in 11

TABLE 9-3. *Certain findings in the 12 patients with massive obesity (> 300 pounds).*

PT SEX	AGE (YR) & SEX	HT in cm	BODY WEIGHT lb	kg	IDEAL BW lb	kg	INCREASE OVER IDEAL WEIGHT (%)	HW (G)*	HW AS % OF BW†	EF (1 +− 3+)‡	SA AND/ OR H	HX OF SH	BP RECORD- ING mm g	RX OF SH	DM	MODE OF DEATH	NARROWING 76–100% OF ≥1 MAJOR CORONARY ARTERY	LV N OR F
1	25F	70	178	425	193	144	65	195	720	0.37	2	−	+	200/110	+	−	AD	0	0
2	26F	66	168	345	157	128	58	169	625	0.40	3	+	−	−	−	−	Sudden	0	0
3	29F	62	158	375	170	113	51	232	380	0.22	1	+	−	−	−	−	CHF	0	0
4	37F	62	158	319	145	113	51	182	430	0.30	3	−	−	−	−	−	Sudden	0	0
5	40F	63	160	370	168	116	53	219	450	0.27	1	−	+	−	+	−	Sudden	0	0
6	25M	69	175	425	193	149	68	185	620	0.32	1	−	+	−	−	−	PO IB	0	0
7	34M	66	168	>500§	>227§	136	62	268	825	0.36	2	0	+	175/110	+	0	CNS Bleed	0	0
8	35M	74	188	358	162	171	78	109	990	0.61	3	−	+	−	−	−	Overdose	0	0
9	42M	73	185	312	142	166	75	88	665	0.47	2	−	−	−	−	−	Sudden	+	+
10	48M	68	173	450	204	145	66	210	560	0.27	2	+	+	140/95	+	+	CHF	0	0
11	48M	71	180	346	157	158	72	119	720	0.46	3	+	+	180/100	+	−	Sudden	0	0
12	59M	−	−	>350§	>159§	−	−	−	410	−	3	0	−	−	−	+	AMI	+	+

* Normal heart weight: ≤350 g in women; ≤400 g in men.
† Heart weight (g) × 100 ÷ body weight (g).
‡ 1+ = mild; 2+ = moderate; 3+ = severe.
§ Body weight exceeded upper limit of available scales and is therefore an approximation.
AD = aortic dissection; BW = body weight; CHF = right-sided congestive heart failure; CNS = central nervous system; DM = diabetes mellitus; EF = epicardial fat; F = fibrosis; H = hypersomnia; HT = height; HW = heart weight; Hx = history; IB = ileal bypass; LV = left ventricle; N = necrosis; PO = postoperative; RV = right ventricle; Rx = treatment; SA = sleep apnea; SH = systemic hypertension; − = no information available; + = present or positive; 0 = absent or negative.

patients and the RV cavity in all 12. Only 2 patients (aged 42 and 59 years) had ≥1 major epicardial coronary artery narrowed >75% in cross-sectional area (XSA) by atherosclerotic plaque, 1 of whom had no symptoms of myocardial ischemia. Of 664 segments of 5 mm from the 4 major epicardial coronary arteries from 11 patients (mean, 60 per patient), 431 (65%) were narrowed 0–25% in XSA, 143 (21%) were narrowed 26–50%, 73 (11%) were narrowed 51–75%, and 17 (3%) were narrowed 76–100%. Thus, these extremely obese patients who died prematurely did not have more coronary atherosclerosis than might be expected at their ages.

Very low caloric food

Kreitzman and associates [22] from Atlanta, Georgia, utilized a 330 calorie per day commercially distributed liquid diet formula (Cambridge Plan International, Monterrey, California) as their sole source of food for 28 days in 27 obese individuals weighing 110 $+$ 26 kg. After 28 days, the weight decreased to 102 ± 25 kg. All 27 subjects were a minimum of 25 kg above ideal body weight or >20% over ideal body weight. Not only did the body weight decrease an average of 9.1 kg (range, 3–19 kg) but the serum total cholesterol level decreased from 204 ± 39–161 ± 31 mg/dl during the 28-day period and the triglyceride level decreased from 150 ± 109–119 $+$ 60 mg/dl during the 28-day period. Of 5 patients with systemic hypertension, the BP returned to normal during the first week on the very low choloric diet. Holter monitor during the study showed no significant disturbances in cardiac rhythm.

Fenfluramine and/or phentermine

Medications used for weight control are often regarded as having only short-term utility because of the purported rapid development of tolerance, rebound increase in appetite with weight gain on cessation, and abuse potential. Anorectic medications frequently are viewed as being similar in both their beneficial and their undesirable effects. Both laboratory and clinical studies, however, have shown important differences between fenfluramine hydrochloride and the traditional stimulant drugs used in treating obesity. The stimulant anorexiants are believed to act via central catecholamine mechanism, and their adverse effects include insomnia, nervousness, increased motor activity, and occasional cardiovascular disturbances, such as increased heart rate and BP. Stimulant anorexiants appear to delay the onset of eating and to shorten its duration. Although chemically related, fenfluramine appears to act via serotonergic mechanisms, and its effects differ considerably from those of the stimulants in various animal models of obesity. Patients taking fenfluramine, for example, have sedative effects often and diarrhea occasionally. Except for decreased BP and potentiation of antihypertensive medications, cardiovascular effects are rare. Weintraub and associates [23] from Rochester, New York, attempted to utilize the differences between available anorexiants to create a treatment regimen with maintained efficacy but fewer side effects, thus providing a superior clinical strategy that would improve long-term acceptance of treatment. They performed a double-blind, controlled clinical trail comparing phentermine resin (30 mg in the morning), fenfluramine hydrochloride (20 mg 3 times a day), and a combination of phentermine resin (15 mg in the morning) and fenfluramine hydrochloride (30 mg before the evening meal), and placebo. They combined low doses of the 2 drugs to maintain efficacy while diminishing adverse effects. Eighty-one people with simple obesity (130–180% of ideal body weight) participated. Individualized diets were prescribed and discussed again during the 24-week study. Weight loss in those receiving the combination (8.4 ± 1.1 kg mean ± SEM) was significantly greater than in those receiving placebo (4.4 ± 0.9 kg; Scheffe's test) and equivalent to that of those receiving fenfluramine (7.5 ± 1.2 kg) or phentermine (10.0 ± 1.2 kg) alone. Adverse effects were less frequent with the combination regimen than with other active treatments. Thirty-seven participants dropped out of the study, 18 for reasons related to drug treatment. Combining fenfluramine and phentermine capitalized on their pharmacodynamic differences, resulting in equivalent weight loss, fewer adverse effects, and better appetite control.

VENTRICULAR FUNCTION
AND ITS ASSESSMENT

Continuous recording of intraventricular electrical impedance had been proposed as a means of instantaneously determining stroke volume and cardiac output. McKay and coinvestigators[24] from Boston, Massachusetts, assessed the feasibility of using continuous on-line recording of intraventricular electrical impedance to measure ventricular stroke volume in 12 patients at cardiac catheterization with a multielectrode impedance catheter. Stroke volumes determined by electrical impedance correlated with stroke volumes determined by the thermodilution technique in 10 patients (r = 0.95). Directional changes in impedance recording throughout the cardiac cycle also were compared with volume curves obtained from 6 patients by radionuclide ventriculography, and in all instances the agreement between the 2 volume recordings was excellent (Fig. 9-6). For all patients, on-line measurements of impedance showed a beat by beat decrease in stroke volume with the Valsalva maneuver and the administration of amyl nitrite and an immediate increase in stroke volume in the contraction after an extrasystolic beat. Similar directional changes in RV and LV stroke volume were recorded. The LV and pressure-volume relations were assessed with simultaneous LV pressure recordings and volume signals recorded from the impedance catheter to determine if impedance measurements of volume can be used clinically. Pressure-volume diagrams were subsequently plotted, and for all patients these diagrams had characteristic isovolumetric contraction and relaxation phases and typical ejection and filling periods. Moreover, beat by beat sequential pressure-volume diagrams constructed for patients during the administration of amyl nitrite had a linear end-systolic pressure-volume relation. The investigators concluded that measurement of intracavitary electrical impedance can be used to monitor instantaneous changes in stroke volume in patients and may be helpful in the construction of pressure-volume diagrams and the assessment of end-systolic pressure volume relations. These techniques offer advantages over previous angiographic techniques, since contrast material will not disturb myocardial properties during the administra-

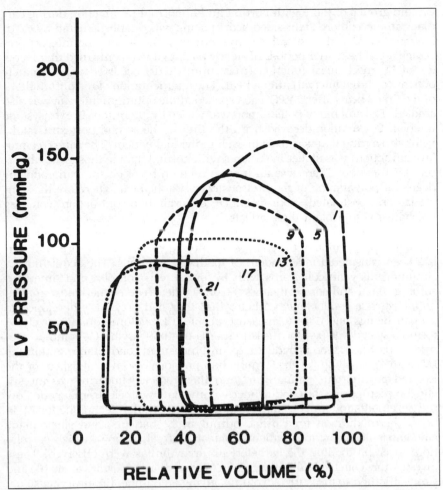

Fig. 9-6. Beat to beat LV pressure-volume diagrams constructed from every fourth beat (no. 1, 5, 9, 13, 17, 21) during the inhalation of amyl nitrite. Reproduced with permission from McKay et al.[24]

tion of drugs and provocative maneuvers to assess sensitive changes in the LV pressure-volume characteristics.

Current theories about excitation-contraction coupling suggest that calcium ions enter myocardial cells during the action potential and those that are taken up from the contractile apparatus during relaxation of contraction enter an intercellular store. Calcium is released on a subsequent depolarization, and thus some of the released calcium is recirculated from the previous beat. Seed and coworkers[25] from Kiel, West Germany, have shown in animals that both the time course of mechanical recovery after a beat (optimal test pulse interval) and the magnitude of this recirculation (recirculation fraction) can be inferred from studies of LV mechanical response during pacing. These investigators classified 26 adult patients by clinical and catheter criteria into groups of those with normal and abnormal LV function during cardiac catheterization. Right-sided heart pacing was established, and LV dP/dt was measured with end-catheter manometers. By varying the interval preceding a test beat after periods of steady pacing, it was confirmed that recovery of LV mechanical function (maximum dP/dt) occurred approximately 800 ms (optimal interval) after a beat. The augmentation of maximum dP/dt of the first 2 beats after a VPC, each spaced at the optimum interval, was also studied. The amount of potentiation was varied by alterations in extrasystolic interval. Potentiation decayed from the first to the second postextrasystolic beat with a ratio that was fixed in each individual patient. The ratio (recirculation fraction) was higher in patients with normal than in those with abnormal LV function. There was an inverse relation between this ratio and the degree of potentiation of the first postextrasystolic beat. Therefore these investigators postulated a disturbance of excitation-contraction coupling mechanisms to explain these effects.

Experimental and clinical studies on LV pressure-volume relations have led to an appreciation of the end-systolic pressure-volume measurement that has been considered independent of loading conditions. The acquisition of simultaneous ventriculograms with LV pressure is complex and time consuming. Baan and coinvestigators[26] from Leiden, The Netherlands, applied an 8-electrode conductance catheter that they had previously developed to human beings and dogs to measure absolute LV volume quantitatively. A formula was developed for measurements of time-varying LV volume, electrode separation, blood conductivity, and measured conductance within the LV cavity. The validity of the formula had previously been established for the isolated postmortem canine heart and the predicted linearity was investigated by comparing the conductance volume data with electromagnetic flow measurements for stroke volume and indicated dilution technique for EF in dogs, thermodilution for cardiac output in 12 patients, and single-plane cineventriculography in 5 patients. Linear regression showed high correlation. After positioning the catheter, no arrhythmias were observed. These investigators concluded that the conductance catheter provides a reliable and simple method to measure LV volume, giving an on-line, time-varying signal that is easily calibrated. Together with LV pressure obtained through the catheter lumen, the instrument may be used for instantaneous display of pressure-volume loops to facilitate assessment of LV pump performance.

Doppler echo measurement of the velocity of blood flow in the ascending aorta is a noninvasive method for determining cardiac output in the critically ill patient. Nishimura and associates[27] from Rochester, Minnesota, in 54 patients in the medical intensive care unit in whom a Swan-Ganz catheter had been inserted measured the cardiac output by a commercially available continuous-wave Doppler echo instrument. The aortic root diameter was measured by M-mode echo. An additional 26 patients (17 men and 9 women; age range, 20–83 years) who had undergone an open heart surgical procedure and had hemodynamic monitoring in the postoperative period also underwent Doppler measurement of cardiac output. In these patients, the aortic root diameter was measured directly intraoperatively. Cardiac output was also determined by thermodilution in both groups. An adequate echo study was possible in 83% of the medical patients but only 27% of the surgical patients. Doppler signals were adequate in 84% of the medical patients and 92% of the surgical patients. The correlation between thermodilution and

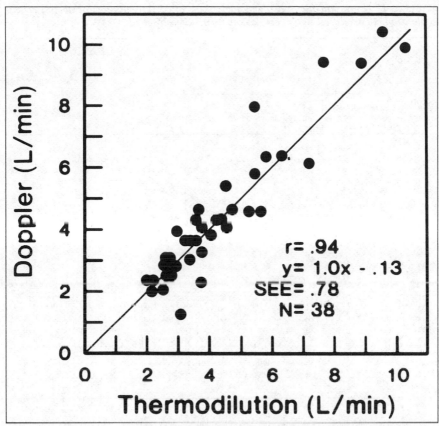

Fig. 9-7. Comparison of cardiac output as determined by thermodilution and Doppler studies in patients in the medical intensive care unit. The diagonal line is the line of identity. Reproduced with permission from Nishimura et al.

Doppler-derived cardiac output was good in both the medical and the surgical group (Fig. 9-7). Doppler echo is a promising noninvasive method for determining cardiac output in critically ill patients.

With the use of 2-D echo, Kaul and associates[28] from Los Angeles, California, analyzed apical and subcostal 4-chamber views for evaluation of RV function in 30 individuals compared with RV EF obtained by RNA. In addition to previously reported parameters of changes in areas and chords, a new simple measurement of tricuspid anular excursion was correlated with RV EF. A close correlation was noted between tricuspid anular plane systolic excursion and RV EF (r = 0.92). The RV end-diastolic area and percentage of systolic change in area in the apical 4-chamber view also showed close correlation with RV EF (r = −0.76 and 0.81); however, the entire RV endocardium could only be traced in about half the patients. The end-diastolic transverse chord length and the percentage of systolic change in chord length in the apical view correlated poorly with RV EF. The correlation between RV EF and both areas and chords measured in the subcostal view was poor. Thus, measurement of tricuspid anular plane systolic excursion offers a simple echo parameter that reflects RV EF. This measurement is not dependent on either

TABLE 9-4. *Radionuclide and physiologic data in 25 patients at initial and repeat evaluation. Reproduced with permission from Kimichi et al.[29]*

			INITIAL STUDY									REPEAT STUDY			RECOVERY FROM SEPTIC SHOCK
PATIENT	AGE (YR) & SEX	PRESENCE OF ARF	RAP	PAP	PCWP	BP	CI	PVRI	RV EF	LV EF	RV EDVI	PRESENCE OF ARF	PAP	Δ RV EF	
1	49F	+	17	22	18	99	1.79	179	22	27	73	−	20	+23	−
2	69F	−	14	17	12	82	2.98	134	54	51	50	−	N/A	−12	+
3	43M	−	5	18	10	77	4.00	160	33	52	115	−	13	+20	+
4	30M	−	15	32	19	70	4.05	257	13	13	238	−	20	−1	+
5	58M	−	12	29	22	90	6.90	81	55	75	125				−
6	81F	−	7	12	8	67	1.91	168	32	36	53	−	33	+13	+
7	77F	−	4	19	9	75	2.82	284	53	37	51	−	14	−2	+
8	44F	+ (PEEP =8)	20	48	16	83	3.00	853	30	65	76				−
9	84F	+	10	22	12	67	2.11	379	41	57	54				
10	25M	+ (PEEP =14)	16	25	24	78	4.48	18	30	43	130	+ (PEEP =11)	28	−1	+
11	31M	−	12	22	20	65	5.58	29	34	35	162	−	22	+8	−
12	80F	+	17	36	18	74	4.90	294	50	75	90				
13	71F	−	8	20	14	99	3.60	133	40	55	113	−	12	+2	+
14	62F	−	20	42	25	69	3.45	394	35	55	100	−	34	+2	+
15	82M	+	11	25	20	73	2.11	190	41	47	56				−
16	69F	−	12	30	20	56	3.13	256	30	49	97	−	27	+2	+
17	54M	−	10	25	16	71	2.99	241	43	63	58	−	18	−1	+
18	74M	+ (PEEP =3)	4	17	11	83	1.86	258	42	41	64	−	24	0	+
19	83M	+	14	37	35	81	2.08	77	10	10	200				−
20	70F	+	8	20	10	107	2.71	295	45	40	42				−
21	74F	−	11	23	18	54	2.54	158	40	50	85	−	30	+1	+
22	83M	+	6	25	18	94	2.53	221	28	30	96	+	15	+13	+
23	74M	+	7	13	9	85	3.14	102	41	41	80				−
24	72F	−	10	18	15	68	3.92	61	34	55	135	−	13	+11	+
25	74F	+	11	28	20	73	3.24	198	37	36	111	+	29	−3	+

ARF = acute respiratory failure; $\overline{BP}$ = mean arterial blood pressure (normal range [NR] 70–105 mmHg); CI = cardiac index (NR: 2.5–4.0 liters/min M^2), LV EF = left ventricular ejection fraction (NR, 48–76%); N/A = not available; $\overline{PAP}$ = mean pulmonary arterial pressure (NR: 9–18 mmHg); $\overline{PCWP}$ = mean pulmonary capillary wedge pressure (NR, 2–12 mmHg); PEEP = positive end expiratory pressure; PVRI = pulmonary vascular resistance index (NR, 69–177 dynes-s-cm^{-5}/M^2); $\overline{RAP}$ = mean right atrial pressure (NR, 2–8 mmHg); RV EDVI = right ventricular end-diastolic volume index (NR, 56–82 ml/m^2); RV EF = right ventricular ejection fraction (NR, 38–58%). ΔRV EF = change in right ventricular ejection fraction (absolute %).

geometric assumptions or traceable endocardial edges. When the endocardial outlines could be traced, the apical 4-chamber view was superior to the subcostal view in assessment of RV function.

Kimchi and coworkers[29] from Los Angeles, California, studied 25 patients with septic shock to determine the role of RV dysfunction. Thirteen patients had a depressed RV EF (<38%) determined by radionuclide ventriculography. The RV dysfunction was found in 4 of 6 patients with elevated cardiac output and in 6 of 19 with normal or low cardiac output and in patients with and without acute respiratory failure. In 8 patients, both RV and LV EF was depressed (<48%), but in 5 patients, RV EF impairment occurred with normal LV EF (Table 9-4). There was no significant correlation between abnormal RV afterload and depressed RV EF. In 17 surviving patients, RV EF improved in 6 and was unchanged in 11. The RV EF improved more frequently in patients without PA hypertension or respiratory distress. Thus, these data suggest that RV dysfunction in septic shock may be more common than previously suspected. These findings indicate that therapeutic interventions that diminish RV afterload and/or increase RV contractility may be of benefit in patients with septic shock and RV dysfunction.

Prostacyclin biosynthesis and platelets

Current concepts of atherogenesis based on animal and human investigations indicate prostaglandins (PGs) as a key factor in atherosclerotic lesions. Jouve and colleagues[30] from Marseille, France, investigated plasma profiles of thromboxane B_2 (TXB$_2$) (metabolite of platelet-derived TXA$_2$), 6-keto-PGF$_{1\alpha}$ (metabolite of endothelium-derived prostacyclin, [PGI$_2$], PGE$_2$ (elevated in experimental atherosclerosis), PGF$_{2\alpha}$, and PGA$_1$ by means of a sensitive radioimmunoassay technique in 40 patients with arteriosclerosis obliterans and in 30 healthy control subjects. Abnormally high levels of TXB$_2$ and PGE$_2$ (223 ± 321 pg/ml [mean ± SD] -vs- 20 ± 2 and 353 ± 235 -vs- 24 ± 3, p < 0.001) were detected in arteriosclerosis obliterans patients. The ratio between TXB$_2$ and 6-keto-PGF$_{1\alpha}$ was increased from 1 in control subjects to 6 in patients. In arteriosclerosis obliterans TXB$_2$ increased in relation to clinical manifestations and to the extension of the vascular damage. In addition, TXB$_2$ was positively related to serum triglyceride content and inversely related to platelet count. This marked imbalance between the stable metabolites of TXA$_2$ and PGI$_2$ in arteriosclerosis obliterans patients provides biologic evidence that is fully consistent with the thrombogenic mechanism of atherogenesis. These results further support the theory that PGs are heavily involved in the atherosclerotic process.

Prostacyclin is a potent vasodilator and platelet inhibitor produced by vascular endothelium. Endogenous production of PGI$_2$ under physiologic conditions is extremely low, far below the capacity of vascular tissue to generate this substance in response to stimulation in vitro. This may reflect a low frequency or intensity of stimulation of PGI$_2$ production. It has been postulated that if PGI$_2$ acts as an endogenous platelet-inhibitory agent, it should be produced in greater amounts in a clinical setting in which platelet-vascular interactions are likely to be increased. To test this hypothesis, Fitzgerald and associates[31] from Nashville, Tennessee, examined PGI$_2$ biosynthesis in patients with severe atherosclerosis and evidence of platelet activation in vivo. Excretion of 2,3-dinor-6-keto-PGF$_{1\alpha}$ a major urinary PGI$_2$ metabolite, was significantly higher in 9 patients with severe atherosclerosis and evidence of platelet activation (251–1859 pg/mg of creatinine) than in 54 healthy volunteers (45–219 pg/mg of creatinine). This difference represented an alteration in biosynthesis rather than in metabolism, since the fractional conversion of infused PGI$_2$ to the dinor metabolite was identical in both groups. Production of PGI$_2$ may be low in healthy persons because there is almost no stimulus for its production, but enhanced in patients with severe atherosclerosis as a consequence of platelet interactions with endothelium or other vascular insults. These observations are compatible with a role for PGI$_2$ as a local regulator of platelet-vascular interactions.

To study the effects of sampling through cardiac catheters on indices of platelet function, Bugiardini and associates[32] from London, England, and

Bologna, Italy, measured the levels of platelet factor 4 (PF4), beta thromboglobulin (BTG), and platelet aggregate ratio (PAR) in 10 patients with AV accessory pathway, 6 patients with primary pulmonary hypertension (PPH), and 6 patients with critical narrowing of the LAD coronary artery. In AV accessory pathway and LAD patients samples were drawn simultaneously from a peripheral vein, coronary sinus, and brachial artery; in AV accessory pathway patients samples also were obtained from the axillary vein before the coronary sinus was entered. In PPH patients samples were drawn from PA, aorta, and a peripheral vein; in these patients the effects of an intravenous infusion of PGI_2 (2–8 ng/kg/min) on PF4, BTG, and PAR also were studied at all sampling sites. In all patients arterial, coronary sinus, PA, and axillary venous levels of PF4, BTG, and PAR significantly exceeded those measured in the peripheral vein. A PGI_2 infusion resulted in a significant decrease of PF4 at all sampling sites, but no consistent BTG changes were observed and PAR levels did not decrease in the peripheral vein. Although a considerable interpatient variability in PF4 levels was observed, a significant correlation was found in patients with AV accessory pathway between simultaneous coronary sinus and arterial PF4 levels. The value of PF4 coronary sinus-arterial difference in LAD patients was consistently higher than that calculated in AV accessory pathway patients (55 ± 29 -vs- 4 ± 4 ng/ml). In conclusion, a considerable and variable degree of platelet activation occurs with catheter sampling, preventing the measurement of absolute levels of platelet metabolites; among the indices examined PF4 appears the most sensitive for detecting changes in platelet activity; and the measurement of coronary sinus-arterial PF4 differences may provide information on directional changes in transcardiac platelet behavior.

Prior studies have indicated that nitroglycerin stimulates PGI_2 release by cultured endothelium and by the coronary vasculature in vivo. The accuracy of such findings in coronary vasculature relies on plasma samples obtained from the circulation via cardiac catheters that have been shown to stimulate PGI_2 release and thereby confounding interpretation of drug action. Fitzgerald and coworkers[33] from Nashville, Tennessee, studied the effects of nitroglycerin and isosorbide dinitrate, short-acting and long-acting nitrates, respectively, on a noninvasive index of PGI_2 synthesis, excretion of urinary 2,3-dinor-6-keto-$PGF_{1\alpha}$. Nitroglycerin was infused into six subjects to either a maximum of 480 μg/minute or until mean arterial pressure decreased 20 mmHg. Urine was collected for negative ion chemical ionization gas chromatographic, mass spectometric analysis before and during the nitroglycerin infusion and for 2 periods of 2 hours after nitroglycerin. The peak nitroglycerin infusion was 387 μg/minute, which caused a decrease in supine BP (systolic/diastolic) of 11/14 mmHg and a 12 beats/minute increase in heart rate. Excretion of 2,3-dinor-6-keto-$PGF_{1\alpha}$ (pg/mg creatinine) was unchanged from control infusion rates, either during or after nitroglycerin infusion. Platelet aggregation to arachidonic acid and epinephrine ex vivo occurred in only 1 subject in whom excretion of 2,3-dinor-6-keto-$PGF_{1\alpha}$ was unaltered. Serum TXB_2 was not changed by nitroglycerin infusion. Similarly, oral administration of isosorbide dinitrate (10–40 mg 4 times a day) failed to alter 2,3-dinor-6-keto-$PGF_{1\alpha}$ excretion from placebo values in patients with angina pectoris. These noninvasive measurements indicate that nitrates failed to stimulate PGI_2 release in vivo and platelet inhibition during infusion of nitroglycerin was unrelated to altered PGI_2 changes in human beings.

Thromboxane A_2 is produced in platelets from arachidonate and is a potent platelet aggregator and vasoconstrictor. Yui and coworkers[34] from Nagano, Japan, studied the effect of selective TXA_2 synthetase inhibitor OKY-1581, a pyridine derivative on TXB_2 and 6-keto-$PGF_{1\alpha}$ levels and platelet aggregation in human volunteers. To clarify its effectiveness as an enzyme inhibitor, the agent was injected intravenously or infused over 3 hours on 3 successive days. The inhibitor was rapidly converted to its main beta oxidized product and subsequently its reduced form. Plasma TXB_2 levels, inhibition of TXB_2 production in serum, and inhibition of rabbit platelet TXA_2 synthetase were monitored continuously. All substances were decreased 25 minutes after the injection of the inhibitor and returned to control levels within 24 hours. Intravenous infusion of the drug reduced platelet aggregation induced by arachidonate significantly. In the serum of incubated whole blood, after the treatment with OKY-1581, serum 6-keto-$PGF_{1\alpha}$ production, a PGI_2 metabolite, increased significantly. The drug caused no untoward symptoms or changes in hemodynamic parameters or ECG or laboratory results, including bleeding time and coagulation. The investigators concluded that in cardiovascular diseases in which TXA_2 may be involved in the pathogenesis, this selective inhibitor of TXA_2 synthetase may become a useful drug because it inhibits TXA_2 production and arachidonate-induced platelet aggregation.

PHARMACOLOGIC TOPICS

Effects of coffee and caffeine

Whitsett and associates[35] from Oklahoma City, Oklahoma, evaluated the cardiovascular effects and elimination kinetics of coffee and caffeine in 54 volunteers selected according to 3 graduations of daily caffeine consumption, cigarette smoking status, and the presence of caffeine intolerance. After 24 hours of caffeine abstinence, subjects received coffee and 2.2 mg/kg of caffeine (equivalent to 2 cups of coffee). Heart rate, BP, systolic time intervals, and plasma concentrations of caffeine were measured before and at timed intervals after coffee and caffeine. There were no differences in response to coffee and caffeine. The average systolic/diastolic BP increased 9/10 mmHg. The maximal decrease in heart rate averaged 10 beats/minute, and there were small increases in the systolic time intervals. There were no cardiovascular differences among the various groups. Caffeine in the smokers and heavy caffeine users had a shorter half-life (3.2 and 4.1 hours) than that in nonsmokers and nonusers (5.1 and 5.3 hours). In the caffeine-intolerant group it had a longer half-life, although the cardiovascular effects were similar to those of the other groups. Thus, irrespective of the amount of daily caffeine consumption, smoking status, or caffeine intolerance, the cardiovascular responses were similar and tolerance, if present, was gone by 24 hours.

Nifedipine's dependence on peripheral responses

Although nifedipine reduces LV and RV end-diastolic pressures in patients with impaired LV function, this calcium blocking agent does not alter the filling pressure in those with normal LV function. To elucidate the mechanisms of reduction of LV end-diastolic pressure by nifedipine in certain individuals, Kurnik and colleagues[36] from St. Louis, Missouri, evaluated cardiac and peripheral hemodynamic responses in 32 patients after they were randomly assigned to nifedipine (20 mg sublingually) or to placebo therapy. Forearm plethysmography was performed during cardiac catheterization with micromanometers. No hemodynamic parameters were changed after placebo. The LV end-diastolic pressure declined by 14% after nifedipine in patients with impaired LV function but was unchanged in those with normal function; indexes of peripheral venous hemodynamics (forearm venous tone, forearm volume change) were not affected. In those patients with abnormal LV function, forearm vascular resistance decreased 36% and forearm blood flow increased 31%, but neither changed in those with normal function. Cardiac output increased by 10% in patients with impaired LV function but was unchanged in the remainder, although calculated total systemic resistance decreased by 24% in those with abnormal LV function. Thus, the results of this study suggest that reduction of LV preload by nifedipine is not attributable to venous pooling, but rather, this beneficial effect appears to be attributable to improved LV systolic function in response to afterload reduction, particularly in patients with impaired LV function.

Anticoagulation clinic

An anticoagulation clinic was established at the University of Massachusetts Medical Center in 1978 to provide a central facility for monitoring long-term outpatient anticoagulation therapy and to facilitate management for referring primary care physicians. Errichetti and associates[37] from Worcester, Massachusetts, reviewed the initial 55 months' experience with 141 patients from inception of the clinic in 1978 through March 1983 (55 months). Warfarin sodium was the only oral anticoagulant prescribed. The 5 mg tablet was routinely used, and dose instructions were generally expressed as half fractions or multiples of 5 mg. Therapy was usually instituted during hospitalization, with 10 mg given daily for 3 days and subsequent dose adjustments dictated by the prothrombin time. The therapeutic value for the prothrombin time was defined as 1.3–2.0 times the control value in seconds. Prothrombin tests were scheduled within 5 days of discharge from the hospital and weekly thereafter, gradually increasing the interval to 4 weeks when the prothrombin time had stabilized on 2 successive visits. Eighty men and 61 women were monitored in the anticoagulation clinic for 144 courses of therapy and a total of 1,264 patient-months. The patients ranged in age from 21–85 years (mean, 59). The indications for anticoagulation therapy were variable but deep venous thrombosis of the lower extremities and cerebrovascular disorders accounted for nearly 50% of the disorders. Only 17 patients had prosthetic cardiac valves; 52 (36%) remained on an anticoagulant regimen at the end of the study period. Warfarin therapy was discontinued in 92 patients (64%): the reasons for stopping therapy included resolution of the indication for therapy (40%), follow-up elsewhere (8%), major complication (5%), treatment failure (3%), death (4%), noncompliance (2%), and development of contraindication (2%). Minor hemorrhagic complications developed in 18% of treatment courses, an incidence of 2% per patient-month. Major complications occurred in 5% of treatment courses, or 0.5% per patient-month. The investigations concluded that to reduce the number of complications, patients and their families should receive comprehensive instruction during their initial and follow-up visits. The following points should be emphasized: the reason for treatment with an anticoagulant; a simplified explanation of how an anticoagulant works; the reason for obtaining a prothrombin time; taking an anticoagulant at a fixed time daily, preferably in the morning on an empty stomach; the effect of alcohol on anticoagulation; the effect of dietary changes, especially foods rich in vitamin K; awareness of drug-drug interactions, including over-the-counter medications containing aspirin; the importance of informing clinic personnel of any changes in medication; commonsense precautions to avoid bleeding complications, and identification of the signs and symptoms of bleeding.

Urokinase for pulmonary emboli

Life-threatening pulmonary emboli associated with shock, RV failure, seizures, or syncope remain a medical emergency and require early, rapid, and effective therapy. To evaluate hemodynamic, angiographic and biologic effects of a single bolus of urokinase Petitpretz and coworkers[38] from Clamart, France, conducted an open descriptive trial in a homogeneous group of 14 patients with acute life-threatening pulmonary emboli and without prior cardiopulmonary disease. For every patient, the efficacy of the treatment was evaluated by comparing control and post-therapeutic values after the bolus

Fig. 9-8. Individual (dotted lines) and mean (continuous heavy line) values from hemodynamic sequential study. Mean pulmonary arterial pressure is expressed as percent of control values (C) in 7 improved patients at 1, 3, 6, and 12 hours after bolus injection of urokinase. Reproduced with permission from Petitpretz et al.[38]

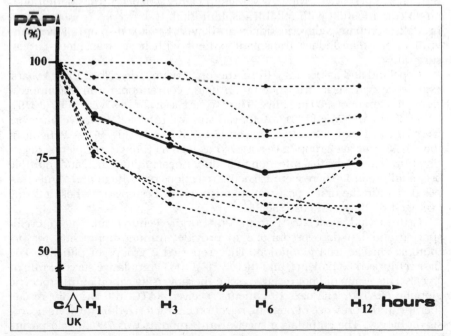

injection of 15,000 IU/kg body weight urokinase administered in 10 minutes in the right atrium followed by continuous intravenous full-dose heparin therapy (Fig. 9-8). In 2 patients clinical status, hemodynamics, vascular obstruction, and biologic parameters of fibrinogen and plasminogen levels remained unchanged. One of 2 patients died, making the mortality rate for the whole group 7%. Twelve of 14 patients had rapid clinical improvement. Evaluation at 12 hours demonstrated significant decreases in pulmonary vascular obstruction, total pulmonary vascular resistances, and fibrinogen and plasminogen levels without any significant change in cardiac index. The hemodynamic sequential measurements performed in 7 of the 12 improved patients showed that the greatest percentage of the total hemodynamic improvement occurred within the first 3 hours after bolus administration of urokinase. No severe hemorrhagic complications were observed. Because of its rapid efficacy and its low cost, the bolus technique appeared particularly useful in the treatment of patients with acute life-threatening pulmonary emboli. Although the patients in this study were diagnosed and monitored with invasive hemodynamic and angiographic studies, the advances in digital subtraction angiography will permit more frequent angiographic studies in patients with suspected pulmonary embolism.

CARDIAC AND/OR PULMONARY
TRANSPLANTATION

Evans[39] from Seattle, Washington, compared cadaveric kidney graft and heart transplant patient survival rates in the USA for patients on conventional immunosuppressive therapy. As shown in Figure 9-9, heart transplantation is on an equal footing with renal transplantation. It, however, is more appropriate to compare cadaveric kidney graft with heart transplant patient survival rather than kidney transplant patient with heart transplant patient survival.

Copeland and associates[40] from Tucson, Arizona, described their 4 years' experience with heart transplantation using conventional immunosuppression. Of 32 patients, 20 are alive. The 1-year survival rates were 75% (1979), 67% (1980), and 75% (1981). Actuarial survival rates for operative survivors were 70% at 1 year, 60% at 2 years, and 51% at 3 years (Fig. 9-10). Patients in the 50–55-year age group have survived as well as younger recipients. Rejection resulted in 6 deaths, infection in 3, donor heart failure in 2, and multiple organ failure in 1. There were 1.5 acute rejections per patient and 1 infection per patient in the first 3 post-transplant months. Postoperative hospital stay averaged 62 days and cost $58,351.

Griffith and associates[41] from Pittsburgh, Pennsylvania, used cyclosporine and low-dose prednisone to provide immunosuppression for orthotopic cardiac transplantation. They reported 2 groups of patients. The first comprised 23 patients, and there was a 61% cumulative survival rate at 1 year. This group did not receive rescue therapy using rabbit antithymocytic globulin (RATG). The next 19 patients received RATG in 6 cases for rescue therapy in the presence of ongoing rejection characterized by myocyte necrosis on biopsy. The cumulative survival at 9 months was 79%. Cyclosporine

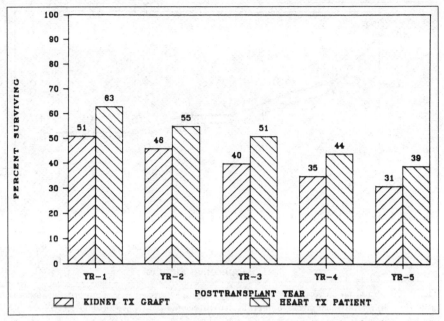

Fig. 9-9 Cadaver kidney and heart transplant survival compared. Reproduced with permission from Evans.[39]

was given at doses between 10 and 17 mg/kg initially and then reduced gradually in each patient. Whole blood levels of cyclosporine were measured by high pressure liquid chromatography (HPLC). Trough values of 250–500 ng/ml were sought. In the first group in whom only methylprednisolone was given for rejection episodes there were 3 acute fatal rejections and 4 chronic fatal rejections. By contrast, in the second group of 19 patients there were no acute fatal rejections. Thus, the Pittsburgh group recommends a modified regimen for cyclosporine immunosuppression. RATG is used in divided doses when there is myocyte necrosis on biopsy. This is an important change suggesting that the cyclosporine immunosuppressive regimen should be and can be altered to produce improved immunosuppression without changing the freedom from injection and other side affects. The units at Cambridge and Alabama now recommend 6–8 days of RATG initially after transplant, assuming that cyclosporine levels are not optimal in this early period. The Stanford group also uses RATG for episodes of important rejection. This is contrasted to the experience at London, Canada, where no RATG has been given. However, their combination cyclosporine and steroid regimen is characterized by higher doses of steroids initially. Finally, it has been suggested by others that azathioprine now be added to the immunosuppressive regimen. In general, this means 5 mg/kg loading dose and 2 mg/kg maintenance dose. The cyclosporine levels are monitored either by HPLC or radioimmunoassay, and blood levels usually vary between 500 and 1,000 ng/dl. It is obvious that cyclosporine has improved survival in cardiac transplantation. However, the optimal immunosuppressive regimen to be used with cyclosporine has not been elucidated.

Lanza and associates[42] from Cape Town, South Africa, performed 54

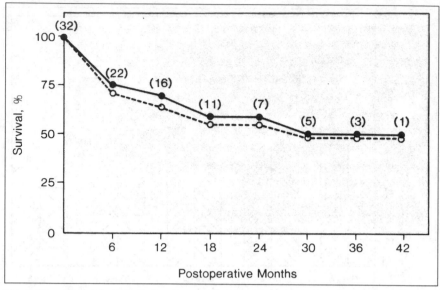

Fig. 9-10. Actuarial survival after heart transplantation. Broken line represents all patients; solid line, all operative survivors. Reproduced with permission from Copeland et al.[40]

human-to-human cardiac transplants (10 orthotopic and 44 heterotopic with donor heart parallel to recipient heart) in 50 patients between December 1967 and December 1981. The underlying cardiac disease was coronary in 29, cardiomyopathy in 17, rheumatic in 4, and mixed or other in 4. Patients with valve disease survived for a mean period (5.2 years), more than 3 times as long as those with either cardiomyopathy (1.2 years, $p < 0.02$) or CAD (1.8 years, $p < 0.05$). Although cardiomyopathy patients were on the average over a decade younger than those in other groups, they had a lower survival rate. There was a higher incidence of death from chronic rejection in patients with CAD, in whom there was also a higher incidence of thromboembolic episodes. Major infections were over twice as frequent in CAD patients than in cardiomyopathy patients ($p < 0.01$). Noncompliance with regard to adherence to instructions and therapy was a significant factor in morbidity and mortality, especially in cardiomyopathy patients. These data suggest that survival and morbidity of recipients of heart transplants may be influenced to some extent by the nature of the underlying primary cardiac condition, valve disease being considered a favorable survival factor compared with CAD, and cardiomyopathy being particularly unfavorable.

Whether lymphoproliferative disorders arising in immunosuppressed recipients of organ transplants are primarily neoplastic or hyperplastic is controversial. Reports of polyclonal B cell proliferations in these lesions suggest the presence of hyperplasia, but these disorders resemble lymphoma histologically and are clinically aggressive and often rapidly fatal, as expected of a malignant neoplastic disease. Cleary and associates[43] from Stanford, California, examined tissue specimens from 10 cases of lymphoproliferative disease that occurred in immunosuppressed recipients of cardiac transplants. Specimens from 9 patients lacked cellular immunoglobulin; however, analysis of DNA extracted from these tissues revealed that each lesion contained large numbers of cells possessing uniform, clonal rearrangements of immunoglobulin-gene DNA. Therefore when first seen clinically, these proliferations contained a notable monoclonal-cell population typical of conventional B cell lymphomas that are not associated with immunosuppression. Thus, lymphoproliferative disorders in recipients of cardiac transplants are neoplastic at the earliest stages of detection.

Cleary and Sklar[44] from Stanford, California, examined tissue specimens from 5 immunosuppressed cardiac transplant recipients with lymphoproliferative disorders for rearrangements in immunoglobulin DNA. In each patient DNA analysis of tissues obtained from several sites or at various times showed different clonal immunoglobulin gene rearrangements for each of the 3 immunoglobulin gene loci. These findings indicate that lymphoproliferative disorders in immunosuppressed cardiac transplant recipients represent multiclonal or oligoclonal B cell lymphomas.

Uys and Rose[45] from Capetown, South Africa, examined 14 donor cardiac transplant hearts with survival in the donor from 1.1–12.5 years. Only 1 of the 14 hearts had no evidence of rejection. The remaining 13 had advanced changes of chronic rejection that was the main cause of death or of graft failure in 11 patients. One patient died of gastric carcinoma, 1 of Kaposi's sarcoma, and 1 of cerebral embolus. The most obtrusive change in the donor hearts was an obliterative arteritis, which in the epicardial coronary arteries mimicked atherosclerosis. Superimposed thrombus often resulted in AMI. These severe vascular lesions bore no constant relation to survival time.

Jamieson and colleagues[46] from Stanford, California, reported results of combined heart and lung transplantation in 17 patients between March 1981 and December 1983. The recipients were between 22 and 45 years old. All patients had end-stage pulmonary hypertension, 10 had Eisenmenger's syndrome, and the remaining 7, primary pulmonary hypertension. Five patients died within the first few postoperative weeks. The remainder are well between 4 weeks and 39 months from operation. The immunosuppressive protocol consisted of cyclosporine and an initial course of rabbit antithymocytic globulin. Azathioprine also was given for the first 2 weeks and then was replaced with prednisone. Rejection occurred in 6 of the 12 survivors. Infections developed in 9 patients but only 1 resulted in a fatal outcome (Legionella). All recipients had PA hypertension; none had obstructive lung disease. Potential donors for heart-lung transplantation should be <35 years old and have compatibility of the ABO blood group and negative crossmatch between recipient serum and donor lymphocytes. There should be a close size match and completely clear roentgenograms for donors. The donor heart and lungs are removed without cardiopulmonary bypass and the heart is preserved with cold cardioplegic solution. The lungs are infused with Collins' solution via the PA. The recipient's heart and lungs are removed separately with care taken to preserve the vagus and phrenic nerves and left recurrent nerve without injury. Implantation involves successive tracheal, atrial, and aortic anastomoses. Immediate postoperative care is similar to that of all patients who have undergone routine cardiopulmonary bypass except for the use of isoproterenol to provide chronotropic support and the strict avoidance of high inspired oxygen concentration. Endomyocardial biopsy is used to monitor rejection; additional techniques to diagnose a pulmonary rejection are lacking. The spectacular results reported by the Stanford group encourage others to examine heart-lung transplantation as a viable clinical procedure. Enthusiasm is tempered, however, by the suggestion that lung rejection may occur in the absence of a positive endomyocardial heart biopsy and that lung function may deteriorate over the long term either due to chronic rejection or in a way as yet unknown in the absence of cardiac rejection.

MECHANICAL HEART

Since the mid-1960s, approximately $160 million in federal funds have been used for research in the development of an artificial heart. DeVries and associates [47] from Salt Lake City, Utah, reported the first initial clinical application of the total artificial heart that was developed at the University of Utah (Fig. 9-11). The patient was a 61-year-old man with chronic CHF secondary to idiopathic dialated cardiomyopathy. He also had chronic obstructive pulmonary disease. Except for dysfunction of the prosthetic mitral valve, which required replacement of the left-heart prosthesis on the 13th postoperative day, the artificial heart functioned well for the entire 112-day postoperative course. The mean BP was 84 ± 8 mmHg, and cardiac output was generally maintained at 6.7 ± 0.8 liters/minute for the right heart and 7.5 ± 0.8 for the left, resulting in postoperative diuresis and relief of CHF. The postoperative course was complicated by recurrent pulmonary insufficiency, several episodes of acute renal failure, episodes of fever of unidentified cause (necessitating multiple courses of antibiotics), hemorrhagic complications of anticoagulation, and 1 generalized seizure of uncertain cause. On the 92nd

Fig. 9-11. Diagrammatic representation of the Utah (Jarvik-7) total artificial heart. Reproduced with permission from DeVries et al.[47]

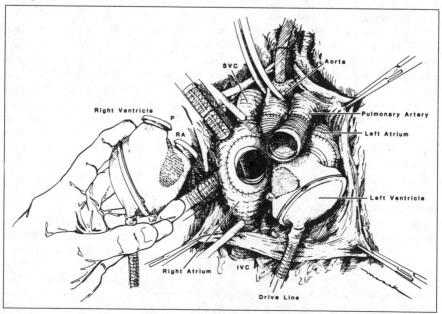

postoperative day, the patient had diarrhea and vomiting, leading to aspiration pneumonia and sepsis. Death occurred on the 112th day, preceded by progressive renal failure and refractory hypotension, despite maintenance of cardiac output. Autopsy revealed extensive pseudomembranous colitis, acute tubular necrosis, peritoneal and pleural effusion, centrilobular emphysema, and chronic bronchitis with fibrosis and bronchiectasis. The artificial heart system was intact and uninvolved by thrombus or infection. This experience will encourage further clinical trials with the artificial heart. This article was followed by an editorial entitled "Replacement of the Heart With a Mechanical Device: The Case of Dr. Barney Clark" by Galletti[48] and also by another article entitled the "Political History of the Artificial Heart" by Strauss.[49]

CARDIOVASCULAR SURGICAL TOPICS

Brain damage in cardiac operations

During the last 15 years, there has been a decrease in both the frequency and severity of brain injury in conjunction with cardiac operations. At the present time the incidence and intensity of subclinical brain injury are unknown. Aberg and colleagues[50] from Uppsala, Sweden, reported investigations on some factors that might reflect cerebral injury. Ninety-four patients were studied after cardiac operation. Cerebrospinal fluid (CSF) was attained 24 hours after bypass and analyzed for adenylate kinase (AK). Psychometry and computed tomography of the brain also were done. In 13% of the patients considerable increase in the CSF-AK was seen. In 46% of patients there was a moderate increase, but in 41% there was no or trivial increase. Psychometry with a test battery measured preoperatively and postoperatively revealed a moderate decrease in intellectual function after operation. There was a significant inverse correlation between CSF-AK and psychometry. Computed tomography in 54 patients showed cerebral infarctions in 2, neither of which had any deviation from a normal postoperative state. Cardiopulmonary bypass was carried out in the usual fashion using a bubble oxygenator, clear fluid prime, a roller pump, nonpulsatile flow, moderate hypothermia, and no arterial filter in the arterial line but a filter in the coronary suction line. The BP was not allowed to decrease below 50 mmHg. Of the 94 patients, 62 had CABG and 24 had cardiac valve replacement. Eight had combined CABG and valve replacement. This study suggests that although the incidence of cerebral injury is low and clinical manifestations are negligible, there is still some subclinical brain injury. The investigators suggest that their psychometrics and CT scanning were sensitive indicators of cerebral function. They also suggest that perhaps the best index of cellular injury in the brain is CSF-AK. Forty-one percent of patients had no elevation of AK. There was no relation of these 3 parameters to duration of bypass, cardiac lesion, BP, or age of the patient. The study does not address the problem of whether the brain lesion is reversible or irreversible. Apparently, it is reversible inasmuch as there were no persisting lesions or functional impairment. Additionally, the investigators suggest that the usual etiology, i.e., microemboli may not be appropriate for these patients inasmuch as 41% of the measurements of AK were normal.

Henriksen[51] from Copenhagen, Denmark, measured by single photon emission computed tomography regional cerebral blood flow (rCBF) in 37 patients after inhalation of xenon-133 before and within the first 10 days after open heart surgery for acquired or congenital heart disease. No patient had a motor deficit postoperatively and no focal abnormalities were disclosed by the rCBF tomograms. The rCBF was generally reduced and mean CBF decreased from a normal value of 54–45 ml/100 g/minute. Changes in rCBF occurred uniformly throughout the brain. The reduction in CBF correlated positively with increasing years, duration of extracorporeal circulation, and low mean arterial BP during the bypass. It was generally more pronounced after valve replacement than after CABG. In 11 patients investigated 1 year after surgery, CBF remained slightly reduced, 51 ml/100g/minute. No CBF reduction occurred in a control group of 15 patients who underwent carotid endarterectomy or extracranial-intracranial shunt operations. The findings are consistent with the suggestion that the extracorporeal circulation causes early postoperative central nervous system dysfunction.

Govier and colleagues[52] from Birmingham, Alabama, examined the relation of rCBF to mean arterial pressure, systemic blood flow, partial pressure of arterial carbon dioxide ($PaCO_2$), nasopharyngeal temperature, and hemoglobin during hypothermic, nonpulsatile cardiopulmonary bypass. The rCBF was measured by clearance of xenon-133 in 67 patients undergoing CABG. There was a significant decrease in rCBF (55% decrease) during cardiopulmonary bypass. Nasopharyngeal temperature and $PaCO_2$ were the only 2 significant factors related to that decrease ($p < 0.05$). In 10 patients variation of pump flow between 1–2 liters/min/M^2 did not significantly affect rCBF. The investigators concluded that cerebral autoregulation is retained during hypothermic cardiopulmonary bypass. Under the usual conditions of cardiopulmonary bypass variations in flow and pressure are not associated with important physiologic or detrimental clinical effects. There are times when adequate surgical exposure may require very low rates of perfusion flow and there has been concern that CBF may drop during these periods. This study underscores the fact that during moderate hypothermia blood flow and arterial perfusion pressure have little or no influence on CBF.

Sternotomy infections

Although wound complications after median sternotomy are rare, infection remains the most threatening difficulty because of the potential for mediastinal sepsis and extension to aortocoronary grafts, cardiotomy incisions, and intracardiac prostheses. Sternal debridement, closed mediastinal antibiotic irrigation, and thoracostomy drainage have significantly improved patient survival. Nevertheless, morbidity and mortality remain high. Pairolero and Arnold[53] from Rochester, Minnesota, reported their experience with recalcitrant infected median sternotomy wounds managed primarily with muscle transposition (Fig. 9-12). During a 7-year period, 38 patients were seen. All required sternal debridement and 17 had resection of bone or cartilage. Reconstruction was done with muscle flaps in 37 patients, omental transposition in 1 and both in 4. The pectoralis major muscle was used in most patients. The mean number of operations for each patient was 3. No deaths occurred within 30 days postoperatively. The mean duration of hospitalization was 25 days. All patients were dismissed with a healed sternum.

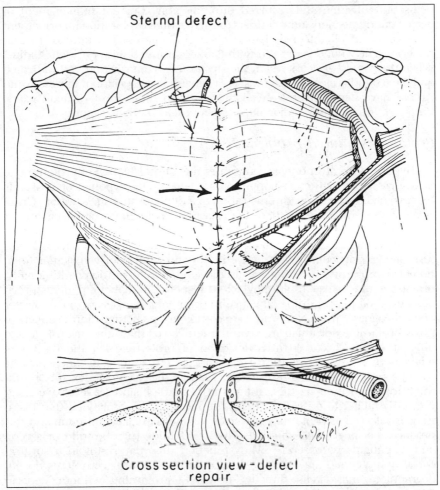

Sternal defect

Cross section view - defect repair

Fig. 9-12. Left (nondominant) pectoralis major muscle is separated from its humeral attachment. Lateral aspect of muscle is left intact to maintain anterior axillary web. Left muscle is "tucked" into sternal (mediastinal) defect and sutured to right (dominant) pectoralis major muscle, which is advanced to midline (inset). Reproduced with permission from Pairolero and Arnold.[53]

Recurrent sternal infection occurred in only 5 patients; 4 of the 5 responded to additional debridement and muscle transposition. In all patients muscle or omental flaps were used either to cover the reconstructed sternum or to obliterate underlying mediastinal dead space if the sternum was resected. Bilateral simultaneous transpositions of the pectoralis major muscle were performed in 29 patients. Wound closure was delayed until the underlying tissue appeared clean and closure occurred at an average of 10 days after the initial debridement. The authors demonstrated that muscle is an ideal tissue to place in contaminated wounds. For the sternotomy the pectoralis major muscle is quite satisfactory. All patients were treated before muscle transposition with mediastinal lavage. That treatment was successful in many patients but infection still recurred unpredictably. Current management of deep wound infections now consists of mediastinal exploration, debridement or resection of all infected tissue, including bone and removal of foreign material. The wound is dressed with gauze, saturated with povidone-iodine. When the wound appears clean, the sternum is reapproximated if indicated and the wound is closed with muscle or omental transposition. Pairolero and Arnold have demonstrated excellent results in these most difficult cases. Early use of pectoralis major flaps is supported by their report.

Protamine-induced problems

Hypotension commonly accompanies the administration of protamine to neutralize heparin after cardiopulmonary bypass. This hypotension is usually best avoided by the slow administration of a dilute protamine solution. Occasionally, severe adverse reactions to protamine, including hypotension and/or generalized urticaria and noncardiogenic pulmonary edema, have occurred. The hypotension together with a presumed elevation of pulmonary vascular resistance is particularly destructive in patients with poor ventricular function or compromised pulmonary circulation before operation. Additionally, protamine may cause an antiphylactoid response in diabetic patients previously exposed to protamine zine insulin or in patients allergic to fish. Frater and colleagues[54] from New York City compared the hemodynamic effects of rapid protamine administration via the left versus the right atrium. No significant change occurred after injection of protamine via the LA route, whereas there was a significant decrease in the systolic BP and systemic vascular resistance with a transient increase in the cardiac index after protamine administration via the right atrium. Plasma histamine levels were significantly higher after RA injection. The investigators concluded that histamine is released as protamine traverses the lungs after RA injection and this produces peripheral vasodilation. The vasodilation may be mild or severe, and in patients with severe LV dysfunction this may result in a surgical catastrophe. Others have found that protamine/heparin complexes do not degranulate mass cells directly; however, protamine without heparin degranulates mass cells and liberates histamine and other vasoactive factors. The investigators suggest in patients suspected of protamine allergy that rapid administration via the left atrium has minimal hemodynamic effect. The advisability of using a histamine antagonist before protamine administration or the use of corticosteroids in critically ill patients was suggested but not proved in this study.

Nonmyxoma cardiac neoplasms

Between 1961 and 1983, 20 patients underwent operations at a Houston, Texas, hospital for primary tumors other than classic benign myxoma. These patients were reported by Reece and colleagues[55]. Total follow-up was 71 patient-years (mean, 3.5 years). There were 10 adults and 10 children. There were 2 operative deaths and 4 late deaths. All pediatric patients had benign lesions (5 fibromas, 5 rabdomyomas) and only 1 patient died (during operation). All operative survivors are alive between 0.9 and 18 years postoperatively, although in 3 cases excision was incomplete. Of the 10 adults, 5 had benign lesions, all were completely excised. In the other 5, unresectable malignant tumors were found, and all 4 operative survivors died of metastases within 8 months. Benign cardiac tumors in childhood have an excellent prognosis when completely excised and appear to have a good short-term prognosis even when excision is incomplete. Although prognosis for benign tumors in adults is good, malignant tumors are associated with very poor survival.

UNCATEGORIZABLE

Reference standards for normal hearts

Patients with normal coronary arteriograms, healthy volunteers, and persons with a low probability of cardiac disease have been used to provide standards in assessing the accuracy of diagnostic tests in cardiology. Each of these 3 populations, however, differ materially from the others. Volunteers are usually selected for youthfulness, the absence of symptoms, and a normal clinical profile. In contrast, patients with normal coronary arteriograms are usually older, and many have symptoms or abnormal test results suggestive of CAD. Despite these differences, some investigators have used these populations interchangeably, presumably on the assumption that they provide equivalent standards of normality. To evaluate each population as a standard of normality relative to the diagnosis of CAD, Rozanski and associates[56] from Los Angeles, California, evaluated the radionuclide ventriculography exercise response in the 3 patient populations: patients with normal coronary arteriograms, healthy volunteers, and uncatheterized patients with a low probability of CAD. Disease probability was determined by Bayesian analysis of age, sex, symptoms, and the results of cardiac fluoroscopy, exercise ECG, or thallium scintigraphy. A wide range of ventriculographic responses was noted in the 62 catheterized normal patients; 21 (34%) had an abnormal EF response and 22 (35%) had an abnormal wall motion response. In contrast, the EF and wall motion responses were normal in the 9 volunteers. In 90 patients (18 catheterized and 72 uncatheterized) who had low disease probability (< 1%), abnormal responses were rare; the EF response was abnormal in only 7% and the wall motion response was abnormal in 8%. Thus, these 3 populations are not equivalent reference standards of normality. Volunteers and patients with low disease probability provide too strict a standard, and their use can overestimate test specificity; catheterized normal patients, on the other hand, provide too lenient a standard, and their use can underestimate test specificity.

ECG criteria for ventricular hypertrophy

Murphy and colleagues[57] from Little Rock, Arkansas, evaluated 30 ECG criteria for LV hypertrophy, 10 for RV hypertrophy, and combinations of both criteria for combined hypertrophy in 323 men whose cardiac chambers were weighed separately at necropsy. Four methods of ECG diagnosis of LV hypertrophy were derived: (1) a modification of the Romhilt-Estes point system; (2) the presence of any 1 of 3 criteria: $SV_1 + RV_5$ or V_6 >35 mm, LA abnormality, or intrinsicoid deflection in lead V_5 or V_6 ≥0.05 second; (3) a combination of any 2 criteria or of 1 criterion plus at least 1 of the following 3 additional criteria: left-axis deviation $> -30°$, QRS duration > 0.09 second, or T-wave inversion in lead V_6 of ≥ 1 mm; and (4) the use of a single criterion— LA abnormality. Sensitivity varied from 57–66% and specificity from 85– 93% among these 4 methods. Acute myocardial infarction increased sensitivity of the foregoing methods, but the specificity was reduced. Method 2 is preferred for the ECG diagnosis of LV hypertrophy. Two methods were useful for RV hypertrophy: (1) the use of any 1 of 4 criteria: R/S ratio in lead V_5 or $V_6 \leq 1$; SV_5 or $V_6 \geq 7$ mm; right-axis deviation of $+90°$, or P pulmonale; and (2) use of any 2 combinations of the foregoing criteria. Sensitivity ranged from 18–43% and specificity from 83–95%. Combined hypertrophy was best diagnosed using LA abnormality as the sole criteria of LV hypertrophy, plus any 1 of 3 criteria of RV hypertrophy: R/S ratio in lead V_5 or $V_6 \leq 1$, SV_5 or $V_6 \geq 7$ mm, or right axis deviation $> +90°$. Sensitivity was 20% and specificity 94%. The ECG diagnosis of RV and combined hypertrophy has low sensitivity but acceptable specificity.

ECG evaluation of ventricular hypertrophy

Echo studies of systolic wall thickening (SWT) of the free wall of the normal human left ventricle have generally yielded values from 40–80%, whereas studies in animals with more direct techniques have produced mean values ranging from 10–30%. To test the validity of echo SWT measurements, the relation between echo-determined end-diastolic and end-systolic LV short-axis myocardial cross-sectional areas (ED Myo CSA and ES Myo CSA, respectively) was assessed by Feneley and Hickie[58] from Sydney, Australia, in 18 normal subjects. Since Myo CSA is a function of wall thickness and wall circumference, overestimation of SWT by echo would be expected to produce an overestimation of ES Myo CSA relative to ED Myo CSA; SWT, as determined by M-mode (52%) and 2-D echo (48%), was consistent with previously reported echo values, but exceeded that reported in animal studies. Statistical correlations demonstrated a close relation in this study between echo-determined ES Myo CSA and ED Myo CSA and was consistent with constant LV myocardial mass throughout the cardiac cycle. Thus, this study did not suggest an overestimation of SWT by echo techniques.

Ventricular function in anemia

The enhanced LV performance in patients with anemia has been attributed to changes in preload and afterload. Whether there is concomitant increase in contractility has been controversial. Florenzano and associates[59] from Santiago, Chile, studied 17 patients with chronic anemia (hematocrit, 17–30%) and 17 control subjects, matched by age and sex. In 10 patients and in 10 control subjects (group I), a noninvasive evaluation of LV function through M-mode echo and cuff BP recording was performed. In patients with anemia, stroke volume increased 43%, fractional shortening, 21%, and mean rate of circumferential shortening, 32%. In patients with anemia, end-systolic stress decreased 27% and diastolic BP, 21%. The effect of serum from these patients and control subjects on the development of isometric tension by isolated cat papillary muscles was assessed compared with the basal (Ringer-Locke bath) values. Anemia serum increased maximal developed tension 21% and maximal rate of tension development 20% relative to basal levels. These changes were significantly higher than the increases produced by control serum (8% and 7%, respectively). In the 7 patients with anemia in group II and their matched controls, the in vitro isometric tension characteristics were assessed before and after blocking beta adrenoreceptors with propranolol, 10^{-6} M. The observed increase in the developed tension persisted after beta blockade, as well as the enhancement of the maximal rate of tension development. Plasma catecholamine levels in group II were within the normal range. Thus, in anemia there is an enhancement of ejection phase indexes of LV performance and in vitro evidence suggesting the existence of a noncatecholamine factor that increases contractility.

Heart in acquired immune deficiency syndrome (AIDS)

A recently described disease, AIDS, that affects primarily homosexuals and intravenous drug abusers has generated considerable interest. At the National Institutes of Health, Silver and associates [60] from Bethesda, Maryland, studied at necropsy 18 patients with AIDS, and of them 5 (28%) had abnormalities in the heart. In each the abnormality consisted of focal deposits of Kaposi's sarcoma. All 5 patients were white men aged 26–52 years and the initial manifestation of AIDS in each was a dermal lesion that, on biopsy, was Kaposi's sarcoma. The interval from the appearance of the dermal lesion to death ranged from 6–22 months. During life, no patient had symptoms attributable to cardiac dysfunction. Thus, asymptomatic cardiac involvement may occur fairly commonly in patients with AIDS.

Fink and associates[61] from Philadelphia, Pennsylvania, studied 15 patients, 14 men and 1 woman, aged 26–49 years with AIDS. Twelve were homosexual or bisexual men and 3 were intravenous drug abusers; the woman was Haitian. Cardiac abnormalities were found by either echo or necropsy or ECG in 73% of the 15 patients. The abnormalities included pericardial effusions, 3 of which resulted in cardiac tamponade, right-sided marantic endocarditis, increased RV size, LV hypokinesia, and MR. Despite the severity of these cardiac abnormalities, they were usually not diagnosed clinically. Because cardiac abnormalities in hospitalized AIDS patients are frequent and may not arouse clinical suspicion, echo assessment may prove helpful in detecting cardiac dysfunction, valvular disease, and cardiac tamponade.

Atrial myxoma and S_1

Gershlick and associates[62] from London, England, studied the interrelation between the loudness of the first heart sound, the time interval from the Q wave to the onset of the first heart sound (QM_1), and the mitral valve closure rate in 9 patients with LA myxoma. In 7 patients the first heart sound was loud preoperatively and was associated with delayed mitral valve closure. After removal of the myxoma, the onset of mitral valve closure returned toward normal. The mitral valve closure rate was reduced, and the first heart sound became softer. In 2 patients the heart sound was normal before and after operation, as were both the time of onset of mitral valve closure and the mitral valve closure rate. In neither of these patients, however, did the myxoma completely fill the mitral orifice during diastole. Thus, the loud first heart sound in LA myxoma is a useful clinical sign and its intensity is directly related to the delay in onset of closure of the mitral leaflets.

Left ventricular function in hemodialysis

Hemodialysis is associated with an improvement in LV contractility but the mechanism or mechanisms responsible for this improvement have not been elucidated. It is known that the increased LV contractility is independent of a change in preload. Henrich and associates[63] from Dallas, Texas, investigated the importance of 3 distinct effects that regularly occur in hemodialysis and could potentially improve LV contractility: the removal of uremic toxins, the increase in the plasma ionized calcium concentration, and the increase in the plasma bicarbonate concentration. Three different dialysates were used for each of 8 stable patients on long-term hemodialysis, and LV contractility was assessed by 2-D echo before and after each dialysis. In the first procedure neither the ionized calcium nor the bicarbonate concentration was allowed to increase, and LV contractility did not improve. In the second procedure, ionized calcium increased (from 4.4–5.4 mg/dl), bicarbonate concentration was held constant, and contractility increased (from 0.74–0.93 circumferences per second). In the third procedure, ionized calcium was kept constant, the bicarbonate concentration was increased (from 19–24 mM/liter), but contractility did not increase. These results suggest that the increase in ionized calcium that occurs in regular dialysis is a key factor in the improvement in LV contractility observed during the procedure.

Nifedipine for Raynaud's phenomenon

Creager and associates[64] from Boston, Massachusetts, studied the effect of nifedipine on fingertip hemodynamics in 10 patients with Raynaud's phenomenon. Fingertip blood flow was determined in a 20°C environment by venous occlusion air plethysmography and fingertip vascular resistance was calculated from the mean BP and the fingertip blood flow. Nifedipine, administered as a 10 mg sublingual dose, increased fingertip blood flow in 8 of the 10 patients. Fingertip vascular resistance for the 10 patients increased 40% from 41 ± 11–24 ± 6 U (p < 0.05). Seven of the 10 patients were followed in a crossover placebo-controlled clinical trial. The frequency and severity of Raynaud's phenomenon was less in all 7 patients when taking nifedipine compared with placebo. Nifedipine-induced fingertip vasodilation may contribute to clinical improvement in some patients with Raynaud's phenomenon.

Angioplasty in leg arteries

Gallino and colleagues[65] from Bern, Switzerland, performed percutaneous transluminal angioplastys (PTA) in the arteries of the legs in 411 patients between 1977 and 1983. The 5-year patency rate in the 482 arteries was 83% for the iliac and 58% for femoropopliteal. Clinical improvement after the procedure was confirmed by a significant drop of the arm-ankle pressure difference: 48 mmHg before -vs- 17 mmHg 2 years after iliac PTA and 73 mmHg before -vs- 28 mmHg after femoropopliteal. Most reocclusions occurred within the first year after angioplasty and patients with stenoses or occlusions of <3 cm had a favorable long-term patency rate of 74%. Conversely, patients with femoropopliteal occlusions presenting with pain at rest, diabetes mellitus, occlusions of >3 cm, or poor distal runoff had an elevated rate of reocclusion. Complications, which occurred in 8% of the patients in whom PTA was attempted, included local hemorrhage, dissection, embolism, and spasm necessitating surgical intervention in 2%. No deaths or amputations were a direct consequence of PTA. Thus, PTA of arteries of the legs may be regarded as a valid complimentary treatment to vascular surgery. With the aging population and increasing incidence of peripheral vascular disease, PTA may enjoy an increasing role in the nonsurgical approach to these individuals.

Symposia on cardiovascular topics in The American Journal of Medicine and in the 4 major USA cardiovascular journals in 1984 and analysis of page utilization and types of articles published in the 4 major USA cardiovascular journals in 1984

Eight symposia on various cardiovascular conditions and therapy for them were published in *The American Journal of Medicine* in 1984. These symposia, along with the guest editors, number of pages, number of articles,

TABLE 9-5. *Symposia on cardiovascular disease published in 1984 in* The American Journal of Medicine.

#	DATE	SUBJECT OF SYMPOSIUM	GUEST EDITOR(S)	# PAGES	# ARTICLES	INDUSTRY SPONSOR
1	2/27	Systemic hypertension therapy	Lennart Hansson, Jerome Lowenstein, Alberto Zanchetti	128	20	Pfizer
2	5/31	Captopril	Norman K. Hollenberg, Elliot Rapaport	128	19	E.R. Squibb & Sons
3	6/22	Nitroglycerin	Robert Roberts	88	12	Marion
4	8/20	Converting enzyme inhibition (enalapril and captopril) for systemic hypertension and congestive heart failure	John H. Laragh	96	12	Merck Sharp & Dohme
5	8/31	Calcium channel blockers for systemic hypertension	Edward D. Frohlich	56	7	Pfizer
6	10/5	Systemic hypertension therapy	Edward D. Frolich	152	20	Marion Laboratories
7	11/5	Electrolytes and cardiovascular disease	Norman K. Hollenberg Robert S. Brown	72	10	Lederle Laboratories
8	12/28	Calcium metabolism and calcium channel blockers for systemic hypertension	John L. Laragh	26	1	Knoll Pharmaceutical Company

TABLE 9-6. *Comparison of the regular issues of the 4 major USA cardiovascular journals for 1984*

	AJC	CIRCULATION	JACC	AHJ
Number pages				
(average/mo)	3,403 (284)	2,413 (201)	2,990 (249)	2,571 (214)
For articles				
(pages/article)				
(avg/month)	3,077 (4.12)	2,252 (7.66)	2,682 (7.23)	2,392 (5.13)
	(256)	(188)	(224)	(199)
For letters (number)				
(no. with replies)	36 (80)(38)	0	30 (31)(21)	21 (21)(14)
For staff,				
editorial board	15	18	39	12
For contents				
in brief	31	26	25	56
For contents				
with abstracts	145	0	98	0
For society news	0	77	15	0
For books	3	0	3	6
For volume indexes	69	30	62	56
For information				
for authors	15	4	28	24
For others	12	6	8	4
Number articles				
(average/mo)	747 (62)	294 (25)	371 (31)	466 (39)
Coronary heart disease	140 (18.7%)	65 (22.1%)	80 (21.6%)	98 (21.0%)
Arrhythmias & CD	76 (10.2%)	37 (12.6%	46 (12.4%)	55 (11.8%)
Systemic hypertension	19 (2.5%)	11 (3.7%)	4 (1.1%)	9 (1.9%)
Congestive heart failure	16 (2.1%)	12 (4.1%)	10 (2.7%)	5 (1.1%)
Valvular heart disease	37 (5.0%)	11 (3.7%)	29 (7.8%)	18 (3.9%)
Cardiomyopathy	18 (2.4%)	9 (3.1%)	8 (2.2%)	7 (1.5%)
Pericardial heart				
disease	3 (0.4%)	2 (0.7%)	1 (0.3%)	1 (0.2%)
Congenital heart				
disease	47 (6.3%)	24 (8.2%)	38 (10.2%)	13 (2.8%)
Cardiovascular				
pharmacology	10 (1.3%)	4 (1.4%)	5 (1.3%)	9 (1.9%)
Miscellaneous	28 (3.7%)	20 (6.8%)	16 (4.3%)	24 (5.2%)
Methods	31 (4.1%)	10 (3.4%)	21 (5.7%)	10 (2.1%)
Experimental studies	64 (8.6%)	66 (22.4%)	50 (13.5%)	33 (7.1%)
Editorials and				
point of view	28 (3.7%)	22 (7.5%)	18 (4.9%)	18 (3.9%)
Brief reports	204 (27.3%)	0	44 (11.8%)	166 (35.6%)
Historical studies	11 (1.5%)	1 (0.3%)	1 (0.3%)	0
From-the-editor				
column	15 (2.0%)	0	0	0

TABLE 9-7. *Symposia published in the 4 major USA cardiovascular journals in 1984*

JOURNAL	MONTH OF PUBLICATION	SUBJECT OF SYMPOSIUM	GUEST EDITOR(S)	# ARTICLES	# PAGES (ARTICLES)	INDUSTRY SPONSOR
AJC	January 27	First-line therapy for systemic hypertension	Norman M. Kaplan	14	64 (58)	Pfizer
AJC	February 27	Flecainide acetate	J. Thomas Bigger	24		
AJC	June 15	Percutaneous transluminal coronary angioplasty	Kenneth M. Kent, Suzanne M. Mullin, Eugene R. Passamani	35	167 (146)	—
AJC	June 25	Metoprolol for acute myocardial infarction	Åke Hjalmarson	9	56 (50)	AB Hässle
AJC	July 30	Bretylium	Lon Castle	6	40 (36)	American Critical Care
AJC	August 13	Lorcainide	John C. Somberg	9	64 (54)	Janssen
AJC	August 27	Cholestyramine	Robert I. Levy	8	56 (41)	Mead Johnson
AJC	November 14	Propafenone	Douglas P. Zipes	12	80 (73)	Knoll
AJC	December 21	Early intervention in acute myocardial infarction	Charles E. Rackley	9	40 (31)	Ciba-Geigy
AHJ	April	Coronary angioplasty	Arthur J. Roberts, C. Richard Conti, Carl J. Pepine	13	58 (58)	15 Sponsors
AHJ	May	Mexiletine	Philip Podrid, Jeremy Ruskin	8	56 (50)	Boehringer Ingelheim
AHJ	July	Transdermal nitroglycerin and clonidine	Peter Goldman	7	42 (42)	Boehringer Ingelheim
AHJ	September	Coronary heart disease in blacks	Katrina W. Johnson, Gerald H. Payne, Richard F. Gillum	34	230 (230)	Schering
AHJ	October	Nadolol	Norman M. Kaplan	21	120 (114)	E.R. Squibb
Circulation	September	Cardiovascular surgery	Floyd D. Loop	35	236 (231)	—

and whether or not the symposium was sponsored by industry are listed in Table 9-5.

The numbers and types of articles and numbers of editorial (nonadvertising) pages published in the 4 major American cardiologic journals in 1984 are summarized in Table 9-6. The 4 journals include *The American Journal of Cardiology* (AJC), *Circulation*, *Journal of the American College of Cardiology* (JACC) and *The American Heart Journal* (AHJ). The subjects presented in 16 symposia published in the AJC, the AHJ and *Circulation* in 1984 are summarized in Table 9-7.

References

1. SINGH S, WANN S, SCHUCHARD GH, KLOPFENSTEIN HS, LEIMGRUBER PP, KEELAN MH, BROOKS HL: Right ventricular and right atrial collapse in patients with cardiac tamponade—a combined echocardiographic and hemodynamic study. Circulation 70:966–971, Dec 1984.

2. MANGA P, VYTHILINGUM S, MITHA AS: Pulsatile hepatomegaly in constrictive pericarditis. Br Heart J 52:465–467, Oct 1984.

3. LOCK JE, BASS JL, KULIK TJ, FUHRMAN BP: Chronic percutaneous pericardial drainage with modified pigtail catheters in children. Am J Cardiol 53:1179–1182, Apr 1, 1984.

4. DE PACE NL, NESTICO PF, SCHWARTZ AB, MINTZ GS, SCHWARTZ JS, KOTLER MN, SWARTZ C: Predicting success of intensive dialysis in the treatment of uremic pericarditis. Am J Med 76:38–46, Jan 1984.

5. WEITZMAN LB, TINKER WP, KRONZON I, COHEN ML, GLASSMAN E, SPENCER FC: The incidence and natural history of pericardial effusion after cardiac surgery—an echocardiographic study. Circulation 69:506–511, March 1984.

6. STEVENSON LW, CHILD JS, LAKS H, KERN L: Incidence and significance of early pericardial effusions after cardiac surgery. Am J Cardiol 54:848–851, Oct 1, 1984.

7. RIBEÍRO P, SAPSFORD R, EVANS T, PARCHARIDIS G, OAKLEY C: Constrictive pericarditis as a complication of coronary artery bypass surgery. Br Heart J 51:205–210, Feb 1984.

8. BATEMAN TM, CZER LSC, GRAY RJ, KASS RM, RAYMOND MJ, GARCIA EV, CHAUX A, MATLOFF JM, BERMAN DS: Detection of occult pericardial hemorrhage early after open-heart surgery using technetium-99m red blood cell radionuclide ventriculography. Am Heart J 108:1198–1206, Nov 1984.

9. RICH S, LEVY PS: Characteristics of surviving and nonsurviving patients with primary pulmonary hypertension. Am J Med 76:573–578, Apr 1984.

10. FUSTER V, STEELE PM, EDWARDS WD, GERSH BJ, McGOON MD, FRYE RL: Primary pulmonary hypertension: natural history and the importance of thrombosis. Circulation 70:580–587, Oct 1984.

11. PACKER M, MEDINA N, YUSHAK M, WIENER I: Detrimental effects of verapamil in patients with primary pulmonary hypertension. Br Heart J 52:106–111, July 1984.

12. PACKER M, MEDINA N, YUSHAK M: Adverse hemodynamic and clinical effects of calcium channel blockade in pulmonary hypertension secondary to obliterative pulmonary vascular disease. J Am Coll Cardiol 4:890–901, Nov 1984.

13. RODEHEFFER RJ, GERSTENBLITH G, BECKER LC, FLEG JL, WEISFELDT ML, LAKATTA EG: Exercise cardiac output is maintained with advancing age in healthy human subjects: cardiac dilatation and increased stroke volume compensate for a diminished heart rate. Circulation 69:203–213, Feb 1984.

14. DIMSDALE JE, HARTLEY LH, GUINEY T, RUSKIN JN, GREENBLATT D: Postexercise peril: plasma catecholamines and exercise. JAMA 251:630–632, Feb 3, 1984.

15. ADES PA, BRAMMELL HL, GREENBERG JH, HORWITZ LD: Effect of beta blockade and intrinsic sympathomimetic activity on exercise performance. Am J Cardiol 54:1337–1341, Dec 1, 1984.

16. SHAPIRO LM: Physiological left ventricular hypertrophy. Br Heart J, 54:130–135, Aug 1984.

17. BALADY GJ, CADIGAN JB, RYAN TJ: Electrocardiogram of the athlete: an analysis of 289 professional football players. Am J Cardiol 53:1339–1343, May 1, 1984.

18. NORTHCOTE RJ, EVANS ADB, BALLANTYNE D: Sudden death in squash players. Lancet 1:148–150, Jan 21, 1984.

19. OSBAKKEN M, LOCKO R: Scintigraphic determination of ventricular function and coronary perfusion in long-distance runners. Am Heart J 108:296–304, Aug 1984.

20. FAGARD R, AUBERT A, STAESSEN J, EYNDE EF, VANHEES L, AMERY A: Cardiac structure and function in cyclists and runners: comparative echocardiographic study. Br Heart J 52:124–129, Aug 1984.

21. WARNES CA, ROBERTS WC: The heart in massive (more than 300 pounds or 136 kilograms) obesity: analysis of 12 patients studied at necropsy. Am J Cardiol 54:1087–1091, Nov 1, 1984.

22. KREITZMAN SN, PEDERSEN M, BUDELL W, NICHOLS D, KRISSMAN P, CLEMENTS M: Safety and effectiveness of weight reduction using a very-low-calorie formulated food. Arch Intern Med 144:747–750, Apr 1984.

23. WEINTRAUB M, HASDAY JD, MUSHLIN AI, LOCKWOOD DH: A double-blind clinical trial in weight control: use of fenfluramine and phentermine alone and in combination. Arch Intern Med 144:1143–1148, June 1984.

24. McKAY RG, SPEARS JR, AROESTY JM, BAIM DS, ROYAL HD, HELLER GV, LINCOLN W, SALO RW, BRAUNWALD E, GROSSMAN W: Instantaneous measurement of left and right ventricular stroke volume and pressure-volume relationships with an impedance catheter. Circulation 69:703–710, Apr 1984.

25. SEED WA, NOBLE MIM, WALKER JM, MILLER GAH, PIDGEON J, REDWOOD E, WANLESS R, FRANZ MR, SCHOETTLER M, SCHAEFER J: Relationships between beat-to-beat interval and the strength of contraction in the healthy and diseased human heart. Circulation 70:799–805, Nov 1984.

26. BAAN J, VAN DER VELDE ET, DE BRUIN HG, SMEENK GJ, KOOPS J, VAN DIJK AD, TEMMERMAN D, SENDEN J, BUIS B: Continuous measurement of left ventricular volume in animals and humans by conductance catheter. Circulation 70:812–823, Nov 1984.

27. NISHIMURA RA, CALLAHAN MJ, SCHAFF HV, ILSTRUP DM, MILLER FA, TAJIK AJ: Noninvasive measurement of cardiac output by continuous wave Doppler echocardiography: initial experience and review of the literature. Mayo Clin Proc 59:484–489, July 1984.

28. KAUL S, TEI C, HOPKINS JM, SHAH PM: Assessment of right ventricular function using two-dimensional echocardiography. Am Heart J 107:526–531, March 1984.

29. KIMCHI A, ELLRODT AG, BERMAN DS, RIEDINGER MS, SWAN HJC, MURATA GH: Right ventricular performance in septic shock: a combined radionuclide and hemodynamic study. J Am Coll Cardiol 4:945–951, Nov 1984.

30. JOUVE R, ROLLAND P-H, DELBOY C, MERCIER C: Thromboxane B_2, 6-keto $PGF_{1\alpha}$, PGE_2, $PGF_{2\alpha}$, and PGA_1 plasma levels in arteriosclerosis obliterans: relationship to clinical manifestations, risk factors, and arterial pathoanatomy. Am Heart J 107:45–52, Jan 1984.

31. FITZGERALD GA, SMITH B, PEDERSEN AK, BRASH AR: Increased prostacyclin biosynthesis in patients with severe atherosclerosis and platelet activation. N Engl J Med 310:1065–1068, Apr 26, 1984.

32. BUGIARDINI R, CHIERCHIA S, CREA F, GALLINO A, WILD S, ROSKOVEC A, LENZI S, MASERI A: Evaluation of the effects of catheter sampling for the study of platelet behavior in the pulmonary and coronary circulation. Am Heart J 108:255–260, Aug 1984.

33. FITZGERALD DJ, ROY L, ROBERTSON RM, FITZGERALD GA: The effects of organic nitrates on prostacyclin biosynthesis and platelet function in humans. Circulation 70:297–302, Aug 1984.

34. YUI Y, HATTORI R, TAKATSU Y, NAKAJIMA H, WAKABAYASHI A, KAWAI C, KAYAMA N, HIRAKU S, INAGAWA T, TSUBOJIMA M, NAITO J: Intravenous infusion of a selective inhibitor of thromboxane A_2 synthetase in man: influence on thromboxane B_2 and 6-keto-prostaglandin $F_{1\alpha}$ levels and platelet aggregation. Circulation 70:599–605, Oct 1984.

35. WHITSETT TL, MANION CV, CHRISTENSEN HD: Cardiovascular effects of coffee and caffeine. Am J Cardiol 53:918–922, March 15, 1984.

36. KURNIK PB, TIEFENBRUNN AJ, LUDBROOK PA: The dependence of the cardiac effects of nifedipine on the responses of the peripheral vascular system. Circulation 69:963–972, May 1984.

37. ERRICHETTI AM, HOLDEN A, ANSELL J: Management of oral anticoagulant therapy: experience with an anticoagulation clinic. Arch Intern Med 144:1966–1968, Oct 1984.

38. PETITPRIZ P, SIMMONEAU G, CERRINA J, MUSSET D, DREYFUS M, VANDENBROEK MD, DUROUX P: Effects of a single bolus of urokinase in patients with life-threatening pulmonary emboli: a descriptive trial. Circulation 70:861–866, Nov 1984.

39. EVANS RW: Heart transplants and priorities. Lancet 1:852–853, 1984.

40. COPELAND JG, MAMMANA RB, FULLER JK, CAMPBELL DW, McALEER MJ, SAILER JA: Heart transplantation: four years' experience with conventional immunosuppression. JAMA 251:1563–1566, March 23, 1984.

41. GRIFFITH BP, HARDESTY RL, BAHNSON HT: Powerful but limited immunosuppression for cardiac transplantation with cyclosporine and low-dose steroid. J Thorac Cardiovasc Surg 87:35–42, Jan 1984.

42. LANZA RP, COOPER DKC, BOYD ST, BARNARD CN: Comparison of patients with ischemic, myopathic, and rheumatic heart diseases as cardiac transplant recipients. Am Heart J 107:8–12, Jan 1984.

43. CLEARY ML, WARNKE R, SKLAR J: Monoclonality of lymphoproliferative lesions in cardiac-transplant recipients. N Engl J Med 310:477–482, Feb 23, 1984.

44. CLEARY ML, SKLAR J: Lymphoproliferative disorders in cardiac transplant recipients are multiclonal lymphomas. Lancet 2:489–493, Sept 1, 1984.

45. UYS CJ, ROSE AG: Pathologic findings in long-term cardiac transplants. Arch Pathol Lab Med 108:112–116, Feb 1984.

46. JAMIESON SW, STINSON EB, OYER PE, REITZ BA, BALDWIN J, MODRY D, DAWKINS K, THEODORE J, HUNT S, SHUMWAY NE: Heart-lung transplantation for irreversible pulmonary hypertension. Ann Thorac Surg 38:554–562, Dec 1984.

47. DEVRIES WC, ANDERSON JL, JOYCE LD, ANDERSON FL, HAMMOND EH, JARVIK RK, KOLFF WJ: Clinical use of the total artificial heart. N Engl J Med 310:273–278, Feb 2, 1984.

48. GALLETTI PM: Replacement of the heart with a mechanical device: The case of Dr. Barney Clark. N Engl J Med 310:312–314, Feb 2, 1984.

49. STRAUSS MJ: Political history of the artificial heart. N Engl J Med 310:332–336, Feb 2, 1984.

50. ABERG T, RONQUIST G, TYDEN H, BRUNNKVIST S, HULTMAN J, BERGSTROM K, LILJA A: Adverse effects on the brain in cardiac operations as assessed by biochemical, psychometric, and radiologic methods. J Thorac Cardiovasc Surg 87:99–105, Jan 1984.

51. HENRIKSEN L: Evidence suggestive of diffuse brain damage following cardiac operations. Lancet 1:816–820, Apr 14, 1984.

52. GOVIER AN, REVES JG, McKAY RD, KARP RB, ZORN GL, MORAWETZ RB, SMITH LR, ADAMS M, FREEMAN AM: Factors and their influence on regional cerebral blood flow during nonpulsatile cardiopulmonary bypass. Ann Thorac Surg 38:592–600, Dec 1984.

53. PAIROLERO PC, ARNOLD PG: Management of recalcitrant median sternotomy wounds. J Thorac Cardiovasc Surg 88:357–364, Sept 1984.

54. FRATER RWM, OKA Y, HONG Y, TSUBO T, LOUBSER PG, MASONE R: Protamine-induced circulatory changes. J Thorac Cardiovasc Surg 87:687–692, May 1984.

55. REECE IJ, COOLEY DA, FRAZIER OH, HALLMAN GL, POWERS PL, MONTERO CG: Cardiac tumors: clinical spectrum and prognosis of lesions other than classical benign myxoma in 20 patients. J Thorac Cardiovasc Surg 88:439–446, Sept 1984.

56. ROZANSKI A, DIAMOND GA, FORRESTER JS, BERMAN DS, MORRIS D, SWAN HJC: Alternative referent standards for cardiac normality: implications for diagnostic testing. Ann Intern Med 101:164–171, Aug 1984.

57. MURPHY ML, THENABADU N, DE SOYZA N, DOHERTY JE, MEADE J, BAKER BJ, WHITTLE JL: Reevaluation of electrocardiographic criteria for left, right and combined cardiac ventricular hypertrophy. Am J Cardiol 53:1140–1147, Apr 1, 1984.

58. FENELEY MP, HICKIE JB: Validity of echocardiographic determination of left ventricular systolic wall thickening. Circulation 70:226–232, Aug 1984.

59. FLORENZANO F, DIAZ G, REGONESI C, ESCOBAR E: Left ventricular function in chronic anemia: evidence of noncatecholamine positive inotropic factor in the serum. Am J Cardiol 54:638–645, Sept 1, 1984.

60. SILVER MA, MACHER AM, REICHERT CM, LEVENS DL, PARRILLO JE, LONGO DL, ROBERTS WC: Cardiac

involvement by Kaposi's sarcoma in acquired immune deficiency syndrome (AIDS). Am J Cardiol 53:983, March 15, 1984.

61. FINK L, REICHEK N, SUTTON MGS: Cardiac abnormalities in acquired immune deficiency syndrome. Am J Cardiol 54:1161–1163, Nov 1, 1984.

62. GERSHLICK AH, LEECH G, MILLS PG, LEATHAM A: The loud first heart sound in left atrial myxoma. Br Heart J 52:403–407, Oct 1984.

63. HENRICH WL, HUNT JM, NIXON JF: Increased ionized calcium and left ventricular contractility during hemodialysis. N Engl J Med 310:19–23, Jan 5, 1984.

64. CREAGER MA, PARISER KM, WINSTON EM, RASMUSSEN HM, MILLER KB, COFFMAN JD: Nifedipine-induced fingertip vasodilation in patients with Raynaud's phenomenon. Am Heart J 108:370–373, Aug 1984.

65. GALLINO A, MAHLER F, PROBST P, NACHBUR B: Percutaneous transluminal angioplasty of the arteries of the lower limbs: a 5 year follow-up. Circulation 70:619–623, Oct 1984.

Author Index

Subject Index